Introduction to Pharmaceutical Biotechnology, Volume 1 (Second Edition)

Basic techniques and concepts

Online at: https://doi.org/10.1088/978-0-7503-5382-3

Introduction to Pharmaceutical Biotechnology, Volume 1 (Second Edition)

Basic techniques and concepts

Edited by
Ahmed Al-Harrasi
Department of Organic Chemistry, University of Nizwa, 616 Birkat Al Maus, Nizwa, Oman

Saif Hameed
Amity Institute of Biotechnology, Amity University Haryana, Gurugram (Manesar) 122413, India

Zeeshan Fatima
Amity Institute of Biotechnology, Amity University Haryana, Gurugram (Manesar) 122413, India

Saurabh Bhatia
Natural and Medical Sciences Research Center, University of Nizwa, 616 Birkat Al Maus, Nizwa, Oman

IOP Publishing, Bristol, UK

ISBN 978-0-7503-5382-3 (ebook)
ISBN 978-0-7503-5380-9 (print)
ISBN 978-0-7503-5383-0 (myPrint)
ISBN 978-0-7503-5381-6 (mobi)

DOI 10.1088/978-0-7503-5382-3

Version: 20240701

IOP ebooks

British Library Cataloguing-in-Publication Data: A catalogue record for this book is available from the British Library.

Published by IOP Publishing, wholly owned by The Institute of Physics, London

IOP Publishing, No.2 The Distillery, Glassfields, Avon Street, Bristol, BS2 0GR, UK

US Office: IOP Publishing, Inc., 190 North Independence Mall West, Suite 601, Philadelphia, PA 19106, USA

Contents

Acknowledgements

We would like to dedicate this book to all students, researchers, academicians, and all the scholars. who have sincerely contributed to the area of Pharmaceutical Biotechnology, depicted in the book, at national as well as international level. We would also like to acknowledge the University of Nizwa, Sultanate of Oman for extending its support in accomplishing this book project successfully. We are grateful to the Natural and Medical Sciences Research Center (NMSRC) housed at the University of Nizwa for providing central resources of advanced analytical instruments for our research work and for promoting interdisciplinary research studies. This centre has given a valuable base to this book project. Thus, authors are thankful to NMSRC for offering excellent facilities required for the completion of this book. Also, I would like to acknowledge School of Health Sciences, University of Petroleum and Energy Studies, Dehradun, Uttarakhand, India, for providing support required for the completion of this book.

Natural and Medical Sciences Research Center, University of Nizwa

Last, but not least, we show our sincere gratitude to the whole team of IOP Publishing for furnishing their active cooperation and support.

Editor biographies

Professor Ahmed Al-Harrasi

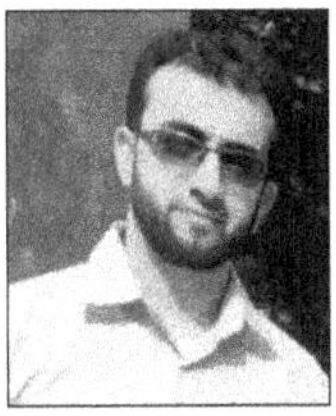

Ahmed Al-Harrasi is a professor of organic chemistry and the vice chancellor for graduate studies, research and external relations at the University of Nizwa. He obtained his BSc in Chemistry from SQU and his MSc and PhD in Organic Chemistry from Free University of Berlin as a DAAD-fellow. Then he received the Fulbright award in 2008 for postdoctoral research in chemical biology from Cornell University. He is a founder and chair of the Natural and Medical Sciences Research Center. He is a member of the Scientific Council of UNESCO. He was named on the list of top 2% scientists for the last three years. He has authored over 800 scientific papers and more than 20 books and book chapters. He received the Order of Royal Commendation from His Majesty, The Sultan of Oman as an outstanding Omani individual for his remarkable contribution and active role in research.

Dr Saif Hameed

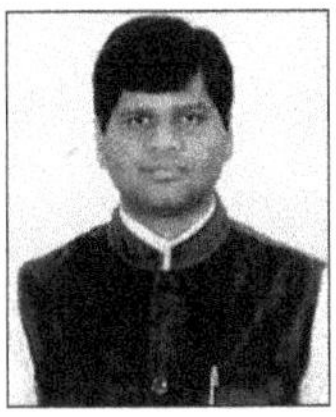

Saif Hameed is currently Associate Professor at Amity Institute of Biotechnology, Amity University Haryana (AUH). He has 70 peer-reviewed papers to his credit in international journals of repute, 26 book chapters and authored 9 books which include 4 from Springer-Nature and 1 from CRC Press, Taylor & Francis. He has supervised 6 PhD students and guided 25 UG & PG level students for their research projects.

Dr Zeeshan Fatima

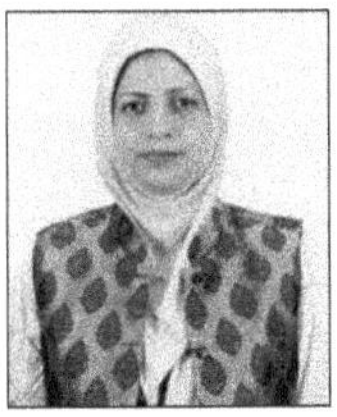

Zeeshan Fatima is currently Associate Professor at Amity Institute of Biotechnology, Amity University Haryana (AUH. She has 65 peer-reviewed papers to her credit in international journals of repute, 24 book chapters and authored 7 books including ones from Springer, Elsevier. She has supervised 5 PhD students and guided 25 UG & PG level students for their research projects.

Dr Saurabh Bhatia

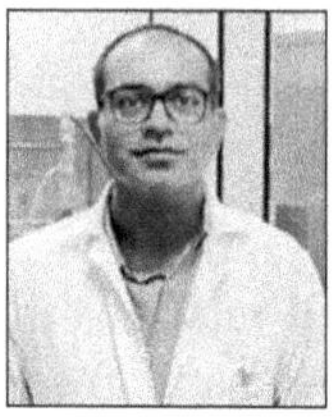

Saurabh Bhatia is an Associate Professor within the Natural and Medical Sciences Research Centre at the University of Nizwa, Oman. He has published 127 referred journal articles and written 94 book chapters. Dr Bhatia has also authored 10 books and is the Associate Editor on several international journals. Currently he is also working as an Adjunct Faculty in School of Health Sciences, University of Petroleum and Energy Studies, Dehradun, Uttarakhand, India.

List of contributors

Sarika Bano
Dr B R Ambedkar Center for Biomedical Research, University of Delhi, Delhi 110007, India

Isha Bansal
Amity Institute of Biotechnology, Amity University Haryana, Gurugram (Manesar) 122413, Haryana, India

Abdullah Faizaan
Biological Sciences, School of Engineering and Sciences, GD Goenka University, Gurugram, Haryana 122103, India

Gajala Deethamvali Ghousepeer
School of Health Sciences and Technology (SOHST), UPES, Dehradun, Uttarakhand 248007, India

Aanvi Goel
Amity Institute of Biotechnology, Amity University Haryana, Gurugram (Manesar)122413, Haryana, India

Vijayshree S Karankar
Department of Biotechnology, National Institute of Pharmaceutical Education and Research-Raebareli, Lucknow 226002, India

Anil Kumar
Biological Sciences, School of Engineering and Sciences, GD Goenka University, Gurugram, Haryana 122103, India

Muskan Kumari
Biological Sciences, School of Engineering and Sciences, GD Goenka University, Gurugram, Haryana 122103, India

Ramendra Pati Pandey
School of Health Sciences and Technology (SOHST), UPES, Dehradun 248007, Uttarakhand, India

Joshma Rasabathina
Amity Institute of Biotechnology, Amity University Haryana, Gurugram (Manesar)-122413, Haryana, India

Syed Shadab Raza
Laboratory for Stem Cell and Restorative Neurology, Department of Biotechnology, Era's Lucknow Medical College and Hospital, Era University, Sarfarazganj, Lucknow 226003, India
and
Department of Stem Cell Biology and Regenerative Medicine, Era's Lucknow Medical College Hospital, Era University, Sarfarazganj, Lucknow 226003, India

Munindra Ruwali
Department of Education in Science and Mathematics (DESM), National Council of Educational Research and Training (NCERT), Sri Aurobindo Marg, New Delhi-110016, India

Sayani Saha
Department of Biotechnology, National Institute of Pharmaceutical Education and Research—Raebareli, Lucknow 226002, India

Tanuja Sarkar
The School of Studies in Neuroscience, Jiwaji University, Sachin Tendulkar Road, Kailash Nagar, Mahalgaon, Gwalior, Madhya Pradesh 474001, India

Sneh Shalini
Clinical Studies and Trials Unit, Division of Developmental Research, Indian Council of Medical Research, New Delhi 110029, India

Prashant Anilkumar Singh
School of Health Sciences and Technology (SOHST), UPES, Dehradun, Uttarakhand 248007, India

Nidhi Srivastava
Department of Biotechnology, National Institute of Pharmaceutical Education and Research—Raebareli, Lucknow 226002, India

Reetika Tandon
Department of Biotechnology, National Institute of Pharmaceutical Education and Research—Raebareli, Lucknow 226002, India

Arshi Waseem
Laboratory for Stem Cell and Restorative Neurology, Department of Biotechnology, Era's Lucknow Medical College and Hospital, Era University, Sarfarazganj, Lucknow 226003, India

IOP Publishing

Introduction to Pharmaceutical Biotechnology, Volume 1
(Second Edition)
Basic techniques and concepts
Ahmed Al-Harrasi, Saif Hameed, Zeeshan Fatima and Saurabh Bhatia

Chapter 1

History, scope and development of biotechnology

Gajala Deethamvali Ghousepeer, Prashant Anilkumar Singh and Ramendra Pati Pandey

Biotechnology refers to implementation of biological systems, species, or processes to create products that are believed to improve human life. This can be broadly described as the engineering of living things for use by humans. We refer to this branch of science as biotechnology. 'The controlled employment of biological agents, e.g. microorganisms or cellular components, for favorable use' is what biotechnology is all about. Over the course of several centuries, biotechnology has made significant advancements and discoveries that have been used in a variety of fields, including industry, agriculture, and medicine. Similar to other cutting-edge technologies, biotechnology can be misused. This chapter examines the development of biotechnology from its inception to its current state of progress.

1.1 Introduction

The utilization of biological processes, organisms or systems to produce products that are anticipated to improve human lives is termed biotechnology. Broadly, this can be defined as the engineering of organisms for the purpose of human usage. It can also be defined as the skill set required for the utilization of living systems or the influencing of natural processes so as to produce products, systems or environments to help human development. Also, the scientific field of biotechnology aims to enhance people's health by integrating technology and biology by utilizing living cells or any of their constituent parts, to create products with targeted functions. It is a multidisciplinary field of study that includes genetics, virology, microbiology, immunology, engineering for the development of vaccines, and a variety of other disciplines. It is essential to health systems, agriculture, soil management, animal husbandry, yield improvement, crop and seed management, cellular processes,

doi:10.1088/978-0-7503-5382-3ch1

biostatistics, and many other areas [1]. Currently biotechnology places more emphasis on the establishment of hybrid genes followed by their transfer into organisms in which some, or all, of the gene is not usually present. In prehistoric times, a primitive form of biotechnology was practised by agriculturalists who established better-quality species of plants and animals by methods of cross-pollination or cross-breeding. Previous forms of biotechnology have included the training and selective breeding of animals, the cultivation of crops and the utilization of microorganisms to produce products such as cheese, yogurt, bread, beer and wine. Early agriculture concentrated on producing food.

The most primitive type of biotechnology is the cultivation of plants and the training (in particular the domestication) of animals. The domestication of animals stretches back over 10 000 years, when our ancestors also started maintaining plants as a reliable source of food. The earliest examples of such domesticated plants were rice, barley and wheat. Wild animals were also controlled to produce milk or meat. The ancient production of cheese, yogurt and bread from microorganisms is also reported. Various alcoholic drinks such as beer and wine were developed during this period, when the process of fermentation was first discovered.

Later, it was discovered that microorganisms, e.g. bacteria, yeast or molds, hydrolyze sugars when they lack oxygen and are ultimately responsible for fermentation. This process results in the formation of products (food and drink). Consequently, fermentation was perhaps first explored by chance, since in earlier times nobody knew how it worked. During the prehistoric era some civilizations considered fermentation to be a gift from their gods. Scientific evidence for fermentation was first described by Louis Pasteur in the late 1800s. He demonstrated a theory known as germ theory, presenting the survival of microorganisms and their further effects on the process of fermentation. Pasteur's efforts contributed towards several branches of science. In earlier times several traditional medicines were used as biotechnology products, such as honey, which could be used to treat several respiratory ailments and as an ointment for wounds. Since honey contains several antimicrobial compounds it is considered to be a natural antibiotic and is effectively used in wound healing. Similarly, in China as far back as 600 BC, soybean curds were used to treat boils. Ukrainian farmers once used utilized moldy cheese to treat infected wounds. It was later observed that antibiotics present in such molds killed bacteria and averted the spread of infection. In 1928 Alexander Fleming extracted penicillin, the first antibiotic, from mold [2]. This discovery revolutionized the available treatments, with antibiotics having more potential and being more effective than earlier medicines. The development of biotechnology in terms of crop rotation (including leguminous crops), vaccinations and animal-drawn technology, was realized between the late eighteenth century and the commencement of the nineteenth century [2]. The late nineteenth century was known to be a milestone in biology. Some of the key developments during this period are highlighted below:

- Structures for examining fermentation and other microbial developments were identified by Robert Koch, Pasteur and Joseph Lister.
- Gregor Mendel's work on genetics was carried out.
- Microorganisms were discovered.

In the 1920s a start was made on the production of useful chemicals through biological processes, when Chaim Weizmann used *Clostridium acetobutylicum* for the conversion of starch into butanol and acetone (the acetone thus produced was used as an essential component of explosives during World War I) [3]. At the beginning of the eighteenth century, developments in biotechnology tended to bring industry and agriculture together. Later, some basic processes of biotechnology such as fermentation were refined to develop paint solvents for the emerging automobile industry and acetone from starch. These processes were promoted during World War I. In the 1930s the processes of biotechnology moved more into utilizing surplus agricultural goods to supply industry as a replacement for imports or petrochemicals.

The advent of World War II brought the manufacture of penicillin. The production of antibiotics from microorganisms became possible when Fleming discovered penicillin, which was later produced at a large scale from cultures of *Penicillium notatum* (this proved useful for the treatment of wounded soldiers during World War II) [2]. The focus of biotechnology shifted to pharmaceuticals. The Cold War years were dominated by work on microorganisms for the preparation for biological products along with antibiotics and fermentation processes [4].

Biotechnology is now being used in numerous disciplines including bioremediation, energy production and food processing agriculture. DNA fingerprinting is often practised in forensics. Insulin production and other biotech-based medicines (biopharmaceuticals) are produced through cloning of vectors with genes of interest (GOIs). Immunoassays are frequently utilized in medicine for drug efficiency and pregnancy testing. In addition, immunoassays are also utilized by farmers to find hazardous levels of pesticides, herbicides and toxins in crops and animal-based products. These tests also offer rapid field tests for the determination of industrial chemicals, in particular, in ground water, sediment and soil. Biotechnology also has vast scope in agriculture for the production of plants that are resistant to insects, weeds and plant diseases. This can be achieved by the introduction of GOIs using genetic engineering.

Selective breeding of plants and animals was practised in the past without awareness of the basic concepts of biotechnology. In this procedure organisms with desirable traits were allowed to mate to further enhance these traits in their offspring. Consequently, it was revealed that selective breeding could improve yields as well as productivity. During this time farmers were not aware that selective breeding innovators were modifying the genetic make-up of organisms. An outstanding example is the corn plant, which has been enriched by selective breeding to develop an improved source of food and has given a platform for plant breeders to develop more hybrid varieties. Regarding animals, dogs are another example of selective breeding. Breeding between different dogs was promoted to improve traits e.g. size, agility, shape and color, resulting in breeds from the tiny Chihuahua to the Great Dane. Another revolutionary development in biotechnology that initiated the era of genetics was started in 1865 by a monk, Gregor Mendel, who recognized genes as the unit of inheritance. It took almost another 90 years of research to determine that genes are made up of DNA. This breakthrough was the beginning of modern biotechnology. Recent developments in biotechnology have led to an expansion in its sophistication, scope and applicability. As mentioned above, the simplest way to define biotechnology is to split this word into its two constituent parts (biotechnology = biology + technology). By considering these two key words we can define biotechnology as a set of techniques that are employed to manipulate living organisms, or utilize biological agents or their components, to produce useful products/services. The vast nature of biotechnology has frequently made a detailed definition of the subject rather difficult. Some definitions of biotechnology are as follows:

- 'Biotechnology means any scientific application that uses biological systems, living organisms or derivatives thereof, to produce or alter products or processes for particular use' [5].
- 'The utilization of living organisms, systems or processes constitutes biotechnology' [6].
- Based on the *Collins English Dictionary* definition [7], biotechnology is the employment of living organisms, their parts or processes, to develop active and useful products and to provide services e.g. waste treatment. The term signifies a broad range of processes, from the use of earthworms as a source of protein to the genetic modification of bacteria to offer human gene products, e.g. growth hormones.
- According to the *Golden Treasury of Science and Technology* [8], biotechnology is a discipline based on the harnessing of life processes which are controlled for the bulk production of valuable substances.

It is obvious from the above definitions that biotechnology includes different technologies that rely on information gained by modern discoveries in biochemistry, cell biology and molecular biology. These technologies are already having a huge impact on diverse areas of life, including agriculture, food processing, medical technology and waste treatment.

- Biotechnology consists of 'the controlled employment of biological agents, e.g. microorganisms or cellular components, for favorable use' [9].
- Biotechnology has been defined as 'Janus-faced' [10]. This means that there are two sides to it. On one side, we know that the technology allows DNA to be modified so that genes can be moved from one organism to another. On the other, it also entails comparatively new techniques whose results are untested and should be met with care.
- Biotechnology is 'the integrated use of microbiology, biochemistry and engineering sciences in production or as service operation' [11].
- Biotechnology is the commercial employment of microorganisms and living plant and animal cells to create substances or effects beneficial to people. It includes the production of antibiotics, vitamins, vaccines, plastics, etc [12].
- 'Bio' refers to life and 'technology' refers to the application of information for practical use, i.e. the application of living organisms to create or improve a product [12].

- It involves the industrial application of living organisms or their products, which entails the intentional manipulation of their DNA molecules. It may mean making a living cell execute a particular task in a predictable and controllable way [12].
- The term biotechnology is occasionally also applied to processes in which microorganisms such as yeasts and bacteria are cultured under strictly controlled environmental conditions. For this reason, fermentation is occasionally called the oldest form of biotechnology. Genetic engineering techniques are frequently, but not always, used in biotechnology [12].
- The *Universities Press Dictionary of Biology* defines biotechnology as 'the application of technology to biological processes for industrial, agricultural and medical purposes' [13].
- The *Oxford Dictionary of Biology* [14] defines biotechnology as 'the development of techniques for the application of biological processes to the production of materials of use in medicine and industry.'
- The employment of cells and biological molecules to explain problems or make valuable products. These biological molecules include DNA, RNA and proteins.
- Biotechnology may be defined as 'the utilization of living organisms in systems or processes for the production of valuable products; it may involve algae, bacteria, fungi, yeast, cells of higher plants and animals or subsystems of any of these or isolated components from living matter' [15].

It may be seen that the diverse definitions of biotechnology above differ in their approach, content and emphasis. But there are two main characteristics common to them all. First, biotechnology involves the exploitation of biological entities (i.e. microorganisms, cells of higher organisms—either living or dead), their components or constituents (e.g. enzymes), in such a way that some functional product or service is generated. Second, this product or service should aim to improve human welfare.

In summary, biotechnology is the '[a]pplication of the theory of engineering and biological science to generate new products from raw materials of biological origin, e.g. vaccines or food', or, in other words, it can also be defined as 'the exploitation of living organism/s or their product/s to change or improve human health and human surroundings' [16].

Hungarian engineer Karl Ereky first coined the term 'biotechnology' in 1919, meaning the production of products from raw materials with the aid of living organisms [17, 18]. As mentioned above, biotechnology is *not* new, since human civilization has been exploiting living organisms to solve problems and improve our way of life for millennia. The production technologies and processes involved in animal husbandry, agriculture, horticulture, etc, utilize plants and animals to produce useful products. However, such technologies are not regarded as biotechnology since they are long recognized and well-established disciplines in their own right. Today, the exploitation of animal and plant cells cultured *in vitro* as well as their constituents for generating products/services is an integral part of biotechnology.

1.2 Branches of biotechnology

The definition of biotechnology can be further divided into different areas. Dr Rita R Colwell originally proposed a color-code method of classification in the field of biotechnology which is one of the many different types of classification known as red, green, blue, white, yellow, brown, grey and gold.

- *Red biotechnology*: This area includes medical procedures such as utilizing organisms for the production of novel drugs or employing stem cells to replace/regenerate injured tissues and possibly regenerate whole organs. It could simply be called medical biotechnology.
- *Green biotechnology*: Green biotechnology applies to agriculture and involves such processes as the development of pest-resistant grains and the accelerated evolution of disease-resistant animals.
- *Blue biotechnology*: Blue biotechnology, rarely mentioned, encompasses processes in the marine and aquatic environments, such as controlling the proliferation of noxious water-borne organisms.
- *White biotechnology*: White (also called grey) biotechnology involves industrial processes such as the production of new chemicals or the development of new fuels for vehicles.
- *Yellow biotechnology*: It focuses on applying biotechnological methods to insects or their cells to produce useful products used by humans. These products are used in industrial biotechnology, medicine, and agriculture [19].
- *Brown biotechnology*: This study aims to establish a connection between the biotechnological developments in desert regions and the contemporary environmental problems of those regions, their ecosystems, and their inhabitants [20].
- *Gray biotechnology*: It is dedicated to environmental applications and is concentrated on implementing biotechnological methods to eliminate pollutants while preserving biodiversity [21].
- *Gold biotechnology*: It has a connection to nanobiotechnology and bioinformatics. In its entirety, it concentrates on creating and sustaining databases for the storage of biological information in addition to the design and manipulation of biological materials and processes at the submicroscopic level [22] (figure 1.1).

A distinction is made between 'non-gene biotechnology' and 'gene biotechnology':

- *Non-gene biotechnology*: Non-gene biotechnology works with whole cells, tissues or even individual organisms. Non-gene biotechnology is the more popular practice, involving plant tissue culture, hybrid seed production, microbial fermentation, production of hybridoma antibodies and immunochemistry.
- *Gene biotechnology*: Gene biotechnology deals with genes, the transfer of genes from one organism to another and genetic engineering.

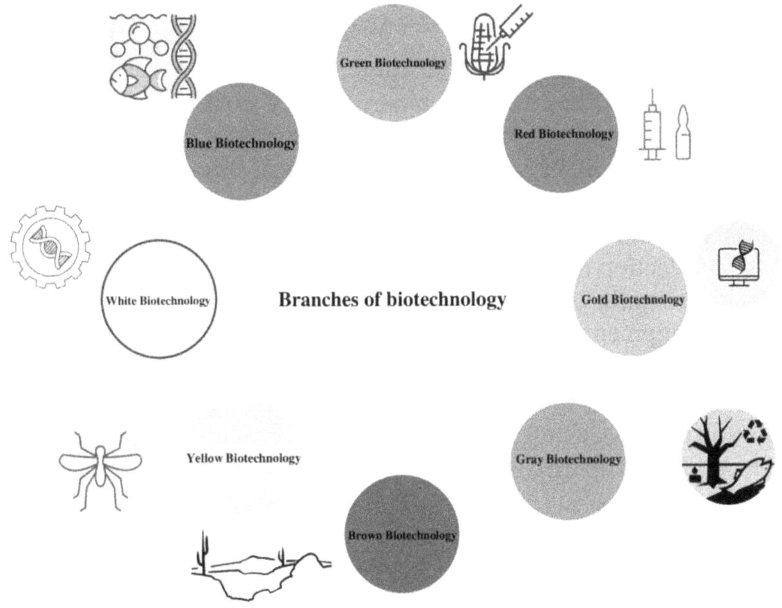

Figure 1.1. Branches of biotechnology.

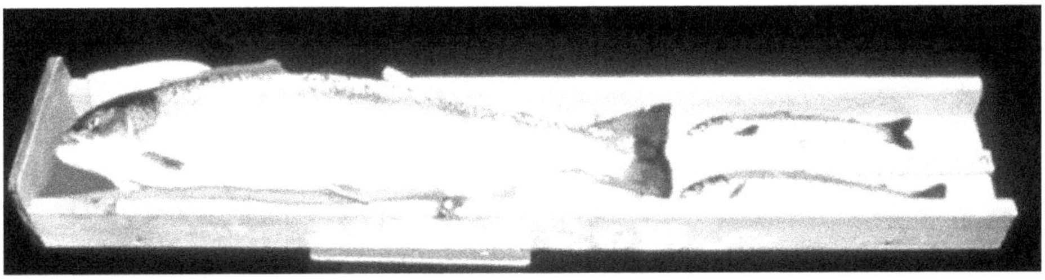

Figure 1.2. Fourteen-month-old genetically engineered ('biotech') salmon (left) and standard salmon (right).

Biotechnology, like other advanced technologies, has the potential for misuse. Concern about this has led to efforts by some groups to enact legislation restricting or banning certain processes or programs, such as human cloning and embryonic stem cell research. There is also concern that if biotechnological processes are used by groups with nefarious intent, the end result could be biological warfare. Apart from their beneficial applications, biotechnological principles also have the potential for destruction, the best example of which is bioterrorism. A representation of the potential pitfalls of biotechnology in fiction can be found in the novel *Frankenstein* [23, 24]. In this science fiction story, the character of Frankenstein has created a human life which becomes a monster; this monster becomes the cause of the destruction of Frankenstein, the creator of human life. The real-life changes that can be brought about by biotechnology can easily be seen in figure 1.2, illustrating a 14-month-old genetically engineered ('biotech') salmon (left) and a standard salmon (right).

1.3 Biotechnology and its various stages of development

It is well known that the technical application of biological material is considered to be biotechnology. To understand how biotechnology works it is important to think about the starting point or material for biotechnology processes. Generally, biotechnology utilizes living material or biological products to generate new products for use in various medical, agricultural, pharmaceutical and environmental applications. The ultimate goal of biotechnology is to benefit humanity by, for example, the production of resistant crops, vegetables, recombinant proteins, higher milk-producing animals, etc.

Different developmental stages have taken place in biotechnology to meet the various needs of humans at the time. Its development was principally based on observations, and the application of these observations to practical scenarios. Owing to the evolution of new technologies and a better understanding of various principles of life science, the complexity of biotechnology has increased. Table 1.1 gives a

Table 1.1. Historical events in biotechnology.

Periods of biotechnology history	Events
Pre-1800 (Early applications and speculation)	**6000 BC**
	Yeast was utilized to prepare beer (Sumerians and Babylonians).
	4000 BC
	In Egypt, a process was discovered to prepare leavened bread by means of yeast.
	420 BC
	Greek philosopher Socrates (470–399 BC) hypothesized on the similar characteristics between parents and their offspring.
	320 BC
	Greek philosopher Aristotle (384–322 BC) theorized that all inheritance originates from the father.
	1000 AD
	Hindus recognized that some illnesses may 'run in the family'. At the same time, the theory of abiogenesis, or spontaneous generation based on the idea that organisms arise from non-living matter, developed. According to this theory maggots could develop from horse hair.
	1630
	William Harvey explained that plants and animals are similar in their reproduction, i.e. they reproduce sexually.

	1660–75 Marcello Malpighi (1628–94) investigated blood circulation in capillaries using a microscope and found that the brain is connected to the spinal cord by bundles of fibers which form the nervous system [25, 26].
	1673 Antonie van Leeuwenhoek (1632–1723) was the first researcher to explain microorganisms such as protozoa and bacteria, and also identify that these microorganisms play an active role in fermentation.
	1701 Giacomo Pylarini found that the deliberate administration of smallpox could prevent its occurrence later in life, especially in children. Later, this procedure was termed 'vaccination' and a process that uses cowpox instead of smallpox was established as the most reliable treatment [27, 28].
1800–1900 (Significant advances in basic understanding)	**1809** Nicolas Appert invent a technique using heat to can and sterilize food.
	1827 In the field of heredity, there had long been a hunt for the so-called mammalian egg. It had proved elusive, however, in 1827 the first report of canine eggs offered a basic clue to major breakthroughs in reproduction, at first in lower animals
	1850 Ignaz Semmelweis utilized epidemiological examinations to suggest the theory that puerperal fever could be transmitted from mother to mother by physicians. He also suggested that all physicians should wash their hands after investigating each patient. For this suggestion he was criticized by medical professionals and ultimately lost his employment.
	1856 Carl Ludwig discovered a procedure for keeping animal organs alive under *in vitro* conditions. This was done by supplying blood to them. In contrast to the concepts of Justus von Liebig, Pasteur (1822–95) suggested that microbes are responsible for fermentation.

(*Continued*)

Table 1.1. (*Continued*)

Periods of biotechnology history	Events
	1859 Charles Darwin (1809–82) speculated that animal populations adapt their forms to eventually best utilize the surroundings, a process he described as 'natural selection'. During his stay in the Galapagos Islands, he saw how the finches' beaks on each island were adapted for the environment, especially regarding food sources.
	1863 Pasteur discovered the method of pasteurization. In this method he heated wine enough to inactivate microbes (that would otherwise convert the 'vin' to 'vin aigre' or 'sour wine') and realized that this procedure did not affect the flavor of the wine [31].
	Heinrich Anton de Bary established that a fungus was responsible for potato blight. A major challenge for researchers during this period was to differentiate whether a microbe was responsible for this or whether it was the outcome of a disease.
	1865 Mendel (1822–84) suggested the laws of heredity to the National Scientific Society (Brunn, Austria). Mendel anticipated that imperceptible core units of information were responsible for noticeable characteristics. He called these 'factors', which were later called genes (units that were inherited by one generation from its parents). The research done by Mendel was overlooked and not acknowledged due to Darwin's more sensational publication five years earlier, until 1900 when Hugo de Vries, Erich von Tschermak and Carl Correns supported Mendel's mechanism of heredity.
	1868 Casimir Joseph Davaine cured plants suffering from bacterial infection by a novel heat treatment. While working in a hospital, Johannes Friedrich Miescher separated nuclein (a compound made of nucleic acid) from pus cells. These pus cells were derived from waste bandages [29].
	1870 Walther Flemming discovered mitosis [30].
	1871 During the period 1873–76 interest in DNA research began. DNA was initially derived from the sperm of trout (found in the river Rhine). During this period Koch investigated

	anthrax and explored certain techniques to identify, culture and stain microorganisms. He also took images of them which were later supported by Gram, Cohn and Weigart [31].
	1880 While working on fowl cholera, Louis Pasteur explored weakened (attenuated) strains of microorganisms that might not be virulent but could nevertheless potentially prevent healthy individuals against severe forms of a similar disease [31].
	1881 Koch explained techniques for harvesting bacterial colonies on potato slices, gelatin and agar medium [31]. For the isolation of pure culture and for distinguishing the nutrients needed for genetic mutations, the agar technique was one of the most common methods. Thomas D Brock considered this breakthrough as the single most important discovery in the development of microbiology. During the same period Pasteur explored the application of the attenuation process in the production of vaccines against certain bacterial pathogens, e.g. fowl cholera and anthrax; this was an early stage in immunology which led to the exploration of areas such as preventive medicine [31].
	1884 Koch established his 'claims' for assessing whether a microbe or another agent is responsible for disease. During the same period Pasteur established a rabies vaccine [31]. Gram described the differential staining technique for cellular peptidoglycan-containing bacteria now known as Gram staining [32]. Mendel passed away after 41 years of predominantly investigating the heredity 'factors' of pea plants. He did not receive any technical support during his lifetime, but said before his death, 'My time will come' [33]
1900–53 (Genetics:converging on DNA)	**1900: Mendel's work finally took on importance** Mendel's work had given birth to genetic science. It was revived again by three researchers, de Vries, von Tschermak and Correns, who were working on the application of original work done by Mendel [34].

(*Continued*)

Table 1.1. *(Continued)*

Periods of biotechnology history	Events
	1902: Human genetics is born Sutton found that chromosomes (paired) contain certain elements which are transferred from one generation to another. During this transfer, traits are transported through carriers called chromosomes. He also advised that Mendel's 'factors' are sited on chromosomes [35].
	1905: X and Y chromosomes related to gender Edmund Beecher Wilson and Nettie Stevens shared the same idea of separating X and Y chromosomes for the determination of sex. They also demonstrated that a single Y chromosome determines maleness, while two copies of the X chromosome decide femaleness [36].
	1905–08 William Bateson and R C Punnett, along with other researchers, found that several genes alter or modify the action of other genes [37].
	1906 Paul Erlich also investigated atoxyl compounds and discovered the important features of Salvarsan (the first chemotherapeutic agent) [38].
	1907 Thomas Hunt Morgan started his investigation into fruit flies that would reveal that chromosomes have a defined role in heredity; additionally, he discovered mutation theory. This resulted in an understanding of the basic concepts and mechanisms of heredity [39].
	1909: Mendel's laws to animals Wilhelm Johannsen used the word 'gene' to mean the carrier/transporter of heredity. He also coined the terms 'genotype' and 'phenotype'; the genotype is the genetic composition/establishment of an organism, whereas the phenotype describes the actual organism or its morphological characteristics, resulting from a blend of the genotype and a range of external/environmental factors [40].
	1910: Basis of modern genetics Morgan also demonstrated that carriers of genetic information, called asor genes, are present on chromosomes, creating the basis for modern genetics. This work later assisted him in utilizing *Drosophila* fruit flies to examine heredity [41].

1911

During the same period Morgan established the separation of certain inherited features that are generally linked to the separation/breaking of chromosomes during the process of cell division. He also investigated the mapping of the genetic sites present on the chromosomes of the fruit fly [41].

1912

Crystallography era: William Lawrence Bragg discovered the application of x-rays in the determination of the molecular structure of crystalline substances [42].

1918

Herbert M Evans stated (mistakenly) that human genetic material is made up of 48 chromosomes [43].

1924: Eugenics in the United States

Several US diplomats, encouraged by the eugenics movement, accepted the US Immigration Act (1924), limiting the admission of illiterate refugees from Southern and Eastern Europe on the basis of their alleged genetic inferiority.

1926

Morgan published *The Theory of the Gene*. This was based on Mendelian genetics (breeding investigations and optical microscopy) [42].

Hermann Joseph Muller discovered that x-rays are responsible for genetic mutations in fruit flies taking place 1500 times faster than under normal conditions. This innovation offered researchers and scientists a procedure to induce mutations. Later, various mutagens were explored to understand the complexity behind different genotypes [44].

1928

Frederick Griffiths observed the 'transforming principle' in which a rough type of bacterium is transformed to a smooth type when a mysterious 'transforming element' from the smooth type is present. After 16 years, Oswald Theodore Avery discovered that 'transforming element' to be DNA [45].

Alexander Fleming studied an old culture of bacteria infected with fungal growth and found that it did not show any bacterial growth in a radius surrounding a piece of mold (fungi) in a petri dish. This breakthrough gave

(*Continued*)

Table 1.1. (*Continued*)

Periods of biotechnology history	Events
	birth to the antibiotics era or penicillin age, and penicillin was accessible to patients 15 years later for therapeutic use [46].
	1938 Proteins and DNA were studied by means of x-rays. This was the dawn of a new age of crystallography in which large molecular weight complex proteins can be studied by x-rays. The term 'molecular biology' was coined.
	1941: One gene, one enzyme George Wells Beadle and Edward L Tatum examined *Neurospora crassa*, a mold that usually invades and grows on bread, and proposed 'one gene, one enzyme' theory: each gene encodes for or is translated into an enzyme to accomplish tasks within an organism [45].
	1943 The Rockefeller Foundation (New York) collaborated with the Mexican government to start the Mexican Agricultural Program [47]. This was the first step toward plant breeding at a global level.
	1943–53 Cortisone (17α,21-dihydroxypregn-4-ene-3,11,20-trione), a pregnane (21-carbon) steroid hormone, was first produced in great amounts. Cortisone is considered as the first biotech product.
	1944 Selman Abraham Waksman (a Ukrainian-American researcher) explored streptomycin, an active antibiotic against TB [48].
	1945 The United Nations Food and Agriculture Organization was established in Quebec, Canada, with the objective of encouraging agricultural practices.
	1945–50 For the first time, animal cell cultures were harvested in laboratories, giving birth to the field of animal tissue culture.
	1947 Barbara McClintock first demonstrated 'transposable elements' known as 'jumping genes' with the capability to move (or jump) from one site on the genome to another

	site. Scientific society did not welcome the implications of her discovery at the time [49].
	1950 Erwin Chargaff discovered that the same levels of adenine and thymine are present in DNA, as are the same levels of guanine and cytosine [50]. These associations were later named 'Chargaff's rules'. Later, Chargaff's rules functioned as an important principle for James Watson and Francis Crick in measuring different models for the structure of DNA.
DNA research, science explodes (1953–76)	**1953–76: Expanding the boundaries of DNA research** The discovery of the structure of DNA finally resulted in an explosion of research into molecular biology and genetics, providing the resources for biotechnology development.
	1953 The journal *Nature* published Watson and Crick's article based on unfolding the double-helix structure of DNA.
	1953 Based on his technical exposure George Otto Gey developed the HeLa human cell line. Cells taken from cancer patient Henrietta Lacks (who died in 1951) became the first immortal human cells and were cultured to develop a polio vaccine [51].
	1957: Central dogma of DNA—how DNA makes a protein Crick and Gamov studied 'central dogma', demonstrating how DNA functions to construct protein [52].
	1959 François Jacob and Jacques Lucien Monod documented the veracity of gene-based regulation. They explained gene mapping with mappable control functions sited on the chromosome in the DNA sequence which they later named the 'repressor' and 'operon' [53].
	1962 Watson and Crick were awarded the Nobel Prize in Physiology or Medicine with Maurice Wilkins. Disappointingly, Rosalind Franklin, who actually contributed to the discovery of the double-helical structure of DNA, died before this date, and Nobel Prize conventions do not permit a prize to be awarded posthumously [54].

(*Continued*)

Table 1.1. (*Continued*)

Periods of biotechnology history	Events
	1966: Genetic code cracked The genetic code was explored by several researchers. Marshall Warren Nirenberg, J Heinrich Matthaei and S Ochoa reported that a genetic sequence of three nucleotide bases (called codons) decides each of 20 amino acids [55].
	1967 Arthur Kornberg reported a study using single-stranded natural viral DNA to assemble 5300 nucleotide building blocks, and at the same time his Stanford group synthesized viral DNA [55].
	1970: Oncogenes Virologists Peter H Duesberg and Peter K Vogt identified the first oncogene in a virus. This gene can be utilized to study various human cancers [56]
	1972: First recombinant DNA molecule Paul Berg, a biochemist, utilized a restriction enzyme to cut DNA into fragments. He employed a ligase enzyme to join two DNA strands concurrently to form a hybrid circular molecule. This was the first recombinant DNA (rDNA) molecule synthesized [57].
	1972: NIH guidelines for rDNA Berg and other researchers at the National Institutes of Health (NIH) worked hard to establish guidelines to sanction the strategy for DNA splicing. Their concerns resulted in the Asilomar Conference (1975).
	1973: Ames test Bruce Nathan Ames, a biochemist at UC Berkeley, developed an investigation to distinguish chemicals that damage DNA. Later, the Ames test became extensively used to identify cancer-causing substances [45].
	1975: rDNA moratorium A global meeting was held in Asilomar, California, with the objective of approving guidelines regulating rDNA experimentation. All the scientists involved discussed the development of 'safe' bacteria and plasmids.
	1976: More about oncogenes J Michael Bishop and Harold Varmus at the University of California, San Francisco (UCSF) established that cancer-causing genes called oncogenes become visible on

	animal chromosomes, and modifications in their structure or expression can result in metastatic growth [58].
	1976: Release of NIH guidelines The NIH released the first set of guidelines for rDNA experimentation. Later, these guidelines restricted several types of trials.
1977–present (modern biotechnology)	**1977–present: The dawn of biotech** With the advent of genetic engineering it was possible to produce human protein in bacteria for the first time. Biotech-based organizations started focusing more on the applications of genetic engineering. In 1978, Herbert W Boyer at UCSF synthesized synthetic human insulin by introducing the insulin gene into the bacterium *Escherichia coli* [59]. This breakthrough opened the gateway for further developments in DNA sequencing and cloning techniques.
	1977 Genentech Inc. was the first organization to achieve the synthesis of a human protein (somatostatin) in a bacterium. Somatostatin is a human growth hormone (hGH)-releasing inhibitory factor. A synthetic, recombinant gene was for the first time employed to clone a protein. Several researchers believed that this was the beginning of the age of modern biotechnology [60].
	1978: Recombinant insulin Genentech Inc. announced that its laboratory had achieved the synthesis of human insulin using rDNA technology [60].
	1980: Patents allowed The US Supreme Court granted that genetically modified living organisms could be patented. According to a Supreme Court decision (1980) the Exxon oil company was allowed to patent an oil-eating micro-organism. Kary Mullis and other researchers at UC Berkeley, California, established a tool for multiplying DNA sequences *in vitro* using the polymerase chain reaction (PCR) [61].
	1982: Site-directed mutagenesis Genentech Inc. signed an agreement from the US Food and Drug Administration (FDA) to further market genetically

(*Continued*)

Table 1.1. (*Continued*)

Periods of biotechnology history	Events
	engineered human insulin. In 1982 the FDA allowed the first genetically engineered drug in the form of human insulin produced by bacteria. Michael Smith at the University of British Columbia, Vancouver, established a procedure for producing precise amino acid changes anywhere in a protein.
	1983: Site-directed mutagenesis Eli Lilly obtained a license to make and sell insulin.
	1985 During this period genetic fingerprinting stepped into the courtroom. Cal Bio produced a gene by a cloning method that encodes human lung surfactant protein, an important step toward reducing premature birth complications. For the first time, genetically modified plants that resistant to insects, viruses and bacteria were examined. The NIH published guidelines for performing experiments in gene therapy on humans.
	1986 Chiron Corp. obtained FDA approval for the production of the first recombinant vaccine for hepatitis. A genetically modified crop (the tobacco plant) was allowed by the Environmental Protection Agency (EPA).
	1987 Calgene Inc. obtained a patent for the tomato polygalacturonase DNA sequence, which was later used to synthesize an antisense RNA sequence that can further extend the shelf life of fruit.
	1988 Harvard molecular geneticists Philip Leder and Timothy A Stewart were granted the first patent based on a genetically modified animal (a mouse that is highly susceptible to breast cancer) [62].
	1990 UCSF and Stanford University achieved their 100th rDNA patent license. At the end of the 1991 financial year, both organizations had received $40 million from the patent.
	1990: Patents and money The first gene-based treatment was performed on a 4-year-old girl suffering from an immunological disorder known

as adenosine deaminase deficiency (ADA) deficiency. Gene therapy emerged, however ethical concerns surrounding gene therapy were highly debated.

Commencement of the Human Genome Project, with the global objective to plot all of the genes in the human body. The expected cost was $13 billion.

Michael Crichton's novel *Jurassic Park* was released, in which bioengineered dinosaurs wander in a paleontological theme park; the project goes wrong, with deadly outcomes.

1992

The US Army started taking blood and tissue samples from all new employees as part of a 'genetic dog-tag'. This course of action was intended for better identification of soldiers killed in battle.

1993

Researcher Kary Mullis won the Nobel Prize in Chemistry for inventing the tool of PCR [63].

1996

A groundbreakingly efficient diagnostic biosensor test allowed for the first time the instant detection of the toxic strain of *E. coli* (strain 0157:H7), the bacteria responsible for several food poisoning outbreaks. The possibility of its use against anthrax and other bioterrorism agents was also assessed.

The discovery of a gene linked to Parkinson's disease offered researchers a significant new chance for the determination of the cause of, and potential treatments for, the incapacitating neurological disorder.

Reports showed that there were public concerns about research into the human genome and gene therapy, with a combination of fear and mistrust.

1997

Researchers at the Roslin Institute in Scotland announced that they had cloned a sheep called Dolly from the cell of an adult ewe. Dolly was the first mammal cloned by a technique called nuclear transfer technology. Nuclear transfer allows the introduction of complete genetic material from one cell into another enucleated unfertilized egg cell.

1998

A group of researchers succeeded in culturing embryonic stem cells. A number of researchers at Japan's Kinki

(*Continued*)

Table 1.1. (*Continued*)

Periods of biotechnology history	Events
	University cloned eight identical calves by means of cells taken from a single adult cow. A rough draft of the human genome map was created, presenting the sites of more than 30 000 genes. **1999** A fatal neurological disease called bovine spongiform encephalopathy (BSE), also known as mad cow disease, that spread from cattle to humans, was diagnosed by a new medical diagnostic examination that facilitated the quick detection of BSE/Creutzfeldt–Jakob disease (CJD).

breakdown of historical events in biotechnology. The development of biotechnology can be divided into broad stages or categories, including:

- Ancient biotechnology (8000–4000 BC): Early history as related to food and shelter; includes domestication of animals.
- Classical biotechnology (2000 BC; 1800–1900 AD): Built on ancient biotechnology; fermentation promotes food production and medicine.
- 1900–53: Genetics.
- 1953–76: DNA research, science explodes.
- Modern biotechnology (1977): Manipulates genetic information in organisms; genetic engineering; various technologies enable us to improve crop yield and food quality in agriculture and to produce a broader array of products in industries.

1.3.1 Old and new biotechnology

While the word biotechnology is of recent origin, the discipline itself is very old. To produce wine, vinegar, curd, leavened bread, etc, humans began employing microorganisms as early as 5000 BC. These processes were commonly employed at a domestic scale and have become such an integral part of normal food processing methods that we may even hesitate to refer to them as biotechnology. Such processes, based on the natural capabilities of microorganisms, are commonly considered to be 'old' biotechnology.

1.3.2 Ancient biotechnology (pre-1800)

Biotechnology's inaugural manifestation is recorded in the domestication of plants and animals. Domestication officially commenced more than 10 000 years ago when our ancestors started cultivating plants as a consistent food source. Wheat, barley, and rice were among the first plants to undergo domestication. The domestication of wild animals followed, serving purposes such as providing meat and milk, aiding in plowing, and contributing to agricultural security. Among the earliest domesticated animals are considered to be goats, sheep, and dogs. The majority of the advancements that took place in ancient times, or before 1800, can be considered 'discoveries' or 'developments', some events that were based on common observations about nature can be categorized as biotechnological developments. Three important basic needs of human civilization are food, clothes and shelter. In the ancient era the paucity of food led to the domestication of food products, formally called 'agriculture'. During ancient times humans understood the importance of water, light and other requirements for the optimal growth of food plants and the domestication of different wild animals, which helped them improve their living conditions and satisfy their hunger. The domestication of wild animals was the beginning of the observation, understanding and applications of animal breeding. This initial period of the evolution of farming led to another development in methods for food preservation and storage. The utilization of cold caves or pots (in the form of leather bags and clay jars) to preserve food for long-term storage began. After discovering the basic facts behind the domestication of food crops and wild animals, human beings moved on to other new inventions such as curd, cheese, etc. Cheese can be considered to be one of the first direct products (or by-products) of biotechnology, since it was prepared by adding rennet (an enzyme found in the stomachs of calves) to sour milk. This is only possible when milk is exposed to microbes (although there was no understanding of this at that time). Among all microbial strains, yeast is one of the oldest microbes to have been exploited by humans for their benefit. This primitive microbe has long been employed for the production of alcoholic beverages such as whiskey, wine, beer, etc. Among the oldest preservatives, vinegar has a significant importance because of its low pH and potential in preventing the growth of certain microbes, which means it can be used successfully in food preservation. These discoveries and their significance allowed people to work on further improvement of the processes involved. However, while processes such as the decomposition of debris or other materials, which was later called fermentation, were powerful tools to improve their living conditions, people were ignorant of the principles behind them.

Among the most primitive examples of cross-breeding for the benefit of humans is the mule. Man started using mules for transportation, carrying loads and farming, before the days of tractors or trucks. Mules are comparatively easier to obtain than hinnies (the offspring of a male horse and a female donkey). Mules and hinnies both have 63 chromosomes, unlike the horse (64) and the donkey (62). Some of the processes and products developed in the ancient period are described in table 1.2.

1.3.3 Classical biotechnology

Classical biotechnology is the second phase of the development of biotechnology. This stage existed from 1800 to almost the middle of the twentieth century. In the classical era different observations started pouring in, supported by scientific evidence. These observations made it possible to solve the puzzles of biotechnology. Each and every observation has made its own contribution in furthering the

Table 1.2. Biotechnological processes and products developed in the ancient period.

Process or product developed	Events that contributed to its development
Domestication	• Food supplies were often seasonal. In winter, food supplies could become quite low. • People came up with ways of capturing fish and small animals. • 15 000 years ago, large animals were difficult to catch. • People may only have had meat when they found a dead animal. • Domestication most likely began 11 000–12 000 years ago in the Middle East. • It involved the adaptation of organisms so they could be cultured. • Seen by scientists as the beginning of biotechnology. • Cattle, goats and sheep were the earliest domesticated food animals.
Food preservation • People knew that some foods rotted, while others changed form and continued to be good to eat. • Foods stored in a cool cave did not spoil as quickly. • Foods heated by fire also did not spoil as quickly. • Immersion in sour liquids prevented food decay. • Food was stored in bags of leather or jars of clay. • Fermentation occurs if certain microorganisms are present, it creates an acid condition that slows or prevents spoilage.	
Cheese	• One of the first food products made through biotechnology. • Strains of bacteria were added to milk, resulting in sour milk. • An enzyme called 'rennet' was added. • Rennet comes from the lining of the stomachs of calves. It is genetically engineered today. • Not all cheese is made from rennet. • It may have been first developed by nomadic tribes in Asia some 4000 years ago.

Yeast	• Long used in food preparation and preservation. • Used in bread baking. • Produces a gas in the dough causing the dough to rise. • Used in fermented products such as vinegar. • Ethanol production require the use of yeast in at least one stage of production.
Vinegar	• Used in pickling. • Keeps foods from spoiling. • Juices and extracts from fruits and grains can be fermented. • Biblical references to wine indicate the use of fermentation some 3000 years ago. • Ancient product used to preserve food.
Fermentation	• Process in which yeast enzymes chemically change compounds into alcohol. • In making vinegar the first product of fermentation is alcohol. • In ancient times, this likely happened by accident. • Advancements occurred in the 1800s and early 1900s.
Fermenters	• Allowed better control, especially with vinegar. • New products such as glycerol, acetone and citric acid resulted.
Antibiotics	• First drug produced by microbes. • Used in both human and veterinary medicine. • Use of fermentation hastened the development of antibiotics. • Penicillin was developed in the late 1920s. • Introduced in the 1940s as a drug used to combat bacterial infections. • Many kinds are available today. • Limitations in their use keep disease-producing organisms from developing immunity to antibiotics. • Some disease organisms are now resistant to certain antibiotics.

exploration of new discoveries. The fundamental idea of the transfer of genetic information from one generation to another forms the core of biotechnology. Information on the transfer of genetic information was first deciphered by Gregor John Mendel (1822–84), an Austrian Augustinian monk. Mendel presented his ideas on the laws of inheritance to the Natural Science Society in Brunn, Austria. He first observed the transfer of genetic information in a plant, *Pisum sativum*, commonly known as the pea plant [16]. Moreover, Mendel also hypothesized that an invisible internal unit of information accounted for observable traits. These 'factors', later called genes, were passed from one generation to the next. Nevertheless, the sad part of his story is that Mendel failed to receive due acknowledgment for his invention for almost 34 years after his death, when other scientists such as Hugo de Vries, Erich von Tschermak and Carl Correns validated his work in 1900. The main reason why Mendel's discovery remained overlooked for such long time was that in the same period Charles Darwin's theory of evolution was so overwhelming that it overshadowed the implications of the work done by Mendel. During this time the nucleus in cells was discovered [16], and Fredrich Miescher, a Swiss biologist, reported the existence of nuclein, a compound that consisted of nucleic acid that he had extracted from pus cells, i.e. white blood cells [16]. These two discoveries gave germination to the DNA era, which became the basis of modern molecular biology, the discovery of DNA as a genetic material and the role of DNA in the transfer of genetic information. Meanwhile the bacterial propagation method was first proposed by Robert Koch (1881), a German physician, who described the bacterial colonies growing on potato slices (the first ever solid medium) [16]. While working on the cause behind the solidification of jelly, Walter Hesse (one of the co-workers in Koch's laboratory) discovered the nutrient agar, the most acceptable and useful medium for obtaining pure microbial cultures, as well as for their identification [16]. He discovered agar when he asked his wife what kept the jelly solid even at high temperatures in summer. She said it was agar, and since then the nutrient has been used for microbial cultures. Heinrich Wilhelm Gottfried von Waldeyer-Hartz, a German scientist in the nineteenth century, coined the term 'chromosome' for an organized structure of DNA and protein present in cells or a single piece of coiled DNA containing many genes, regulatory elements and other nucleotide sequences [16]. Among various other prominent discoveries during this period, vaccinations against smallpox and rabies were developed by Edward Jenner, a British physician, and Louis Pasteur, a French biologist, respectively. The development of biological sciences seemed to be reaching an exponential phase. During this period the principle of genetics in inheritance was redefined by T H Morgan. He showed inheritance, and the role of chromosomes in inheritance, using fruit flies (*Drosophila melanogaster*). Later, in 1926, this work was published in Morgan's book *The Theory of the Gene.* Prior to Morgan's 1909 work, the term 'gene' had already been coined by Wilhelm Johannsen (1857–1927). He described the gene as the carrier of heredity. Afterwards Johannsen coined the terms 'genotype' to describe the genetic constitution of an organism, and 'phenotype' to describe the actual organism. After this exploration genetics started gaining importance. This led to the beginning of the eugenics movement in the USA (1924). At the same time, Alexander Fleming, a

British physician, discovered antibiotics when he observed that one micro-organism can be used to kill another micro-organism. The basic idea behind it was a true representation of the 'divide and rule' policy of humans. He noticed that all bacteria (*Staphylococci*) died when a mold was growing in a petri dish. Afterwards he discovered penicillin, the antibacterial toxin from the mold *P. notatum*, which could be used against many infectious diseases. He wrote 'When I woke up just after dawn on September 28, 1928, I certainly didn't plan to revolutionize all medicine by discovering the world's first antibiotic, or bacteria killer' [16]. He also concluded that vaccines and antibiotics would turn out to be the best saviors of humanity: 'Can we attribute these two discoveries for the ever increasing population as well the ever ageing population of the world?'

1.3.4 Modern biotechnology

A major obstacle to scientific discoveries was the Second World War. After the war, some essential discoveries were explored. These discoveries form the basis for modern biotechnology and have brought this field to its current status. Some of the prominent events of the modern age of biotechnology are highlighted in table 1.3.

Table 1.3. Historical and current events that form the basis of modern biotechnology.

Year	Discoveries
The 1950s	
1952	• George Otto Gey created a continuous cell line taken from a human cervical carcinoma. This cell line, known as HeLa, is still used in therapeutic research.
1953	• Watson and Crick explored DNA as a genetic material, and discovered its structure, called the double-helix.
1954	• Joseph Murray carried out the first kidney transplant between identical twins.
1957	• Scientists revealed that sickle-cell anemia occurs due to an alteration in a single amino acid in hemoglobin cells.
1958	• Arthur Kornberg created DNA in a test tube for the first time. The first mechanical protein sequencer, the Moore–Stein amino acid analyzer, is developed.
The 1960s	
1960	• A French researcher discovered messenger RNA (mRNA).
1961	• François Jacob and Jacques Monad demonstrated the concept of Operon.

(*Continued*)

Table 1.3. (*Continued*)

Year	Discoveries
1962	• Osamu Shimomura explored the green fluorescent protein in the jellyfish *Aequorea victoria*. He afterward developed it into a technique for examining formerly invisible cellular processes [64].
1963	• Samuel Katz and John F Enders developed the first vaccine for measles [65].
1963	• Autonomous groups in the USA, Germany and China produced insulin, a pancreatic hormone.
1964	• The existence of reverse transcriptase was predicted.
1967–71	• Maurice Hilleman made the first American vaccine for mumps [66]. • The first vaccine for rubella was developed. • Rubella was combined with the measles and mumps vaccines to yield the measles/mumps/rubella (MMR) vaccine.
1968	• How the arrangement of nucleotides in nucleic acids regulates the cell's synthesis of proteins was discovered.
The 1970s	
1970	• Restriction enzymes were discovered.
1972	• DNA ligases, which join DNA fragments together, were used for the first time. • The DNA composition of humans was discovered to be 99% similar to that of chimpanzees and gorillas. • The purified enzyme reverse transcriptase was first employed to prepare complementary DNA from purified messenger RNA in a test tube.
1973	• Stanley Cohen and Herbert Boyer used bacterial genes to perform the first successful rDNA experiment [67]. • Sir Edwin Mellor Southern developed a blotting technique for DNA called the Southern blot.
1974	• The NIH formed a Recombinant DNA Advisory Committee to supervise recombinant genetic research. • The first vaccine for chicken pox was developed in Japan.
1975	• Colony hybridization and Southern blotting were explored for identifying specific DNA sequences. • The first monoclonal antibodies were prepared. • César Milstein, Georges Jean Franz Kohler and Niels Kaj Jerne explored the monoclonal antibody technique by fusing immortal tumor cells with antibody-producing B-lymphocyte cells to generate hybridomas that constantly produce identical antibodies.

1975 • The theory of cytoplasmic hybridization was proposed, and the first ever monoclonal antibodies were synthesized [68].

1976 • The NIH published the first guidelines for rDNA research.
• Molecular hybridization was employed for the prenatal diagnosis of alpha thalassemia. Yeast genes were expressed in *E. coli* bacteria.

1977 • Procedures were developed to swiftly sequence long sections of DNA. Genetically engineered bacteria were employed to manufacture the human growth protein somatostatin, marking the first time a synthetic recombinant gene was employed to clone a protein. Several believed this to be the arrival of the 'age of biotechnology'.
• R Austrian *et al* at the University of Pennsylvania developed the first vaccine for pneumonia [69].

1978 • Boyer synthesized the human insulin gene (i.e. a synthetic version of it) and inserted it into the bacterium *E. coli*, allowing the bacterium to produce human insulin.
• Louise Brown, the first test tube baby, was born in the UK. The first vaccine for meningococcal meningitis was developed.

The 1980s

1980 • According to US Supreme Court, genetically altered life forms could be patented, creating vast possibilities for commercially exploiting genetic engineering.
• The first patent of this nature was awarded to the Exxon oil company to patent an oil-eating micro-organism, which would afterward be employed in the 1989 cleanup of the Exxon oil spill at Prince William Sound, Alaska. S Cohen and D H Boyer received a US patent for gene cloning.
• The first automatic gene machine was developed in California.
• Launch of Amgen, which would grow to become the world's largest biotechnology medicines company.

1981 • Baruch Blumberg and Irving Millman developed the first vaccine for hepatitis B [70].
• Researchers in Switzerland cloned mice.
• The first transgenic animals were produced by transforming genes from other animals into mice.

1982 • The FDA supported the first recombinant protein.

1983 • Luc Montagnier of the Pasteur Institute in Paris isolated the AIDS virus.
• Kary Mullis discovered the polymerase chain reaction (PCR), a technique for multiplying DNA sequences.
• PCR was identified as the most innovative molecular biology technique. The FDA sanctioned a monoclonal antibody-based diagnostic analysis to identify *Chlamydia trachomatis*.
• The first artificial chromosome was produced and the first genetic markers for specific inherited diseases were discovered.

(*Continued*)

Table 1.3. (*Continued*)

Year	Discoveries
1984	• The DNA fingerprinting technique was discovered. When a restrictive enzyme is applied to DNA from various individuals, the ensuing sets of fragments sometimes vary noticeably from one person to the next. Such differences in DNA are called restriction fragment length polymorphisms and are particularly helpful in genetic investigations. • The first genetically engineered vaccine was discovered for hepatitis B. The whole genome of the human immunodeficiency virus (HIV) virus was cloned and sequenced.
1985	• Genetic fingerprinting stepped into the courtroom. • Genentech became the first biotechnology organization to launch its own biopharmaceutical product. • Genetically engineered plants resistant to viruses, insects and bacteria were field-tested for the first time. • Cloning of the gene that encodes human lung surfactant protein was achieved. This was a major step toward reducing premature birth problems. • The NIH sanctioned guidelines for executing trials of gene therapy on humans.
1986	• Peter G Schultz from UC Berkeley explained how to conjugate antibodies and enzymes (abzymes) to create therapeutics [71]. • The automated DNA sequencer was discovered in California. The FDA sanctioned the first monoclonal antibody treatment to fight kidney transplant rejection. • The FDA sanctioned the first biotech-derived interferon drugs to treat cancer. Drugs to treat Kaposi's sarcoma, a complication of AIDS, were discovered. • The FDA sanctioned the first genetically engineered human vaccine to avert hepatitis B.
1987	• The FDA sanctioned a genetically engineered tissue plasminogen activator to treat heart attacks. • Maynard Olson and colleagues at Washington University discovered yeast artificial chromosomes, which are expression vectors for large proteins. • Reverse transcription and the PCR were linked to augment messenger RNA sequences. DNA microarray technology, the use of a set of various DNAs in arrays for expression outline, was first explained. • The collection of DNA was used to recognize genes whose expression is altered by interferon. • The FDA sanctioned a diagnostic serum tumor marker test for ovarian cancer.
1988	• Congress financed the Human Genome Project, a huge international attempt to map and sequence the human genetic code as well as the genomes of other species. • The first contract between two organizations with parallel patents for cross-licensing of biotech products occurred and became the example.
1989	• The FDA sanctioned Amgen's first biologically derived human therapeutic. • Oil-eating bacteria were employed to clear up the Exxon Valdez oil spill. • A gene responsible for cystic fibrosis was explored.

The 1990s

1990
- The first nationally sanctioned gene therapy treatment was executed effectively on a four-year-old girl suffering from an immune disorder called adenosine deaminase deficiency.
- The Human Genome Project was launched.
- The FDA approved the first hepatitis C antibody test, which helped to guarantee the purity of blood bank products.
- The FDA sanctioned a bioengineered form of the protein interferon gamma to treat chronic granulomatous disease.
- The FDA sanctioned a modified enzyme for enzyme replacement therapy to treat severe combined immunodeficiency disease. It was the first successful application of enzyme replacement therapy for an inherited disease.

1992
- The US Army accumulated blood and tissue tests from all new recruits as part of a genetic dog-tag plan intended to achieve better recognition of soldiers killed in combat.
- The FDA sanctioned the first genetically engineered blood-clotting factor—a recombinant protein used to treat hemophilia A.
- The FDA sanctioned a recombinant protein to treat renal cell cancer. American and British researchers revealed a technique for analyzing embryos *in vitro* for genetic abnormalities, e.g. cystic fibrosis and hemophilia.

1993
- The FDA approved a recombinant protein to treat multiple sclerosis—marking the first new multiple sclerosis treatment in 20 years.
- A global research team, led by Daniel Cohen from the Center for the Study of Human Polymorphisms, Paris, created a rough map of all 23 pairs of human chromosomes.
- Two minor trade organizations merged together to form the Biotechnology Industry Organization, an international biotechnology support group.

1994
- The FDA sanctioned a recombinant protein to deal with growth hormone (GH) deficiency.
- Mary-Claire King at UC Berkeley explored the first breast cancer gene, BRCA1 [72]. The FDA sanctioned a modified enzyme to deal with Gaucher's disease.
- A number of genes, human and otherwise, were identified and their functions explained. These comprised: Ob, a gene inclining to obesity; BCR, a breast cancer receptiveness gene; BCL-2, a gene linked to apoptosis (programmed cell death); Hedgehog genes (named because of their shape), which synthesize proteins that direct cell differentiation in complex organisms; and Vpr, a gene regulating the reproduction of the HIV virus.
- Genetic linkage studies recognized the role of genes in a variety of disorders, including bipolar disorder, cerulean cataracts, melanoma, dyslexia, prostate cancer, thyroid cancer, hearing loss, sudden infant death syndrome and dwarfism.
- The FDA sanctioned a genetically engineered description of human DNase, which breaks down protein accretion in the lungs of cystic fibrosis patients. This corresponded to the first new therapeutic drug for treating cystic fibrosis.

(*Continued*)

Table 1.3. (*Continued*)

Year	Discoveries
1995	• The first baboon-to-human bone marrow transplant was executed on an AIDS patient. • The first vaccine for hepatitis A was explored. • The NIH, the US Army and the Centers for Disease Control and Prevention were considerably involved in the growth and clinical testing of the vaccine. • Researchers at the Institute for Genomic Research completed the first full gene sequence of a living organism for the bacterium *Haemophilus influenzae*. • A European study group determined a genetic defect that turned out to be the most frequent cause of deafness.
1996	• Researchers at the Department of Biochemistry at Stanford University and Affymetrix developed the gene chip, a small glass or silica microchip that contains thousands of individual genes that can be examined simultaneously. This symbolized a scientific breakthrough in gene expression and DNA sequencing technology. • Research groups sequenced the complete genome of a complex organism, *Saccharomyces cerevisiae*, otherwise known as baker's yeast. The accomplishment symbolizes the entire sequencing of the largest genome to date. A novel, economic diagnostic biosensor test was developed to hasten the detection of a toxic strain of *E. coli*, the bacteria responsible for several food poisoning outbreaks.
1997	• The first human artificial chromosome was discovered. • A mixture of natural and synthetic DNA was used to synthesize a genetic cassette that could possibly be adapted and employed in gene therapy. • The FDA sanctioned a recombinant follicle stimulating hormone to deal with infertility. • The FDA permitted the first bloodless HIV-antibody analysis, which used cells from patients' gums. Researchers at the Institute for Genomic Research sequenced the entire genome of the Lyme disease pathogen, *Borrelia burgdorferi*, along with the genome for the organism associated with stomach ulcers, *Helicobacter pylori*. • Researchers at the University of Wisconsin–Madison sequenced the *E. coli* genome. • The FDA permitted the first therapeutic antibody to treat cancer in the USA. It was employed for patients with non-Hodgkin's lymphoma.
1998	• Human skin was created in the laboratory for the first time. • Two research groups cultured embryonic stem cells. • Embryonic stem cells were employed to regenerate tissue and produce disorders mimicking diseases. • Researchers at the Sanger Institute in the UK and at the Washington University School of Medicine in St Louis, USA, sequenced the first whole animal genome for the *Caenorhabditis elegans* worm. • A rough draft of the human genome map was created, displaying the sites of more than 30 000 genes. • The first vaccine for Lyme disease was discovered. • The FDA sanctioned a novel monoclonal antibody to treat Crohn's disease.

- A monoclonal antibody therapy employed against breast cancer had positive outcomes, indicating a new age of management based on the molecular targeting of tumor cells.
- Support for using the HER2 inhibitor for the management of breast cancer in patients who had tested positive for the HER2 mutation brought personalized medicine to oncology.

The 2000s

2000
- Har Gobind Khorana synthesized DNA in a test tube [16].
- Kary Mullis added value to Har Gobind Khorana's findings by amplifying DNA in a test tube, to create a thousand times more than the original amount of DNA [16].
- Sir Ian Wilmut cloned an adult sheep and called the cloned sheep 'Dolly' [16].
- Craig Venter sequenced the human genome; the first publicly accessible genomes would later be those of James Watson and Ventor.
- Researchers at Celera Genomics and the Human Genome Project successfully completed a rough draft of the human genome [16].

2001
- The journals *Science* and *Nature* reported the human genome sequence, making it feasible for researchers all over the world to start investigating innovative treatments for diseases that have genetic origins, e.g. heart disease, cancer, Parkinson's and Alzheimer's.

2002
- An era of very rapid shotgun sequencing of major genomes was completed. Included were the mouse, chimpanzee, dog and hundreds of other species.

2003
- Celera and the NIH successfully finished the sequencing of the human genome.

2004
- The FDA supported the first monoclonal antibody (i.e. antiangiogenic, inhibiting blood vessel formation or angiogenesis) for cancer therapy.
- The FDA approved a DNA microarray analysis system, which helped in selecting medications for different conditions. This was a significant step toward modified medicine.

2006
- The FDA sanctioned a recombinant vaccine against human papillomavirus, which causes genital warts and cervical cancer.
- Researchers established the three-dimensional (3D) structure of HIV, which causes AIDS.

2007
- Researchers discovered how to use human skin cells to produce embryonic stem cells.

2008
- Venter replicated a bacterium's genetic structure completely from laboratory chemicals, taking a step nearer to generating the world's first living artificial organism [16].

2008
- Japanese chemists developed the first DNA molecule made nearly entirely of artificial parts. The finding could be used in areas of gene therapy.

(*Continued*)

Table 1.3. (*Continued*)

Year	Discoveries
2009	• Former US President Barack Obama signed an administrative order releasing national funding for broader research on embryonic stem cells. • Scientists identified three new genes connected with Alzheimer's disease, paving the way for possible new diagnostics and therapeutics. • Geron commenced the first FDA approved clinical trial by means of embryonic stem cells.
2010	• The FDA sanctioned a modified prostate cancer medicine that improves a patient's immune cells to distinguish and attack cancer cells. • The FDA sanctioned an osteoporosis treatment that was one of the first medicines based on genomic investigations. • Craig Venter showed that a synthetic genome could duplicate alone.
2011	• A trachea developed from stem cell was transplanted into a human recipient. Progress in 3D printing technology resulted in 'skin-printing'. • The FDA sanctioned the first cord blood therapy to be employed in hematopoietic stem cell transplantation protocols in patients with disorders influencing the hematopoietic system.
2012	• The FDA issued draft regulations for biosimilar drugs.

In the modern era, researchers had almost all the basic tools available to them for their applications. With these tools the majority of basic concepts were elucidated, which fast-forwarded the path to important scientific discoveries. These studies and discoveries have unlimited implications and applications. Conclusively, biotechnology has brought humanity to this level of comfort; looking ahead, the next question is, where will it take us? Biotechnology has both beneficial and destructive potential. It is we who should now decide how to use this technology to help humanity rather than to destroy it.

1.4 Scope and importance of biotechnology

Biotechnology is the science of the controlled application of biological agents for beneficial use. Since biotechnology is not an independent discipline, its well-known integration with allied fields such as biochemistry, molecular biology and microbiology facilitates the technological application of biological agents. Therefore, modern biotechnology has developed as a science with enormous potential for human welfare in areas ranging from food processing to human health and environmental protection. The major significance of this field of science in different fields will be evident from the following examples.

1.4.1 Biotechnology in medicine

One of the major areas in biotechnology is the medical sector. The branch of medicine known as 'medical biotechnology' undertakes research on living cells and cell components in order to create pharmacological and diagnostic products. This is the field in which most of the research is taking place and several breakthroughs have been made. The scope of biotechnology in medicine is to utilize techniques in living systems to produce therapeutic proteins, which are usually called biopharmaceuticals or recombinant proteins. These products can aid in both disease prevention and treatment. Medical biotechnology has assisted millions of people and made tremendous advances in a variety of fields, including agriculture, human DNA mapping, and the development of the Ebola vaccine. Artificial tissue growth, medication therapies, and gene sequencing are some of the most modern applications of biological technology. Products such as monoclonal antibodies, DNA and RNA probes are produced for the diagnosis of various diseases. Additionally, therapeutic protein-based drugs such as insulin and interferon have been synthesized with bacteria for the treatment of human diseases. As a result of numerous advances in medical biotechnology, new worries have emerged. In this quick-paced profession, there are a lot of factors to decide upon and control, ranging from funding to ethics and legal issues.

Medical biotechnology offers multiple prospective possibilities for technological innovation that could benefit a large number of people, including agriculture along with breakthroughs in cancer research. As previously mentioned, the use of biotechnology in the field of medicine is also known as 'red' biotechnology. It deals with many major and minor aspects of human life, from making medicines more effective in terms of cost and efficiency, to tackling one of the most difficult branches of medicine, curing genetic diseases. Red biotechnology covers various potential medicines for diseases such as cancer and AIDS. It can be divided into four main areas: biopharmaceuticals, gene therapy, pharmacogenomics and genetic testing.

As described above, red biotechnology deals with production of medicinal drugs that can be proteins (including antibodies that fight infection) or nucleic acids (DNA or RNA). There is no involvement of chemicals in the synthesis process since they are derived from microorganisms which synthesize them naturally. The first approved product for therapeutic use was biosynthetic 'human' insulin made via rDNA technology. Human insulin replaced the pig insulin that had been previously used and revolutionized the industry with its success. This human insulin, sometimes called rHI, or the trade name Humulin, was developed by Genentech but licensed to Eli Lilly and Company, which manufactured and marketed the product starting in 1982.

The second major field of red biotechnology is gene therapy, which deals with the diagnosis and treatment of genetic diseases and some other diseases such as cancer. This therapy encompasses the manipulation of genes and the correction of defective genes. During this process genes are inserted, deleted or modified. One of the most common forms of gene therapy is the incorporation of functional genes into an unspecified genomic location in order to replace a mutated and dysfunctional gene.

Pharmacogenomics and genetic testing both use techniques of red biotechnology that are individual-specific. In pharmacogenomics the genetic information of the individual is derived, and drugs are developed that can be inserted into that particular individual, whereas in genetic testing different tests are conducted among family members to determine genetic diseases, sex and carrier screening. It can also be used in paternity disputes. Monoclonal antibodies, DNA and RNA probes are used for the diagnosis of various diseases and valuable drugs such as insulin and interferon have been synthesized by bacteria for the treatment of human diseases. DNA fingerprinting is utilized for the identification of parents and criminals. The development of recombinant vaccines for diseases such as human hepatitis B using genetically engineered microbes is one of the lists of notable achievements.

Major biotechnology advancements such as tissue nano-transfection, CRISPR, the HPV vaccine, recombinant DNA technology and stem cell research have revolutionized the area of biotechnology. Significant advances over the past ten years have impacted the CRISPR which is called clustered regularly interspaced short palindromic repeats and Cas (CRISPRassociated) toolbox for modifying genes. The CRISPR-Cas approach is often used for targeting, regulating, and editing genomic sequences, it is a potential technique for producing genetically modified animals. The CRISPR Cas system provides microorganisms along with RNA-guided adaptive immunity for foreign gene components by guiding nucleases to attach and alter selective nucleic acid sequences [73]. Yoshimi *et al* developed two new gene modification methods: lsODN (long single-stranded oligodeoxynucleotide) and 2H2OP (two-hit two-oligo with plasmid). These approaches use clustered, regularly interspaced, short palindromic repeats (CRISPR) Cas systems (associated proteins) and single-stranded oligodeoxynucleotides (ssODN). The application of CRISPR-Cas-based technology offers a versatile and easily accessible way to modify, control, and display genomes, facilitating biological investigations and biotechnological uses across numerous domains. Research has advanced significantly, through the use of CRISPR-Cas tools, which have made it possible to identify genes that directly cause disease as well as understanding the biological processes of organisms that were previously unknown. With several Cas9-based clinical studies underway or shortly to start, the area of Cas-based biotechnology is expanding quickly. The outcomes of these trials will probably influence the direction of somatic cell editing in the future, both *ex vivo* and in patients. With its ever-growing range of uses, the CRISPR-Cas toolbox is unquestionably at the forefront of genetic engineering and genome editing.

The use of recombinant DNA technologies (RDT) is prevalent. In the field of medical biotechnology, RDT was merely a theory a century ago, based on the idea that target gene expression might be controlled to enhance desired traits in living cells. But in the last several years, this field has shown that it can have a special influence on improving life for humans. Innovative approaches for medicinal applications, including diabetes, cancer treatment, hereditary diseases, and many plant disorders, particularly fungal and viral resistance, have been made possible by

RDT. Recombinant technology is assisting in the treatment of a number of diseases that are in incurable under normal circumstances, despite the fact that the immune system prevents effective outcomes [74]. Microbes have been employed to generate various human proteins through the utilization of cloned complementary DNA. Thorough testing in humans has proven successful for both growth hormone and insulin, leading to the marketing approval of insulin. Through large-scale production of bacterial and viral antigens, recombinant DNA technology holds the promise of delivering safe and efficient vaccinations for diseases that currently lack treatment [75]. Biotechnology in the field of medicine has developed many products which are mentioned in figure 1.3 (table 1.4).

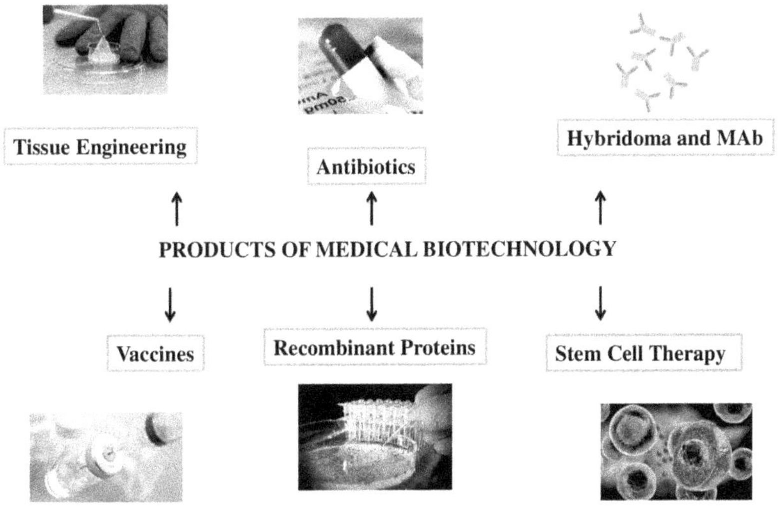

Figure 1.3. Products of medical biotechnology.

Table 1.4. Advanced techniques in medical biotechnology [73–75].

Techniques	Application
Polymerase chain reaction	Amplification of DNA strands
Fluorescence *in situ* hybridization	Identifying a specific DNA sequence's positioning on a chromosome.
Sequencing	Determining the order of nucleotides within a DNA molecule.
Microarrays	A multiplexed lab-on-a-chip that uses high-throughput screening to assess vast volumes of biological material.
Cell culture	The controlled growth of living cells outside of the body.
Interference RNA	mRNA molecule degradation.
Genome editing	To use modified nucleases to alter a gene's or genome's structure.
Recombinant DNA technology	It is possible to identify, cut, and insert one or more genes into the genome of another organism.

1.4.2 Industrial biotechnology

Industrial biotechnology—also called 'white biotechnology'—uses live cells and/or their enzymes to apply contemporary biotechnology to the environmentally friendly production of nutrients, biofuels, and chemicals from renewable energy sources. Industrial biotechnology was established for the large-scale production of alcohol and antibiotics by microorganisms. Currently, various pharmaceutical drugs and chemicals such as lactic acid, glycerine, etc, are being produced by genetic engineering for better quality and quantity. Biotechnology has provided us with a very efficient and economical technique for the production of a variety of biochemicals, e.g. immobilized enzymes. The most significant tool of industrial biotechnology is protein engineering where the proteins that already exist along with the enzymes are designed for a particular function or to maximize the efficiency of their function. A wild-type enzyme found naturally is typically not appropriate to use in an industrial process. To make the enzymatic process commercially feasible, it is crucial to engineer and optimize enzyme performance with respect to activity, selectivity on thermo stability, organic solvent tolerance, non-natural substrates, enantio-selectivity, and substrate/product inhibition [76].

Despite the fact that protein engineering along with metabolic engineering have made major advancements in the field of industrial biotechnology, a new field called synthetic biology, which is generally basic genetic components along with modules that are integrated into a synthetic biological circuit, holds great promise for understanding, designing, and developing customized gene expression networks. Synthetic biology allows scientists to develop synthetic networks at the signal transduction, translation and transcription levels by modifying and assembling modular biological components such as promoters, repressors, and RNA translational control devices [77].

The profitability of particular procedures determines the viability of industrial biotechnology. The following aspects would have a significant impact on the rise of industrial biotechnology: global warming, price of feedstock, policies run by the government, consumer awareness, dwindling fossil fuel reserves, and rising costs of other fuels, and further technological advancement. A growing number of chemical and pharmaceutical industrial processes will be biotechnologically driven due to the greater availability of genetic information as they are sequenced and form an expanding toolkit for manipulating metabolic pathways [78]. It appears from the current surge of innovative applications that we have barely discovered in-depth.

1.4.3 Biotechnology and the environment

A body of scientific and engineering knowledge known as environmental biotechnology deals with the use of microorganisms and the results of their metabolic processes, which can actively participate in the biotreatment of different waste, contribute to the bioremediation of contaminated environments, and monitor the environment and treatment procedures to prevent pollution. Environmental problems such as pollution control, the depletion of natural resources for non-renewable energy, conservation of biodiversity, etc, are being dealt with using biotechnology. The following are some benefits of treating waste biotechnologically: the capacity of a variety of biotechnological techniques to completely destroy hazardous waste; the availability of a wide range of biodegradation conditions; and natural microorganisms exhibit the potential to biodegrade or detoxify a vast array of hazardous compounds. For example, bacteria are being utilized for the detoxification of industrial effluents, to combat oil spills, for treatment of sewage and for biogas production. Biopesticides offer an environmentally safer alternative to chemical pesticides for control of insect pests and diseases.

The biodegradation of organic wastes in municipal wastewater and the biodegradation/detoxication of hazardous chemicals in industrial wastewater are among the primary uses of environmental biotechnology. Environmental biotechnology encompasses diverse sectors, including pathogenicity and toxicity testing, the application of biosensors and biochips for monitoring environmental quality, the creation of biotechnological analogues to curb the production of hazardous waste, the formulation of biodegradable materials for environmental sustainability, the production of fuel from biomass and organic wastes, and the bioimmobilization of hazardous substances to decrease toxicity.

Both aerobic and anaerobic treatment of waste comes under environmental biotechnology. Microorganisms can be classified as either obligatory aerobic, microaerophilic, facultative anaerobic, or anaerobic. As a terminal acceptor of electrons given by organic or inorganic materials, oxygen is necessary for aerobic microbes to function. One source of energy that is available to biology is the movement of electrons from donor to acceptor. The efficiency of aerobic microorganisms extends to the effective handling of various xenobiotics, including but not limited to azo dyes, chlorinated aliphatic compounds, aliphatic hydrocarbons and their derivatives, polycyclic aromatic hydrocarbons, aromatic hydrocarbons, organophosphate waste, halogenated aromatic compounds, and compounds containing nitrogroups [79].

Tolerant anaerobes are a subclass of anaerobic microorganisms that possess defence mechanisms against oxygen exposure. Others, referred to as obligatory anaerobes, lack these defenses and may perish after being exposed to aerobic conditions for a few seconds. Fermentation and anaerobic respiration employing electron acceptors, such as anoxygenic or oxygenic photosynthesis, are the two ways whereby obligatory anaerobes generate energy. Anaerobic treatment, however, operates more slowly than aerobic treatment, and it might produce a significant quantity of dissolved organic fermentation products or anaerobic respiration energy [80].

Heavy metal-containing liquid and solid waste, which is considered harmful for the environment can be effectively handled using biotechnological techniques. Certain metals can be reduced or oxidized by bacteria that contain particular enzymes. Products from microbial metabolism, such as hydrogen, oxygen, and H_2O_2, can be utilized to oxidize or reduce metals. Metal solubilization or precipitation typically occurs together with metal reduction or oxidation. Metal solubilization or precipitation can also be facilitated by metabolites produced by microorganisms [81].

Biomonitoring, which includes monitoring of biodegradability, toxicity, mutagenicity, concentration of toxic compounds, and concentration and pathogenicity of microbes in waste and the environment, is a significant application of environmental biotechnology. Enzymes or entire bacterial cells can be used by biosensors to identify particular hazardous chemical compounds. Specially designed for toxicity monitoring, whole-cell sensors can have their bioluminescence inhibited in the presence of hazardous substances [82].

1.4.4 Biotechnology and agriculture

Due to developments in the area of molecular biology, various researchers were able to alter DNA, at the molecular level in the 1970s, which is called genetic engineering. Additionally, it permits DNA transfer between organisms that are more genetically related than could be achieved through conventional breeding methods. Due to technological progress, scientists can now move specific genes from nearly any organism, such as bacteria, viruses, plants, and animals, into another organism. A genetically modified organism, commonly referred to as a transgenic organism, is an organism that has been subject to genetic engineering. Genetic engineering is not excluded from the risks and rewards that come with life. Although there has been a lot of discussion over the possible problems associated with genetic engineering technologies, there is currently little proof from scientific research to support these claims. Benefits from transgenic organisms extend beyond those that resulted from advancements in conventional agricultural biotechnology.

Many discovered vital tools in the field of biotechnology are used in the agricultural sector, and are given in table 1.5. Currently, the potential of plant tissue culture is widely utilized for the rapid and economic clonal multiplication of fruit and forest trees, for the production of virus-free genetic stock and planting material, as well as in the creation of novel genetic variations through somaclonal variation. With the aid of rDNA technology, it has now become possible to produce transgenic plants with desirable genes such as herbicide resistance, disease resistance, increased shelf life, etc. The enhancement of crop yields is attributed to biotechnology, which imparts characteristics such as disease resistance and improved drought tolerance to crops. Scientists now possess the ability to transfer genes responsible for disease resistance from other species to important crops. Techniques such as molecular breeding have been employed to accelerate the process of crop improvement. For instance, molecular markers, such as restriction fragment length polymorphism (RFLP), and simple sequence repeats (SSRs) provide potential tools for the indirect selection of both qualitative and quantitative traits, and also for studying genotypic diversity. Farmers employ crop-protection technologies because they provide low-cost solutions to pest problems that, if left untreated, would drastically lower harvests. As was previously noted, a few crops such as cotton, potatoes, and corn have been successfully modified through genetic engineering to create a protein that kills particular insects when they feed on the plants. The protein

Table 1.5. Vital tools used in agricultural biotechnology.

Genetic engineering	• Tissue culture is employed to reconstruct cells into a complete organism with a genetic make-up distinct from the original cells. This is achieved by inserting DNA fragments into the chromosomes of the cells. Referred to as rDNA technology, this approach results in the creation of transgenic animals
Tissue culture	• In order to either create fully formed, developing organisms or allow them to endure for extended periods of time in a laboratory, this involves manipulating cells, anthers, pollen grains, or other components. Genetically modified cells can become genetically modified organisms through tissue culture.
Embryo rescue	• To finish developing into whole organisms involves implanting embryos with transplanted genes into tissue cultures. Embryo rescue is often used to facilitate 'wide crossing,' creating complete plants from embryos that are the result of crossing two plants that would not normally produce progeny.
Somatic hybridization	• By breaking down the cell walls of various species and causing the DNA of the treated cells to combine directly. The treated cells are then used in tissue culture to regenerate into entire creatures.
Marker-aided genetic analysis	• It analyses DNA sequences to determine the identities of genes, quantitative trait loci, and other genetic markers and links them to the functions of the organism.
Marker-aided selection	• It is the recognition and generation-by-generation tracking of previously recognized DNA segments.
Genomics analyses	• The entire genomes of species along with additional biological information about the species to comprehend which features of the creatures are inherited from their DNA. Proteomics, in a similar vein, examines the proteins inside a tissue to determine the expression of specific genes and the precise roles played by the proteins. These are subfields of bioinformatics, together with metabolomics (metabolites) and phenomics (phenotypes).

is derived from the soil bacterium *Bacillus thuringiensis*, which has long been the active ingredient in a number of 'natural' insecticides.

The development of molecular techniques that are DNA-based and their widespread use in agriculture have had significant consequences. These include the broad commercial use of agricultural biotechnology in just a few nations, the substantial financial contributions made by the private sector to biotechnology research, the ongoing debate over the technology's effects on the environment, the proliferation of national and international regulations resulting from the technology and property rights, fluctuating public opinion, and the technology's relatively small contribution to improving food production, nutrition, or farm incomes in less developed nations [83].

1.5 Biotechnology techniques

Some of the basic tools that are frequently experimented with in biotechnology to explore surrounding applications are listed in table 1.6.

Table 1.6. Basic techniques used in biotechnology.

Techniques	Description
Genetic engineering (rDNA) technology	The use of cellular enzymes to manipulate DNA; transferring DNA between unrelated organisms
Protein engineering technology	Used to improve existing/create novel proteins to make useful products
Antisense or RNAi technology	Can block or decrease the production of certain proteins
Cell and tissue culture technology	Growing cells/tissues under laboratory conditions to produce an entire organism, or to produce new products
Bioinformatics technology	Computational analysis of biological data, e.g. sequence analysis macromolecular structures, high-throughput profiling data analysis
Protein separation and identification techniques	Contour-clamped homogeneous electric field gel electrophoresis
	Agarose gel electrophoresis
	Vertical pulse field gradient electrophoresis
	Pulsed field electrophoresis
	Polyacrylamide gel electrophoresis
	Microarray
	Isoelectric focusing
	Field inversion gel electrophoresis
	Two-dimensional (2D) gel electrophoresis
Blotting techniques	Nucleic acid blotting
	Southern blot analysis
	Protein blotting
	Northern blot analysis
	Dot blot technique
	Autoradiography
Sterilization techniques	Steam sterilization
	Ultraviolet sterilization
	Flame sterilization
	Filter sterilization
	Dry sterilization
	Chemical sterilization

	Alcohol sterilization
PCR-based techniques	Single-nucleotide polymorphism
	Targeted PCR and sequencing
	SSRs or microsatellites
	Sequence-targeted microsatellites
	Sequence-related amplification polymorphism
	Sequence-characterized amplified regions
	Sequence-specified amplified polymorphism
	Selective amplification of microsatellite polymorphic loci
	Retrotransposon-based markers
	Retrotransposon microsatellite-amplified polymorphism
	Retrotransposon-based insertional polymorphism
	Random amplified polymorphic DNA
	Random amplified microsatellite polymorphism
	Microsatellite-directed PCR: unanchored primers
	Microsatellite-directed PCR: anchored primers
	Inter-retrotransposon amplified polymorphism
	DNA amplification fingerprinting
	Cleaved amplified polymorphic sequences
	Arbitrarily fragmented length polymorphism
Gene transfer techniques	• Chemical methodsCalcium phosphate co-precipitation
	• Polycation-DMSO technique
	• PEG-mediated transformation
	• DEAE-dextran procedurePhysical methods
	• Ultrasound-mediated gene transformation
	• Silicon carbide fiber-mediated transformation
	• Microinjection
	• Macroinjection
	• Liposome-mediated method
	• Electroporation
	• Biolistics/particle bombardment/microprojectile
	• Virus-mediated gene transfer
	• Bacteria-mediated gene transfer
	• Agrobacterium-mediated gene transfer
Miscellaneous techniques	Protoplast fusion techniques, transposon tagging in heterologous species, techniques used for single-cell cultures (Bergmann cell plating technique), immobilization techniques, artificial seed technology, chromosome elimination techniques, rDNA technology, spectrophotometry (quantitation, enzyme kinetics), nucleic acid purification and molecular weight determinations, cell separation methods, protein separation and quantitation, liquid scintillation (double label) counting, autoradiography (cellular and gross), restriction enzyme mapping, gene expression and oligonucleotide synthesis.

1.5.1 Bioreactors

In earlier times bioreactors were used for centuries to make wine and beer. The bioreactor is possibly the most important single piece of equipment used in biotechnology. Bioreactors are the containers or vessels that allow biological processes to take place under optimum conditions. These reactors, in controlled environments, will yield a useful substance in large amounts. The initial feedstock and the end result are connected centrally through the bioreactor. Because productivity is frequently influenced by process technology, biochemical reaction engineering serves as a bridge between biologists and engineers. The biocatalyst determines the reaction yield and selectivity. Advances in bioreactor design, such as continuous reaction, immobilized enzymes, whole-cell immobilization, and process control, will progressively mirror the biochemical process industry's demand for interdisciplinary collaboration.

1.5.2 Cell fusion

Two different perspectives have been used to study and advance the biological phenomena of cell fusion. The function that biological membrane fusion may play in typical cellular processes including plasma membrane synthesis and vesicle movement during endocytosis and exocytosis has aroused the interest of biochemists and cell biologists. This technique involves the fusion of two cells to make a single cell that contains all the genetic material of the original cells. So far, this technique has been employed to create new plants by fusing cells from species that do not naturally hybridize (from a cross-breed) and then generating whole plants from the fused cells.

1.5.3 Liposome-based delivery

When it comes to treating diseases, biological medications are receiving a lot of attention. Nevertheless, their applicability is significantly constrained due to intrinsic characteristics such as low stability, poor membrane permeability, excessive hydrophilicity, and larger size. Because liposome-based drug delivery methods optimize administration to the precise target site, they can increase bioavailability, improve therapeutic efficacy, and reduce toxicity. As a result, they are emerging as promising techniques to improve drug delivery.

Liposomes are microscopic spherical structures that develop when lipids form a suspension in water. Long-chain fatty acids, membrane proteins, cholesterol, glycolipids, sphingolipids, and non-toxic surfactants are the basic components used for producing liposomes. These spherical vesicles arrange themselves so as to generate a tiny space inside the center of the liposome. Such space can potentially be exploited to deliver/transport another substance, such as a drug. Liposomes have important applications in biotechnology since they may offer novel means of transporting certain drugs to particular parts of the body across the biological membranes, e.g. peptides could be encapsulated in liposomes and transported across biological membranes.

Serving as a highly effective drug delivery platform for biological therapeutics, liposomes offer advantages like enhanced drug stability and superior encapsulation performance. Despite the widespread utilization of catalytic liposomes in biological drug delivery, their systemic toxicity poses a hindrance to translation. A promising approach to tackle this issue is the integration of ionizable cationic lipids. This allows liposomes to attain a positive charge in low pH environments, ensuring effective encapsulation of biopharmaceuticals within their cores. Under normal physiological conditions, they exhibit an anionic surface charge or a net neutral charge, facilitating endosomal escape for intracellular delivery [84].

1.5.4 Cell or tissue culture

Tissue culture has been a widely used method in morphological research. Today's animal cell culture technology is essential to the life sciences since it gives researchers a foundation for studying differentiation, proliferation, and control as well as for altering genes. To do it successfully, specialized technical skills are required. But since it was not adapted to the needs of such types of investigations, its application to physiological problems was long delayed. The initial method, which was developed from Ross Harrison's work and is still often employed, just required hanging a piece of tissue in a sealed hollow slide with a drop of lymph, plasma, serum, saline solution, or another medium. The cells must contend with complex and elusive requirements to survive under these conditions, including those from necrotic cells of the same kind, other types of cells, both dead and living and a medium that quickly declines on its own [85]. This method is used extensively in biological laboratories, for example, in cancer research, plant breeding and routine analysis of chromosome karyotopes. The whole process is conducted in an *in vitro* environment by providing a suitable culture medium that contains a mixture of nutrients either in solid form or in liquid form.

1.5.5 Genetic engineering

The manipulation of a genome's DNA sequence(s) using diverse techniques and molecular biology technologies is known as genetic engineering. The basis of genetic engineering is the alteration of genetic material (hereditary material) or the combination of genes in an organism. By modifying the organism, genetic researchers give the organism and its descendants different traits. While homologous recombination can identify specific sequences in cultured cells such as mouse embryonic stem cells, it is a laborious and ineffective process that depends on pharmacological positive/negative selection in cell culture. This technology was practiced in earlier times by breeding plants and animals to produce favorable combinations of genes. By using this technology, 'genetic engineers' have produced most of the economically important varieties of flowers, vegetables, grains, cows, horses, dogs and cats. During the 1970s and 1980s, researchers established ways to isolate individual genes and reintroduce them into cells or into plants, animals or other organisms. Other widely used approaches for creating transgenic mice and rats through genetic engineering encompass random integration of DNA through direct transfection (microinjection), DNA insertion facilitated by transposons, and DNA insertion mediated by viral vectors. There are numerous methods for inserting additional genetic material into an animal and cell's chromosome. The most desirable technique at the moment is single-copy gene insertion at a specific location. In terms of repeatable transgenic expression, this method offers many benefits. In mouse models, random insertion transgenesis has proven to be an efficient method for examining gene function. These are the advancements that have supported by genetic engineering [86].

1.5.6 DNA fingerprinting

DNA fingerprinting is a technique that is employed for identifying the components of DNA (the material of the genes) that are unique to a particular individual. It uses DNA analysis and comparison to establish identity, resolve legal issues like paternity tests and inheritance matters, and identify missing people and mass disaster victims from human remains. While all population members share 99.1% of the human genome, 0.9% of human DNA varies throughout individuals. These varying DNA sequences, known as polymorphic markers, can be utilized to associate and distinguish between people. Variations in DNA among different individuals can be used for identification purposes. This small section of the DNA of an organism uniquely distinguishes that particular organism from all others. Such varying bits of genetic material take the form of sequences of DNA called mini-satellites, which are repeated several times. The number of repetitions of mini-satellites per region of a gene can vary enormously between unrelated individuals.

1.5.7 Cloning

An animal or human has the same entire set of genes in every body cell. Any of these cells could potentially be used to create a new embryo. In typical sexual reproduction, half of the genes are contributed by each parent; but, in a cloning process, all of the genes are passed on by one parent. The method of production of identical animals, plants or microorganisms from a single individual is known as cloning. In other words, it is a process by which an organism is derived from a single parent through non-sexual reproduction. Cloning is gifted in nature to those organisms that reproduce asexually and produce their own clones, e.g. plants, microorganisms and simple animals such as corals. However, mammals reproduce sexually, and cannot clone naturally since the descendant of a mammal inherits its genetic material not from one parent but half from each parent. Hence, the offspring produced is never an identical copy of either of its parents. In nature, clones from mammals are confined to the production of identical twins.

Many individuals were introduced to the concept of cloning in 1997 with the arrival of Dolly the sheep. In laboratory settings, there are two methods to create a genetically identical clone of an organism: somatic cell nuclear transfer and artificial embryo twinning. The latter, artificial embryo twinning, is a relatively low-tech approach that mimics the natural process leading to the formation of identical twins. Twinning occurs in the initial days following the union of the egg and sperm, when the embryo consists mostly of unspecialized cells. The embryo's two halves continue to divide independently and eventually separate into fully formed humans. The progeny are genetically similar because they grew from the same fertilized egg. The process of artificial embryo twinning is similar; however, it takes place outside of the mother's body in a Petri dish. An early-stage embryo undergoes division into individual cells, each allotted a brief time in a Petri dish for maturation. Following this, the embryos are introduced into a surrogate mother for the completion of their development. Notably, each embryo is genetically identical, originating from the same fertilized egg. Another laboratory technique for generating a genetically identical replica of an organism is somatic cell nuclear transfer (SCNT), commonly known as nuclear transfer. Unlike artificial embryo twinning, this method results in a clone, an exact genetic duplicate of an individual. Dolly the sheep was created using this process [87].

1.5.8 Artificial insemination and ET technology

Development in the study of embryology, urology and urogenitology has led to progress in the area dealing with artificial insemination. Artificial insemination (AI) has been studied for more than 200 years, and it has been used commercially for 75 of those years. Artificial insemination allows the artificial introduction of semen into the reproductive tract of a female animal, and is extensively used in breeding animals, such as sheep and cattle. Males with dominant and desirable hereditary traits/characteristics are selected for semen collection. Collected semen from males with desirable traits can be frozen and transported long distances to fertilize female animals. It is appropriate to consider the impact of this potent gene-dissemination method. Artificial insemination is also employed to help women who wish to conceive where normal conception is not possible. One of the key technologies for assisted reproduction is still artificial insemination. Its three main applications are that it is successful, affordable, and easy to use. In the coming decades, there will be challenges to the significance of artificial insemination. There is a chance that the amazing advancements in other assisted reproductive technologies will produce children quickly. The challenge for any of these reproductive technologies to become widely used is to be as successful, affordable, and straightforward as artificial insemination.

1.5.9 Stem cell technology

With the advancement of biotechnology, it is now possible to utilize the potential of stem cells for beneficial purposes. Stem cells are undifferentiated and can mitotically divide to create mature functional cells, e.g. bone marrow stem cells can give rise to the entire range of immune system blood cells. Stem cells are found in most organisms, but are usually found in multicellular organisms. In 1908 Alexander Maksimov coined the term 'stem cell', and later stem cell research work was continued by Canadian scientists Ernest A McCulloch and James E Till in the 1960s. During this period two extensive types of mammalian stem cells were discovered: embryonic stem cells that are isolated from the inner cell mass of blastocysts, and adult stem cells that are found in adult tissues. During the development of embryos, stem cells can differentiate into all of the specialized embryonic tissues whereas in adult organisms, stem cells and progenitor cells act as a repair system for the body, replenishing specialized cells, but also maintaining the normal turnover of regenerative organs, such as blood, skin or intestinal tissues. Current research utilizes highly plastic adult stem cells from a variety of sources, including umbilical cord blood and bone marrow, for various medical therapies. Advancements in therapeutic cloning allow the development of embryonic cell lines and autologous embryonic stem cells more conveniently and offer promising candidates for future therapies.

The classical definition of a stem cell requires that it possesses two properties:

- Self-renewal or the ability to go through numerous cycles of cell division while maintaining an undifferentiated state.
  - Potency or the capacity to differentiate into specialized cell types. Stem cells can be of the following types:Totipotent (in other words, omnipotent) stem cells can differentiate into any kind of cell type. Such cells can construct a complete, viable, organism. They are produced from the fusion of an egg and sperm cell.
  - Pluripotent stem cells come from totipotent cells and can differentiate into almost all cells, i.e. cells derived from any of the three germ layers. Pluripotent adult stem cells are rare and usually small in number but can originate in a number of tissues including umbilical cord blood. In mice, pluripotent stem cells are directly produced from adult fibroblast cultures. Regrettably, mice do not live long with stem cell organs. Most adult stem cells are lineage-restricted (multipotent) and are normally referred to by their tissue origin.
  - Multipotent stem cells can differentiate into a number of cells, however only into those of a closely connected family of cells. Multipotent stem cells are also originated in amniotic fluid. These stem cells are very active, expand broadly without feeders and are not tumorigenic. Amniotic stem cells are multipotent and can differentiate into cells of osteogenic, myogenic, endothelial, adipogenic, hepatic and also neuronal lines.
  - Oligopotent stem cells can be distinguished into only a few cells, such as lymphoid or myeloid stem cells.
  - Unipotent cells can offer only one cell type, their own; but they have the property of self-renewal.

The potential of stem cells can be demonstrated *in vitro* by means of methods such as clonogenic assays, in which single cells are characterized by their ability to differentiate and self-renew. Also, stem cells can be isolated based on a distinctive set of cell surface markers. However, *in vitro* culture conditions can alter the behavior of cells, making it unclear whether the cells will behave in a similar manner *in vivo*. Considerable debate exists as to whether some proposed adult cell populations are truly stem cells. The term 'adult stem cell' refers to any cell which is found in a developed organism that has the properties of a stem cell. Also known as somatic stem cells and germ line (giving rise to gametes) stem cells, they can be found in children, as well as adults. Adult stem cell treatments have been successfully used for many years to treat leukemia and related bone/blood cancers through bone marrow transplants. Adult stem cells are also used in veterinary medicine to treat tendon and ligament injuries in horses. Stem cell transplantation was first used in the treatment of blood disorders and it was a breakthrough. Conventionally known as bone marrow transplantation, the stem cells responsible for the production of blood cells reside in the bone marrow, a special tissue inside the cavity of the bones. The blood cells originate in the bone marrow from a parent cell or the 'stem cell'. The blood stem cell is given simply as an intravenous infusion like a blood transfusion. The stem cells will automatically find their way home to the bone marrow. They will replace the patient's diseased marrow to give healthy blood cells. The best donors would be siblings of the patient, a twin or extended family members. Unrelated donors may also be used.

1.6 Applications of biotechnology

The enormous potential of biotechnology is exploited to yield high therapeutic compounds (table 1.7).

Table 1.7. List of biotechnological products explored from 1938 to 1998.

Year	Product
1938	Howard Florey/Ernst Chain, Oxford University, England, isolated penicillin.
1940–45	Large-scale production of penicillin.
1943–53	Cortisone first manufactured in large amounts.
1977	Genentech produced somatostatin (human GH-releasing inhibitory factor), manufactured in bacteria. A recombinant gene was used to clone a protein for the first time.
1978	Harvard researchers produced rat insulin by rDNA.
1982	The FDA approved genetically engineered human insulin.
1986	Orthoclone OKT3 (Muromonab-CD3) approved for reversal of kidney transplant rejection.
1986	First recombinant vaccine approved—hepatitis.
1987	Genentech obtained approval for rt-PA (tissue plasminogen activator) for heart attacks.
1990	Actimmune (interferon 1b) approved for chronic granulomatous disease.
	Adagen (adenosine deaminase) approved for severe combined immunodeficiency disease.
1994	First genetically engineered food, the Flavr Savr tomato, was approved.
1994	Genentech's Nutropin was approved (GH deficiency).
1994	Centocor's ReoPro approved for patients undergoing balloon angioplasty. Genzyme's Ceredase/Cerezyme was approved for Gaucher's disease (inherited metabolic disease).
	Recombinant GM-CSF was approved (chemotherapy induced neutropenia).
1998	Centocor's Remicade was approved (monoclonal antibody for Crohn's disease).

1.6.1 Basic applications of biotechnology

There are numerous established applications of biotechnology that are segregated according to their respective defined areas, as shown in table 1.8.

Table 1.8. Applications of biotechnology in different areas.

Area	Applications
Plant biotechnology	Transgenic plants, production of secondary metabolite, production of pathogen-free plants or crop improvement, production of herbicide-resistant crops, pest-resistant ('Bt concept' pest-resistant transgenic) plants, drought resistance, flood resistance, salt tolerance, high-yielding GM crops, nitrogen fixing ability, acidity and salinity tolerance, *in vitro* germplasm conservation, genetic variability, *in vitro* pollination, induction of haploidy, somatic hybridization, genetic transformation, molecular pharming, somatic embryogenesis, organogenesis, phytoremediation, *in vitro* plant germplasm conservation, mutant selection, somaclonal variation, plant genome analysis, hybrid seeds, artificial seeds
Animal biotechnology	Biopharmaceuticals: Production of hormones, growth factors, interferons, enzymes, recombinant proteins, vaccines, blood components, oligonucleotides, transcription factor-based drugs, oligonucleotides
	Antibiotics
	Replacement therapies: Lack of production of normal substances (factor VIII—missing in hemophilia, insulin)
	Diagnostics: antibodies, biosensors, PCR, therapeutics, vaccines, medical research tools, human genome research, development of biosensors
	IVF, ET
	Gene therapy
	Stem cell therapy
	Animal tissue culture: Cell, tissue and organ culture
	Gene cloning: rDNA technology, genetic engineering, transgenic animals, antibiotics, DNA markers, animal husbandry, xenotransplantation, medical biotechnology
	Therapeutics: Natural products such as from the foxglove (*Digitalis*, heart conditions) and yew tree (cancer agent, taxol) for breast and ovarian cancers, endogenous therapeutic agents i.e. proteins produced by the body that can be replicated by genetically engineering, tPA—tissue plasminogen factor (dissolves blood clots), biopharmaceuticals (drug or vaccine developed through biotechnology), therapeutants, i.e. products used to maintain health or prevent disease, biopharming, i.e. production of pharmaceuticals in cultured organisms, certain blood-derived products needed in human medicine can be produced in the milk of goats
	Biopolymers and medical devices: natural substances useful as medical devices: hyaluronate, an elastic, plastic-like substance used to treat arthritis, prevent post-surgical scarring in cataract surgery, used for drug delivery, adhesive substances to replace stitches

	Designer drugs: Using computer modeling to design drugs without the lab-protein structure Evolutionary and ecological genomics: Finding genes associated with ecological traits and evolutionary diversification. Common goals are health and productivity
Agricultural biotechnology	The applications of animal biotechnology, crop biotechnology, horticultural biotechnology, tree biotechnology, food processing, plant biotechnology (photosynthesis improvers, bio-fertilizers, stress-resistant crops and plants, bio-insecticides and biopesticides), food biotechnology Food: Increased milk production, leaner meat in pork, growth hormones in farm-raised fish that result in earlier market-ready fish Pharmaceuticals: Animals engineered to produce human proteins for drugs, including insulin and vaccines Breeding disease tolerance, exact copies of desired stock, increased yields Health: Microorganisms introduced into feed for beneficial purposes, diagnostics for disease and pregnancy detection, animals engineered to produce organs suitable for transplantation into humans
Environmental biotechnology	Environmental monitoring: Diagnosis of environmental problems via biotechnology Waste management: Bioremediation is the use of microbes to break down organic molecules or environmental pollutants Pollution prevention: Renewable resources, biodegradable products, alternative energy sources
Fuel and fodder	Provides a clean and renewable alternative to traditional fossil fuels, the burning of which contributes to global warming Tissue culture technique offers rapid afforestation of degraded forests and regeneration of green cover Biotechnology could play an important role in three ways in the productivity of biomass Can be used to generate methane
Industrial biotechnology	Metabolite production (acetone, butanol, alcohol, antibiotics, enzymes, vitamins, organic acids), anaerobic digestion (for methane production), waste treatment (both organic and industrial), production of bio-control agents, fermentation of food products, bio-based fuel and energy, industrial microbiology, biotechnology in the galvanizing industry, recovery of metals and minerals, bioethanol, bioconversion of synthesized gas to liquid fuels such as methanol, using bacteria to remove by-products, pulp and paper, sugars from starches, animal feed, food, textiles and leather, pharmaceuticals, an enzymatic process for producing antibiotics
Aquatic biotechnology	Aquaculture, restoring and protecting marine ecosystems, improving seafood quality, environmental remediation, marine by-products for human health, biomaterial and bioprocessing, marine molecular biotechnology

1.6.2 Most common applications

Some of the most common applications of biotechnology are highlighted below.

1.6.2.1 Cloning

The term cloning describes a number of different processes that can be used to produce genetically identical copies of a biological entity. The copied material, which has the same genetic make-up as the original, is referred to as a clone. Various historical events that led to the development of cloning are listed in table 1.9.

Table 1.9. The timeline of cloning.

Year	Cloning event
1885	First ever display of artificial embryo twinning.
1901	Cloning hypothesized: Hans Spemann splits a two-celled newt embryo into two parts, effectively producing two larvae. (Later, in 1938, Spemann hypothesized that animals could be cloned by fusing an embryo with an egg cell.)
1902	Artificial embryo twinning in a vertebrate achieved.
1928	It was found that the cell nucleus regulates embryonic development.
1952	First thriving nuclear transfer (frog).
1958	Nuclear transfer from a differentiated cell (frog).
1963	Term 'clone' coined: John Burdon Sanderson Haldane used 'clone' in his speech on the biological potential for the human species over the next ten thousand years.
1963	First cloned fish: Tong Dizhou, an embryologist from China, developed the world's first cloned fish by incorporating the DNA from a cell of a male carp into an egg from a female carp.
1973	Stanley Norman Cohen and Herbert Boyer discovered the tool of DNA cloning, which copies genes to facilitate their transplantation between various biological species.
1975	First mammalian embryo produced by nuclear transfer (rabbit).
1980	First transgenic (genetically modified) mouse.
1982	Giant mouse created by transferring GH genes from a rat.
1984	First mammal produced by nuclear transfer (sheep).
1985	First transgenic domestic animal, a pig.
1987	A sequence of transgenic mice developed carrying human genes.
1987	Nuclear transfer from an embryonic cell (cow).
1995	Transgenic pig hearts made: researchers discover transgenic pig hearts that endure up to 30 h when transplanted to baboons. The FDA sanctions the use of transgenic pig livers as bridge organs for transplant candidates awaiting organs.
1996	Nuclear transfer from laboratory cells (sheep).
1996	The birth of the first cloned animal, Dolly the sheep, was proclaimed.
1997	First primate engineered by embryonic cell nuclear transfer (rhesus monkey).
1997	Cloning of a transgenic lamb (Polly) from cells engineered with a marker gene and a human gene was announced. In this fashion, the genetic alteration of a lamb was combined with the techniques of cloning, thereby generating animals that produce a new protein.

1997	Nuclear transfer from genetically engineered laboratory cells (sheep).
1998–99	Additional mammals cloned by somatic cell nuclear transfer (mice, cows and goats).
2000	First pigs cloned: PPL Therapeutics clones the first pigs, engineered to create organs for human transplant.
2000	First transgenic pigs cloned: Infigen clones the first transgenic pigs, as a potential source of organs and tissues for transplant for humans.
2000	The Raelian sect claimed it would clone a human within the year.
2001	Endangered animals cloned by somatic cell nuclear transfer.
2001	A patent was approved to the University of Missouri for a technology for cloning mammals; the University then licensed the patent to Massachusetts company Biotransplant. Critics were troubled since the patent application did not prohibit humans, and specifically mentioned human eggs. Others challenged that the patent was for just the process and not the product, although the patent says it covers 'cloned products'.
2001	Human clones banned in England: the Human Reproductive Cloning Act was passed, barring the implanting of cloned embryos in the womb.
2001	Researchers produced the first clone of an endangered species: a type of Asian ox known as a guar. Sadly, the baby guar, which had developed inside a surrogate cow mother, died just a few days after its birth.
2002	US President Bush set up the Council on Bioethics to advise him on issues such as stem cell research and cloning.
2002	Cloning to make body parts: Advanced Cell Technology proclaimed that cells from cloned cow embryos were employed to cultivate kidney-like organs.
2002	CC (Carbon Copy), the first cloned pet: CC is not a phenotypic copy of the animal she was cloned from. A number of people have expressed interest in having their deceased pets cloned in the hope of getting a similar animal to replace the dead one. But as demonstrated by CC the cloned cat, a clone may not turn out precisely like the original pet whose DNA was employed to create the clone.
2003	Cloning approved for research purposes: the Kentucky House Judiciary Committee banned reproductive cloning but permitted cloning for research purposes. The bill would make the shipping or use of cloned embryos for reproductive purposes a crime punishable by 10–20 years in prison, as well as requiring those conducting cloning research to record it with the state Cabinet for Health Services 30 days before commencement of research.
2003	An endangered type of ox, called the Banteg, was successfully cloned.
2006	A pig was developed to generate omega-3 fatty acids via the incorporation of a roundworm gene.
2007	Primate (rhesus monkey) embryonic stem cells developed by somatic cell nuclear transfer.
2013	Human embryonic stem cells developed by somatic cell nuclear transfer.

1.6.2.1.1 Reproductive cloning

This involves constructing an egg using genetic material from another source. The egg then develops into an embryo, before being planted in a female host's uterus to continue to develop. Reproductive cloning produces copies of whole animals.

1.6.2.1.2 DNA/gene cloning

DNA cloning is a simpler method, whereby DNA is extracted from a host then replicated using plasmids. Even individual genes can be cloned in this manner. Gene cloning produces copies of genes or segments of DNA. A simple demonstration of gene cloning is shown in figures 1.4 and 1.5.

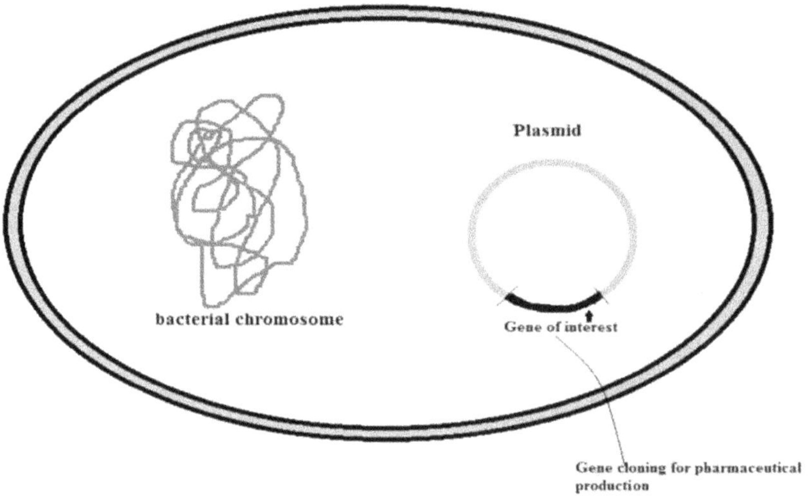

Figure 1.4. Gene cloning for the production of pharmaceutical compounds.

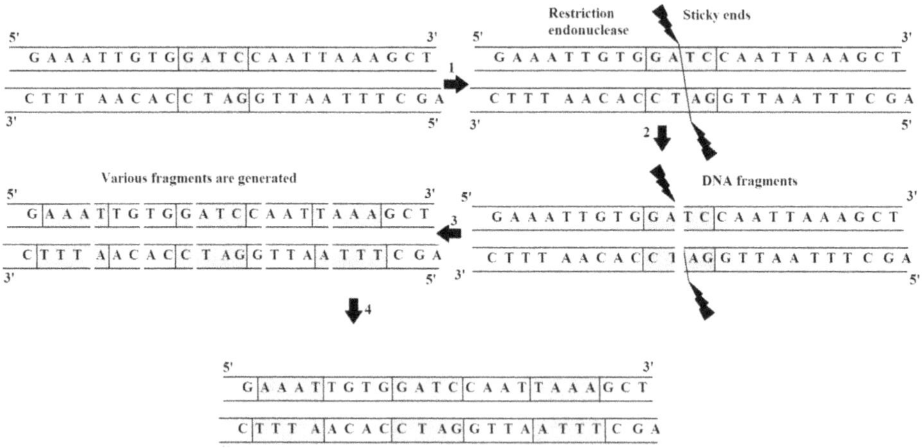

Figure 1.5. rDNA, gene cloning and pharmaceutical production. In this mature and widely utilized biotechnology, DNA can be cut at specific sequences using restriction enzymes. This creates DNA fragments useful for gene cloning. Restriction enzymes are enzymes that cut DNA only at particular sequences. Different restriction enzymes have different recognition sequences. This makes it possible to create a wide variety of different gene fragments. Then, DNA cut by a restriction enzyme can be joined together in new ways. These are known as rDNAs and they often are made of DNAs from different organisms. Ultimately this results in new recombinant DNA with different sequences.

1.6.2.1.3 Therapeutic cloning

This type of cloning is similar to reproductive cloning, except that stem cells are extracted from the embryo and used to treat the host. This type of cloning has many medical benefits for treating all sorts of diseases but is highly controversial because of the destruction of the embryo following stem cell extraction. A simple demonstration of therapeutic cloning is shown in figure 1.6. Therapeutic cloning produces embryonic stem cells for experiments aimed at creating tissues to replace injured or diseased tissues. The inner cell mass (ICM) is the source of embryonic stem cells. The embryo is destroyed by separating it into individual cells for the collection of ICM cells. Stem cells are found in adults, but the most promising types of stem cells for therapy are embryonic stem cells.

In the context of cell replacement therapy, therapeutic cloning holds huge potential for *de novo* organogenesis and the permanent treatment of incurable diseases such as Parkinson's disease, Duchenne muscular dystrophy and diabetes mellitus, as shown by *in vivo* studies. Major obstacles obstructing advancement in therapeutic cloning are tumorigenicity, epigenetic reprogramming, mitochondrial heteroplasmy, interspecies pathogen transfer and low oocyte availability. Moreover, therapeutic cloning is also often tied to ethical considerations concerning the source, destruction and moral status of IVF embryos based on the argument of potential. Legislative and funding issues also need to be addressed. Future considerations would include a distinction between therapeutic and reproductive cloning in legislative formulations.

1.6.2.1.4 Applications

Reproductive cloning may enable researchers to make copies of animals with potential benefits for the fields of medicine and agriculture. Since the announcement of Dolly the sheep by Scottish researchers, other sheep have been genetically modified to produce milk that contains a human protein essential for blood clotting. This research was conducted to derive the protein from the milk for humans whose blood does not clot properly. This, along with many other studies, exemplifies the

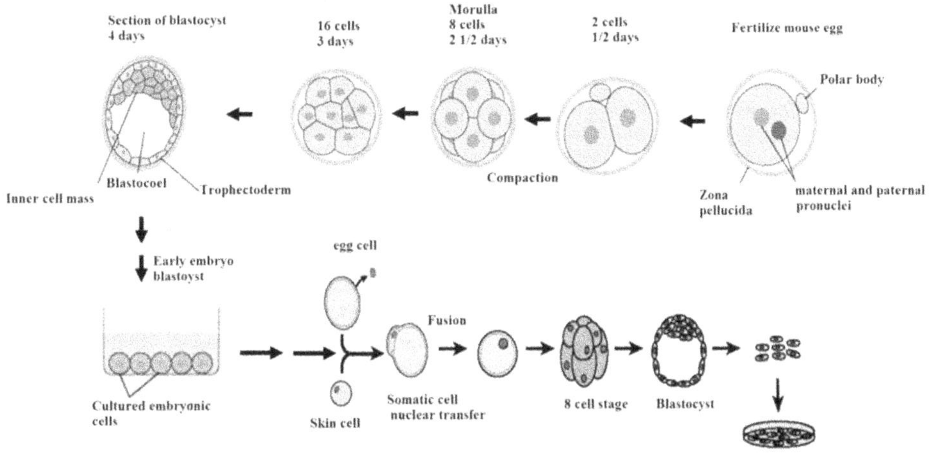

Figure 1.6. Therapeutic cloning from embryonic cells.

possibilities of cloned animals for testing of new drugs and treatment strategies. The main motivation for using cloned animals for drug testing is that they are all genetically identical. This means their responses to the drugs should be uniform rather than variable as seen in animals with different genetic make-ups.

In 2008, the FDA decided that meat and milk from cloned animals, such as cattle, pigs and goats, are as safe as those from non-cloned animals. This decision means that researchers are now free to use cloning methods. These methods can be used to make copies of animals with desirable agricultural traits, such as high milk production or lean meat. However, because cloning is still very expensive, it will likely take many years until food products from cloned animals actually appear in supermarkets. Moreover, cloning can also be utilized to create clones to build populations of endangered, or possibly even extinct, species of animals. During the era of genetic engineering most of the research has been focused towards transgenesis using rDNA and cloning as a basic tool for the procurement and maximum utilization of elite traits.

1.6.2.2 DNA fingerprinting

Different individuals carry different alleles. Most alleles useful for DNA fingerprinting differ on the basis of the number of repetitive DNA sequences they contain. If DNA is cut with a restriction enzyme that recognizes sites on either side of the region that varies, DNA fragments of different sizes will be produced. A DNA fingerprint is made by analyzing the sizes of DNA fragments produced from a number of different sites in the genome that vary in length. The more common the length variation at a particular site and the greater the number of sites analyzed, the more informative the fingerprint. A simple demonstration of DNA fingerprinting is illustrated in figure 1.7.

The techniques used in DNA fingerprinting also have applications in paleontology, archaeology, various fields of biology and medical diagnostics. In biological classification, it can help show evolutionary change and relationships on the molecular level, and it has the advantage of being useable even when only very small samples, such as tiny pieces of preserved tissue from extinct animals, are available. In criminal investigations, the DNA fingerprint of a suspect's blood or other body material is compared to that of the evidence from the crime scene to see how closely they match. The technique can also be used to establish paternity. DNA fingerprinting is generally regarded as a reliable forensic tool when done properly, but some scientists have called for wider sampling of human DNA to ensure that the segments analyzed are indeed highly variable for all ethnic and racial groups. It is possible to create false genetic samples and use them to misdirect forensic investigators, but if those samples have been produced using gene amplification techniques they can be distinguished from normal DNA evidence.

1.6.2.2.1 Applications

Personal identification. This is the idea of keeping everyone's DNA on a computer as a bar code. This concept has been discussed and has been decided to be impractical and very expensive. It is very unlikely to become a system in general use. Photo

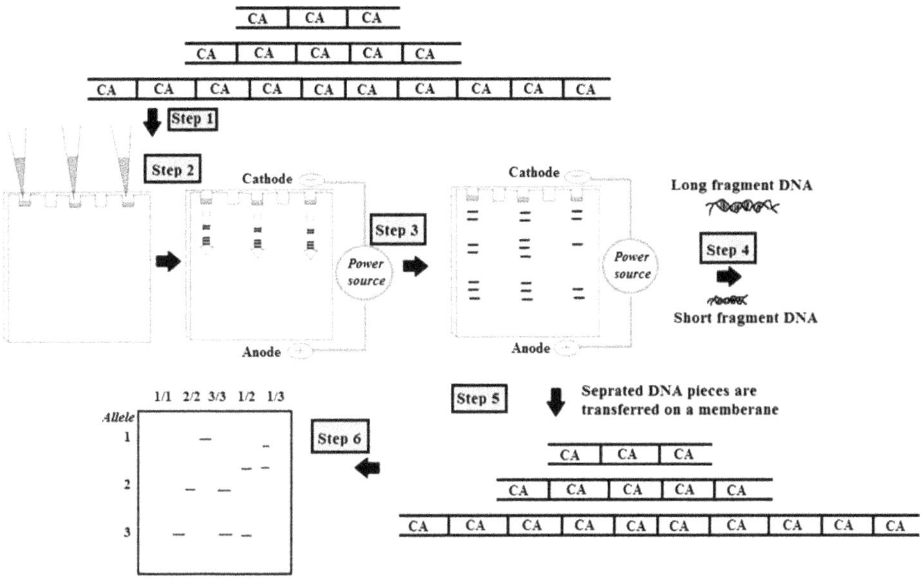

Figure 1.7. DNA fingerprinting. Step 1: A site is chosen with three alleles useful for DNA fingerprinting. DNA fragments of different sizes will be produced by a restriction enzyme that cuts at the points shown by the arrows. Step 2 to step 4: The DNA fragments are separated on the basis of size. The technique is gel electrophoresis. Step 5: Separated DNA pieces are transferred on a membrane. Step 6: Six diploid genotypes are present in the population, possible patterns for a single 'gene' with three alleles: in a standard DNA fingerprint, about a dozen sites are analyzed, with each site having many possible alleles.

identification cards and social security numbers, for instance, are much more efficient methods of identification and are not likely to change.

Paternity and maternity: This is also a well-known application of DNA fingerprinting. This is the test used to find out who is the father of a baby or child. Every individual has a variable number tandem repeat (VNTR) pattern which is inherited from their parents. The pattern in each individual is different but it is similar enough to reconstruct the parents' VNTR. This method can also be used to ascertain the real biological parents of an adopted child or determine legal nationality. Individuals should be careful when using a test like this because it may have surprising results that could cause distress.

Criminal identification and forensics. This is a very famous field of DNA fingerprinting. It has become popularly known because of the hit TV series *CSI: Crime Scene Investigation*. It is a very important use of DNA fingerprinting because it can prove an individual's innocence or guilt of committing a crime. To be used, a sample of DNA has to be obtained from the scene of the crime and matched with the suspect in question. The two pieces of DNA are then compared through VNTR patterns.

Diagnosis and cures for inherited diseases. DNA fingerprinting can also be used to detect and cure genetically inherited diseases. Using DNA fingerprinting one can detect genetic diseases such as cystic fibrosis, hemophilia, Huntington's disease and many others. If the disease is detected at an early age it can be treated and there is a greater chance that it can be defeated. Some couples who are carriers of a disease seek out genetic counsellors who can use a DNA fingerprint to help them understand the risks of having an affected child and give them information and assistance. The fingerprints can be used by researchers to look for patterns that specific diseases have and try to figure out ways that they can cure them.

1.6.2.3 rDNA technology
Restriction enzymes are enzymes that cut DNA only at particular sequences (figures 1.8 and 1.9). Different restriction enzymes have different recognition

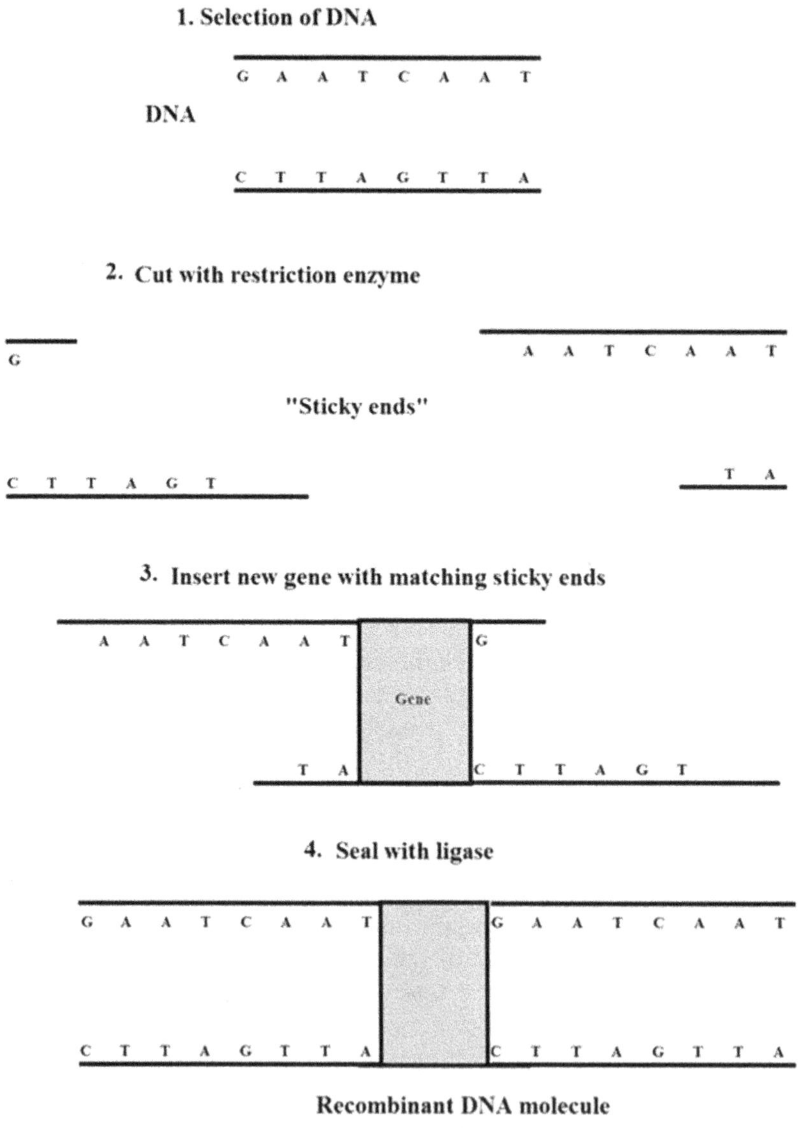

Figure 1.8. Role of restriction enzyme in rDNA technology.

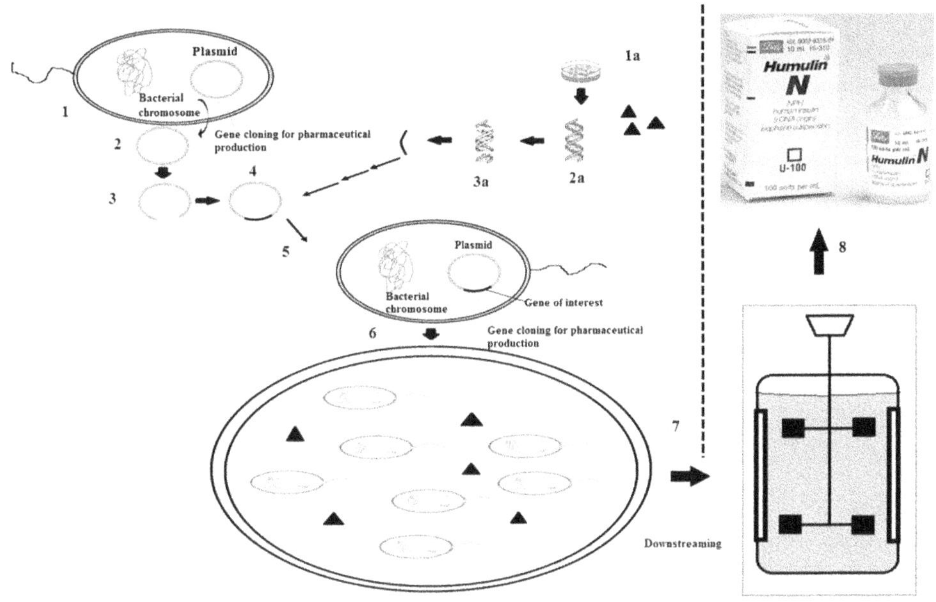

Figure 1.9. rDNA technology. Step 1: Select specific strains of bacteria. Step 2: Isolate the plasmid from the bacteria. Step 3: Cut with restriction enzyme. Step 1a: Isolate human cells containing GOI that codes for the synthesis of protein of interest and grow in tissue culture. Step 2a: Isolate DNA from human cells, cut with same restriction enzyme. Step 3a: Allow the insertion of GOI into plasmid to form recombinant plasmid. Step 4: Transformation of plasmid in bacteria. Step 5: Allow to grow them on culture medium. Step 6: Multiple bacterial clones are screened for their GOI expression to produce protein. Step 7: Allow mass propagation of the new bacteria. Step 8: Isolate and purify human protein such as insulin and develop formulations such as Humulin.

sequences. This makes it possible to create a wide variety of different gene fragments. To harness the power of rDNA technology, human insulin produced by bacteria plasmids is used to replicate rDNA. Plasmids are small circles of DNA found in bacteria which replicate independently of the bacterial chromosome. Pieces of foreign DNA can be added within a plasmid to create a recombinant plasmid. Replication often produces 50–100 copies of a recombinant plasmid in each cell. The route to the production of human insulin by bacteria is shown in figure 1.9.

Genetically modified plants have generated a large amount of interest in recent years and continue to do so. In spite of this, the general public remains largely uninformed of what a genetically modified (GM) plant actually is or what merits and demerits the technology has to offer, particularly with a view to the range of applications for which it can be used. From the first generation of GM crops, two major areas of concern have appeared, specifically danger to the environment and hazards to human health. Since GM plants are steadily being established in the European Union (EU) there is the possibility of increased public concern regarding potential health issues. While it is now routine for the press to espouse 'health campaigns', the information they publish is often unpredictable and unreliable

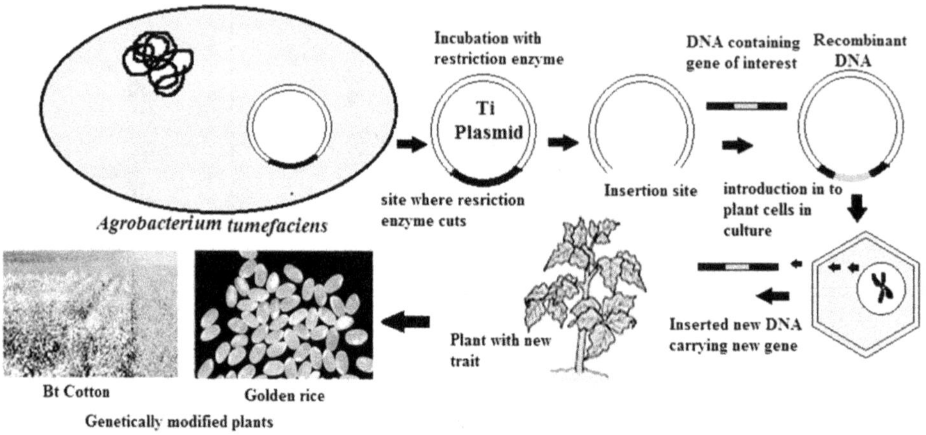

Figure 1.10. rDNA technology-based production of transgenic plant.

compared to the available scientific proof. It is essential to understand the rDNA-technology-mediated production of transgenic plants (figure 1.10).

1.6.2.4 Stem cell therapy

A stem cell is an undifferentiated, dividing cell that gives rise to a daughter cell like itself and a daughter cell that becomes a specialized cell type (figure 1.11).

1.6.2.4.1 Applications

Stem cells can be used to study development, i.e. they may help us understand how a complex organism develops from a fertilized egg. In the laboratory, scientists can follow stem cells as they divide and become increasingly specialized, making skin, bone, brain and other cell types. Identifying the signals and mechanisms that determine whether a stem cell chooses to carry on replicating itself or differentiates into a specialized cell type, and into which cell type, will help us understand what controls normal development. Some of the most serious medical conditions, such as cancer and birth defects, are due to abnormal cell division and differentiation. A better understanding of the genetic and molecular controls of these processes may yield information about how such diseases arise and suggest new strategies for therapy. This is an important goal of stem cell research.

Stem cells have the ability to replace damaged cells and treat disease. This property is already used in the treatment of extensive burns, and to restore the blood system in patients with leukemia and other blood disorders. Stem cells may also hold the key to replacing cells lost in many other devastating diseases for which there are currently no sustainable cures. Today, donated tissues and organs are often used to replace damaged tissue, but the need for transplantable tissues and organs far outweighs the available supply. Stem cells, if they can be directed to differentiate into specific cell types, offer the possibility of a renewable source of replacement cells and tissues to treat diseases including Parkinson’s, stroke, heart disease and diabetes.

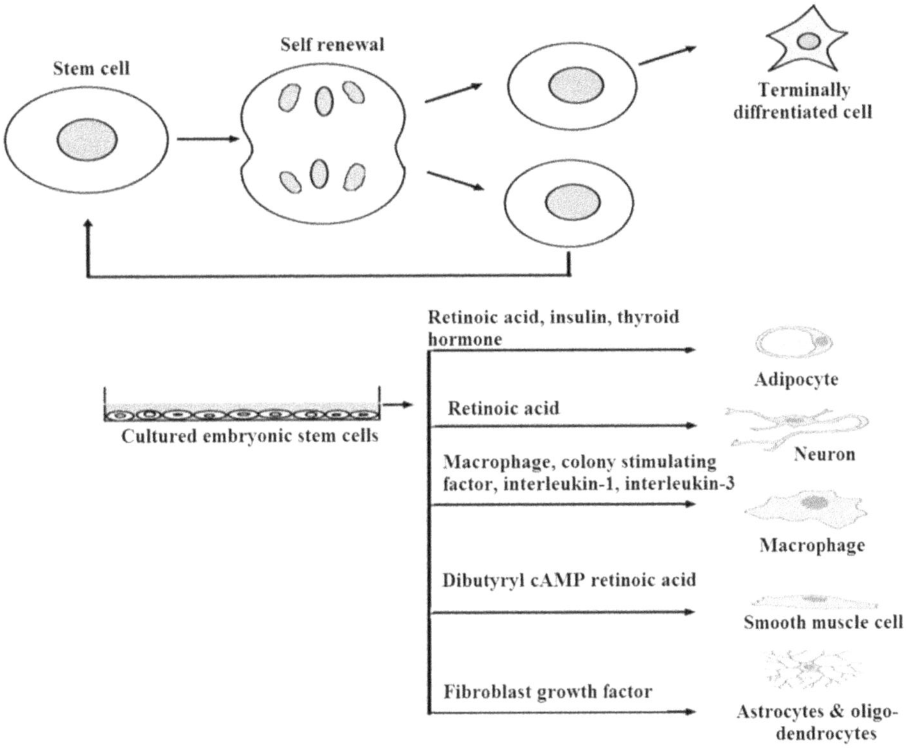

Figure 1.11. Stem cell and its development.

This prospect is an exciting one, but significant technical hurdles remain that will only be overcome through years of intensive research.

Stem cells can be used to study disease. In many cases it is difficult to obtain cells that are damaged by a disease and to study them in detail. Stem cells, either carrying the disease gene or engineered to contain disease genes, offer a viable alternative. Scientists could use stem cells to model disease processes in the laboratory, and better understand what goes wrong.

Stem cells could provide a resource for testing new medical treatments. New medicines could be examined for safety on specialized cells generated in large numbers from stem cell lines—reducing the requirement for animal testing. Various types of cell lines are already used in this way. Cancer cell lines, for example, are used to screen potential anti-tumor drugs.

1.7 Biotech research: 2015–16

There now follows an overview of the most recent discoveries in biotechnology.

Genetic modification is an alternative for incorporating new traits or producing elite varieties, particularly in crops and trees. These superior varieties of plants have socio-economic and environmental advantages. However, complex and lengthy EU protocols are delaying their introduction to the market [88]. Considering GM development, scientist's state that Europe has not acquired a leading position in the global GM market and that Europe is lagging behind in worldwide GM developments, and they call for a more technically authentic decision-making process.

In another study scientists have produced microbes that cannot 'run away from home'. Swarmbots are the microbes engineered by rDNA technology from genetically engineered bacteria, and could be useful in various fields. Current reports suggest a platform technology (microbial swarmbot) which employs a spatial arrangement to regulate the growth dynamics of engineered bacteria. This scheme can stop GM organisms from escaping into the surrounding environment and additionally it can often encourage colonies of bacteria to react to changes against surrounding environment [89].

Current researchers have also discovered an effective method of gene transfer which involves culturing and transfecting of cells with genetic material on an array of carbon nanotubes. This innovation has overcome the drawbacks of other gene editing techniques. In this study researchers were more focused on the structure of regulatory sequences in DNA is packaged in a cell [90].

Recent transfection approaches have considerable limitations, as most of them are time consuming, cytotoxic, have inefficient introduction of test molecules into target cells and are limited by the size of the genetic cargo. Golshadi *et al* [70] developed a novel approach of inserting genes and biomolecules into tens of thousands of mammalian cells. This was achieved using hollow carbon nanotubes, manufactured by template-based nanofabrication processes, to achieve rapid high-efficiency transfer with low cytotoxicity, which will ultimately overcome the molecular weight limits of recent approaches. In addition to nucleic acids this approach can be utilized to deliver drugs or proteins. We have hypothetically demonstrated this approach in figure 1.12.

Wrapping of histone by nuclear DNA to form nucleosomes limits the binding of transcription factors to gene regulatory sequences. Iwafuchi *et al* used low and high levels of micrococcal nuclease digestion to evaluate the nucleosomal configuration in mouse liver and finally discovered that MNase-accessible nucleosomes are present more at liver-specific enhancers than at promoters and ubiquitous enhancers (figure 1.13) [91]. They have concluded that as pioneer factor FoxA displaces linker histone H1, nucleosomes are not solely repressive to gene regulation when they are retained with, and exposed by, pioneer factors [91].

In another study, a comprehensive molecular investigation (transcriptional mapping of human embryo) of the embryo's first week of development has been carried out [92]. In this study transcriptional mapping of human embryo development, including the sequenced transcriptomes of 1529 individual cells from 88 human preimplantation embryos, are presented. They report that there are considerable differences in embryonic development between humans and mice.

The *Hydra* (freshwater polyp) is capable of restructuring a complete creature from any piece of its body. It has been observed that *Hydra* remains alive when all its neurons have gone. *Hydra* constantly differentiate a sophisticated nervous system made of interstitial stem cells. Wenger *et al* describe the impact of the loss of neurogenesis in *Hydra* by performing transcriptomic profiling at five positions along

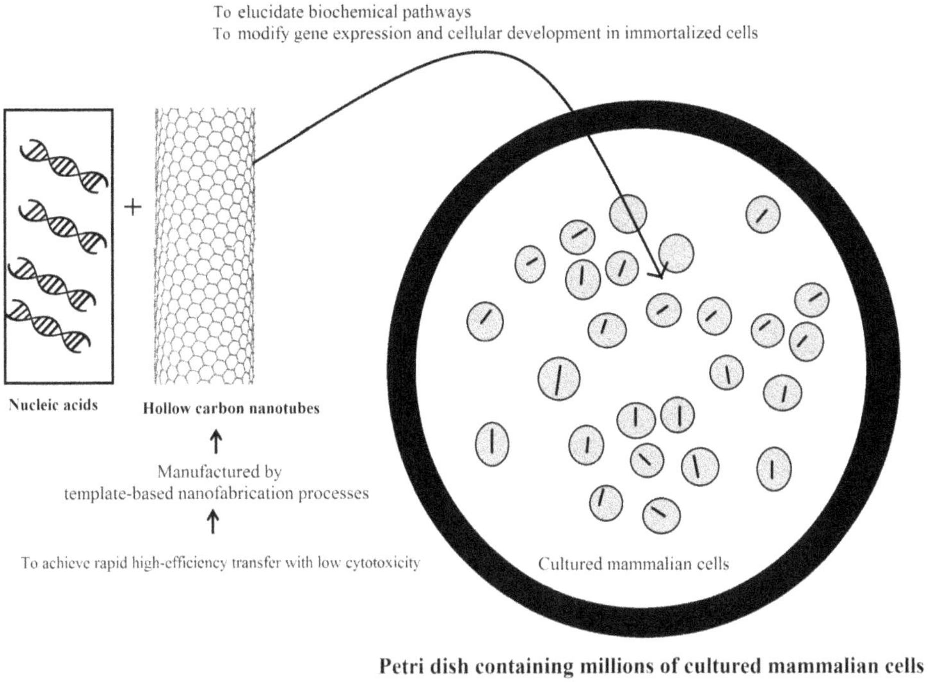

Figure 1.12. Novel approach of incorporating nucleic acids in ten thousand mammalian cells [90].

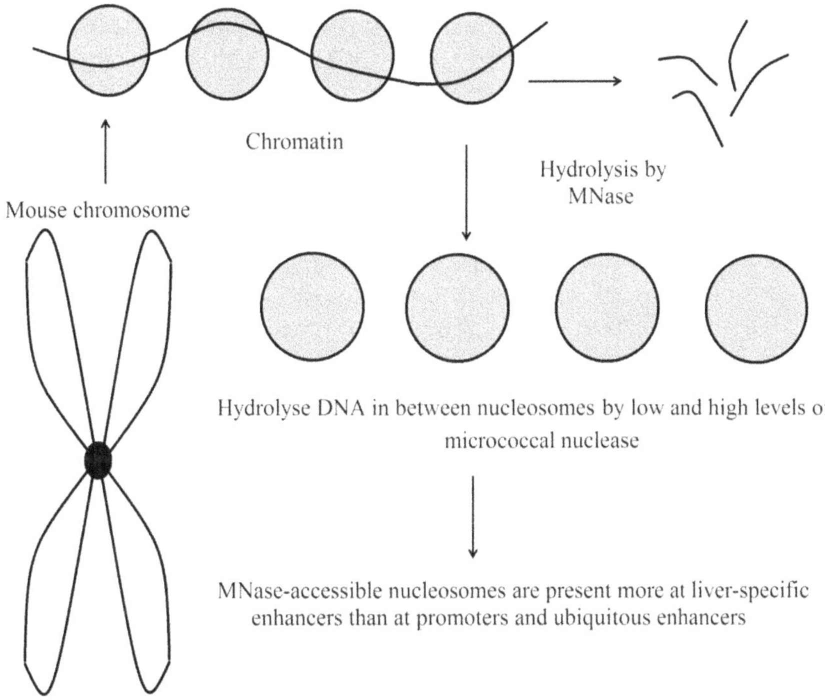

Figure 1.13. MNase-accessible nucleosomes to assess the nucleosome configuration in mouse liver [88].

the body axis [93]. They have concluded from their study how epithelial cells alter their genetic program by overexpressing a sequence of genes, of which some are related to various nervous functions. These epithelial cells improve their sensing ability when neurogenesis is compromised. This unknown plasticity may represent the potential of epithelial-like cells in early Planulozoa development [93].

Schaumberg *et al* have taken genetic engineering to a more advanced level. Currently, various researchers a are developing modular, programmable genetic circuits that control specific plant functions [94]. Plant synthetic biology ensures enormous scientific benefits, containing the possible advancement of a sustainable bio-based economy by the prognostic design of synthetic gene circuits. These circuits are generated from quantitatively characterized genetic parts; nevertheless, this approach has considerable obstacles in work with plants as it requires time for stable transformation. Schaumberg co-workers described the quantitative characterization of genetic parts and circuits for plant synthetic biology, describing how genetic circuits control specific plant functions [94].

Another breakthrough was based on the determination of microbial growth using GM fluorescing *E. coli* cells. This approach works in a similar way to the method that is adopted to determine population levels of animals in the particular environments [95]. The growth dynamics of microbes is characteristically determined after observing them directly, or when death is rare. In mammalian gut microbiota, neither of these conditions holds, thus typical tactics cannot exactly determine the microbial growth under an *in vivo* environment. To determine microbial growth dynamics, Myhrvold *et al* explored a novel approach, by using distributed cell division counting (DCDC), that uses the precise segregation at cell division of genetically encoded fluorescent particles [95]. DCDC can allow the measurement of microbial growth during antibiotic therapy, gut dysbiosis, infection, or other situations relevant to human health. GM fluorescing *E. coli* measures gastrointestinal microbe growth rates (the population) that lives inside mammalian gastrointestinal tracts.

Another major breakthrough was achieved in the field of optogenetics, in regulating the movement of proteins. Protein regulation in eukaryotes is a very complex process. One of the key mechanisms for protein regulation is active nucleocytoplasmic transport. LEXY is a potential optogenetic toolbox with various applications in synthetic and cell biology. With the help of optogenetic tools it is possible to control the import of nuclear protein and several reports are already available on this. Optogenetics is the approach to control well-defined events within specific cells of living tissue by using genetics and optics. In 2016 Niopek *et al* for the first time, evidenced an approach for spatiotemporal regulation of the export of a tagged protein using a light-inducible nuclear export system (LEXY) [96]. In this study light can be utilized to regulate the import/export of proteins from the cell nucleus and also the activity of proteins in mammalian cells [96] (see figure 1.14).

Tissue engineering is an emerging area that has been attracting considerable attention from researchers. In an effort to create artificial cartilage tissue, researchers from Umea University have used cartilage cells from cow knee joints [97]. This novel approach can be utilized to develop healthy cartilage tissue, and further researchers

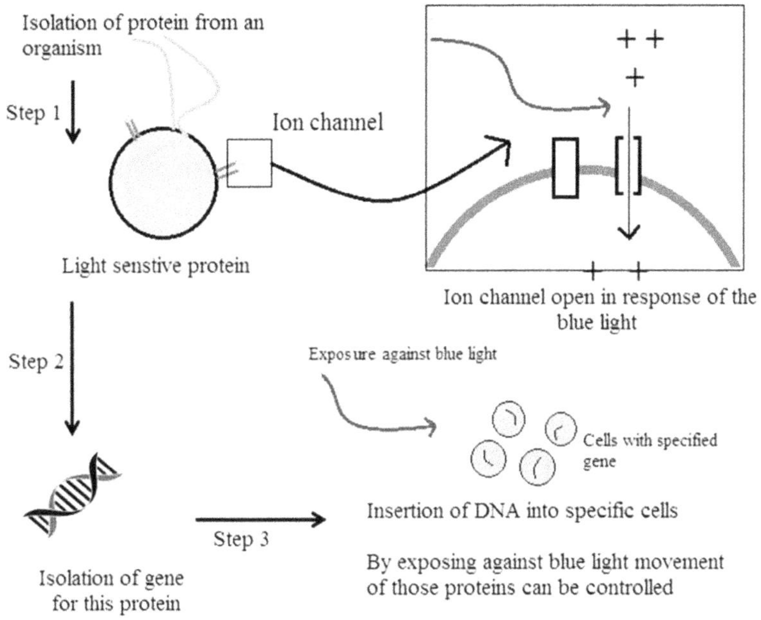

Figure 1.14. Application of optiogenetics in regulating the movement of proteins [96].

could use the findings to develop a treatment, or cure, for osteoarthritis using stem-cell-based tissue engineering. In this study, scientists have investigated how cells (primary bovine chondrocytes), signaling molecules and the artificial support material for the cartilage-like tissues (neotissues) can collectively work to encourage tissue regeneration at an injured joint site. This approach offers treatment against osteoarthritis by using healthy cartilage tissue which contains stem cells [97]. The next breakthrough was made by researchers at the Harvard Wyss Institute for Biologically Inspired Engineering and Harvard Medical School, which was based on R-bodies (retractable protein polymer) polymeric protein inclusions synthesized inside the cytoplasm of bacteria. One of the most important features of these proteins that they show structural variation at different pH. At high pH R-bodies resemble a coil of ribbon whereas at lower pH they undergo a conformational change and convert themselves into pointy hollow tubes. These hollow tubes are capable of puncturing through membranes, rupturing the cell membrane and releasing material present inside. This could offer applications in new drug delivery and other applications in biotechnology and medicine [98].

Cellular reprogramming is an excellent approach to renew the capacity of selected tissue to synthesize useful biochemicals inside the body. Scientists have invested many years to replace the beta cells (insulin-producing pancreatic cells) that are lost in diabetes. In 2016, Ariyachet *et al* showed the potential of antral stomach cells (cells derived from the lower stomach) after reprogramming to produce functional insulin-secreting cells [99]. In this study Ariyachet and co-workers separated tissue from mice and after reprogramming cultured them into 'mini-organs'.

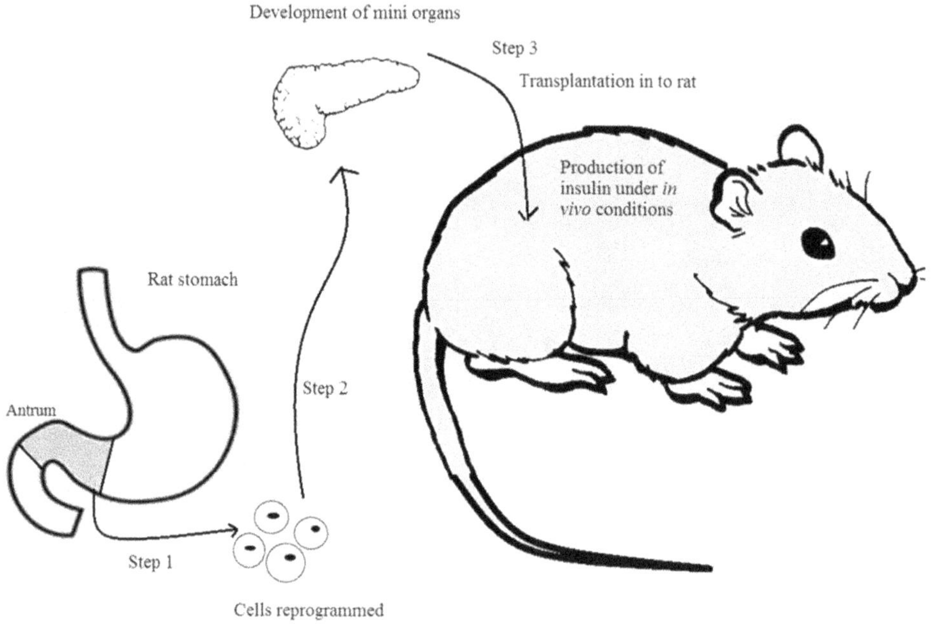

Figure 1.15. Cellular reprogramming and development of mini-organs for the efficient production of biochemicals [99].

These mini-organs produced insulin when transplanted back into the animals under *in vivo* conditions (see figure 1.15) [99].

In another study scientists have argued for the compulsory labeling of genetically modified foods, which is essentially required to let the community, especially consumers, to know what they are eating. This is based on a broad evaluation of the global scientific and legal frameworks associated with genetically modified organisms [100]. Certain producers and manufacturers are afraid of a negative consumer response to GM labeled products.

Opiates have been used from historical times as pain-relieving agents and are mainly derived from opium poppies. Modification of the alkaloid biosynthetic pathway to increase the productivity of these alkaloids is difficult as regulation of biosynthetic pathways in plants is complex. Therefore, current researchers used a step-wise fermentation approach using engineered strains of *E. coli* to trigger the production of thebaine up to a 300-fold increase. According to these researchers, this enhancement is may be due to the presence of strong activity of enzymes related to thebaine synthesis from (R)-reticuline in *E. coli.* These developments in opiate production using genetically modified *E. coli* system signify a key step towards alternative opiate production systems [101].

Emerging novel proteins can be a lead source in the drug delivery industry. The recent discovery of R-protein in the cytoplasm of bacteria that live inside *Paramecia* (tiny aquatic organisms) can possibly be utilized to deliver drugs [100]. To understand this phenomenon, it is essential to understand the role of R-bodies in

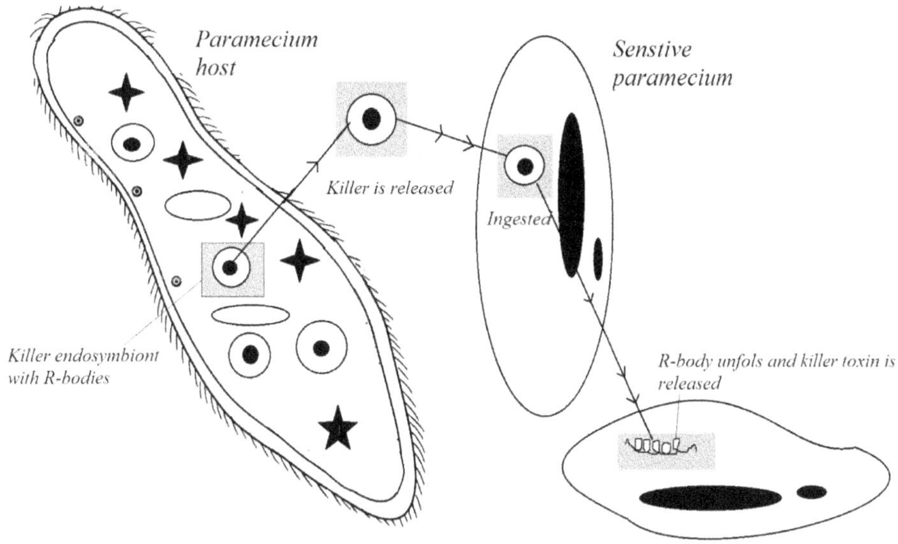

Figure 1.16. The role of R-bodies in *Paramecia.*

Paramecia, as shown in figure 1.16. Recently researchers have identified that the response of R-bodies present in *Paramecia* can be manipulated in a pH-dependent manner. These proteins are capable of selectively rupturing membrane compartments, thus may be important for programming cellular compartmentalization [100].

Another work synthesized genetically encoded biosensors for intracellular concentration of a target metabolite. These biosensors are synthesized from transcription factors conjugated with a fluorescent substance to track product formation. By tracking pathways researchers are engineering microbes in highly creative factories to produce products such as fine chemicals, therapeutics and biofuels [103].

Intestinal parasites infect more than one billion people worldwide, resulting in malnutrition and developmental issues [104]. Currently two benzimidazoles and two nicotinic acetylcholine receptor agonists are approved by the WHO. They are available on the market, however, the development of resistant strains against these agents urgently required new anthelminthics. Researchers made efforts to develop *B. thuringiensis* (Bt) crystal (Cry) proteins to treat intestinal nematode infections in humans. Cry proteins have been considered as safe for humans. We have used these proteins from over 50 years as crop insecticides [102].

For the production of these insecticidal proteins (Bt proteins), researchers inserted genes in the non-toxic bacteria *Lactococcus lactis* (figure 1.17). This can further help in integration of this protein in to dairy products, or in the form of probiotics to further deliver the protein to the intestines of affected people.

Another major breakthrough in the year 2015 was that the Joint Research Centre (JRC) developed a new database called the bioinformatics pipeline or JRC GMO-Amplicons, which includes the more than 240 000 DNA sequences emerging in GMOs [105]. This database will offer a complete source for the detection of DNA

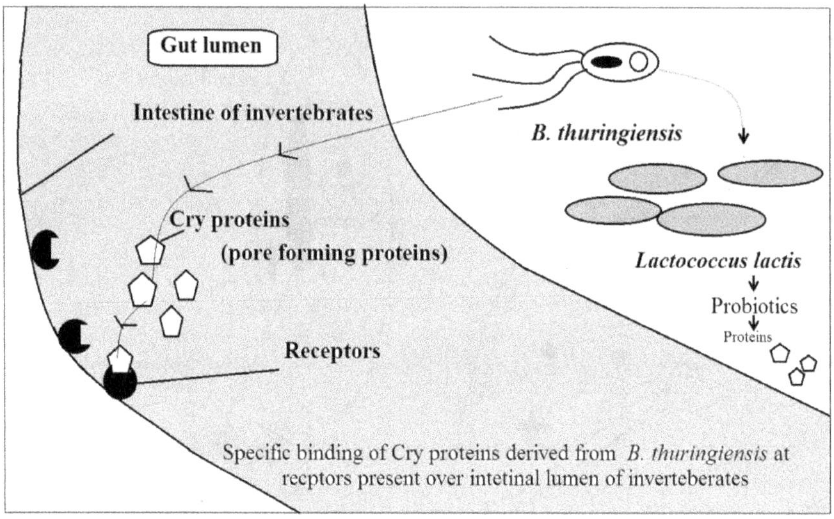

Figure 1.17. Specific binding of Cry proteins derived from *B. thuringiensis* and expression of Bt protein gene in *L. lactis*.

target sequences and also assist in checking the presence of GMOs in food, feed and the environment. This record is the broadest source of information available and can help in developing approaches for identifying GMOs in food and feed [106]. DiCarlo *et al* in their study 'Safeguarding CRISPR-Cas9 gene drives in yeast' described an effective safeguarding mechanisms for working with gene drives and unveiled a first-of-its-kind approach for reversing the changes they spread [107].

It was observed that heat shock response is a type of stress which is important in understanding the biogenesis and degradation of proteins inside the body and it is equally important to understand cellular death [108]. It is well-known that aging can increase the risk for protein conformational disease. It was observed that during the onset of reproductive maturity HSR declines quickly. The suppression was because of the increase in H3K27me3 marks at stress gene loci. In adult cells, genes start aging by turning off cell stress responses [108]. These responses protect the cell by keeping potential proteins folded and functional. During early maturity germ line stem cells throw the switch and individual cells retain their reproductive capability [108]. Based on similar work, Yang *et al* investigated the minimal set of gene functions required to sustain life in *E. coli.* This study covers the set of genes required to sustain life [109]. By using a comparative genomics-based core proteome, minimal gene lists have been suggested.

Embryonic stem cell development is an area of heightened attention today. Recently, several scientists discovered an approach to control embryonic stem cell differentiation with the help of beams of light. This approach allows them to be transformed into neurons in reaction to an accurate external sign. In another study, the complete pathway of endocytosis was described by a team of researchers. In particular, they studied how cells perform endocytosis by absorbing molecules which can result in rapid embryonic healing. Considering this factor, the outcomes of the study can be employed to design better treatments for wounds in adults [110].

Researchers have engineered the cassava plant to offer higher levels of vitamin B6 in its storage roots and leaves. This could help guard millions of people in Africa against serious deficiencies [111].

Several reports are available on target-based mutagenesis mediated by Cas9 (RNA-guided DNA endonuclease enzyme). Woo *et al* [112] reported genomic editing in plants without insertion of foreign DNA into cells. They introduced the Cas9 protein to guide RNA into protoplasts of several plants and achieved targeted mutagenesis at frequencies of up to 46%. This study may alleviate regulatory concerns related to genetically modified plants, as the researchers used the Cas9 protein and did not insert foreign DNA.

Several reports were published in 2012 and while it is not possible to describe all of these, some promising research cannot be skipped, such as the research based on the revolutionary tool for editing DNA (CRISPR), which could replace all medicine with better treatments. This research was discovered by Jennifer A Doudna, a biochemist at UC Berkeley, and her collaborator, Emmanuelle Charpentier of the Helmholtz Centre.

In general, CRISPR allows scientists to change DNA and it could allow scientists to cure diseases. This technology came from a project studying how bacteria fight against viruses. Some bacteria have an adaptive immune response called CRISPR that allows then to detect viral DNA and destroy it (figure 1.18). One of the parts of the CRISPR system, called Cas9, is able to seek out, cut and eventually degrade viral DNA in a specific way. Doudna and colleagues realized that they could harness its functions as a genetic engineering tool. Currently this technology is being used in many parts of the world which Their work suggests that this tool will perhaps fundamentally change both medicine and agriculture. A number of studies have repaired defective DNA in mice, e.g. treating genetic disorders. Furthermore, plant-based researchers have used CRISPR to manipulate genes in crops, raising hopes that it could lead to a better food supply. In 2014, *MIT Technology Review* called CRISPR ‘the major biotech discovery of the century’ [113].

Now pharmaceutical companies are showing interest in taking CRISPR to the next level to produce new drugs in the form of therapeutic proteins. Using CRISPR-based technology can create animal models, treat blood related disorders (easy to deliver in the blood), correct mutations and have certain clinical applications which will be seen in future. However, CRISPR technology raises many ethical issues, so discussion continues on validation and safety concerns. In January 2016, Novartis declared that it would be using Doudna’s CRISPR technology for its study into cancer treatments. It intends to manipulate the genes of immune cells so that they will attack tumors (figure 1.19). Microbes have been using CRISPR to alter their own DNA for millions of years, and currently they continue to do so all over the planet, from the bottom of the sea to the recesses of our own bodies. They utilize it as a complicated immune system, permitting them to learn to identify their enemies. Now researchers are discovering that microbes use CRISPR for other purposes as well (figure 1.19).

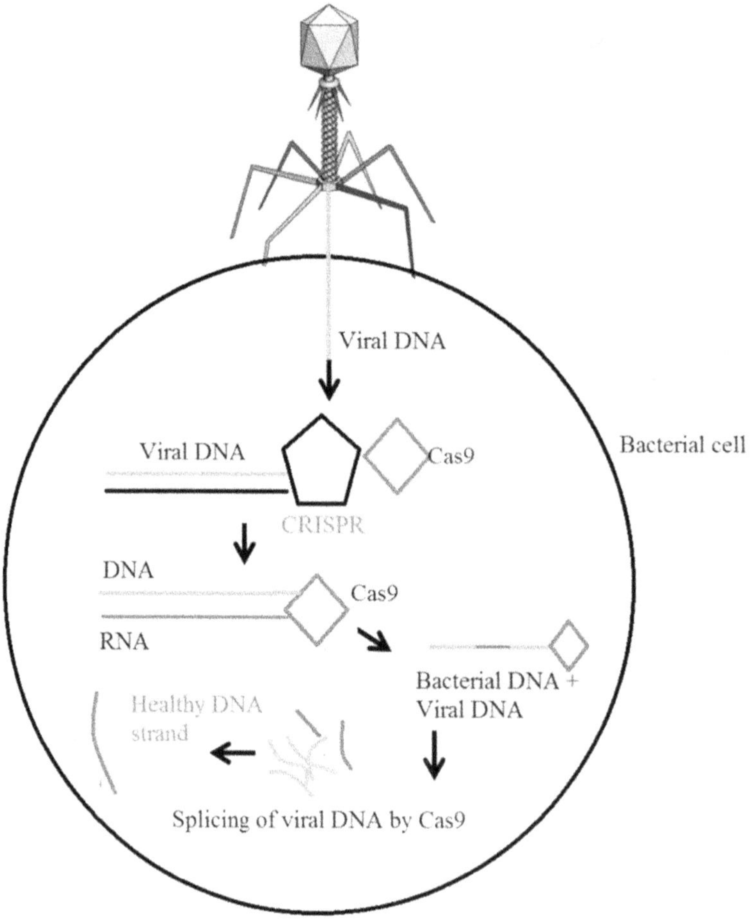

Figure 1.18. CRISPR technology. The virus incorporates DNA and inserts its DNA into the bacterial DNA, where the bacterial immune response CRISPR identified this insertion and cut the DNA wherever an insertion was made, and finally converted it back to healthy DNA.

1.7.1 Artificial intelligence and biotechnology

Due to its highly computational intelligence, artificial intelligence (AI) is expanding quickly throughout the world. When biotechnology and AI combine, new opportunities arise that have the ability to be beneficial in a various fields, including energy, clean water, agriculture, and medicine. In the realm of the biological sciences, AI has become widespread today. Various topics are addressed, such as biomedical ontologies, temporal and spatial representation and inference, natural language processing, knowledge-based reasoning, the analytics of Big Data, and machine learning. Additionally, methodological aspects of explainable AI (XAI) are explored, with applications in biotechnology, along with reasoning under uncertainty.

"CRISPR DISCOVERY FOUND IT BY ACCIDENT IN DNA RESEARCH" HBCJHDCCC CW CNC M X M MN C CMNC D CD CD C C C CC CHJCDCDWCDNJCJKWNDCSDC S C NKS FSF F C F FF F , WMDM DCM , NXX VSCGXVGS QXVSQ DCEDCDC **"BITTER FIGHT OVER THE PATENTS FOR CRISPR, A BREAKTHROUGH NEW FORM OF DNA EDITING"** HBXHSB SXVJAS VCJDAVVVJ SBXAJ XCC XXJSAXJSAXJS **"DOUDNA J AND CHARPENTIER E SHOWED UP IN BLACK GOWNS TO RECEIVE THE $3 MILLION BREAKTHROUGH PRIZE, A GLITZY AWARD PUT ON BY INTERNET BILLIONAIRES"** NNNN HBJHBCDDXJ X BBCBDBDB BDCBDCBDCBDC BCHDBCHDBCHSC BWBW BBBBBSXX SXB **"THEY'D WON FOR DEVELOPING CRISPR-CAS9, A "POWERFUL AND GENERAL TECHNOLOGY"** XNNSXNS SJNWJNSJNSKJN SJWHD WH SWUD SJSJS JWJKWDDDWDJDD GVWSXVS

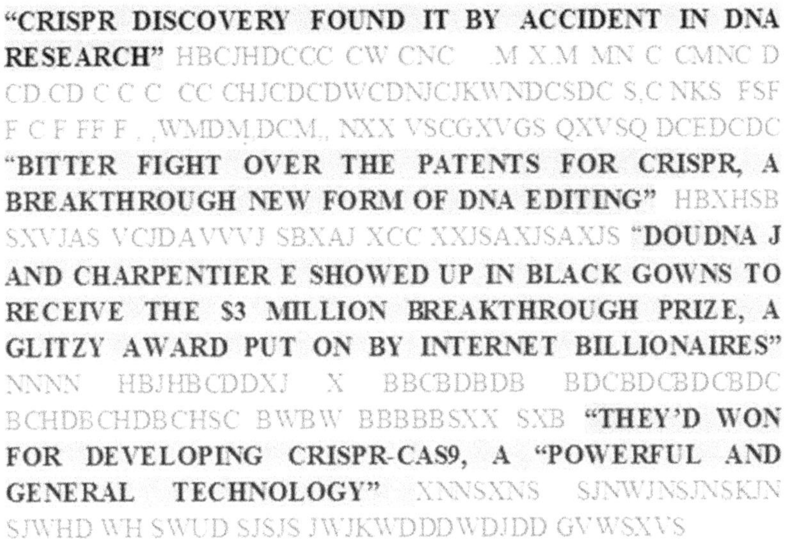

Figure 1.19. Out of thousands of studies in 2016, few headlines made such a remarkable contribution to biotechnology.

AI in agricultural biotechnology—agricultural biotechnology mainly involves genetically modifying crops to increase their yield and resistance to diseases and various climatic conditions. The agriculture sector can be transformed with the help of AI in various areas such as crop management, soil management, pesticide and fertilizer management, crop monitoring and yield prediction etc [114]. Biotech firms use various sophisticated manufacturing techniques, which involves use of autonomous robots. These robots handle various agricultural tasks such as much faster harvesting compared to traditional methods. Data collected by drones equipped with computer vision is evaluated and processed by various algorithms of machine learning and deep learning that are used to evaluate health of plants and soil. For example, EfficientNetV2 is AI-based drone technology used to detect plant diseases with accuracy of ~99%. Also, machine learning algorithms track and predict environmental changes to assess the impact of climate change on crop yield [115]. In the agricultural sector by adjusting agricultural management to a changing climate, artificial intelligence can offer a solution for food security [116] (figure 1.20 and table 1.10).

In the field of medicine, medical biotechnology with DNA research and genetically modified cells are used to enhance human health via drugs production, antibiotics and other therapeutic agents. Target identification for biological molecule or various cellular pathways that can be modulated by drugs for therapeutic potential is a crucial aspect of modern drug discovery. Over the past few decades, innovation in experimental and various omics technologies has been increased significantly (figure 1.21). The amalgamation of AI algorithms with multi-omics

Figure 1.20. AI in agriculture.

Table 1.10. AI-based algorithms in the agricultural sector [116].

Study	Objective	Method	Sample Size	Findings	References
1	Predicting *Salmonella* in agriculture streams	k-Nearest Neighbors, Support Vector Machines, Artificial Neural Networks	400	Accuracy: 58.15%–59.23%	[117]
2	Modeling rice growth rate	Regression (REG), Artificial Neural Networks (ANN), Gene Expression Programming (GEP)	95	Better prediction with ANN and GEP	[118]
3	Identifying seed germination	Convolutional Neural Network (CNN)	16	97% seed recognition accuracy	[119]
4	Detecting tomatoes and mass	Mask-RCNN, ResNet101-FPN, Region Proposal Network (RPN)	—	Accuracy: 99.02%, precision: 99.7%	[120]

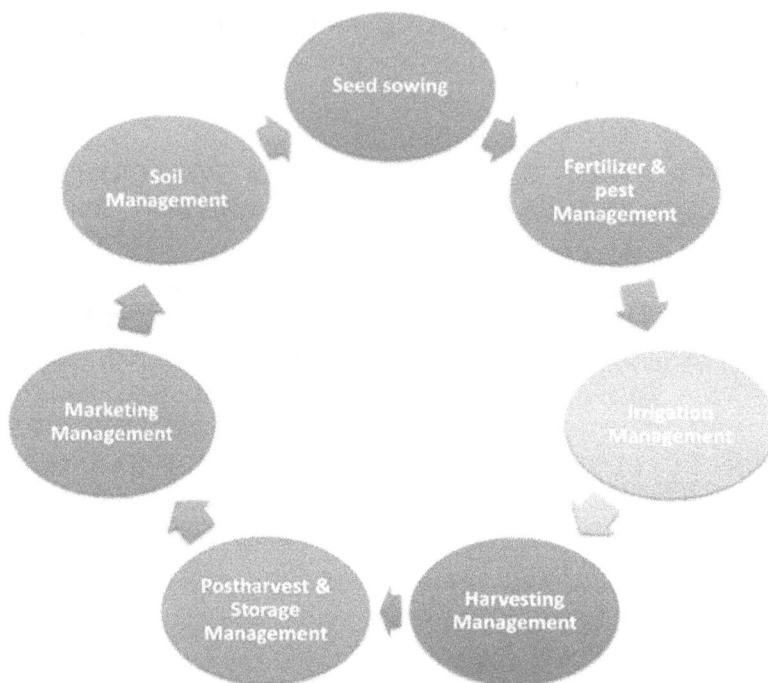

5	Smart tree crop sprayer design	LiDAR, machine vision, GPS, Convolutional Neural Network (CNN)	—	Tree classification accuracy: 84%, reduced chemical spraying by 28%	[121]

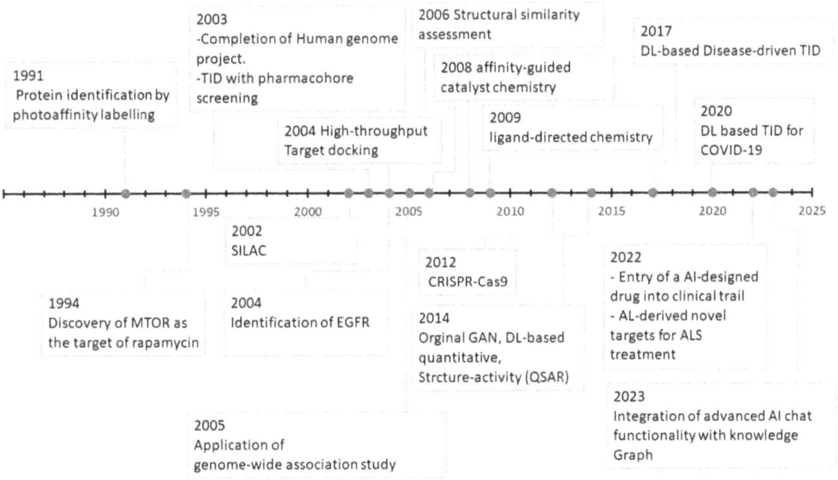

Figure 1.21. Timeline for emergence of AI in early drug development [129].

data holds immense promise for target identification. AI can be used to diagnose as it would be assisted in providing software for data analysis and also for finding potential targets for drugs through the analysing genomic data so that the potential therapeutic target can be identified while these drugs can be screened to find their effect and the data can be analyzed by different software assisted by AI [122] (table 1.11). AI can be used to evaluate individual genetic information as well as other forms of health data to create personalized treatment programmes that are catered to their unique requirements. This is called personalized medicine. These developments are still in the beginning of the developmental stage with no end in sight [123].

1.7.2 Use of biotechnology in advancements of plant metabolite extraction and identification techniques

Secondary metabolites in plants due to their diverse application in various industries are of great importance. The need for extraction and identification of these compounds in their pure form requires use of various advanced techniques that use different extraction methods depending on their chemical nature, such as solubility and distribution coefficient. Extraction method can be categorized into

Table 1.11. Examples of AI in medical biotechnology.

Disease	Algorithm	Findings	References
Age related macular degeneration	Machine learning based predictive mode	The AI prediction algorithm demonstrated a high degree of accuracy in forecasting the course of age related macular degeneration.	[124]
Alzheimer's	SHAP, RF	An AI model with 93.95% accuracy in the first layer and 87.08% accuracy in the second layer was able to detect and to identify and predict Alzheimer's disease.	[125]
COVID-19	PA	An accuracy of 70%–80% was achieved in predicting severe COVID-19 cases	[126]
Ovarian cancer	ANN	An accuracy of 93% was achieved in predicting the survival of ovarian cancer patients, and 77% accuracy was achieved in predicting the surgical outcome	[127]
Pulmonary cancer	LCP-CNN, Brock	LCP-CNN was able to predict the malignancy of pulmonary nodules with higher accuracy and lower false negative results than the Brock model	[128]
Influenza	IAT-BPNN	IAT-BPNN was able to predict influenza-like illness in large population size with a high accuracy	[129]

Abbreviations: AGC chemistry, affinity-guided catalyst chemistry; ALS, amyotrophic lateral sclerosis; DL, deep learning; EGFR, epidermal growth factor receptor; GAN, generative adversarial network; GWAS, genome-wide association study; LD chemistry, ligand-directed chemistry; MTOR, mammalian target of rapamycin; NSCLC, non-small cell lung cancer; SILAC, stable isotope labeling with amino acids in cell culture; TID, target identification.

three types liquid–liquid extraction, solid–liquid extraction and supercritical fluid extraction.

Liquid–liquid extraction: this is the most widely used extraction method for recovery and purification. Choice of solvent is the most crucial aspect depending upon the polarity and selectivity; the method involves a delicate balance between mixing and phase separation to prevent unwanted emulsion formation

Solid–liquid extraction—This includes methods like Soxhlet extraction, percolation, infusion, decoction, maceration and ultrasound-assisted extraction. These methods mainly involve penetration of solvent into solid matrix. The efficacy of this method depends on factors like temperature, extraction time and particle size. Alcohols like universal solvent like methanol and ethanol are commonly used for the extraction purpose.

Supercritical fluid extraction—A newer technique which involves using supercritical fluid as a solvent. This gives favorable transport properties for extracting sensitive and valuable compounds. This technique is considered to be faster than conventional methods and is most suitable for the extraction of thermolabile compounds. But the method involves high operational cost compared to traditional methods.

Isolation and identification techniques—Secondary metabolics present in the plant matrices complex at very low concentration. Isolation and identification is influenced by compound characteristics like solubility, stability, molecular size and acid base properties etc. It is the most commonly used technique for the separation of the compound to its pure form mixture in the plant via chromatography. Chromatography techniques are characterized by their flexibility and adaptability to meet analytical needs.

Chromatography techniques are classified on various ways, one of which is based on the shape of the chromatographic bed, which is further classified into flat chromatography which involves paper chromatography and thin layer chromatography.

Flat chromatography involves the use of a support matrix i.e., cellulose, alumina or silica gel. Paper chromatography is the simplest and cost-effective technique using cellulose as the stationary phase. If further analytes are not visible, the leaf is treated with reagent for additional confirmation and accurate identification. Thin layer chromatography involves the use of alumina or silica gel on an aluminum or glass plate and is similar to paper chromatography. The separation of the component is measured by the distribution factor (Rf). The unknown sample retention value is compared with the known sample to confirm its identity. Further, additional confirmation can be done my measuring the retention value of an unknown sample and known sample in different chromatographic conditions such as various columns or mobile column/phase combination [131] (table 1.12).

Table 1.12. Plant metabolite obtained employing varied extraction method [130].

Metabolite	Source	Biotech application	Yield
Piperine	Derived from Piper nigrum	Medicinal use: anti-tumor, bioinsecticide, nutraceutical	Extracted with an EAU yield of 14.83 g/20 g (74.1%)
Capsaicin	Obtained from Capsicum annuum L and Capsicum frutescens	Food application: flavoring	Extracted with a FSC of 2.10% (p/p), EAM yield of 5.28 mg g^{-1}, and EAU yield of 4.01 mg g^{-1}
Resveratrol	Sourced from polygonum cuspidatum	Medicinal use: anti-inflammatory, antioxidant	Extracted with an ELL yield of 11.47 mg g^{-1} and EAU yield of 3.82 mg g^{-1}
Steviosides	Derived from Stevia rebaudiana	Food application: Sweetener	Extracted with an EAU yield of 68.3 mg g^{-1} and EAM yield of 70.5 mg g^{-1}

(*Continued*)

Table 1.12. (*Continued*)

Metabolite	Source	Biotech application	Yield
Menthol	Obtained from Mentha arvensis and Mentha piperita	Food application: flavoring	Extracted with an EAU yield of 14.83 g/20 g (74.1%)
Ascorbic acid (Vitamin C)	Sourced from Myrciaria dubia, Rough rose Thunb, and Clinacanthus nutans	Medicinal use: vitamin	Extracted with a UHPLC-DAD yield of 1.297 g/100 g (92.81%), EAU yield of 6.38 mg g^{-1}, and EAM yield of 0.166 mg g^{-1}
Ergosterol	Derived from Agaricus blazei Murrill	Medicinal use: antineoplastic	Extracted with a MAE yield of 25.44 ± 5.1 mg/100 g
Vanillin	Obtained from Vanilla planifolia	Food application: flavoring	Extracted with a FSC of 19.6808 g $K^{-1}g^{-1}$, ED yield of 5.3 mg g^{-1}, EAU yield of 5.1 mg g^{-1}, and EAM yield of 6.7 mg g^{-1}
Lycopene	Sourced from Solanum lycopersicum	Food application: nutraceutical, antioxidant	Extracted with a UAE yield of 94.3 mg kg^{-1}
Camptothecin	Derived from Nothapodytes nimmoniana	Medicinal use: antineoplastic	Extracted with an EAU yield of 78% and EAM yield of 95%
Vinblastine	Obtained from Catharanthus roseus	Medicinal use: antineoplastic	Extracted with a FSC of 92% and EAU yield of 90.9% ± 1.06%
Paclitaxel	Derived from Taxus chinensis and Taxus wallichiana	Medicinal use: antineoplastic	Extracted with an EAM yield of 99% and EAU yield of 93.1% ± 4.4%

Abbreviations: EAU: ultrasound-assisted extraction, EAM: microwave assisted extraction, FSC: Supercritical fluids, ELL: Liquid–liquid extraction, UHPLC-DAD: Ultra high-performance liquid chromatography coupled to photodiode array, ED: Solvent extraction, DPV: steam distillation, ESX: Soxhlet extraction, SPM: membrane separation.

References

[1] Dundar M and Akbarova Y 2011 Current state of biotechnology in Turkey *Curr. Opin. Biotechnol.* **22** S3–6

[2] Steinberg F M and Raso J 1998 Biotech pharmaceuticals and biotherapy: an overview *J. Pharm. Pharm. Sci.* **1** 48–59

[3] Weizmann C and Rosenfeld B 1937 The activation of the butanol-acetone fermentation of carbohydrates by *Clostridium acetobutylicum* (Weizmann) *Biochem.* J. **31** 619–39

[4] Kuiper-Goodman T, Scott P M and Watanabe H 1987 Risk assessment of the mycotoxin zearalenone *Regul. Toxicol. Pharmacol.* **7** 253–306

[5] Secretariat of the Convention on Biological Diversity; UNEP 1992 *Convention on Biological Diversity Handbook* (UNEP) 3rd edn https://cbd.int/doc/handbook/cbd-hb-01-en.pdf (accessed 29 September 2015)

[6] Sreenivasulu N S 2008 *Biotechnology and Patent Law: Patenting Living Beings* (Noida: Manupatra) vol 13 p 249

[7] Collins 2017 *Collins English Dictionary* (www.collinsdictionary.com/dictionary/english/biotechnology)

[8] CSIR/NISCAIR 2013 *Golden Treasury of Science and Technology* (New Delhi: CSIR/NISCAIR) pp 9–11

[9] Gupta R and Rajpal T 2012 *Concise Notes in Biotechnology* (Tata/McGraw-Hill Education) ch 1

[10] Mathuriya A S 2010 General introduction to biotechnology *Industrial Biotechnology* (New Delhi: Ane Books Pvt Ltd) p 2

[11] Bu'lock J D and Kristiansen B 1987 *Basic Biotechnology* (London/Orlando: Saunders College Publishing/Harcourt Brace)

[12] Samiksha S 2017 Biotechnology: meaning, technologies and applications in India (www.yourarticlelibrary.com/biotechnology/biotechnology-meaning-technologies-and-applications-in-india-8617-words/11249)

[13] Demain A L and Dana C A 2007 The business of biotechnology *Comp. Ind. Biotechnol.* **3** 269–83

[14] Doelle H W, Rokem J S and Berovic M 2009 Biotechnology: fundamentals in biotechnology *EOLSS Publ* **1** 325–9

[15] Gibbs D F and Greenhalgh M E 1983 *Biotechnology, Chemical Feedstocks, and Energy Utilization: Report Prepared for the Commission of the European Communities, Directorate-General for Research and Development, as Part of the FAST Programme* (Dover, NH: Pinter)

[16] Verma A S, Agrahari S, Rastogi S and Singh A 2011 Biotechnology in the realm of history *J. Pharm. Bioallied Sci.* **3** 321–3

[17] Ereky K 1919 *Biotechnologie der Fleisch-, Fett-, und Milcherzeugung im landwirtschaftlichen Grossbetriebe: für naturwissenschaftlich gebildete Landwirte verfasst* (Berlin: Parey)

[18] Fári M G and Kralovánszky U P 2006 The founding father of biotechnology: Karl Ereky *Int. J. Hort. Sci.* **12** 9129–12

[19] Ejiofor A O 2015 Insect biotechnology *Short Views on Insect Genomics and Proteomics* (Springer) 11 pp 185–210

[20] Rodríguez-Núñez K, Rodríguez-Ramos F, Leiva-Portilla D *et al* 2020 Brown biotechnology: a powerful toolbox for resolving current and future challenges in the development of arid lands *SN Appl. Sci.* **2** 1187

[21] Adepoju F O, Ivantsova M N and Kanwugu O N 2019 Gray biotechnology: an overview *AIP Conf. Proc.* **vol 2174** (AIP Publishing LLC) 020199

[22] Kanwugu O N, Ivantsova M N and Chidumaga K D 2018 Gold biotechnology: development and advancements *AIP Conf. Proc.* **vol 2015** (AIP Publishing)

[23] Campbell C S 2003 Biotechnology and the fear of Frankenstein *Camb. Q. Healthc. Ethics* **12** 342–52

[24] Belt H 2009 Playing God in Frankenstein's footsteps: synthetic biology and the meaning of life *Nanoethics* **3** 257–68

[25] Daston L 2011 *Histories of Scientific Observation* (Chicago, IL: University of Chicago Press) p 440

[26] Eknoyan G and Santo N G D (ed) 1997 *History of Nephrology 2: Reports from the First Congress on the International Association for the History of Nephrology (Kos, 1996)* (Basel: Karger) p 198

[27] Porter R 2001 *The Cambridge Illustrated History of Medicine* (Cambridge: Cambridge University Press) p 375

[28] Belongia E A and Naleway A L 2003 Smallpox vaccine: the good, the bad, and the ugly *Clin. Med. Res.* **1** 87–92

[29] Dahm R 2005 Friedrich and the discovery of DNA *Dev. Biol.* **278** 274–88

[30] Paweletz N 2001 Walther Flemming: pioneer of mitosis research *Nat. Rev. Mol. Cell Biol.* **2** 72–5

[31] Smith K A 2012 Louis Pasteur, the father of immunology? *Front. Immunol* **3** 68

[32] Coico R 2005 Gram staining *Curr. Protoc. Microbiol.* **App.3C** A.3C.1–2

[33] Richter F C 2015 Remembering Johann Gregor Mendel: a human, a Catholic priest, an Augustinian monk, and abbot *Mol. Gen. Genom. Med.* **3** 483–5

[34] Keynes M and Bateson W 2008 The rediscoverer of Mendel *J. R. Soc. Med.* **101** 104

[35] Hegreness M and Meselson M 2007 What did Sutton see? Thirty years of confusion over the chromosomal basis of Mendelism *Genetics* **176** 939–44

[36] Mittwoch U 2013 Sex determination *EMBO Rep.* **14** 588–92

[37] Edwards A W F 2012 Reginald Crundall Punnett: first Arthur Balfour professor of genetics, Cambridge, 1912 *Genetics* **192** 3–13

[38] Boscha F and Rosicha L 2008 The contributions of Paul Ehrlich to pharmacology: a tribute on the occasion of the centenary of his Nobel Prize *Pharmacology* **82** 171–9

[39] Kenney D E and Borisy G G 2009 Thomas Hunt Morgan at the Marine Biological Laboratory: naturalist and experimentalist *Genetics* **181** 841–6

[40] Roll-Hansen N 2014 Commentary: Wilhelm Johannsen and the problem of heredity at the turn of the 19th century *Int. J. Epidemiol.* **43** 1007–13

[41] Másová H 2008 Thomas Hunt Morgan (1866–1945) *Cas. Lek. Cesk.* **147** 72

[42] William D J and Bragg L 2008 Father and son: the most extraordinary collaboration in science *J. Clin. Invest.* **118** 2371

[43] Evans H M and Swezy O 1928 A sex difference in chromosome lengths in the mammalia *Genetics* **13** 532–43

[44] Crow J F 2006 H J Muller and the 'Competition Hoax' *Genetics* **173** 511–14

[45] Griffiths A J F 2000 *An Introduction to Genetic Analysis* 7th edn (New York: Freeman)

[46] Tan S Y and Tatsumura Y 2015 Alexander Fleming (1881–1955): discoverer of penicillin *Singap. Med. J.* **56** 366–7

[47] Harwood J 2009 Peasant friendly plant breeding and the early years of the green revolution in Mexico *Agric. Hist.* **83** 384–410

[48] Woodruff H B and Waksman S A 2014 Winner of the 1952 Nobel Prize for Physiology or Medicine *Appl. Environ. Microbiol.* **80** 282–8

[49] Ravindran S 2012 Barbara McClintock and the discovery of jumping genes *Proc. Natl Acad. Sci. USA* **109** 20198–9

[50] Manchester K L 2008 Historical opinion: Erwin Chargaff and his 'rules' for the base composition of DNA: why did he fail to see the possibility of complementarity? *Trends Biochem. Sci.* **33** 65–70

[51] Gey G O, Coffman W D and Kubicek M T 1952 Tissue culture studies of the proliferative capacity of cervical carcinoma and normal epithelium *Cancer Res.* **12** 264–5

[52] Crick F H 1970 Central dogma of molecular biology *Nature* **227** 561–3

[53] Lodish H 2000 *Molecular Cell Biology* 4th edn (New York: Freeman)

[54] Sulek K 1969 Nobel prize for J D Watson, F H C Crick and M H F Wilkins in 1962 for discoveries of the molecular structure and their role in the organism *Wiad Lek* **22** 695–7

[55] Baldwin R L 2008 Recollections of Arthur Kornberg (1918–2007) and the beginning of the Stanford Biochemistry Department *Protein Sci.* **17** 385–8

[56] Vogt P K 2010 Oncogenes and the revolution in cancer research: homage to Hidesaburo Hanafusa (1929–2009) *Genes Cancer* **1** 6–11

[57] Berg P and Mertz J E 2010 Personal reflections on the origins and emergence of recombinant DNA technology *Genetics* **184** 9–17

[58] Larsen C J 1989 The Nobel Prize in physiology and medicine 1989. J Michael Bishop and Harold E Varmus *Pathol. Biol.* **37** 1077–8

[59] Rosenberg N, Gelijns A C and Dawkins H 1995 *Sources of Medical Technology: Universities and Industry. Institute of Medicine (US) Committee on Technological Innovation in Medicine* (Washington DC: National Academies Press)

[60] Reh C S and Geffner M E 2010 Somatotropin in the treatment of growth hormone deficiency and Turner syndrome in pediatric patients: a review *Clin. Pharmacol.* **2** 111–22

[61] Garibyan L and Avashia N 2013 Research techniques made simple: polymerase chain reaction (PCR) *J. Invest. Dermatol.* **133** e6

[62] Resnik D B 2007 Embryonic stem cell patents and human dignity *Health Care Anal.* **15** 211–22

[63] Chan c c, Shen D and Tuo J 2005 Polymerase chain reaction in the diagnosis of uveitis *Int. Ophthalmol. Clin.* **45** 41–55

[64] Brejc K 1997 Structural basis for dual excitation and photoisomerization of the *Aequorea victoria* green fluorescent protein *Proc. Natl Acad. Sci. USA* **94** 2306–11

[65] Katz S L 2009 John F Enders and measles virus vaccine—a reminiscence *Curr. Top. Microbiol. Immunol* **329** 3–11

[66] Newman L 2005 Maurice Hilleman *Brit. Med. J.* **330** 1028

[67] Cohen S N, Chang A C Y, Boyer H W and Helling R B 1973 Construction of biologically functional bacterial plasmids *in vitro Proc. Natl Acad. Sci. USA* **70** 3240–4

[68] Sullivan M, Kaur K, Pauli N and Wilson P C 2011 Harnessing the immune system's arsenal: producing human monoclonal antibodies for therapeutics and investigating immune responses *F1000 Biol. Rep.* **3** 17

[69] Austrian R, Douglas R M, Schiffman G, Coetzee A M, Koornhof H J, Hayden-Smith S and Reid R D 1976 Prevention of pneumococcal pneumonia by vaccination *Trans. Assoc. Am. Physicians* **89** 184–94

[70] Blumberg B S, Millman I, Venkateswaran P S and Thyagarajan S P 1990 Hepatitis B virus and primary hepatocellular carcinoma: treatment of HBV carriers with *Phyllanthus amarus Vaccine* **8** S86–92

[71] Friboulet A, Izadyar L, Avalle B, Roseto A and Thomas D 1994 Abzyme generation using an anti-idiotypic antibody as the 'internal image' of an enzyme *Appl. Biochem. Biotechnol.* **47** 229–39

[72] Knott G J and Doudna J A 2018 CRISPR-Cas guides the future of genetic engineering *Science* **361** 866–9

[73] Khan S, Ullah M W, Siddique R, Nabi G, Manan S, Yousaf M and Hou H 2016 Role of recombinant DNA technology to improve life *Int. J. Genomics* **2016** 2405954
[74] Luetz S, Giver L and Lalonde J 2008 Engineered enzymes for chemical production *Biotechnol. Bioeng.* **101** 647–53
[75] Agapakis C M and Silver P A 2009 Synthetic biology: exploring and exploiting genetic modularity through the design of novel biological networks *Mol. Biosyst.* **5** 704–13
[76] Tang W L and Zhao H 2009 Industrial biotechnology: tools and applications *Biotechnol. J.* **4** 1725–39
[77] Ivanov V and Hung Y T 2010 Applications of environmental biotechnology *Environmental Biotechnology. Handbook of Environmental Engineering* (Springer) pp 1–7
[78] McCarty P L 2001 The development of anaerobic treatment and its future *Water Sci. Technol.* **44** 149–56
[79] Gupta A, Joia J, Sood A, Sood R, Sidhu C and Kaur G 2016 Microbes as potential tool for remediation of heavy metals: a review *J. Microb. Biochem. Technol.* **8** 364–72
[80] Reuschenbach P, Pagga U and Strotmann U 2003 A critical comparison of respirometric biodegradation tests based on OECD 301 and related test methods *Water Res.* **37** 1571–82
[81] Wieczorek A 2003 *Use of Biotechnology in Agriculture—Benefits and Risks* (Honolulu (HI): University of Hawaii) 6 (Biotechnology; BIO-3)
[82] Magar K T, Boafo G F, Li X, Chen Z and He W 2022 Liposome-based delivery of biological drugs *Chin. Chem. Lett.* **33** 587–96
[83] Carrel A 1924 Tissue culture and cell physiology *Physiol. Rev.* **4** 1–20
[84] Lanigan T M, Kopera H C and Saunders T L 2020 Principles of genetic engineering *Genes* **11** 291
[85] University of Utah n.d. What is Cloning https://learn.genetics.utah.edu/content/cloning/whatiscloning
[86] Welcsh P L and King M C 2001 BRCA1 and BRCA2 and the genetics of breast and ovarian cancer *Hum. Mol. Genet.* **10** 705–13
[87] Custers R, Bartsch D, Fladung M, Nilsson O, Pilate G, Sweet J and Boerjan W 2016 EU regulations impede market introduction of GM forest trees *Trends Plant Sci.* **21** 283–5
[88] Huang S, Lee A J, Tsoi R, Wu F, Zhang Y, Leong K W and You L 2016 Coupling spatial segregation with synthetic circuits to control bacterial survival *Mol. Syst. Biol.* **12** 859
[89] Golshadi M, Wright L K, Dickerson I M and Schrlau M G 2016 High-efficiency gene transfection of cells through carbon nanotube arrays *Small* **12** 3014–20
[90] Zaret K S 2016 The pioneer transcription factor foxa maintains an accessible nucleosome configuration at enhancers for tissue-specific gene activation *Mol. Cell.* **62** 79–91
[91] Petropoulos S 2016 Single-cell RNA-seq reveals lineage and X chromosome dynamics in human preimplantation embryos *Cell* **165** 1012–26
[92] Wenger Y, Buzgariu W and Galliot B 2015 Loss of neurogenesis in *Hydra* leads to compensatory regulation of neurogenic and neurotransmission genes in epithelial cells *Phil. Trans. R Soc.* **371** 0040
[93] Schaumberg K A 2015 Quantitative characterization of genetic parts and circuits for plant synthetic biology *Nat. Methods* **13** 94–100
[94] Myhrvold C, Kotula J W, Hicks W M, Conway N J and Silver P A 2015 A distributed cell division counter reveals growth dynamics in the gut microbiota *Nat. Commun.* **6** 10039
[95] Niopek D, Wehler P, Roensch J, Eils R and Ventura B D 2016 Optogenetic control of nuclear protein export *Nat. Commun.* **7** 10624

[96] Umeå University 2016 Cells from cow knee joints used to grow new cartilage tissue in laboratory *ScienceDaily* www.sciencedaily.com/releases/2016/01/160121093155.htm (accessed 21 January 2016)
[97] Polka J K and Silver P A 2016 A tunable protein piston that breaks membranes to release encapsulated cargo *ACS Synth. Biol.* **5** 303–11
[98] Ariyachet 2016 Reprogrammed stomach tissue as a renewable source of functional beta-cells for blood glucose regulation *Cell Stem Cell* **18** 410–21
[99] ResearchSEA 2016 Pros and cons of mandatory GMO labeling *ScienceDaily* www.sciencedaily.com/releases/2016/04/160401092125.htm (accessed 1 April 2016)
[100] Yoshimi K, Kunihiro Y, Kaneko T, Nagahora H, Voigt B and Mashimo T 2016 ssODN-mediated knock-in with CRISPR-Cas for large genomic regions in zygotes *Nat. Commun.* **7** 10431
[101] Nakagawa A, Matsumura E, Koyanagi T, Katayama T, Kawano N, Yoshimatsu K, Yamamoto K, Kumagai H, Sato F and Minami H 2016 Total biosynthesis of opiates by stepwise fermentation using engineered *Escherichia coli Nat. Commun.* **7** 10390
[102] Polka J K and Silver P A 2016 A tunable protein piston that breaks membranes to release encapsulated cargo *ACS Synth Biol.* **5** 303–11
[103] Rogers J K and Church G M 2016 Genetically encoded sensors enable real-time observation of metabolite production *Proc. Natl. Acad. Sci. U.S.A.* **113** 2388–93
[104] Durmaz E, Hu Y, Aroian R V and Klaenhammer T R 2015 Intracellular and extracellular expression of *Bacillus thuringiensis* crystal protein Cry5B in *Lactococcus lactis* for use as an anthelminthic *Appl. Environ. Microbiol.* **82** 1286–94
[105] European Commission, Joint Research Centre (JRC) 2015 DNA sequences in GMOs: largest database now publicly available *ScienceDaily* www.sciencedaily.com/releases/2015/11/151126104207.htm (accessed 1 July 2017)
[106] DiCarlo J E, Chavez A, Dietz S L, Esvelt K M and Church G M 2015 Safeguarding CRISPR-Cas9 gene drives in yeast *Nat. Biotechnol.* **33** 1250–5
[107] Labbadia J and Morimoto R I 2015 Repression of the heat shock response is a programmed event at the onset of reproduction *Mol. Cell* **59** 639–50
[108] Yang L 2015 Systems biology definition of the core proteome of metabolism and expression is consistent with high-throughput data *Proc. Natl. Acad. Sci. U.S.A.* **112** 10810–5
[109] Sokolik C 2015 Transcription factor competition allows embryonic stem cells to distinguish authentic signals from noise *Cell Syst.* **1** 117–29
[110] Hunter M V, Lee D M, Harris T J C and Fernandez-Gonzalez R 2015 Polarized E-cadherin endocytosis directs actomyosin remodeling during embryonic wound repair *J. Cell Biol.* **210** 801–16
[111] Li K T 2015 Increased bioavailable vitamin B6 in field-grown transgenic cassava for dietary sufficiency *Nat. Biotechnol.* **33** 1029
[112] Woo J W 2015 DNA-free genome editing in plants with preassembled CRISPR-Cas9 ribonucleoproteins *Nat. Biotechnol.* **33** 1162–4
[113] Beale K 2015 The CRISPR patent battle: who will be 'cut' out of patent rights to one of the greatest scientific discoveries of our generation? *Boston Coll. Intell. Prop. Technol. Forum* **2015** 1–24 https://lira.bc.edu/work/sc/c26e4d7a-f4d7-4bf3-918e-6875274d9fe5
[114] Bhardwaj A, Kishore S and Pandey D K 2022 Artificial intelligence in biological sciences *Life* **12** 1430

[115] Vaish S, Agarwal A and Raheja R 2022 Role of artificial intelligence in biotechnology *Int. Res. J. Modern. Eng. Technol. Sci.* **4** 670–4
[116] Holzinger A, Keiblinger K, Holub P, Zatloukal K and Müller H 2023 AI for life: trends in artificial intelligence for biotechnology *New Biotechnol.* **74** 16–24
[117] Polat H, Topalcengiz Z and Danyluk M D 2020 Prediction of *Salmonella* presence and absence in agricultural surface waters by artificial intelligence approaches *J. Food Saf.* **40** e12733
[118] Liu L W, Lu C T, Wang Y M, Lin K H, Ma X and Lin W S 2022 Rice (*Oryza sativa* L.) growth modeling based on growth degree day (GDD) and artificial intelligence algorithms *Agriculture.* **12** 59
[119] Shadrin D, Menshchikov A, Somov A, Bornemann G, Hauslage J and Fedorov M 2019 Enabling precision agriculture through embedded sensing with artificial intelligence *IEEE Trans. Instrum. Meas.* **69** 4103–13
[120] Lee J, Nazki H, Baek J, Hong Y and Lee M 2020 Artificial intelligence approach for tomato detection and mass estimation in precision agriculture *Sustainability.* **12** 9138
[121] Partel V, Costa L and Ampatzidis Y 2021 Smart tree crop sprayer utilizing sensor fusion and artificial intelligence *Comput. Electron. Agric.* **191** 106556
[122] Schmidt-Erfurth U, Waldstein S M, Klimscha S, Sadeghipour A, Hu X, Gerendas B S, Osborne A and Bogunović H 2018 Prediction of individual disease conversion in early AMD using artificial intelligence *Invest. Ophthalmol. Vis. Sci.* **59** 3199–208
[123] Schork N J 2019 Artificial intelligence and personalized medicine *Cancer Treat. Res.* **178** 265–83
[124] El-Sappagh S, Alonso J M, Islam S R, Sultan A M and Kwak K S 2021 A multilayer multimodal detection and prediction model based on explainable artificial intelligence for Alzheimer's disease *Sci. Rep.* **11** 2660
[125] Jiang X *et al* 2020 Towards an artificial intelligence framework for data-driven prediction of coronavirus clinical severity *Comput. Mater. Continua* **63** 537–51
[126] Enshaei A, Robson C N and Edmondson R J 2015 Artificial intelligence systems as prognostic and predictive tools in ovarian cancer *Ann. Surg. Oncol.* **22** 3970–5
[127] Baldwin D R *et al* 2020 External validation of a convolutional neural network artificial intelligence tool to predict malignancy in pulmonary nodules *Thorax.* **75** 306–12
[128] Hu H, Wang H, Wang F, Langley D, Avram A and Liu M 2018 Prediction of influenza-like illness based on the improved artificial tree algorithm and artificial neural network *Sci. Rep.* **8** 4895
[129] Pun F W, Ozerov I V and Zhavoronkov A 2023 AI-powered therapeutic target discovery *Trends Pharmacol. Sci.* **44** P561–72
[131] Ramirez-Estrada K, Vidal-Limon H, Hidalgo D, Moyano E, Golenioswki M, Cusidó R M and Palazon J 2016 Elicitation, an effective strategy for the biotechnological production of bioactive high-added value compounds in plant cell factories *Molecules* **21** 182

Chapter 2

Modern DNA science and its applications

Vijayshree S Karankar, Sayani Saha, Reetika Tandon and Nidhi Srivastava

2.1 Introduction

Deoxyribonucleic acid, more often known as DNA, is a multifarious molecule that comprises all of the information required to create and conserve an organism. All living organisms contain DNA within their cells; as a matter of fact, almost every cell in a multicellular biological organism has the whole set of DNA required for that organism. Nevertheless, DNA does more than controlling the structure and purpose of biological components. It also offers the primary unit of heredity in organisms of all kinds. In other words, when organisms replicate, a fragment of their DNA is transferred to their offspring. This genetic communication of the entirety or a fragment of an organism's DNA facilitates a certain level of stability from one generation to another. The evitable nature of base paring based in the Watson–Crick model of DNA allows us to genetically modify it with ease [1]. However, it still allows for minor alterations that add to the variety of life. So, what exactly is DNA, what minor components make up this multifaceted molecule, how are these elements organized and how is information extracted from them? This chapter answers each of these questions and provides other critical information related to DNA science, and it also offers an important plan for the path to DNA invention.

2.1.1 Genes: units of inheritance

The gene is the basic unit of inheritance, establishing the elementary physical and functional units of heredity. Genes encompass information as messages that are represented by nucleic acid base pair sequences or codons. Further, these codons are well organized in the form of DNA, and act as directives to create molecules known as acting proteins in the form of enzymes. British biologist Richard Dawkins, in his famous book *The Selfish Gene* (1989), explained that 'They are in you and me; they created us, body and mind; and their preservation is the ultimate rationale for our

doi:10.1088/978-0-7503-5382-3ch2

existence … they go by the name of genes, and we are their survival machines' [2]. Thus, the precise definition of genes usually overlays molecular genetics onto Mendelism. The study of genetics has seen persistent growth and has explored several modern concepts which determinedly aim to honor the gene as a 'unit' of structure and/or function, language that offers multiple meanings for the term but fails to recognize the diversity of gene architecture. Generally, any biological organism genotype comprises a set of units of inheritance called genes which functions by storing and expressing the genetic information encrypted within its DNA as messages. DNA is a systematically structured biologically active element that not only stores genetic information, but also expresses it by transmitting the message or instructing essential proteins to initiate biological responses. So, DNA is a multifarious organic chemical that conveys genetic information and forms the chromosomes existing in the nucleus of most cells. The gene is an element of inheritance, and different forms of similar genes are called alleles. Generally, alleles are established as pairs of genes that appear at a specific site on a particular chromosome and regulate similar characteristics, e.g. blood type or color blindness. Alleles are also known as allelomorphs. Certain genes have a variety of different forms, which are sited at the same position (or genetic locus) on a chromosome. Higher animals are diploid organisms as their genetic make-up encompasses two alleles at each genetic locus, with one allele inherited from each parent. Both pairs of alleles link to the genotype of a specific gene. Genetic construction is based on the resemblance and the variance between two alleles, e.g. in homozygous genotypes there are two of the same allele at a specific locus and in heterozygous genotypes the two alleles vary. Phenotypic features, or the external appearance of the organism, are always contributed to by alleles, depending upon their dominant or recessive features; an organism is heterozygous at a precise locus and transmits one dominant and one recessive allele. In such cases the creature will express the dominant phenotype; nonetheless, alleles can also contribute to minor DNA sequence alterations between alleles that do not fundamentally affect the gene's phenotype. In cases where one of the alleles is dominant and the other allele is recessive, the phenotype of the heterozygous organism is denoted by the dominant allele. Phenotype in heterozygous organisms is governed by the interaction of two alleles. DNA structures the genetic material for most biological organisms; nevertheless, the genetic material of some viruses is ribonucleic acid (RNA). In such viruses the RNA is transformed into DNA copies within a multiple infected cell, so it could be assumed that the majority of genes are demarcated as messages or code 'transcribed' in DNA. DNA in the form of X-shaped chromosomes is present in the nucleus of most cells. Long strands of DNA act as the building blocks for chromosomes. These chromosomes are twisted in a rope-like manner and transmit the genetic information for creating a specific protein called a gene (figure 2.1). The gene, or 'unit of inheritance', is present in numbers of several thousands in all chromosomes. These elements of inheritance are responsible for the transformation of inherited features from one generation to another. Human beings receive particular chromosomes from the egg of the mother and sperm of the father. These inborn chromosomes transmit genetic code that regulates our phenotype or physical characteristics, which are a mixture of those of our two parents. Genes operate by base pair expression present in the DNA, which conveys the different codes essential for different amino acids. The code for a

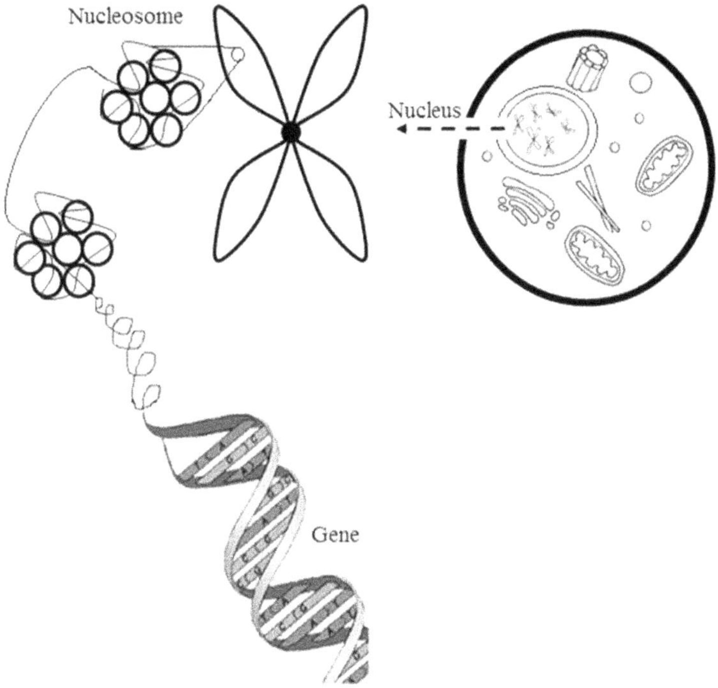

Figure 2.1. Nucleus, chromosome and gene.

specific amino acid is prepared from three bases in a particular arrangement. The principle of inheritance states that you inherit one allele for each gene from your father and one allele for each gene from your mother, e.g. the gene for eye color has alleles for blue eye color and alleles for brown eye color. That is, the expression of a trait (e.g. eye color) will depend on the combination of alleles you have inherited from your parents.

A biological organism's phenotype refers to the recognizable characteristics of that organism. This originates from the interaction of the organism's genes with the surrounding environment. Genes are very stable in their role, otherwise it would not be possible for genetic information to be passed accurately from generation to generation. Genetic stability is not absolute, however, and erratic modifications in genetic architecture cause drastic alterations in the function of genes, which is called mutation. After modification, mutant genes also develop into stable units and are inherited in the same way as normal, wild-type genes. Phenotypic alterations in the organism occasionally direct the occurrence of a mutation. Several human disorders are triggered by single mutations in a single gene. However, some mutations do not alter the function of the protein made by the gene. Different phenotypic features are regulated by more than one gene or set of genes.

2.2 The human genome project

The Human Genome Project (HGP) was launched at the end of the 20th century. Twenty years ago, the White House hosted a momentous event where the world witnessed the simultaneous release of the initial human genome sequences. The groundbreaking findings emerged from two distinct sources: the publicly funded International Human Genome Project (HGP) Consortium and Celera Genomics. Subsequently, the results were published in prestigious scientific journals, with *Nature* and *Science* carrying the respective publications. Although the analyses conducted at that time may seem rudimentary when compared to today's advanced standards, they marked a pivotal moment in scientific history, offering thrilling initial insights into the complete human genome. The announcement was celebrated as 'the conclusion of the initial phase' and a catalyst for a fresh era of discovery. Fast forward two decades, and it is evident that the ambitious goals of the Human Genome Project (HGP) have undeniably been achieved. In fact, the idea of not having ready access to the human genome today is as inconceivable as living without computers or the internet, highlighting the transformative impact of this monumental endeavor. Skeptics point to the HGP's inability to fulfill the most extravagant expectations as evidence that it has fallen short of its grandiose promises. In its initial conception, the project held more realistic expectations, focusing on the potential advantages of a comprehensive cancer genome, advancements in genetics, and the refinement of technological capabilities [3]. The shift in rhetoric towards grandiose claims of revolutionizing biology, biotechnology, drug development, and society did not occur until closer to the launch of the program in 1990 and at various significant points during its progression. Human genetic make-up differs in size from a few hundred DNA bases to more than two million bases. As discussed in the previous chapter, the genetic material in a living organism is called its genome. Owing to several biotic and abiotic features this genetic material is affected and displays dissimilarity/variation, sometimes manifested in the form of a syndrome or sometimes appearing to have no effect. The HGP projected that humans carry between 20 000 and 25 000 genes. It was very ambitious and had several objectives, including:

- To identify genetic variation by recognizing the sequences of defective and altered genes.
- To explore quicker methodologies for sequencing DNA.
- To develop the order or sequence of all the three billion base pairs in the human genome.
- Identification of all the genes.

The sequencing assignment was accomplished in 2001, and the effort continues to identify all the genes in the human genome. The HGP used the DNA of some people to obtain an approximately average sequence, although each individual has a unique sequence (unless they have an identical twin).

2.3 DNA synthesis begins at replication origins

As stated above, the DNA double-helix molecule is usually very stable. Eukaryotic cell DNA replication necessitates the precise generation of substantial DNA quantities. Furthermore, for the development of an adult organism from a single fertilized oocyte, the DNA must undergo multiple rounds of replication, resulting in the creation of the approximately 4×10^{13} DNA copies that constitute the human body. Mistakes in DNA replication can undergo amplification and accumulate gradually, resulting in genome instability. This instability has adverse repercussions for organs and tissues and is a defining characteristic of cancer. Eukaryotic cells have evolved multiple mechanisms to safeguard genome stability, and one of these mechanisms involves maintaining the accuracy of DNA replication at replication forks. It is now well-established that the regulation of DNA replication origin activation plays a pivotal role in allowing eukaryotic cells to respond to their surroundings, adapt to tissue-specific transcriptional programs, and address the challenges posed by the intricate structures and diverse conformations of chromosomes. Both DNA strands are sealed together tightly by various hydrogen bonds formed between the bases on each strand. The double-helix structure must first be unzipped or opened up by unraveling the two strands separately to reveal unpaired bases. This is accomplished to discover the structural features of the DNA template. The process of DNA replication is activated by distinctive initiator proteins that bind to double-stranded DNA (dsDNA) and pry the two strands apart by splitting the hydrogen bonds between the bases. The junctions at which the DNA helix is first unzipped are known as the replication origins (figure 2.2). In prokaryotic organisms such as bacteria, the origins of replication are stated by DNA sequences which are usually several hundred nucleotide pairs in length. This type of DNA configuration contains short sequences that entice initiator proteins and sections of DNA that are mainly easy to expose. As illustrated in figure 2.2, the A-T base pair is held together by fewer hydrogen bonds than the G-C base pair. Therefore, DNA rich in A-T base pairs is relatively easy to separate, and sections of DNA enhanced in A-T pairs are typically found at replication origins.

Figure 2.2 shows the most essential steps involved in the origination of replication forks at replication origins. DNA configuration formed at the last step, in which both strands of the parental DNA helix have been detached from each other and function as templates for DNA production, is known as the replication bubble.

2.4 Gene expression

2.4.1 One gene, one product

In 1908 Sir Archibald Garrod [4] suggested that certain human ailments were owing to 'inherited errors of metabolism'. Additionally, he demonstrated that these errors are caused by the absence of specific enzyme to execute a specific biochemical reaction. This kind of defect in genetic expression resulted in enzyme dysfunction which results in metabolic syndrome followed by any specific disease. Thus, according to this theory, inheritance of a faulty gene is responsible for flaws in offspring by dominant interference in its phenotypic traits. After Garrod's claims, in 1941 Beadle and Tatum [5] stated interrelated work on fungus *Neurospora*. In this investigation they exposed *Neurospora* to x-rays to induce mutations that usually would have been lethal. This x-ray induced mutation enabled them to recognize *Neurospora* cells that would only propagate when the development medium was added with vitamin B6 synthesis. This investigation showed that a specific gene

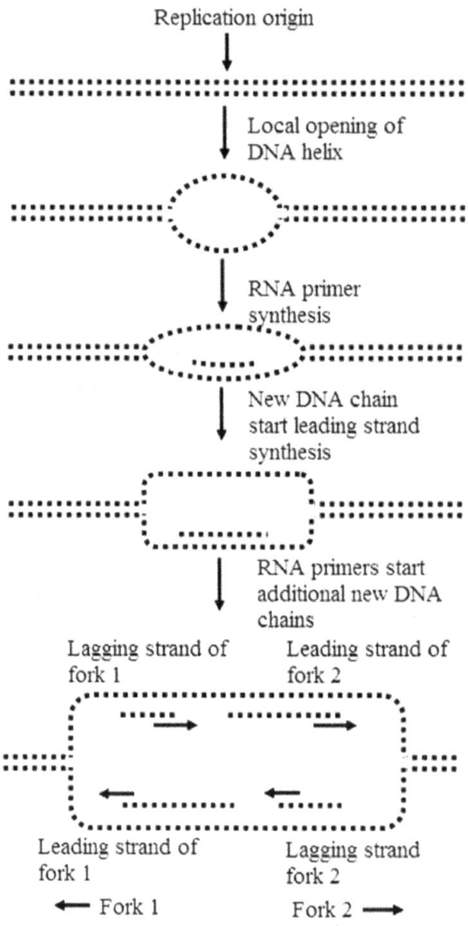

Figure 2.2. A replication bubble formed by replication fork initiation.

coded for the production of one enzyme, which undoubtedly established the 'one gene, one enzyme' theory [6]. Later various genetic and biochemical information was acquired in its support, and the theory was subsequently changed to 'one gene, one protein' [7]. Later the 'one gene, one protein' hypothesis was again reformed when it was demonstrated that various proteins consist of two or more separate polypeptide chains that are encoded by different genes. Next to this theory a more accurate description of the association between a gene and its product was developed: 'one gene, one polypeptide'. Still this description is not entirely correct since not all genes encode proteins, e.g. some translate polynucleotide RNA species such as transfer RNA and ribosomal RNA. Eventually the most stringently precise expression was proven to be 'one gene, one product'. This innovation of the relationship between gene and gene product recognized the key connection between conventional genetics and biochemistry. This was a sensational time in biochemistry as metabolism could now be acknowledged as the most likely tool of genetics.

2.4.2 Genetic regulation of worldwide gene expression

Even over a century following the rediscovery of Mendel's work, the genetic foundations of complex and quantitative traits continue to elude easy categorization. Fundamental questions persist without clear answers, such as how many genetic loci contribute to variations in inheritable characteristics, the range of their impact, their molecular properties, modes of operation, interplay, and their reliance on environmental factors. These inquiries lie at the heart of crucial concerns in the fields of medical and agricultural genetics, as well as in fundamental evolutionary biology. A prominent unresolved issue in the latter pertains to the factors responsible for generating, preserving, and organizing inheritable variations in phenotypes. Currently, a burgeoning method known as genetic mapping of genome-wide gene expression is gradually furnishing the essential empirical data necessary to address these inquiries. Since the inception of the first empirical linkage study on global transcript levels in 2002 [8], numerous fundamental principles have been established, providing a robust foundation upon which further research can be constructed. While small-scale investigations into the genetics of gene expression have a lengthy and storied history, the advent of modern large-scale studies can be largely attributed to the emergence of microarray technology in the mid-1990s. In the year 2000, microarrays were initially utilized to explore genetic variation. These groundbreaking studies unveiled distinctions in gene expression among different strains in both yeast and mice [9, 10] demonstrating that such disparities are inherited in genetic crosses [11, 12]. Following investigations provided substantial evidence of inheritable variations in gene expression in both *Drosophila melanogaster* [13] and killifish [14]. At the point when Jansen and Nap [15] put forth the concept of genetic mapping for genome-wide gene expression, numerous research groups had already made significant progress in this area. The first empirical study mapping global gene expression in yeast cross was published shortly thereafter, early the following year.

2.5 Structure of DNA

Many people are not aware of the true story of DNA as they still think that James Watson (an American biologist) and Francis Crick (an English physicist) discovered DNA in the 1950s. However, this is not the case. Rather, DNA was first discovered in the late 1860s by Friedrich Miescher (a Swiss chemist). Then, subsequent to Miescher's discovery, the investigators Phoebus Levene and Erwin Chargaff undertook a series of studies that exposed further information about the DNA molecule, comprising its primary chemical components, their organization and the ways in which they linked together. Without the scientific efforts contributed by these investigators, Watson and Crick may never have accomplished their revolutionary breakthrough in 1953 that led to their announcement 'that the DNA molecule exists in the form of a 3D double helix' [16, 17].

DNA is a molecule that encloses hidden information in the form of the essential instructions for an organism to develop, live and reproduce (figure 2.3). These

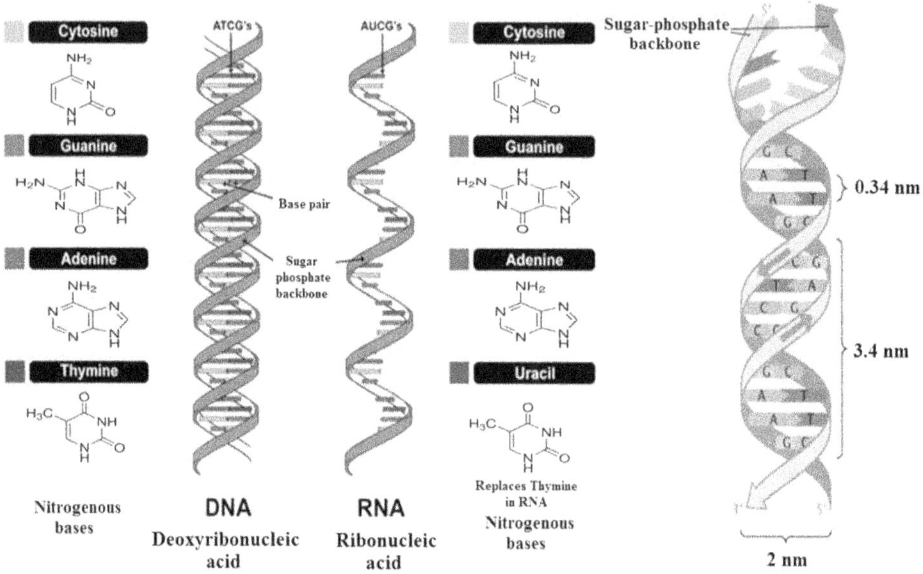

Figure 2.3. The double helical structure of DNA.

hidden codes or instructions are present inside every cell and are transferred from one generation to another.

DNA is made up of fragments called nucleotides. The building blocks of nucleotides are a phosphate group, a sugar group and a nitrogen base. The four basic types of nitrogen bases are adenine (A), guanine (G), thymine (T) and cytosine (C). The order or arrangement of these bases controls the DNA's instructions, or genetic code. The systematic organization of these alphabets present in the nucleotides forms genes, in a similar fashion to the arrangement of the letters of the alphabet can be utilized to form a word. Then the words assemble to form a sentence and are considered to take the form of language; correspondingly, the arrangement of nitrogen bases in a DNA sequence forms genes. This language of the cell directs cells in how to manufacture proteins. DNA transmits genetic information to another type of nucleic acid known as RNA to synthesize essential proteins. These proteins are called acting proteins, since they are active biomolecules (such as enzymes) essential for commencing any specific biochemical reaction. Once RNA converts the genetic information from DNA into proteins, essential proteins are produced to either initiate or regulate any biological reaction, or sometimes these proteins abort biological reactions. Nearly 3 billion bases and around 20 000 genes exist in the entire human genome. In DNA, nucleotides are well organized and connected together to form two long strands that are coiled to produce a biological structure called a double-helix 3D structure. If you imagine this double-helix configuration as a ladder, the bases would be the steps and the phosphate and sugar molecules would be the edges. Bases form the links between two discrete strands. These bases on one strand connect with the bases on another strand, i.e. adenine pairs with thymine, and guanine pairs with cytosine. The double-helix configuration of DNA fragments is very lengthy, so lengthy that they cannot even fit conveniently into cells without the right packing. Thus, to appropriately fit this long double-helix chain inside a cell, DNA is tightly packed and twisted firmly to form structures known as chromosomes. Every chromosome is made up of a single DNA molecule and there are 23 pairs of chromosomes found inside the human cell nucleus. DNA is conformationally not a homogenous molecule, it tends to change its structure based on conditions, functions. Some of the unusual structures of DNA are left-handed Z and recently reviewed P DNA. Of the different conformations of DNA, it is believed that B-DNA is one of the most stable forms and tends to be stable in living cells within the environmental conditions. Gene regulation is the result of interaction of DNA with other biological regulatory proteins. In comprehension to the molecular details it is important to understand the DNA–protein interactions to understand the normal and diseased states.

2.6 DNA replication

In 1993, Nobel laureate Kary Mullis described the procedure of replication of DNA [18]. Correct genetic transformation of information inherited from generation to generation facilitates correct copying of the DNA nucleotide sequence from the original parenteral DNA molecule to two daughter molecules. Secret evidence for this copying lies in the double helical structure of DNA molecules. In the double-helix configuration of DNA, two free stands are held together by hydrogen bonding and their separation can be readily achieved for the production of complimentary strands. Replication involves movement of the replication fork along the parental DNA, so that there is continuous denaturation of the parental strands and formation of daughter duplication. The synthesis of DNA is aided by specific enzymes (DNA polymerases) that recognize the template strand and catalyze the addition of nucleotide subunits to the polynucleotide chain that is being synthesized. Once strands are separated, each strand functions as a template for the creation of a complimentary copy to form two similar daughter duplex molecules. Therefore, these two molecules are developed from the original DNA duplex in the replication process. During this process one strand of a daughter molecule has been freshly synthesized while the other strand is preserved from the original parenteral duplex. This kind of replication is thus called semi-conservative; nevertheless, semi-conservative replication encompasses strand separation, the interference of the double helical structure occurs only momentarily and only a small portion of a chromosome is single-stranded at any specific time. The replicated region appears as a replication bubble when viewed under an electron microscope within the non-replicated DNA. The great intricacy of DNA replication at the molecular level includes the management and involvement of many proteins with several enzymatic processes. The following steps are involved in this process (figure 2.4).

- The first stage in DNA replication is to 'unzip' the double-helix structure of the DNA molecule.
- The uncoiling process is carried out by an enzyme known as *helicase.* This enzyme disrupts the hydrogen bonds holding the complementary bases of DNA together (A with T, C with G).

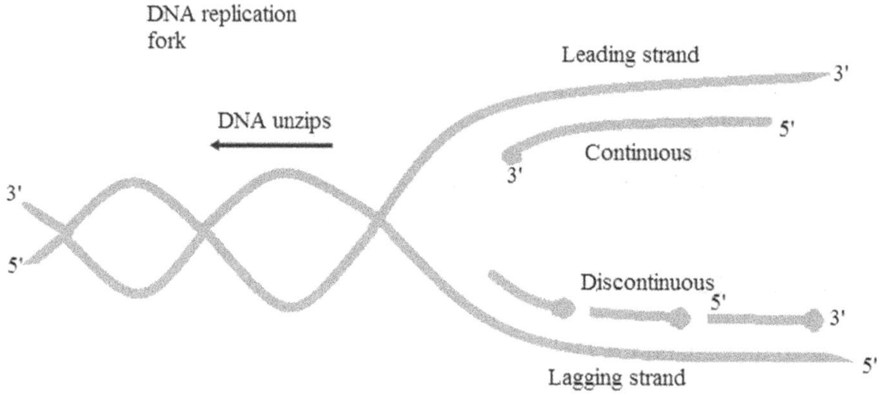

Figure 2.4. An illustration of the replication of the leading and lagging strands of DNA.

- Uncoiling of the DNA is further progressed by the separation of the two single strands of DNA to form the 'Y' shape known as the replication 'fork', which facilitates the production of new strands from DNA templates (two separated strands).
- In the replication process one of the strands is leaning in the 3′–5′ direction (towards the replication fork); this is called the leading strand. The other strand is leaning in the 5′–3′ direction (away from the replication fork); this strand is known as the lagging strand. Conferring to their different placements, the two strands are replicated inversely.
- Different activities are involved in the stages of initiation, elongation, and termination. Before initiation can occur, however, the supercoiled chromosome must be relaxed.
- Initiation involves recognition of an origin by a complex of proteins. Before DNA synthesis begins, the parental strands must be separated and stabilized in the single-stranded state, creating a replication bubble.
- Elongation is undertaken by another complex of proteins. The replisome exists only as a protein complex associated with the particular structure that DNA takes at the replication fork. It does not exist as an independent unit, but assembles *de novo* at the origin of each replication cycle. As the replisome moves ahead, the parental strands unwind and synthesize daughter strands.
- At the end of termination process, the duplicate chromosomes must be separated from one other, which requires a higher order complex DNA structure formation.

2.6.1 Leading strand

At the end of the leading strand, a short piece of RNA known as the primer (the primer functions as the initial point for DNA production) comes along and binds. This primer is synthesized by an enzyme known as primase. Once the enzyme adds the RNA primer to the 3′ end of the leading strand, DNA synthesis continues from the 3′–5′ direction in respect to the lagging strand behind without interruption.

Later, an enzyme known as DNA polymerase ε attaches to the leading strand and then 'walks' along it. During its steering movement through the template, DNA polymerase supplements new complementary nucleotide bases (A, C, G and T) to the strand of DNA in the 5′–3′ direction. This sort of replication is known as 'continuous'.

2.6.2 Lagging strand

In this strand, the primase enzyme produces several RNA primers and fixes at different points along the lagging strand.

Pieces of DNA called Okazaki fragments are then added to the lagging strand, also in the 5′–3′ direction. This kind of replication is called 'discontinuous' as the Okazaki fragments will need to be attached later.

At the end of these Okazaki fragments, DNA polymerase runs through the 5′ of the previous fragments that contains RNA primer with a small segment of DNA attached to it. This results in production of RNA–DNA single-strand flap, that must be cleaved using DNA ligase-I.

2.7 DNA supercoiling

DNA supercoiling is defined as the over- or underwinding of a DNA strand and is an expression of the strain on that strand. Supercoiling is significant in a number of natural processes, for example compacting DNA, and by regulating access to the genetic code. DNA supercoiling intensely influences DNA metabolism and perhaps gene expression. Moreover, certain enzymes such as topoisomerases are able to alter DNA topology to allow functions such as DNA replication or transcription [19]. Mathematical languages are employed to define supercoiling by relating different coiled states to relaxed B-form DNA. The noun form 'supercoil' is frequently used in the context of DNA topology.

Most DNA fragments do not have free/open ends, however; they exist as closed (circular) structures under *in vivo* conditions. The winding of a circular DNA duplex about its axis promotes supercoiling in the DNA, in the same manner as when a rubber band is twisted. The number of times one strand is linked with another strand is described as a fundamental property of DNA fragment called linking number. Linking number is defined as the sum of twists (rotation of strands along one another) and writhes (measures the path of helix within the space of the strands) with the two complementary strands. When the reverse forces are utilized to coil DNA, it results in negative supercoils which allows the DNA molecule to minimize the twisting force by slackening the twisting of the two strands around each other. Only a closed circular structure encourages super winding, and the higher the number of supercoils the more the twisting in the closed duplex. As the DNA molecule cannot form a supercoil if one or both strands are wrecked, if this happens, the DNA supercoil unwinds to a relaxed form. Therefore, super winding is categorized in two different ways: as negative and positive supercoils. Positive supercoils coil the DNA in the same direction as the right-handed helix, while negative supercoils coil the DNA about its axis differing from the direction of the turn's right-handed helix. It is believed that only negative supercoiled DNA exists *in vivo*, however positively supercoiled DNA may be produced *in vitro*. Negative supercoils encourage resident relaxing of the DNA, allowing genetic processes such as transcription, DNA replication and recombination to happen. In addition, negative super twisting also promotes development and controls the interactions of the DNA-binding proteins involved in gene regulation.

Topoisomerases are the enzymes maximally found in all the replicating cells, which regulates the DNA supercoiling. They alter the DNA structure by creating a transient break in the sugar phosphate backbone. DNA topoisomerase type-1 is the main class of topoisomerase enzyme that is mainly responsible for creating single-stranded transient breaks within the strands of the DNA. Within them there are two subclasses, topoisomerase IA and topoisomerase IB, which utilize different mechanisms to alter the super helical structure of DNA. Type II topoisomerase acts by creating double-strand breaks in the structure of DNA through which it passes as a sperate intact double helix. DNA gyrase and topoisomerase II are the two different enzymes that are produced by the type 2 class. Most of the type 2 class enzymes act on both positive and negative supercoiling. Among all the topoisomerases, DNA gyrase is a unique enzyme that negatively coils the DNA helix. Type II enzymes not only remove the supercoils but also topological structures such as knots and tangles. In comparison to negative supercoiling, positive supercoiling makes it harder to pull the double helical structure and sometimes it also regulates the normal cellular functions. Because of this underwinding or overwinding, DNA experiences the torsion force. Underwinding coiling is responsible for negative supercoiling in which a smaller number of base pairs are twisted per helix, while overwinding includes positive supercoiling in which a greater number of base pairs are involved per helix. DNA globally from all species of bacteria and eubacteria underwinds to about ~6% and this plays a significant role in the function of double strands. And in order to replicate and transcribe, two strands of double helix must be separated, which also includes supercoiling of strands. Negative supercoiling includes more energy compared to positive supercoiling, which makes it underwind through the length of the double strand, thus it increases the rate of replication and transcription.

Supercoiling mainly plays a role in DNA packaging within the cells, as the length of genetic material is larger in size to fit within the cell it would be a difficult feat. Supercoiling exits on various levels such as solenoid supercoiling, plectonemic supercoiling. Of these, solenoid supercoiling provides the most effective DNA packaging. Solenoid supercoiling includes a 30 nm fiber densely packed chromatin coiled upon itself several times. Packaging increases the nuclear divisions during several stages of the cell cycle (i.e., mitosis and meiosis). Some special proteins such as condensins and cohesins are important as structural maintaince of chromosomes (SMC) proteins, and are involved in the condensation of sister chromatids and conjoining of the centromeres within the sister chromatids. They are mainly responsible for positive supercoiling in the double-stranded DNA. Supercoiling is also important in the synthesis of nucleic acids (DNA and RNA), as unwinding of DNA is mainly required during the RNA or DNA polymerization action. This creates a stress during unwinding and involves positive supercoiling of double strands. It is also important to note that Topoisomerase II (DNA Gyrase) causes rewinded and generates stress during DNA and RNA synthesis.

2.8 Repair and recombination

As DNA is the storeroom of genetic information in each living cell, its reliability and stability are vital to life. DNA is not an inactive fragment; rather, it is a vigorous chemical unit vulnerable to attack from the environment. Thus, any injury, if not healed, can result in mutation and probably disease [20]. Environmentally stimulated skin cancer after extreme exposure to UV radiation in the form of sunlight is perhaps the best-known instance of the connection between environmentally stimulated DNA damage and disease. Numerous environmental factors are known to encourage mutation or sometimes act as mutants themselves, such as the fact that tobacco smoking can result in mutations in lung cells and then cancer of the lung. In addition to being affected by environmental factors, DNA is also vulnerable to oxidative injury from byproducts of metabolism, e.g. free radicals. In fact, it has been shown that a human cell can experience up to one million DNA changes per day [21]. In addition, it is also evidenced that each of the $\sim 10^{13}$ cells within the human body experiences tens of thousands of DNA-injuring events per day [22]. Human body cells are constantly exposed to attacks from endogenous and exogenous agents which can cause injury to our DNA and cause genomic variability. Most of this damage affects the structural features of DNA and can alter or stop basic cellular processes, e.g. DNA transcription or replication. DNA damage usually comprises base and sugar alterations, DNA–protein cross-links, double-strand breaks and base-free sites. Cells have their own specialized DNA repair systems to neutralize the effects of DNA damage. This DNA restoration system can be subcategorized into different mechanisms based on the type of DNA injury. These repair-based procedures include mismatch repair, base excision repair (BER), nucleotide excision repair (NER) and double-strand break repair. These procedures encompass both homologous recombination (HR) and non-homologous end-joining (NHEJ). Both prokaryotic and eukaryotic organisms have DNA repair mechanisms controlled by different biological proteins and many of the proteins involved have been exceptionally conserved during growth.

Cellular systems employ various mechanisms to identify and repair the different types of injury that can occur to DNA. These cellular mechanisms capably recognize injury produced by the environment or by faults in replication. DNA molecules play a dynamic and vital role in cell division. DNA controls these cellular mechanics stimulated biological responses to regulate DNA repair, which is closely tied to regulation of the cell cycle. During the cell cycle, checkpoint machinery assures that a cell's DNA is safe before permitting DNA replication and cell division to take place. Errors in this checkpoint machinery can lead to accumulation of damage, which may further result in mutations. Lack of DNA repair encourages several human genetic diseases that affect a wide variety of body systems, but have an assembly of common traits, particularly an inclination to cancer [23]. These ailments include xeroderma pigmentosum (XP), a disorder defined by sensitivity to sunlight and associated to a fault in an important ultraviolet injury repair pathway, and ataxia-telangiectasia, a progressive motor disorder caused by incapability to repair oxidative damage in the cerebellum. In addition, various genes that have been involved in cancer, e.g. the restriction-associated DNA (RAD) group, have also been examined to encode proteins critical for DNA damage repair.

Current research. The 2015 Nobel Prize in Chemistry was awarded to Tomas Lindahl, Paul Modrich and Aziz Sancar 'for mechanistic studies of DNA repair'. Lindahl presented that DNA is inherently unstable and involves active repair, and recognized the function of DNA glycosylase enzymes in base excision repair. Modrich was influential in understanding a process called mismatch repair that is involved in repairing errors caused by the DNA replication machinery, and Sancar established biochemically how enzymes repair damage to DNA from ultraviolet rays, by a process called nucleotide excision repair.

2.9 Types of DNA damage

DNA is a genetic chemical/molecule which regulates several biological reactions, like any other biomolecule. There are different *in vivo* and *in vitro* intrinsic or extrinsic agents that may cause injury to DNA. Generally, most of the DNA alterations are endogenous in origin and the simplest form of endogenous DNA injury is impulsive hydrolysis [24]. DNA is also susceptible to different chemical alterations by reactive molecules produced through the redox mechanism or normal cellular metabolism. Most of these reactive molecules are reactive oxygen species which include O^{2-}, H_2O_2 and •OH and are responsible for advanced aging in human beings [25, 26]. These reactive oxygen species are involved in the usual aging process via extreme production of intrinsic/extrinsic stress-causing agents. This produces a large amount of reactive oxygen species which may form the basis of severe injury to biological tissue, instigating inflammation at the initial stages, and finally may result in cancer or other disorders. These reactive oxygen species generate more than 100 diverse oxidative DNA adducts in the form of deoxyribose oxidation, single- or double-strand damage, base alteration and DNA-protein cross-links [27].

Correspondingly reactive oxygen species generate endogenous reactive nitrogen species, chiefly nitric oxide (NO•) and its end-products, and can also produce similar oxidative adducts [28]. Sometimes noticeable errors caused by biological DNA processing reactions can result in endogenous genomic injury, for instance as a consequence of misincorporation of base pairs by replicative DNA polymerases, DNA mismatches comprising insertions and deletions are sometimes presented at a frequency of 10^{-4}–10^{-6} [29]. In addition to several endogenous sources of DNA injury, cellular DNA is also under consistent attack from exogenous or environmental DNA-damaging agents. These surrounding DNA-damaging agents comprise physical stresses, mainly radiation, e.g. ultraviolet light or x-rays. Ultraviolet light from the Sun mainly acts as a source of two types of DNA injuries, namely 6–4 pyrimidone and cyclobutane pyrimidine dimers photoproducts. Each of them involves various covalent bonds between neighboring pyrimidine bases [30].

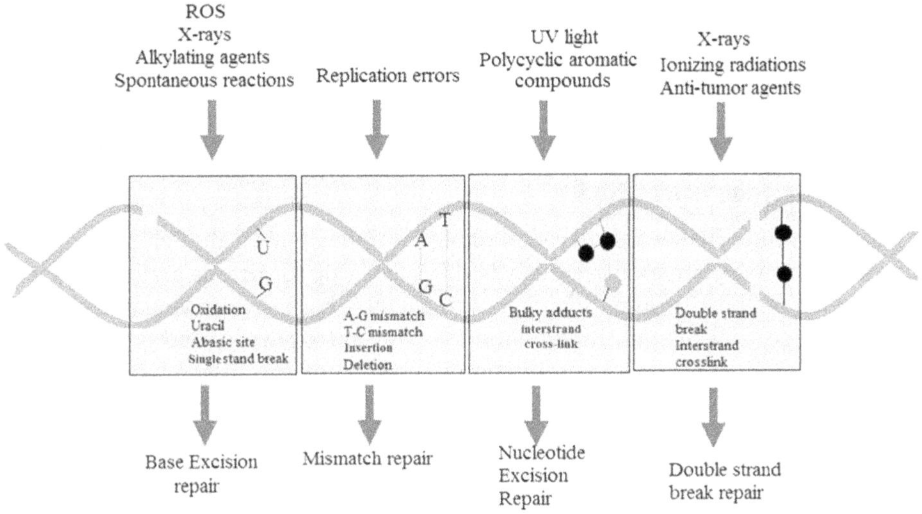

Figure 2.5. Various types of DNA repair.

Ionizing radiation is one of the most damaging physical causes of DNA harming agents which can originate from both artificial (e.g. medical treatments, such as x-rays and radiotherapy) and natural sources (e.g. cosmic and gamma radiation) (figure 2.5). Among different DNA injuries stimulated by ionizing radiation, the most damaging of these is double-strand breaks. DNA can directly or indirectly be damaged by ionizing radiation via the production of reactive oxygen species (ROS) [31]. In addition to physical assaults, the cell must also be confronted with different chemical sources of DNA damage [32, 33] such as various chemical agents in the form of clinical drugs that have been produced to target DNA as an option to treat cancer or other ailments. Chemical agents that attack DNA include mainly alkylating agents, e.g. temozolomide and methyl methanesulfonate, which trigger alkylation of the DNA bases. Moreover, these also encompass bifunctional alkylating agents, e.g. nitrogen mustards, platinum compounds and the natural product mitomycin C (figure 2.5). These agents affect DNA in the form of intrastrand and interstrand cross-links [34] that lead to DNA injury. Various anticancer drugs, e.g. topoisomerase I or II inhibitors, cause single-strand or double-strand breakdowns by deceiving topoisomerase–DNA covalent complexes, respectively [35]. Furthermore, well studied environmentally existing DNA-damaging chemicals comprise heterocyclic amines, N-nitrosoamines and polycyclic aromatic hydrocarbons, which are usually found in the diet, and are also generated in air emissions, such as cigarette smoke and vehicle exhaust. Usually these sorts of chemically active compounds covalently attach to different sites on the DNA bases to form the so-called bulky DNA adducts. Different other similar adducts are generated between DNA and aflatoxins, which are naturally occurring toxins formed by fungi (genus: *Aspergillus*) that grow in several types of food crops [36].

Cells have developed multiple repair mechanisms to compensate for the many types of DNA damage. Different types of biomechanisms are involved in repair mechanisms wherein each corrects a different subset of lesions. There are five basic DNA repair mechanisms usually adopted by mammalian cells, such as mismatch repair (MMR), BER, NER and double-strand break repair, which includes both HR and NHEJ [37].

2.9.1 Base excision repair (BER)

Broadly speaking, BER (base excision repair) is a mechanism that eliminates DNA damage that may occur spontaneously within a cell due to various hydrolytic events. These events include deamination or loss of a DNA base, oxidative damage caused by oxygen free radicals, and methylation of ring nitrogens by endogenous agents [38]. Hence, BER serves as an indispensable DNA repair pathway crucial for the maintenance of genetic material. The pivotal step in BER involves the cleavage of the N-glycosyl bond that connects a modified base to the deoxyribose-phosphate chain, thereby removing the base residue in its liberated form. Every DNA glycosylase exhibits specificity for a distinct range of lesions, and each enzyme type is examined individually. The subsequent formation of an apurinic or apyrimidinic site is addressed through cleavage by an AP endonuclease. Since the total absence of BER would be incompatible with an organism's survival, a backup system or one of various alternative pathways is frequently available to repair a particular lesion. However, inherited syndromes may manifest with modifications in the enzymes within the BER pathway. Base excision repairs the main machinery responsible for the repair of damaged DNA bases, and unlike NER, does not significantly change the complete structural features of the DNA helix [39]. Significant genes and their five major DNA repair mechanisms are listed in table 2.1.

2.9.1.1 Mechanisms for the conclusion of base excision repair

The final stages of BER involve the elimination of the 5′ terminal deoxyribose-phosphate residue produced by the AP endonuclease, followed by DNA synthesis for repair and subsequent ligation. In human cells, an enzyme activity with a

Table 2.1. Important genes and their five major DNA repair mechanisms. Base excision repair (BER); mismatch repair (MMR); nucleotide excision repair (NER); homologous recombination (HR); non-homologous end-joining (NHEJ).

Mechanisms	Processes
NHEJ	XRCC4-DNA ligase IV, XLF, Ku70-Ku80, DNA-PKc,
NER	DNA polymerase δ or ε, RPA, XPG, XPD, XPA, UV-DDB (DDB1-XPE), CSA, CSB, TFIIH, XPB, ERCC1-XPF, XPC-Rad23B-CEN2,
MMRBER	MutLγ (MLH1-MLH3), MutLα(MLH1-PMS2), MutSα (MSH2-MSH6), MutSβ (MSH2-MSH3), Exo1, PCNA-RFC MutLβ (MLH1-PMS2)
HR	CtIP, Mus81/Eme1BRCA2, Exo1, GEN1-Yen1, Slx1-Slx4, Mre11-Rad50-Nbs1, BLM-TopIIIα, Rad52, BRCA1, RPA, Rad51,
BER	PARP, PCNA-RFC, APE1, DNA glycosylase, XRCC1, FEN1, PNKP, APTX, DNA polymerase β, Tdp1, DNA polymerase δ or ε

molecular weight of approximately 50 kDa, capable of excising sugar phosphate residues from double-stranded DNA, has been recognized and is denoted as DNA deoxyribophosphodiesterase (dRPase).

2.9.2 Mismatch repair (MMR)

DNA damage, if unrepaired, has the possibility to induce mutations in somatic or germline cells, which can alter cellular phenotype and cause dysfunction and disease. To prevent such damaging effects and shield the integrity of the genome, cells adopt several mechanisms to repair DNA injury and therefore avoid mutations. One such scheme is the important path called DNA mismatch repair [40]. The mismatch repair system plays a significant role in post-replication repair of mis incorporated bases that have skipped the correcting activity of replication polymerases. Moreover, for mismatched bases, mismatch repair proteins also rectify insertion/deletion loops caused by polymerase slippage during replication of repetitive DNA sequences. Mismatch repair corrects DNA mismatches generated in DNA replication, therefore preventing mutations from becoming steady in dividing cells. As mismatch repair reduces the number of replication-linked errors, faults in mismatch repair enhance the spontaneous mutation rate. Mismatch repair inactivation in human cells is associated with hereditary and recurrent human cancers and the mismatch repair system is obligatory for cell cycle detention and/or programmed cell death in response to definite types of DNA damage. Thus, mismatch repair actively plays a significant role in the DNA injury retort pathway that eliminates severely damaged cells and prevents both mutageneses in the short term and tumorigenesis in the long term.

2.9.3 Nucleotide excision repair (NER)

NER is a multistep process. It identifies and eradicates a range of damage causing significant modifications in the DNA configuration, e.g. UV-induced damage and bulky chemical adducts. Its extremely multipurpose repair pathway can identify and eliminate a broad diversity of bulky, helix-distorting lesions from DNA. The most imperative case among these injuries is pyrimidine dimmers (e.g. cyclobutane pyrimidine dimmers and 6–4 photoproducts), which are produced by UV light. A further significant substrate of NER is cisplatin–DNA intrastrand cross-links. NER is intervened by the systematic assembly of repair proteins at the site of the DNA lesion [41, 42].

2.9.4 Double-strand break (DSB) repair

DSBs are the most naturally destructive sort of DNA injury, e.g. a single unrepaired double-strand breakdown is frequently sufficient to cause cell death. Moreover, incorrect repair can also result in deletions or chromosomal aberrations. These actions can grow into the development of cancer or other genomic instability syndromes. Mammalian cells repair DSBs by two main mechanisms: HR and NHEJ. These sorts of repair machineries differ in their need for a homologous template DNA and in the reliability of DSB repair. Double-strand DNA break takes place once the individual strand of the DNA duplex creates a break in one or both of the strands, often by ionizing radiation or by certain chemicals. However, it can also break by mechanical stress or any sort of cytotoxic lesion. Homology directed repair is a type of repair mechanism existing in the cell to heal double-strand DNA lesions. It is similar to single-strand breaks (SSBs) in which in one strand of the DNA double-helix results in by loss of a single nucleotide.

2.10 DNA recombination

DNA recombination encompasses the splitting and covalent assembly of DNA sequences. Recombination can occur between two locations of a single DNA molecule (intramolecular recombination) or two dissimilar DNA molecules (intermolecular recombination). Intermolecular recombination can occur with multiple types of DNA templates. The DNA templates may be linear DNA developed via transduction, linear chromosomes or conjugation, transformation and plasmids. In bacteria with circular or dsDNA chromosomes, circular plasmids, the recombination can take place between linear and circular dsDNA templates or between two circular dsDNA templates. Via recombination and transposition, the DNA sequence of a chromosome can modify in large segments as well. Recombination is defined as the generation of new DNA molecule(s) from two parental DNA molecules or different segments of the same DNA molecule. Transposition is the main form of recombination in which DNA sections translocate from one location to another, either on the same type of chromosome or a different chromosome.

2.10.1 Types and examples of recombination

In biological organisms four kinds of recombination have been identified (figure 2.6).

2.10.1.1 General or homologous recombination

This kind of recombination occurs between DNA molecules of very similar sequence (e.g. homologous chromosomes) and takes place through the genome of diploid organisms. The entire natural process is attained by using one or a small number of common enzymatic pathways [43]. Illegitimate recombination (IR) is the interchange of genetic information by the formation of connections between non-homologous chromosome segments and it takes place in sections where no large-scale sequence resemblance is obvious. For example, translocations between various chromosomes or deletions that eliminate some genes along a chromosome. However, when the sequences of DNA at the divisions for these events are studied, short sections of sequence connection are found in several circumstances, such as recombination between two similar genes that are quite a few million base pairs apart can have consequences in the deletion of the intervening genes in somatic cells.

2.10.1.2 Site-specific recombination

Site-specific recombination, also called conventional site-specific recombination, is a kind of genetic recombination in which DNA strand altercation occurs between

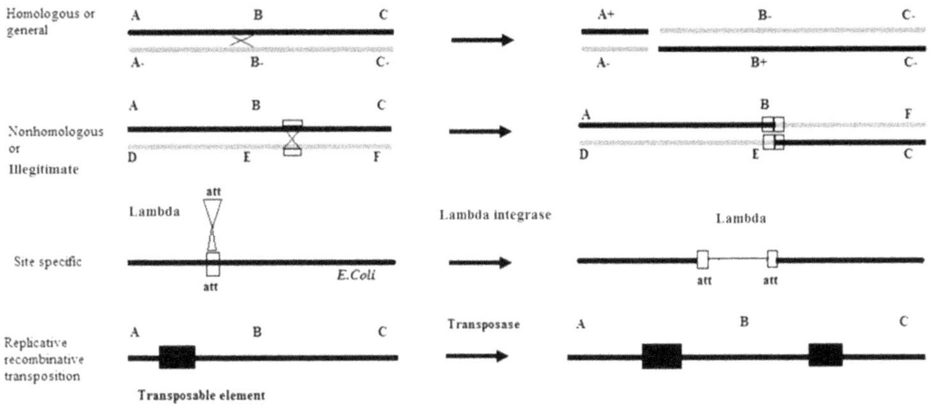

Figure 2.6. Types of biological recombination. In this illustration every line symbolizes a chromosome or segment of a chromosome; hence a single line corresponds to both strands of duplex DNA. For homologous or general recombination, each homologous chromosome is shown as different shades, with different alleles for each of the three genes on each. Exchange of genetic information occurs by recombination between genes A and B which results in changing the arrangement of alleles on the chromosomes. In the case of non-HR two different chromosomes recombine, e.g. gene C so that it is now on the same chromosome as genes D and E. Nevertheless, sequences of the two chromosomes differ for most of their lengths and the segments at the sites of recombination may be related. Site-specific recombination results in arrangement of two dissimilar DNA molecules and the whole process was catalyzed by a specific enzyme. This enzyme identifies a short sequence present in both the phage DNA and the target site in the bacterial chromosome, called att. Replicative recombination is seen for some transposable elements using a specific enzyme, encoded by the transposable element.

fragments holding at least a certain degree of sequence homology, i.e. recombination takes place between particular short sequences present on otherwise dissimilar parental molecules [44]. This type of recombination encompasses a specific enzymatic mechanism, primarily one enzyme or enzyme system for each specific site such as the integration of some bacteriophage, e.g. λ, into a bacterial chromosome and the reorganization of immunoglobulin genes in vertebrate animals.

2.10.1.3 Replicative recombination

In this category of recombination a new copy of a fragment of DNA is generated. Different transposable elements exploit this process of replicative recombination to produce a new replica of the transposable element at a new site (figure 2.6) [45].

rDNA technology exploits two more kinds of recombination: *restriction endonuclease* and *DNA ligase* based site-specific cutting and retorting of various DNA molecules *in vitro*. After cutting at particular junctions/ends these rDNA molecules are then introduced into the host organism, generally into a bacterium. In circumstances where the rDNA is a plasmid, phage or other molecule capable of replicating in the host it will remain extrachromosomal. This recombinant is DNA presented into a host where it cannot replicate, for instance an animal cell in culture, a plant or a fertilized mouse egg. To facilitate stable transformation, the DNA is transformed into a host chromosome. This course can ensue by HR in bacteria and yeast, at a practically high frequency. However, this does not occur in plant or animal cells.

In contrast, at a low incidence rate, some of these transformed DNA molecules are introduced at random sites in the chromosomes of the host cell. Therefore, random recombination into chromosomes facilitates the stable transfection of cells leading to the best transgenic plants and animals. The recombination mechanism has not apparently been studied during transformation or transfection, nevertheless it is usually used in the laboratory.

2.11 DNA isolation is the commencement of molecular marker analysis

A molecular marker is nucleic acid or proteins present in organism used to study, control, and explore genetic composition of living organisms. It is different in individual organisms or species but closely linked to a target gene expressing a specific trait. They are classified by the nature of analyzing molecules such as peptides, DNA, RNA. Primarily, DNA molecular markers are used in the field of identification of genetically engineered organisms as well as identifying traceability of molecules. RNA is more challenging as a molecular marker because of its liability and susceptibility to degradation. It has been utilized in techniques such as Northern blot analyses and various PCR-based approaches such as RNA Arbitrarily Primed-PCR (RAP-PCR) and Restriction Fragment Differential Display-PCR(RAP-PCR). This RNA marker analysis can be performed using microarray and transcriptome sequencing [46]. DNA (i.e. nuclear, mitochondrial and/or chloroplast DNA) isolation from the specimen to be studied is the first step for all molecular marker types. There are different sources of DNA (i.e. lyophilized, preserved, fresh or dried samples), but a fresh sample is suitable for receiving high-quality DNA. Genomic DNA refers to the total DNA content of organism, including both organellar and nuclear genome. This isolated gDNA is then cut with two restricted enzymes, followed by ligation of adapter to restricted fragment. The adapter attached fragments are amplified by PCR. The resulting PCR product is analyzed by denaturing polyacrylamide gel electrophoresis to reveal the existing genetic polymorphism. It can be analyzed using various molecular markers such as, AFLP, RAPD, microsatellite. Mitochondrial genomes are smaller than nuclear genomes and provide insights of maternal lineages. They contain genes involve in energy production and gene flow patterns in population. Nuclear DNA contains genetic information that determines an organism's traits and characteristics. It can be analyzed using techniques such as AFLP, ISSRs and SSRs to investigate genetic diversity and the phylogenetic relationship among species. chloroplast DNA (cp DNA) is relatively conserved and evolves slowly. It is found in the plant cell and inherited maternally. It comprises an intergenic spacer and a non-coding region that has repetitive genomic sections, i.e., microsatellites. These reveal higher allelic variation, often targeted for genetic diversity characterization [47]. Different protocols exist for the DNA isolation and selection of the procedure depends upon the type of sample, the superiority and quantity of DNA required, and the existence of natural substances that may obstruct the extraction procedures and successful investigation. This collection of extraction methodologies ranges from easy and quick approaches [48–50] that yield low-quality DNA suitable enough for consistent study, to lengthy and time-consuming standard protocols [51, 52] that typically produce high-quality and adequate amounts of DNA.

2.11.1 DNA extraction protocols

The high quality and quantity of DNA isolation is necessary for reliable genotyping data, long-time DNA preservation, and cost- and time-saving. DNA extraction methods are categorized based on chemical and physical methods. Phenyl-chloroform and isoamyl alcohol are organic solvent-based DNA extraction methods. SDS, CTAB, Proteinase-K, salting out and silica-gel-based DNA extractions are inorganic solvent methods. Physical extraction methods include magnetic-bead-based and chromatography-based DNA extraction methods. Each of these methods has its own advantages and limitations, and choice of sample is based on type of sample, desired yield, and purity of DNA. For bacteria and plant DNA isolation, CTAB method and the phenol-chloroform method are commonly preferred. These methods are more effective in precipitating DNA and separating it from other cellular components. Along with CTAB method, chromatography-based DNA isolation methods including size exclusion chromatography, ion exchange chromatography are also used for fungal DNA isolation [53]. The most commonly used DNA extraction protocols include breaking (via grinding) or digesting away cell walls and membranes so as to release the cellular/subcellular components. Various detergents, e.g. cetyl trimethylammonium bromide (CTAB), sodium dodecyl sulfate (SDS) or mixed alkyl trimethylammonium bromide are used to eliminate the lipids of membranes. These detergents allow the release of DNA, which should be protected from endogenous nucleases. For this purpose, ethylenediaminetetraacetic acid (EDTA) is often supplemented in the extraction buffer to chelate magnesium ions which is an important co-factor for nucleases. An enormous quantity of biomolecules, e.g. RNA, proteins, polysaccharides, tannins and pigments, impede the extraction of DNA, therefore different procedures are used to eliminate these biomolecules without influencing the integrity of DNA. Most of the proteins are removed by adding a protein-degrading enzyme (proteinase-K), followed by denaturation at 65 °C and precipitation using chloroform and isoamyl alcohol. RNA-degrading enzyme (RNase A) is frequently exploited to eliminate RNA. High molecular weight polysaccharide-like impurities are, on the other hand, very challenging to eliminate. Hydrolyzing agent, e.g. NaCl, in combination with CTAB is documented to eliminate polysaccharides [54]. In different methodologies NaCl is substituted by KCl [55]. High-speed centrifugation at suitable temperature, generally at low temperature, is required to isolate DNA from other compounds, e.g. proteins, carbohydrates, lipids and/or phenols. Once all debris/undesirable material are eliminated, then DNA in the aqueous phase will then be moved into fresh tubes, followed by precipitated in salt solution (e.g. sodium acetate) or alcohol, and lastly redissolved in sterile water or buffer. Finally, the ultimate amount of DNA needed is measured via either 1% agarose gel electrophoresis or spectrophotometer. The aim of this procedure is to determine DNA concentration by virtually investigating band intensities of the isolated DNA with a molecular ladder of hypothetical concentration and agarose gel is suitable for examining whether the DNA is degraded or not. From spectrophotometer examination the intensity of absorbance of DNA solution at 260 nm wavelength can be examined, and moreover it also shows the occurrence of protein impurities; nevertheless, it does not analyze whether the DNA is degraded or not. After completion of DNA extraction there are three main possibilities:

- No DNA.
- The DNA appears as broken/sheared (too fragmented), which is an indication of degradation for different reasons.
- The DNA appears as whitish thin threads (good-quality DNA) or brownish thread (DNA in the presence of oxidation from contaminants such as phenolic compounds).

Therefore, scientists need to study various methodologies in order assess the most appropriate or best one that works for the sample under consideration.

2.12 Types of molecular markers

Methods involved in cloning and PCR amplification of small DNA fragments to derive millions of copies of each fragment are explained in this section. These methods are now widely used for different purposes in the extensive field of biotechnology. One of the main uses of these techniques is the development and use of DNA-based molecular markers for different purposes. These molecular markers are based on the polymorphism noted at the level of small fragments of DNA. Over a period of two decades (1980–2000), an extensive range of molecular markers became accessible which are being used in a diversity of ways. A large number of abbreviations for these molecular markers are in common usage now. The main use of these molecular markers is the improvement of molecular maps for human and animal systems. On the basis of the principles and approaches utilized, DNA-based molecular markers can be generally categorized into the following four groups:

- Hybridization-based markers.
- Molecular markers based on PCR followed by hybridization.
- PCR-based markers.
- Sequencing and DNA-based markers.

One of the main difficulties is thus to associate the purpose(s) of a particular project with the various molecular marker types. The different molecular markers can be categorized into different groups based on:

- Method of gene investigation: hybridization-based or PCR-based markers.
- Mode of gene action: co-dominant markers or dominant.
- Mode of transmission: maternal organelle inheritance, or paternal organelle inheritance, biparental nuclear inheritance, maternal nuclear inheritance.

Different types of molecular markers (table 2.2) have been defined and are recorded in alphabetical order in the table.

Table 2.2. List of acronyms for different DNA markers with references.

DNA markers	Acronyms	Reference
Allele-specific associated primers	ASAP	[56]
Allele-specific oligo	ASO	[57]
Allele-specific PCR	AS-PCR	[58]
Amplified fragment length polymorphism	AFLP	[59]
Anchored microsatellite primed PCR	AMP-PCR	[60]
Anchored SSRs	ASSR	[61]
Arbitrarily primed PCR	AP-PCR	[62]
Cleaved amplified polymorphic sequence	CAPS	[63, 64]
Degenerate oligonucleotide primed PCR	DOP-PCR	[65]
Diversity arrays technology	DArT	[66]
DNA amplification fingerprinting	DAF	[67]
Expressed sequence tags	EST	[68]
Inter-simple sequence repeat	ISSR	[60]
Inverse PCR	IPCR	[69]
Inverse sequence-tagged repeats	ISTR	[70]
Microsatellite primed PCR	MP-PCR	[71]
Multiplexed allele-specific diagnostic assay	MASDA	[72]
Random amplified microsatellite polymorphisms	RAMP	[73]
Random amplified microsatellites	RAM	[74]
Random amplified polymorphic DNA	RAPD	[75]
Restriction fragment length polymorphism	RFLP	[76]
Selective amplification of microsatellite polymorphic loci	SAMPL	[77]
Sequence-characterized amplified regions	SCAR	[78]
Sequence-specific amplification polymorphisms	S-SAP	[79]
Sequence-tagged microsatellite site	STMS	[80]
Sequence-tagged site	STS	[81]
Short tandem repeats	STR	[82]
Simple sequence length polymorphism	SSLP	[83]
Simple sequence repeat	SSR	[84]
Single-nucleotide polymorphism	SNP	[85]
Single primer amplification reactions	SPAR	[86]
Single-stranded conformational polymorphism	SSCP	[87]
Site-selected insertion PCR	SSI	[88]
Strand displacement amplification	SDA	[89]
Variable number tandem repeat	VNTR	[90]
Others	Similar types (e.g. ASAP, ASO and AS-PCR), some synonymous (e.g. ISSR, RAMP, RAM, SPAR, AMP-PCR, MP-PCR and ASSR); and some identical (e.g. SSLP, STMS, STR and SSR) [91].	

2.12.1 Hybridization-based molecular markers

RFLP is the most broadly applied hybridization-based molecular marker which is based on polymorphisms arising due to base insertion, substitution and translocation that might have taken place in the past in specific regions of genomic DNA. Such alterations on a particular region results in variation in the size of the restriction fragments achieved due to digestion with definite restriction enzymes. These markers were initially utilized in 1975 to identify DNA sequence polymorphisms for genetic mapping of a temperature-sensitive mutation of adenovirus serotypes [92]. The method is more reliable yet recognizes variation only in the parts of these fragments that are linked with each other via homology with the molecular probe employed for hybridization. It was employed for human genome mapping after mapping of the adenovirus [76], and later was accepted for plant genomes [93]. RFLP is completely based on restriction enzymes that uncover a pattern variation among DNA fragment sizes in individual organisms. However, two individuals belonging to the same species have nearly the same genomes; they will differ by a few nucleotides for several reasons, e.g. translocation, point mutation, insertion/deletion, inversion and duplication. A number of variations in DNA sequences at the restriction sites can result in the loss, gain or relocation of a restriction site. Thus, DNA digestion with a restriction enzyme produces different fragments whose amount and size can vary between individuals, populations and species. The principles and processes of using RFLP markers are shown in figure 2.7.

- Digestion of DNA with one or more restriction enzyme(s).
- Separation of restriction fragments in agarose gel.
- Southern-blotting-based shifting of separated fragments from the agarose gel to a filter.
- Identification of individual fragments by nucleic acid hybridization with a labeled probe.
- Autoradiography ([94–96]).

Bacterial-enzyme-derived restriction enzymes (endonucleases, e.g. MseI, EcoRI, PstI, etc) are enzymes that recognize specific four, six or eight base pair (bp) sequences in DNA, and cut dsDNA when these sequences are found. For example, EcoRI has six bp recognition sequences, so it cuts between G and A whenever the sequences 5′...GAATTC...3′ or 3′...CTTAAG...5′ exist together. Depending upon the resolution required and the existing electrophoresis facility, a choice between using enzymes for four, six or eight bp can be made. It has been found that optimum and maximum resolution is attained by using 'four-cutters' (enzymes recognizing a four bp sequence) as there are different such locations in the genome. Fragments derived by these specific cutting agents are relatively small, which offers a better chance of identifying single-base alterations. In contrast, the utilization of enzymes that recognize an eight bp sequence will include fewer probes, because bigger fragments of the genome are inspected at one time. Therefore, simply bulky alterations of the DNA will be inspected with the help of complex electrophoresis

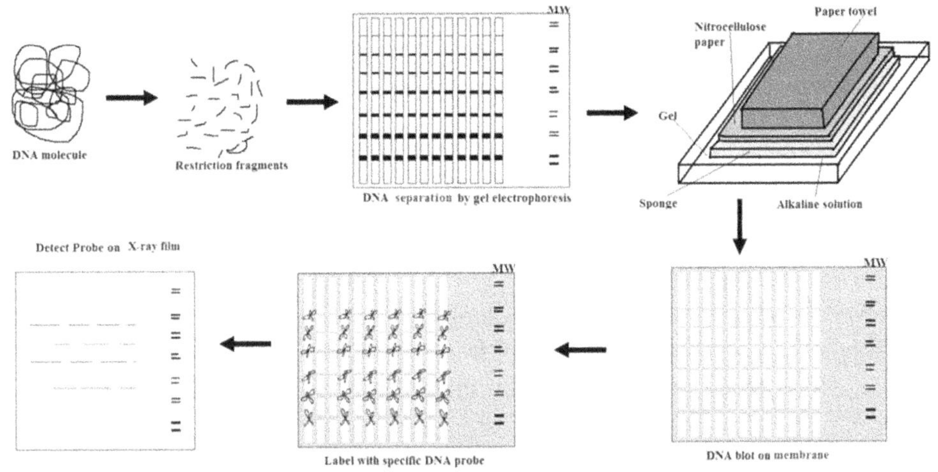

Figure 2.7. Protocol including various steps of RFLP markers. With the help of gel electrophoresis, dsDNA fragments produced by restriction enzymes are separated according to their length. This step is followed by laying a nitrocellulose or nylon paper (membrane) sheet over the gel. Then the separated DNA fragments are relocated to the sheet by blotting (Southern transfer). On a thick layer of sponge in a bath of alkali solution the gel is supported and then suction of the DNA from the gel to the nitrocellulose paper is induced by heaping paper towels on top of the nitrocellulose sheet. Once the buffer is absorbed through, it allows the denaturation of the DNA and relocates the single-stranded fragments from the gel to the periphery of the nitrocellulose sheet, where they stick tightly. This relocation is essential to keep the DNA firmly in place as the hybridization procedure is carried out. Then the nitrocellulose sheet with the bound single-stranded DNA fragments is cautiously peeled off the gel. Subsequently this sheet is transferred into a sealed plastic bag that contains a radioactively labeled DNA probe for hybridization. Later, the sheet is removed from the bag and carefully washed, so that just those probe molecules that are hybridized to the DNA on the paper remain fixed. Then, with the aid of autoradiography, the DNA that has hybridized to the labeled probe will show up as bands on the autoradiograph.

to arrange the fragments into separate bands. Thus, for settlement, ‘six-cutter’ enzymes are principally utilized for RFLP studies as they are cost-effective, readily accessible and usually offer DNA fragments in the size range of 200–20 000 bp. This size range can be simply segregated on agarose gels After the DNA molecule is digested by restriction enzymes, it is accessible as a combination of linear double-stranded molecules of varying lengths. Later, these are segregated by electrophoresis using agarose or polyacrylamide gels. The assortment of the gel is based on the restriction enzymes selected. For example, four-cutters produce fragments that are too small to be resolved by agarose gels; therefore, polyacrylamide gels are essential. In contrast, polyacrylamide gels cannot generally be exploited to control the fragments produced by six-cutters, so agarose gels must be utilized in that circumstance. These investigative concerns led most scientists to employ six-cutter enzymes, as agarose gels are more suitable for handling [97]. After the segregation of DNA fragments by gel electrophoresis, they are suitable for denaturing to single strands and then moving to a solid support (‘nylon membranes’ or ‘filters’). This method is called 'Southern blotting' or 'Southern hybridization' [98]. The complete basis of this method is the transfer of the DNA from a gel to a solid support which facilitates the conservation of the fragments as they were existent in the gel, but allowing hybridization reactions to be carried out. DNA immobilized on filter paper is then used to hybridize to labeled probe DNA. The DNA probes engaged for hybridization are generally single-locus and mostly species-specific probes of about 500–3000 bp in size [99]. There are two types of probes which are employed to identify particular DNA fragments by hybridization: cDNA clones (DNA copies of mRNA molecules) and genomic clones (fragments of nuclear DNA). Gene libraries and their respective databanks are simple to generate and comprise various similar probes as repetitive sequences include the main part of plant genomic DNA. These probes will hybridize into different fragments on the filters and produce very sophisticated prototypes. It is very tough to build cDNA libraries as they typically encompass unique or low copy number sequences, suggesting expressed genes, and usually produce fewer bands on the filter. Nevertheless, application of cDNA probes facilitates the identification of small alterations, although if the genomes protected by each probe are relatively small various other probes must be used [97]. Consequently, the selection of the appropriate source for an RFLP probe varies with the necessities of the specific purpose under consideration. To allow hybridization of the probe to mark sequences, denatured probe solution is left in contact with the filter. Through hybridization the labeled probe binds to complementary DNA on the filter, allowing imaging of particular DNA fragments. Radioactive labeling has been attained conventionally via radioactive nucleotides, although other radioactive methodologies are currently accessible [96, 100]. Then labeling is followed by washing off non-specific hybridization under more simple circumstances than those used for primary hybridization. In circumstances where radioactive probes are employed, the filter paper is positioned adjacent to photographic film facilitating the disintegration from the probe which may affect the results in visible bands. An autoradiography of photographic film will reveal the set of fragments analogous to the probe. With the aid of non-radioactive probes such as digoxigenin, antibodies and enzymatic reaction, it is also suitable to demonstrate the set of fragments directly on the membrane [96]. Information derived from the RFLP technique depends on both the quantity of probes and the kind of restriction enzymes used in this process. In this process every diverse probe hybridizes with a singular set of genomic DNA fragments and each distinct enzyme slices out a fragment of genomic DNA at different points [101]. The basic merits of RFLP markers are their reproducibility, high co-dominant inheritance, good transferability between laboratories, locus-specific markers that allow synteny investigations, no requirement for sequence information and relative simplicity of scoring due to the great size difference among various fragments. There are, on the other hand, several disadvantages to RFLP investigation:

- It depends on the development of specific probe libraries for the species.
- It generally requires radioactively labeled probes.
- It is time-consuming, laborious, and costly [102].
- It necessitates the presence of a high quantity and quality of DNA [103].

- The level of polymorphism is low, and few loci are identified per assay.
- The technique is not responsive to automation.

2.12.2 PCR-based markers

PCR is one of the most consistent and advanced scientific techniques of all historical innovations. It is a molecular biology-based technique intended for enzymatically replicating (amplifying) a very small quantity of DNA without using a living organism. PCR is frequently utilized to amplify a short, i.e. typically up to 10 kilobases (kb), distinct part of a DNA strand from a single gene or simply a part of a gene. PCR was developed by Kary Mullis in 1983 and this technology has led to the growth of different types of PCR-based techniques (and a Nobel Prize for Mullis in 1993). However, the basic PCR protocol was previously described by Kjell Kleppe (1971) and his co-researchers in Khorana's group, and it has been questioned whether the key input of Mullis was the thermostable DNA polymerase or if he actually knew of this paper. This situation has been important in stimulating the PCR patent. The basic process involved in PCR is very simple:

- In the initial step of PCR dsDNA is denatured at a high temperature (92 °C–95 °C) to produce single strands (templates).
- These short single fragments of DNA primer attach at a lower annealing temperature to the single-stranded complementary templates at ends flanking the target sequences.
- In the next step the temperature is raised, generally to 72 °C (sometimes 68 °C), for the DNA polymerase enzyme to catalyze the template-directed production of new dsDNA molecules that are similar in structure to the first material.
- Later, the newly produced dsDNA target sequences are denatured at high temperature and the cycle is again repeated.

The amplification of target DNA can be exponential in every cycle. This augmentation has the potential to double the amount of target DNA from the previous cycle, as long as there is an acceptable quantity of primers, DNA polymerase and deoxynucleotide triphosphates (dNTPs) in the reaction solution. Nevertheless, the basic protocol of PCR is very simple, and each analysis entails manipulation of the various factors for the sample to be studied. In old-style PCR, the DNA polymerase would need to be added fresh to the reaction at each and every temperature progression as thermostable (high-temperature tolerant) DNA polymerases were not available commercially. There were no thermocycles so transferring the tubes from one temperature bath to another for several hours was an effort that was restricted to graduate students and/or technicians. The invention of Taq DNA polymerase, which is utilized by the *Thermus auquaticus* bacterium in hot springs, was very significant for the enormous effectiveness and approval of PCR-based techniques. The exclusive role of this enzyme was to permit the *in vivo* replication of DNA in thermophilic bacteria. Thus, this enzyme was able to work at the high temperatures compulsory for *in vitro* replication. The main benefit of this enzyme is its stability at the high temperatures needed to perform the amplification, where other DNA polymerases become denatured. Recently, PCR technology has become more developed with the accessibility of thermostable DNA polymerases (e.g. Pfu, Taq or Vent polymerase). Moreover, computerization of PCR-based reactions can be accomplished by a PCR machine (thermocycler) that has found its way into nearly every molecular biology lab in the world. The main advantages of PCR-based techniques in contrast to hybridization-based methods include:

- A small quantity of DNA is needed.
- Suitability for small labs in terms of equipment, facilities and cost.
- Exclusion of radioisotopes in most practices.
- High polymorphism that makes it possible to yield various genetic markers within a short time.
- No earlier sequence information/data is compulsory for various purposes, e.g. AP-PCR, AFLP, DAF, RAPD and ISSR.
- The ability to amplify DNA sequences from preserved tissues.
- The ability to screen various genes simultaneously either for direct collection of information or as an exploratory study prior to nucleotide sequencing efforts [104].

These benefits, on the other hand, can fluctuate depending on the exact technology selected by the operator. Various PCR-based techniques are classified into two types depending on the primers employed for amplification:

- Site-targeted PCR-based techniques that developed from known DNA sequences (e.g. CAPS, EST, STS SSR, SCAR).
- Arbitrary or semi-arbitrary primed PCR methods that developed without prior sequence information (e.g. DAF, RAPD, AP-PCR, AFLP, ISSR).

2.12.2.1 Arbitrarily amplified DNA markers

Random amplified polymorphic DNA (RAPD), arbitrarily primed PCR (AP-PCR) and DNA amplification fingerprinting (DAF) have been collectively described as multiple arbitrary amplicon profiling (MAAP) [105]. The key objective of these three PCR-based techniques is primarily to amplify DNA fragments from any samples lacking previous sequence information. There are various dissimilarities among MAAP-based techniques which include:

- Annealing temperatures.
- Methods of fragment separation.
- Enzyme-based digestion of template DNA or amplification products.
- The number of PCR cycles employed in a reaction [106].
- The thermostable DNA polymerase used [107].
- Variations in amplification profiles by altering primer sequence and length.

Most of these procedures offer markedly diverse amplification profiles, changing from quite simple (RAPD) to highly complex (DAF) arrangements. Application of a single arbitrary oligonucleotide primer to amplify template DNA, deprived of prior data of the target sequence is the important revolution of RAPD, AP-PCR and DAF. Nucleic acid augmentation with arbitrary primers is mainly evaluated by the interaction between template annealing sites, primers and enzymes, and also motivated by complex kinetic and thermodynamic procedures. A different PCR product is produced when, at an appropriate annealing temperature, the individual primer attaches to positions on complimentary strands of the genomic DNA that are within an amplifiable distance, generally <3000 bp. During most of these procedures polymorphisms (band presence or absence) result from changes in the DNA sequence that impede primer binding or hinder amplification of a specific marker in some individuals; as a result, they can be easily identified as DNA fragments that are augmented from one individual but not from another. Usually the RAPD technique at 34 °C–37 °C uses a 10 bp arbitrary primer at continuous low annealing temperature. The primers that are employed through this approach can be derived as sets or separately from various sources (e.g. Operon Biotechnologies www.operon.com, or the University of British Colombia www.michaelsmith.ubc.ca/services/NAPS/Primer_Sets). However, although the sequences of RAPD primers are arbitrarily chosen, two important conditions stated in 1990 by Williams *et al* must be considered: the absence of palindromic sequences (a base sequence that reads precisely the same from right to left as from left to right) and a minimum amount of 40% GC (50%–80% GC is generally used) [108]. Since the G-C bond contains three hydrogen bridges and the A-T bond contains only two, a primer–DNA hybrid with less than 50% GC will perhaps not tolerate the 72 °C temperature at which DNA elongation occurs by DNA polymerase. The subsequent PCR products are usually determined on 1.5%–2.0% agarose gels and stained with ethidium bromide (EtBr). In this process polyacrylamide gels in combination with either $AgNO_3$ staining [109], radioactivity [110] or fluorescently labeled primers or nucleotides [111] are sometimes used. Regardless of its low resolving potential, the ease of handling and low cost of agarose gel electrophoresis has made RAPD a more widespread and rapid process than AP-PCR and DAF. A maximum of RAPD fragments results from the augmentation of one locus, and two types of polymorphism take place. In the first type the band may be present or absent, and in the other case the intensity of the band may be altered. These band brightness (intensity) differences might result from copy number or relative sequence abundance [112]. This can help to distinguish homozygote dominant individuals from heterozygotes, since more intense (bright) bands are found for the former. However, one group of scientists [119] found no association between copy number and band intensity. The reality is that brighter (more intense) bands are generally less robust in RAPD tests [113]. This suggests that fluctuating degrees of primer incompatibility may indicate various band intensity alterations. Since the main cause of band intensity dissimilarities is doubtful (copy number or primer mismatch), most studies avoid counting variations in band intensity; nevertheless, some scientists have used up to a seven-state scale of band intensity. RAPD has three major disadvantages:

- Dominant inheritance.
- Homology.
- Reproducibility.

There are countless factors that have been shown to influence the reproducibility of RAPD reactions: the amount of template DNA, PCR buffer, quality, primer to template ratio, annealing temperature, concentration of magnesium chloride, thermal cycler brand and Taq DNA polymerase brand or source [114]. Issues related to the reproducibility of RAPD markers can be overcome by:

- Selection of an appropriate DNA isolation procedure to eradicate any impurities [115].
- Optimizing the factors used [116].
- Investigating different oligonucleotide primers and rating only the reproducible DNA fragments [117].
- Using an appropriate DNA polymerase brand.

The presence of false positive bands associated with reorganized fragments produced by nested primer-binding sites [118] and intra strand annealing and communications during PCR [119] have also been found to influence the reliability of RAPD data. The presence of both false negatives and false positives could, if regularly occurring, critically restrict the reliability of RAPD for numerous purposes, e.g. genetic diversity and mapping studies. Each pairwise mapping of RAPD fragments with samples starts with the assumption that co-migrating bands (i.e. bands that migrate an equal distance) represent homologous loci. This means bands that migrate an equal distance relative to homologous loci.

On the other hand, as in any study based on electrophoretic determination, the theory that equal length equals homology may not be fundamentally correct, especially in polyploid species. For example, certain RAPD bands have been recorded as analogous (equal in length) but have been found not to be homologous [119] (see figure 2.8). More ideal resolution of fragment size by polyacrylamide gels

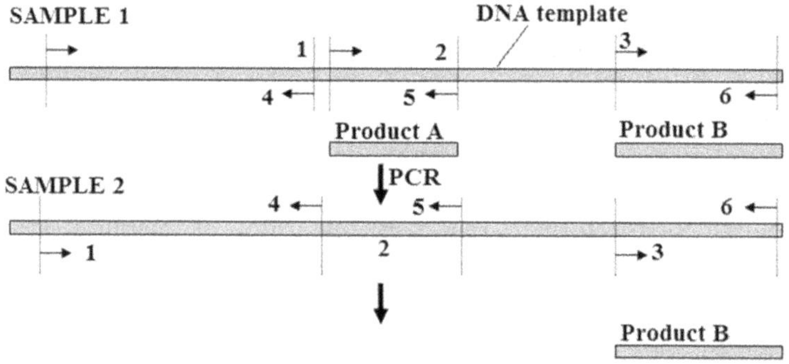

Figure 2.8. Representation of reaction conditions for RAPD. In the first stage primers must anneal in specific alignment (such that they point towards each other) and within a reasonable distance of one another. The bold arrows indicate multiple copies of a single primer and the direction of the arrows indicates the direction in which DNA synthesis will occurs. The numbers relate to primer annealing regions on the DNA template. For sample one, primers anneal to locations one, two and three on the top strand of the DNA template and to locations four, five and six on the bottom strand of the DNA template. In this diagram, only two RAPD products are produced for sample one:

and $AgNO_3$ staining has been studied to reduce such faults [105]. A further drawback of RAPD markers is that most of the alleles separate out as dominant markers. Thus, the method does not help in identifying dominant homozygotes from heterozygotes. The RAPD assessment produces fragments from homozygous dominant or heterozygous alleles. No fragment is produced from homozygous recessive alleles as amplification is disturbed in both alleles. The exclusive DAF protocol is usually dissimilar to RAPD in that it operates with short primers (not less than 5 bp), two-temperature cycles in place of three-temperature cycles, high primer concentrations and identification of amplification product on $AgNO_3$ stained polyacrylamide gel. The main characteristics of the AP-PCR procedure compared with RAPD and DAF are:

- The whole amplification reaction is separated into three steps, each with different rigors and concentrations of constituents.
- Primers of 20 or more nucleotides, initially designed for other purposes (e.g. sequencing primers), are chosen randomly.
- High primer concentrations are employed in the first cycles.
- Investigation of amplification products encompasses radioactivity and auto-radiography [120].
- Product A is formed by PCR amplification of the DNA sequence which lies in between the primers bound at positions two and five.
- Product B is formed by PCR amplification of the DNA sequence which lies in between the primers bound at positions three and six.

No PCR product is produced by the primers bound at positions one and four as these primers are too far apart to allow the successful completion of the PCR reaction. Also, no PCR products are produced by the primers bound at positions four and two or positions five and three as these primer pairs are not directed towards each other. For sample two, the primer failed to anneal at position two and the PCR product was finally achieved only for primers bound at positions three and six.

2.12.2.2 Amplified fragment length polymorphism (AFLP)

The AFLP procedure combines the potential of RFLP with the agility of the PCR-based technique by ligating primer recognition sequences (adaptors) to the restricted DNA. The significant feature of AFLP is its potential for 'genome representation': the simultaneous assortment of characteristic DNA regions dispersed randomly all over the genome. AFLP markers can be generated for DNA of any individual devoid of original outflow in primer/probe growth and sequence investigation. Correspondingly high-quality and partly degraded DNA can be employed for digestion; however, the DNA should be free from restriction enzyme and PCR inhibitors. Complete reports of the AFLP technique have been evidenced by several workers [121]. The preliminary step in AFLP analysis involves restriction digestion of genomic DNA (about 500 ng). This is attained by a blend of occasional cutter (EcoRI or PstI) and regular cutter (MseI or TaqI) restriction enzymes (figure 2.7). Then double-stranded oligonucleotide adaptors are created in such a way that the primary restriction site is not re-established after ligation. These double-stranded oligonucleotide adaptors are ligated to both ends of the fragments to present identified sequences for PCR amplification. As stated by [122], CR amplification will only occur where the primers are able to anneal to fragments with the adaptor sequences, and the complimentary base pairs to the further nucleotides called selective nucleotides. Afterwards an aliquot is permitted to two successive PCR amplifications in very harsh conditions with primers complimentary to the adaptors and retaining 3′ selective nucleotides of 1–3 bases (figure 2.9) [122]. The first PCR (pre-amplification) is performed with primer combinations with a single bp extension while final (selective) amplification is performed through primer pairs with up to 3 bp extension. Due to the high selectivity, primers fluctuating by only a single base in the AFLP extension augment a different subset of fragments. Generally, primer extension of one, two or three bases reduces the number of amplified fragments by factors of 4, 16 and 64, respectively.

Suitable primer extension lengths will vary with the genome dimension of the species and will result in an optimal number of bands. This means not too many bands are available to cause high levels of band co-migration during electrophoresis, nevertheless it is sufficient to produce adequate polymorphism [122]. With the assistance of autoradiography AFLP fragments are identified either on agarose gel or on denaturing polyacrylamide gels. This can be attained by $AgNO_3$ staining (figure 2.9) or automatic DNA sequencers. Polyacrylamide gel electrophoresis (PAGE) presents the utmost resolution of AFLP banding arrangements to the level of single-nucleotide length differences, while fragment length differences of less than ten nucleotides are challenging to score on agarose gels. To facilitate automatic AFLP product separation through fluorescent detection systems on DNA sequences, such as the ABI Prism (genetic analyzer), one of the selective primers must be labeled with multiple colored dyes (e.g. fluorophore) at the 5′ end, such as tetrachloro-6-carboxy-fluorescine, hexachloro-6-carboxy-fluorescine, 6-carboxy-fluorescine, etc. Only fragments holding a priming site analogous to the fluorophore labeled primer will be observed by the sequencers. Generally, there are four basic elements of fluorescence detection systems:

- A detector that records emission photons and produces a recordable output, usually as an electrical signal or a photographic image.
- A fluorophore.
- An excitation source.
- Wavelength filters to separate emission photons from excitation photons.

Albeit its potential uses, the compatibility of these four elements is compulsory for manipulating fluorescence recognition. From three to nine different reactions labeled with different dyes can be multiplexed and loaded in a single lane or in a single injection for attaining high-throughput investigation. To govern the size of AFLP amplification fragments using computer programs, an internal size standard labeled in a different color must be loaded (e.g. GeneScan and GeneMapper software from PE Applied Biosystems). AFLP investigation is not that much

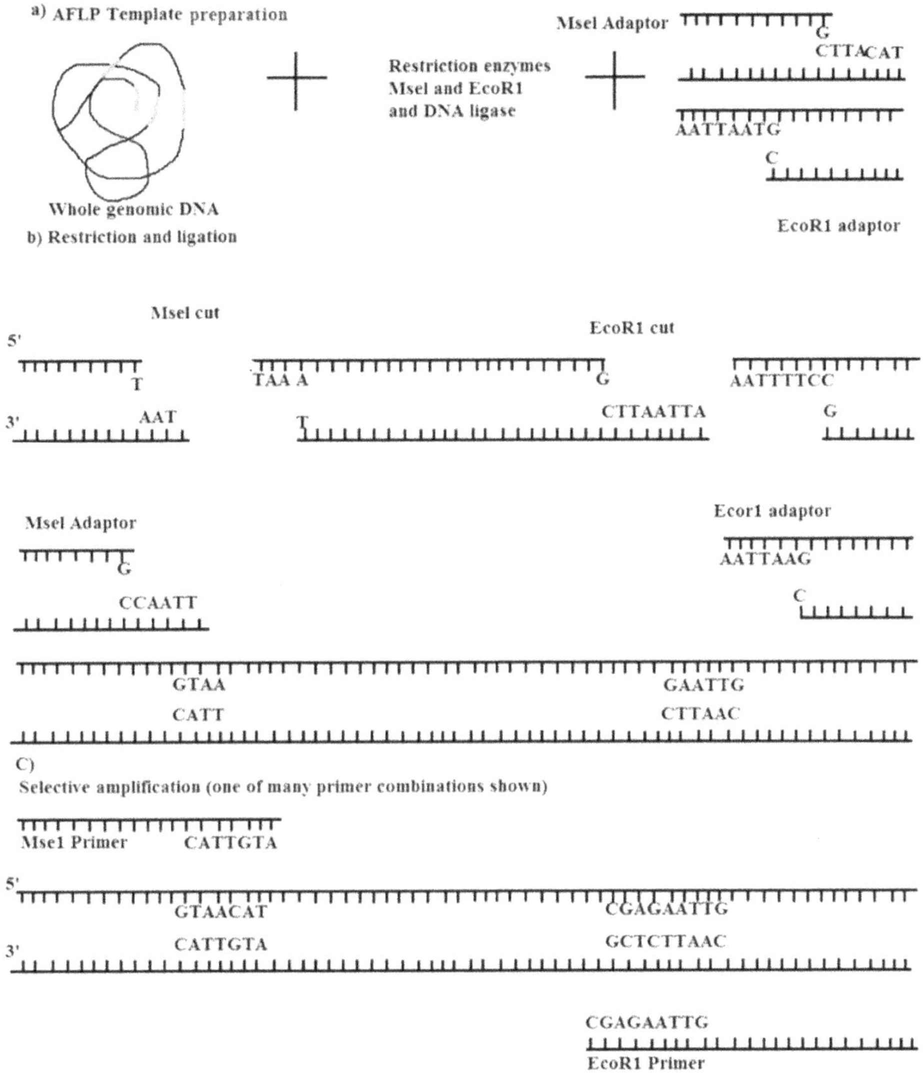

Figure 2.9. Sequential events involved in AFLP analysis. First, a small amount of DNA is digested with two restriction enzymes this is followed by ligating with adaptors to these ends. The end sequences of each adapted fragment consist of the adaptor sequence and rest portion of the restriction sequence. Primers are extended into the anonymous part of the fragments (highlighted base pairs) to accomplish amplification of a subset of these fragments. This extension is generally accomplished by one to three random assortments of bases ahead of the restriction site. Initial PCR (pre-amplification) is achieved by single-bp extension, followed by a more selective primer with up to a 3 bp extension [123].

simpler to accomplish than RAPD but is more capable than RFLP. AFLP has some basic benefits such as:

- Co-migrating AFLP amplification products are characteristically homologous and locus-specific [124], with exceptions in polyploidy species.

- It does not require any DNA sequence data from the individual under investigation.
- It is highly consistent and reproducible [125].
- It is information-rich due to its capability to study a huge number of polymorphic loci at the same time (effective multiplex ratio) with a single primer combination on a single gel in contrast to microsatellites, RAPD and RFLP [126].

2.12.2.3 Inter-simple sequence repeat (ISSR)

The ISSR method involves the amplification of DNA segments existing at an amplifiable distance between two similar microsatellite replicate regions aligned in opposite directions (figure 2.10). ISSR exploits microsatellites as primers in single-primer PCR reactions, pinpointing multiple genomic loci to amplify principally inter-SSRs of different sizes. In this procedure microsatellite recurrences exploited as primers for ISSRs can be dinucleotide, trinucleotide, tetranucleotide or pentanucleotide. The primers engaged can both be unanchored [70] or more usually anchored. These primers are anchored at the 3′ or 5′ end with 1–4 degenerate bases extended into the flanking sequences [60], see figure 2.10. ISSRs favor longer primers (15–30 mers) unlike RAPD primers (10 mers), which allows the consecutive utilization of a high annealing temperature resulting in higher inflexibility. The annealing temperature is dependent on the GC content of the primer employed and ranges from 45 °C–65 °C. The amplified fragments obtained are usually 200–2000 bp long and open to investigation by both polyacrylamide and agarose gel electrophoresis. ISSRs disclose the specificity of microsatellite markers; however, they require no sequence information for primer creation aided by the benefit of random markers [127]. It is widely acknowledged that primers are not registered and can be produced by any person. This method is simple and rapid, and the use of radioactivity is not essential. Unlike the other approaches, ISSR markers usually validate high polymorphism [128], but the phase of polymorphism has been found to differ depending on the detection methodology utilized. As demonstrated by recent developments in DNA marker science, polyacrylamide gel electrophoresis (PAGE) together with radioactivity was shown to be the most sensitive, followed by PAGE with $AgNO_3$ staining, followed by agarose gel with the EtBr system of detection.

Comparable to RAPD, the homology of co-migrating amplification products, dominant inheritance and reproducibility are the main limitations of ISSR. A reproducibility level of more than 99% after executing consistent examinations for ISSR markers was reported by Fang and Roose (1997) [129]. This was accomplished by using DNA specimens of the same cultivar developed in diverse locations. In this study DNA was initially separated from different aged leaves of the comparable individual, and by performing distinct PCR runs, while in another study the reproducibility of ISSR amplification products varied from 86%–94%, with the maximum individual, when polyacrylamide gel electrophoresis and $AgNO_3$ staining were employed and weak bands excluded from counting [130]. ISSRs separate typically as dominant markers [131], but co-dominant separation has been studied in

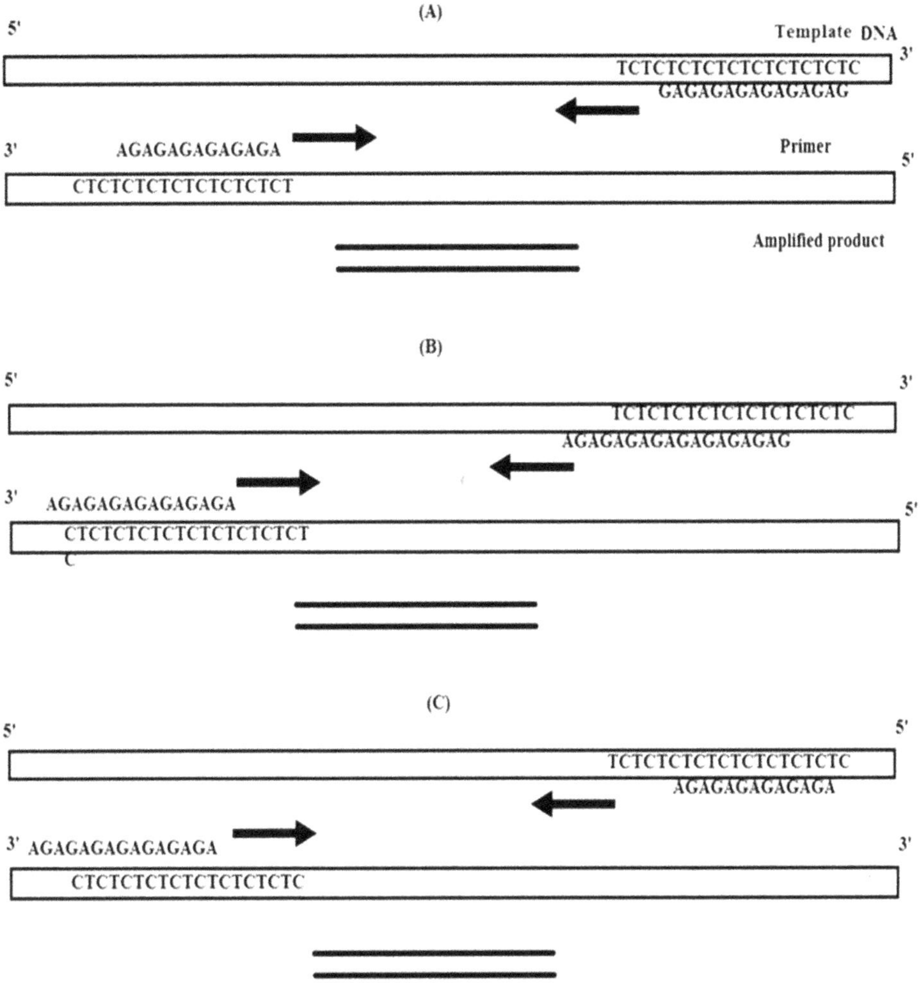

Figure 2.10. A plan illustration of ISSR-PCR with a single primer (AG)8, unanchored (A), 3′-anchored (B) and 5′-anchored (C) targeting a (TC)n repeat used to augment an inter-simple sequence repeat region flanked by two inversely oriented (TC)n sequences [91].

some cases [132]. One more alternative lies in RAPD, that fragments with the same mobility are instigated from non-homologous regions [133].

2.12.2.4 Microsatellites

A higher organism's genome contains three types of copies of simple repeated DNA sequences (mini-satellites, satellite DNAs and microsatellites) organized in a range of markedly varying size [91]. Microsatellites [134], also known as short tandem repeats (STRs) or simple sequence length polymorphisms (SSLPs) [135], SSRs, are the smallest class of simple repetitive DNA sequences. Some scientists [136] describe microsatellites as 1–6 or even 1–5 bp repeats [137], others [138] as 2–8 bp repeats. Throughout their investigation, Chambers and MacAvoy (2000) established a strict description of 2–6 bp repeats, in line with parameters used by scientists [139]. Microsatellites are described as originating from sites in which variants of simple repetitive DNA sequence subjects are over characterized [140]. Recent DNA research has found that the principal mutation mechanism in microsatellite tracts is 'slipped-strand mispairing' [141]. Slipped-strand mispairing was well described by Eisen (1999), who said that when slipped-strand mispairing is present within a microsatellite range during DNA production, it can result in either the gain or loss of one or more repeat units depending upon whether the newly produced DNA chain loops out or the template chain loops out, correspondingly [142]. This sort of relative inclination for either chain to loop out seems to depend in part on the sequences structuring the collection, and in part on whether the incident occurs on the lagging (discontinuous DNA synthesis) or leading (continuous DNA synthesis) strand [143]. Thus, SSR allelic variations are the result of differing quantities of repeat units within the microsatellite structure and this repeated sequence is often simple, containing two, three or four nucleotides. A superlative case of a microsatellite is a dinucleotide repeat $(CA)n$, where n signifies the whole number of repeats that lie between 10 and 100. These markers often present high levels of inter- and intra-specific polymorphism, particularly while the tandem repeat number is ten or greater [144]. Due to the repetitive nature of microsatellite markers, they are prone to causing errors during sequencing. They are preferentially used for high resolution genetic analysis as a molecular marker widely used for genetic analysis of cultivated plants. They can detect a large number of alleles in a population, thus they can be used for studying genetic diversity, population structure, relatedness among individuals or population. There has been advancement in analysis and characterization of microsatellite markers. The traditional Sanger's method and use of genomic libraries enriched with microsatellite sequence are replaced with *in-silico* analysis and next-generation sequencing [145].

2.12.2.5 Expressed sequence tags (EST)

It is widely acknowledged that every gene must be transcribed into messenger RNA (mRNA) that functions as a pattern for protein synthesis. During this procedure the mRNA guides subsequent protein synthesis through a process called translation. One obstruction of this biological process is that messenger RNA is very unstable outside of a cell, therefore scientists employ an enzyme called reverse transcriptase to translate mRNA to complementary DNA (cDNA). Complementary DNA production is the reverse of the biological process of transcription in cells, as this natural process employs messenger RNA as a pattern rather than DNA. Complementary DNA is a stable compound and presents only the expressed DNA sequence as it is produced from mRNA that presents exons by splicing introns. After the separation of cDNA representing an expressed gene, scientists can sequence a few hundred nucleotides from both the $5'$ or $3'$ end to create $5'$ expressed sequence tags (ESTs) and $3'$ ESTs, correspondingly. A $5'$ EST is obtained from the segment of a transcript (exons) that is usually programmed for a protein and sites that have a tendency to be conserved across species and do not change a lot inside a gene family. The $3'$ ESTs are anticipated to come under non-coding (introns) or untranslated regions (UTRs), and therefore have a tendency to establish less cross-species preservation than do coding sequences. EST sequencing is mainly used to identify and sequence the expressed gene in an organism. In plant genomics, it provides valuable insights into gene expression pattern, functional annotation, transcriptome analysis and molecular marker development. To generate ESTs the cDNA libraries are prepared. Each cDNA clone is sequenced using automated sequence, typically from one end of the clone. The resulting short nucleotide DNA sequence represents a portion of a transcribed region of the corresponding gene [146]. The main challenge associated with recognizing genes from genomic sequences is variation between organisms which is dependent upon genome size as well as the presence or absence of introns. These introns are the dominant DNA sequences disrupting the protein coding sequence of a gene.

2.12.2.6 Cleaved amplified polymorphic sequence (CAPS)

The cleaved amplified polymorphic sequence (CAPS) procedure is a combination of PCR and RFLP techniques and was previously called PCR-RFLP [147]. This method comprises amplification of a target DNA through PCR, later pursued by digesting with restriction enzymes [148]. Thus, CAPS markers rely on differences in restriction enzyme digestion patterns of PCR fragments caused by nucleotide polymorphism among different specimens. The main stages involved in the CAPS marker methodology are DNA isolation followed by PCR and the quantity or allocation of polymorphic sites. To perform cleaved amplified polymorphic sequence protocol, one needs to design a primer pair that amplifies fragments ranging from 1000 bp to 1500 bp consisting of sequence-tagged sites (STSs). After PCR amplification, screening and detection of the polymorphism can be performed using a different combination of STSs and restriction endonuclease. The resulting CAPS markers can be used for construction of linkage mapping that shows the position of the CAPS marker location on chromosomes. The analysis of polymorphism helps in understanding functional diversity and genetic aspects of the CAPS marker [149]. The CAPS marker method displays several merits: it is much simpler and less time-consuming in comparison to examining other types of markers including Southern hybridizations. Moreover, CAPS primers produced from ESTs are more important as genetic markers for relative mapping studies than those markers derived from non-functional sequences, e.g. genomic microsatellite markers. In addition to its afore mentioned advantages, CAPS markers are inherited mainly in a co-dominant manner [150]. Nevertheless, the potential of CAPS to identify DNA polymorphism is not as high as with SSR and AFLP, as nucleotide differences influencing restriction sites are required for the evaluation of DNA polymorphism by CAPS. Additionally, the development of CAPS markers is only possible where mutations interject or produce a restriction enzyme recognition site. Some researchers have produced auxiliary markers termed derived-CAPS (dCAPS) that eliminate the problem linked with CAPS markers by generating mismatches in a PCR primer, which are subsequently employed to produce a polymorphism based on the target mutation [151].

2.12.2.7 Sequence-characterized amplified region (SCAR)
SCAR is a genomic DNA fragment which is identified by PCR amplification by means of a pair of specific oligonucleotide primers [77]. SCARs are acquired by cloning and sequencing the two ends of RAPD markers that seem to be relevant for particular uses, such as a RAPD band present in disease-resistant lines that is not present in susceptible lines. SCARs are advantageous over RAPD markers as their amplification is not very sensitive to reaction conditions, they can possibly be transformed into co-dominant markers and can recognize only a single locus [77]. SCAR is highly efficient and sensitive; it requires only a small amount of DNA samples to develop the marker. SCAR markers allow for effective and reliable differentiation of plant species that are morphologically similar. It also can be used in traditional medicine to detect specific species in both homogeneous and heterogeneous formulations. These markers can correlate DNA fingerprinting data with quantity of selected phytochemical marker associated with a specific medicinal herb. SCAR markers are a qualitative and quantitative diagnostic tool for quality control of active phytochemicals in plant material for pharmaceutical purpose [152]. SCAR primers are used to identify and quantify specific bacteria in the plant rhizosphere. These primers are designed to target specific DNA sequences that are unique to desired strains [153].

2.12.2.8 Sequence-tagged site (STS)
The STS is a short stretch of DNA ranging from 200–300 base pairs in length, that has unique sequences and can be amplified using PCR. This region has numerous applications in genetic research and analysis. It can be used to detect microdeletions in specific genes, and to identify the genetic variation within and between populations. It serves as reference points for physical mapping data and contributes to construct a genetic map. It is used in genome analysis to map a gene of interest, and analyze structure and organization of the genome. The technique has wide use in forensic analysis, which involves a unique STS pattern of each individual [154]. Previous researchers [80] reported STSs as DNA markers in the corporal mapping of the human genome, and later they were identified in plants. An STS is a small, elite sequence whose correct sequence is found nowhere else in the genome. Two or more clones with related STSs must overlap and the overlap must contain STSs.

2.12.2.9 Single-nucleotide polymorphism (SNP)
According to previous studies SNP is the most common type of genetic variation between different individuals. Every SNP presents an alteration in a single DNA building block, known as a nucleotide. The best example is an SNP that substitutes the nucleotide cytosine (C) with the nucleotide thymine (T) in a definite stretch of DNA. SNPs take typically place throughout an individual's DNA. This occurs in every 300 nucleotides on average, i.e. there are approximately 10 million SNPs in the human genome. Most often, these variations are reported in the DNA between genes. They can function as biological markers, helping scientists locate genes that are linked with ailments. When SNPs take place within a gene or in a monitoring region near a gene, they can display a direct role in a syndrome by manipulating the gene's function.

Most SNPs have no effect on health or growth. Several genetic variations, however, have been found to be very important in the study of individual health. Researchers have exposed SNP's potential to support forecasting of an individual's response to specific drugs, their susceptibility to environmental factors, e.g. toxins, and their threat of developing certain diseases. SNPs can also be employed to track the inheritance of disease genes inside families. Future investigations will try to identify SNPs associated with complex diseases, e.g. heart disease, diabetes and cancer. A few methods that are used for determining individual SNPs' genotyping are gel-based assays such as AFLP and RFLP based assay, single-strand conformation polymorphism (SSCP) assay. Allele-specific amplification of SNP genotyping and non-gel-based assays are based on the SNP site present in amplicon for that direct DNA sequencing and variant detector arrays techniques are used [155].

2.12.2.10 Diversity arrays technology (DArT)

Diversity arrays technology (DarT) is one of the most newly established molecular methods and its discoverers promoted it as an open source (non-exclusive) technology with great potential for genetic assortment and mapping investigations in several 'orphan' crops applicable in Third World countries. A DArT marker is a DNA fragment, existing or absent in a demarcated genomic representation, relying on the individual genotype. It is a microarray hybridization-based procedure that allows the concurrent inputting of several hundred polymorphic loci distributed over the genome [65]. The particulars of the procedure for DArT were initially explained by Jaccoud *et al* in 2001 (figure 2.11) [65]. Genomic demonstration is completed by a

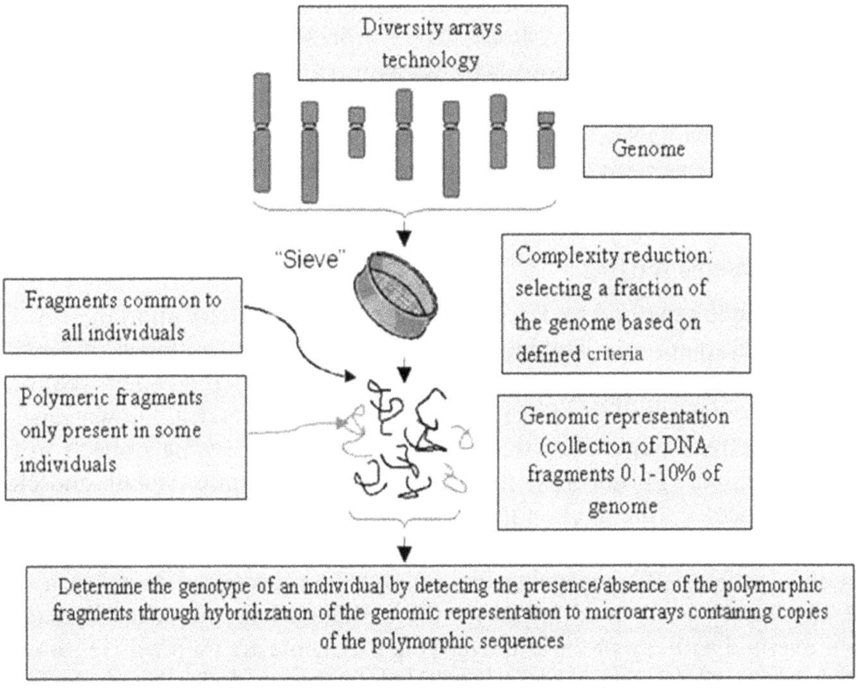

Figure 2.11. Principle of DArT.

precise fraction of the genome, formed in a reproducible fashion by applying to the genome a complexity reduction technique. For each person's DNA specimen being typed, genomic representations are organized by restriction enzyme digestion of genomic DNA, followed by joining of restriction fragments to adapters. Genomic representations employed in DArT generally contain 0.1%–10% of the genome relying on the initial complexity of the organism. There are various potential procedures to offer a genomic representation of suitable complexity.

2.13 Genomic library screening methods

Genetic broadcast is one of the most potent methodologies accessible for gaining insights into complex biological processes [65]. The main use of the cloning technique is to separate a specific gene from the complete genome. For a 99% possibility of attaining one fragment for each clone, 1500 cloned fragments are required with *Escherichia coli*, 4600 with yeast, and 800 000 with mammals. Procedures such as chromosomal walking and colony hybridization [156] are usually utilized for choosing a specific genome as follows.

2.13.1 Colony hybridization

This is a type of DNA hybridization in which a radioactive probe is used to detect a DNA sequence on a nitrocellulose filter. Sometimes this is also called a 'colony filter' because in this process a filter is placed on the surface of agar plate and bacterial colonies are transferred to grow on the filter. In this method there is no need to purify the DNA from bacterial cells as bacterial colonies are directly grown and lyse on the nitrocellulose filters [156]. During lysing (alkali hydrolysis) DNA is denatured and binds directly to the filter. Radioactive probes are added to the filter disks. Hybridization takes place followed by washing of the filter to remove unbound probes [156]. The colonies that contain sequences complementary to the probe will bind the radioactive DNA. Hybridized probes can be visualized when the resulting filters are exposed to x-ray film. Finally, the desired colonies will be lit up on the autoradiograph.

2.13.2 Chromosome walking

Primer walking is a method to determine the sequence of DNA up to the 1.3–7.0 kb range, while chromosome walking is employed to generate clones of previously known sequences of the gene. Chromosome walking is a method employed to clone a gene (e.g. disease genes) from its identified closest markers (e.g. known genes) and thus is used in reasonable alterations in cloning and sequencing projects in fungi, plants and animals. Particularly, it is employed to recognize, isolate and clone a specific sequence existing in close proximity to the gene to be mapped. Libraries of bulky fragments, mostly bacterial artificial chromosome libraries, are typically used in genomic projects. To recognize the anticipated colony and to select a certain clone, the library is screened initially with a preferred probe. After selection, the clone is overlaid with the probe and overlying fragments are mapped. These sections are then employed as a new probe (short DNA fragments derived from the 39 or 59

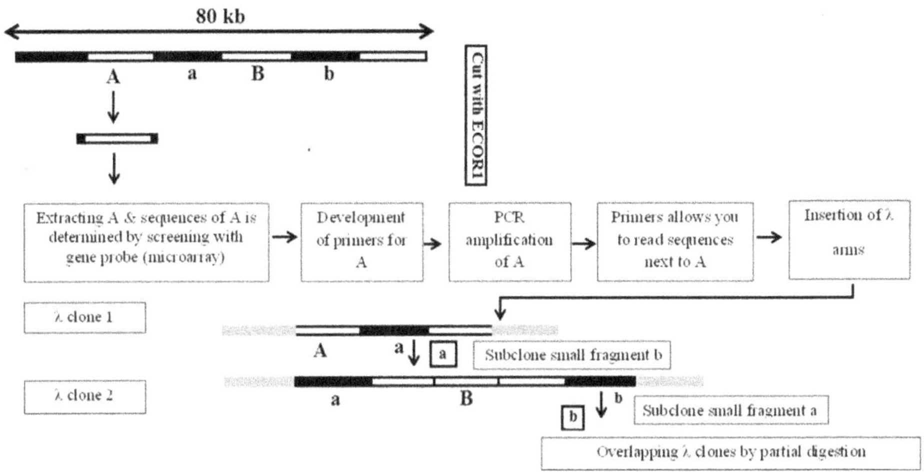

Figure 2.12. Protocol for chromosomal walking of DNA.

ends of clones) to recognize other clones. A library consists of 96 clones and each clone covers a different insert. Probe one recognizes λ1 and λ2 as it overlays them (figure 2.12). Probe two obtained from λ2 clones is employed to recognize λ3, and so on. Placement of the clones is evaluated by restriction mapping of the clones. Therefore, new chromosomal regions existing in the locality of a gene can be identified. The procedure for chromosomal walking of DNA is explained in figure 2.12. As chromosomal walking is very monotonous, chromosome landing is favored for gene documentation. This strategy entails the recognition of the marker that is closely associated with the mutant locus [157].

2.13.3 Blotting techniques

In molecular biology and genetics, a blot is the process of transporting proteins, DNA or RNA, on a carrier (nitrocellulose polyvinylidene fluoride or nylon membrane). Blotting includes four main steps:

- Immobilization of samples (nucleic acid, proteins) on a solid support (nylon or nitrocellulose membranes).
- Electrophoretic identification of nucleic acids in a gel.
- Allocation of the separated components to a membrane.
- Detection of particular sequences by probing the membrane.

Transfer and immobilization on the membrane make the nucleic acids accessible to probes used for recognition, which do not freely enter the gel. Southern and Northern blotting are the two most common nucleic acid blotting methods. Southern blotting is used to distinguish a sequence in a DNA mixture, and Northern blotting identifies a sequence in an RNA mixture. By contrast, western blotting is employed for the identification of proteins.

2.13.4 Southern blot analysis

British biologist Edwin Southern [98] developed a technique for identifying DNA fragments in an agarose gel by blotting on a nylon or nitrocellulose membrane followed by detection with a probe of complementary DNA or RNA sequence [98]. In this technique, DNA molecules are fragmented by restriction endonucleases and DNA sections are segregated on the basis of their size by agarose gel electrophoresis. DNA sections are denatured by alkali action and relocated to a nitrocellulose filter after their immobilization by heat treatment. Filter paper containing DNA fragments is incubated with radiolabeled probes in a buffer solution. Hybridized DNA can be visualized by autoradiography. The blotting procedure has not changed since it was first described, except for the accessibility of increasingly sophisticated blotting membranes, kits for labeling and apparatus for electrophoresis transfer. Membranes initially employed for DNA transfer were made of nitrocellulose. Owing to their high nucleic-acid-binding capacity and physical strength, nylon-based membranes are preferred.

2.13.4.1 Principle

For many years, scientists have been aware of the DNA-binding properties of nitrocellulose powder and sheets. This knowledge was put to practical use in the 1950s and 1960s for various nucleic acid hybridization studies. During these early techniques, the DNA that was immobilized on nitrocellulose was unsorted and essentially consisted of total DNA that had been either bound to nitrocellulose powder or applied as spots on nitrocellulose sheets.

In the early 1970s, the introduction of gel electrophoresis methods allowed for the separation of DNA restriction fragments based on their size. This advancement prompted the development of techniques for transferring these separated DNA fragments in bulk from the gel to a nitrocellulose support. The method described by Southern in 1975 involved the capillary transfer of DNA from the gel to a nitrocellulose sheet placed on top of it. This method was straightforward and efficient. Although it has been refined over the years, the original procedure remains largely unchanged and is still commonly employed in many molecular biology laboratories [158].

2.13.4.2 Methodology

The original technique for Southern blotting, as depicted in figure 2.13, involves several key steps. An agarose electrophoresis gel containing the separated restriction fragments is positioned on a filter paper wick that acts as a bridge between the gel and a reservoir of high-salt buffer. On top of the gel, a nitrocellulose membrane is carefully placed, and the entire setup is covered with a stack of paper towels secured by a weight.

Capillary action comes into play as the high-salt buffer travels through the filter paper wick, the gel, and eventually reaches the nitrocellulose membrane, continuing its path into the layers of paper towels. During this process, the DNA

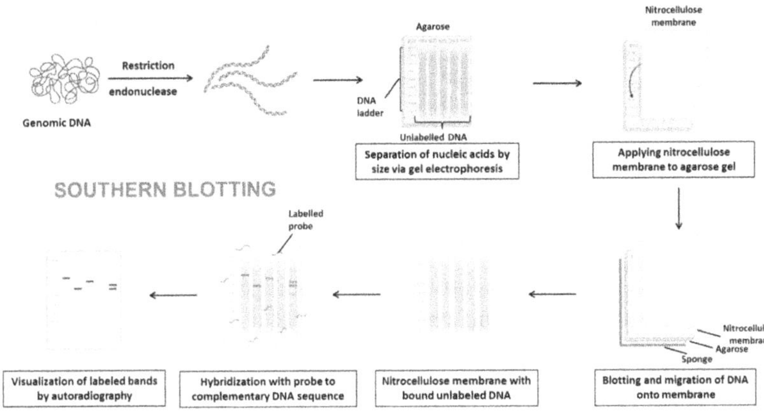

Figure 2.13. Diagrammatic representation of Southern blotting technique.

fragments are carried along with the buffer and become firmly bound to the nitrocellulose membrane.

The effective transfer of DNA fragments, even those as long as 15 kilobases (kb), typically requires approximately 18 h, which is roughly equivalent to leaving the setup to work overnight. The primary technical concern to address is the potential for the buffer to bypass the gel and travel directly from the wick to the paper towels. However, this can be minimized by assembling the setup with care to ensure proper capillary transfer [159].

2.13.4.3 Recent modifications in Southern blotting

Recent advancements in Southern blotting have introduced several modifications to improve the technique's efficiency and sensitivity. Some of these include:

1. Transfer methods: While the original Southern blotting technique relied on capillary action, newer methods, such as vacuum blotting or electroblotting, have been developed. These techniques offer faster and more controlled transfer of DNA fragments from the gel to the membrane.
2. Membrane options: Traditional nitrocellulose membranes have been supplemented with alternatives like nylon membranes. Nylon membranes are more robust and offer increased binding capacity, allowing for better retention of DNA fragments.
3. Probe labeling: Enhanced probe labeling techniques, such as using non-radioactive labels like biotin or digoxigenin, have gained popularity. These labels provide a safer and more environmentally friendly alternative to radioactive labeling while maintaining high sensitivity.
4. Hybridization methods: Hybridization conditions have been optimized to increase the specificity of probe binding. Stringency washes can be adjusted to reduce non-specific binding, resulting in cleaner and more accurate results.
5. Detection systems: Newer detection systems, such as chemiluminescent or fluorescent detection, have largely replaced autoradiography. These methods are more sensitive and allow for the quantification of signal intensity.

6. Automated systems: Automation has streamlined the Southern blotting process, reducing the risk of human error and increasing throughput. Automated systems can perform the various steps of Southern blotting, from gel preparation to detection, with greater efficiency.
7. Computer analysis: Advances in computer software have enabled the digital analysis of Southern blots. Quantification and data analysis can be done with greater precision and speed, reducing the need for manual interpretation.
8. Multiplexing: Researchers can now perform multiplex Southern blotting, allowing the simultaneous analysis of multiple DNA targets in a single experiment, saving time and resources.

These recent modifications have made Southern blotting more reliable, faster, and adaptable to a wider range of applications, making it a valuable tool in molecular biology and genetic research.

2.13.4.4 Applications of Southern blotting

Southern blotting is a versatile molecular biology technique with several valuable applications:

1. Gene identification: It is used to identify specific genes in complex genomes. Researchers can probe DNA samples to locate genes of interest and study their organization.
2. Genomic mapping: Southern blotting assists in mapping the arrangement of genes or specific DNA sequences within a genome. This aids in understanding gene order and organization.
3. Copy number variation analysis: Southern blotting can be employed to determine the copy number of a specific DNA sequence, which is crucial in studies related to gene dosage and gene amplification.
4. DNA methylation analysis: It can be used to assess DNA methylation patterns, helping in the study of epigenetic modifications and their role in gene regulation.
5. Genetic testing: Southern blotting is utilized in medical genetics for detecting genetic mutations and identifying carriers of certain genetic disorders.
6. Forensic analysis: In forensics, it can be applied to identify individuals through DNA fingerprinting, which relies on variable number tandem repeats (VNTRs).
7. Transgene detection: Southern blotting can be used to confirm the integration of transgenes in genetically modified organisms.

2.13.4.5 Limitations of Southern blotting

Despite its utility, Southern blotting has some limitations:

1. Time-consuming: The technique is relatively time-consuming, taking up to two days to complete, which can hinder rapid analysis.
2. Radioactive labels: The use of radioactive probes in traditional Southern blotting poses safety and disposal issues. Although non-radioactive labels are available, they may be less sensitive.

3. Low sensitivity: In some cases, Southern blotting may lack the sensitivity required to detect low-abundance DNA sequences, especially when dealing with small sample amounts.
4. Fragment size: The method is not ideal for very large DNA fragments, and the transfer efficiency may vary for different-sized fragments.
5. High DNA purity: Southern blotting necessitates high-quality DNA samples, and impurities can interfere with the results.
6. Semi-quantitative: It provides a qualitative or semi-quantitative assessment of DNA, making it less suitable for precise quantification.
7. Labor-intensive: The technique demands careful handling and multiple steps, which can lead to experimental errors if not executed meticulously.

Despite these limitations, Southern blotting remains a fundamental tool in molecular biology and genetics for its ability to provide valuable insights into DNA structure and organization. Researchers often use it in conjunction with other, more rapid techniques to complement its strengths and overcome its limitations [160]. A diagrammatic representation of Southern blotting is given in figure 2.13.

2.13.5 Northern blot analysis

This methodology was explored by James Alwine *et al* in 1977 [161] at Stanford University. The procedures used in Southern and Northern blotting studies are similar, except that RNA rather than DNA is blotted on the membrane. Northern blot includes the blotting of RNA separated by gel electrophoresis on nylon or nitrocellulose membranes followed by hybridization with nucleic acid (RNA or DNA) sequences. Blotting is executed in such a way that the maximum sum of RNA sequences is bound covalently on chemically sensitive paper. The RNA was blotted/immobilized on diazotized cellulose. As with Southern blotting, Northern hybridization does not require denaturation of DNA before blotting, this makes the procedure less time-consuming.

2.13.5.1 Principle

The principle of northern blotting is to analyze and study RNA molecules based on their size, abundance, and specific sequences [162]. This technique is named after its similarity to Southern blotting, which is used for DNA analysis. Northern blotting involves several key steps:

1. RNA isolation: The first step is to extract the RNA of interest from a biological sample. This can be total RNA or specific RNA fractions, depending on the research question. The RNA is typically isolated using methods like phenol-chloroform extraction or commercially available RNA isolation kits.
2. RNA denaturation and gel electrophoresis: The extracted RNA is denatured (heated to break the secondary structure) and then separated by size through gel electrophoresis. Agarose or denaturing polyacrylamide gels are

commonly used, with the choice depending on the size range of RNA molecules being analyzed.
3. Transfer to membrane: After electrophoresis, the separated RNA molecules are transferred from the gel onto a solid support membrane. Nitrocellulose or nylon membranes are commonly used for this purpose. This transfer can be achieved through capillary action, using a method similar to Southern blotting.
4. Hybridization with probe: A labeled RNA probe, which is complementary to the RNA sequence of interest, is used to detect and bind specifically to the target RNA molecules on the membrane. The probe is typically labeled with radioactive, fluorescent, or non-radioactive markers.
5. Washing and detection: After hybridization, the membrane is washed to remove any unbound probe. The presence of the labeled RNA probe bound to the RNA molecules of interest is then detected, depending on the type of label used. For radioactive probes, autoradiography is commonly employed, while non-radioactive labels may require chemiluminescence or fluorescence detection.
6. Analysis and interpretation: The resulting image or data reveals the size and abundance of the target RNA molecules. By comparing the position and intensity of the bands on the membrane to a standard ladder or control samples, researchers can determine the size and relative expression levels of specific RNA species.

The key principle of northern blotting is to provide information about the RNA molecules in a sample, including their size and expression patterns. This technique has been widely used in molecular biology for gene expression analysis, RNA splicing studies, and other applications that require the characterization of RNA molecules in a biological sample.

2.13.5.2 Applications of northern blotting

1. Gene expression analysis: Northern blotting is used to determine the expression levels of specific genes in different tissues, developmental stages, or under varying experimental conditions. It provides valuable information about which genes are transcribed and to what extent.
2. RNA splicing studies: Researchers can investigate alternative splicing patterns of pre-mRNA by examining the size and abundance of different RNA isoforms. This helps in understanding how different protein variants are produced from the same gene.
3. Post-transcriptional modifications: Northern blotting can reveal information about post-transcriptional modifications and processing of RNA molecules, such as precursor and mature forms, which is essential for understanding RNA maturation processes.
4. Validation of RNA sequencing (RNA-Seq) data: Northern blots can be used to validate the results of high-throughput techniques like RNA-Seq,

providing a more direct confirmation of the presence and size of specific RNA species.

5. Quantitative analysis: Although it is generally less quantitative than modern methods like quantitative PCR (qPCR) or RNA-Seq, Northern blotting can still provide some semi-quantitative data on the relative abundance of specific RNA molecules.

2.13.5.3 Limitations of northern blotting

1. Time-consuming: Northern blotting is a time-consuming process, often taking one to two days to complete, which makes it less suitable for high-throughput applications.
2. RNA quality: The technique requires high-quality RNA samples, and RNA degradation can affect the results. Contaminants, such as DNA or proteins, can also interfere with the analysis.
3. Sensitivity: While it is suitable for the detection of abundant RNA species, northern blotting may lack the sensitivity to detect low-abundance RNA molecules, especially when dealing with small sample amounts.
4. Labor-intensive: The method involves multiple steps, each of which requires careful handling and attention to detail, increasing the risk of experimental errors.
5. Radioactive probes: While non-radioactive probes are available, the use of radioactive probes (such as 32P-labeled probes) in traditional northern blotting poses safety and disposal concerns.
6. Semi-quantitative: Although it provides some quantification, northern blotting is not as precise as qPCR or RNA-Seq for measuring RNA expression levels.

Despite these limitations, northern blotting remains a valuable tool for studying RNA molecules and gene expression, especially when used in conjunction with other complementary techniques. Researchers often choose northern blotting for its specificity and ability to provide insights into RNA processing and alternative splicing patterns [162]. A diagrammatic representation of northern blotting is given in figure 2.14.

2.13.6 Western blot analysis

This technique was introduced by Harry Towbin at the Friedrich Miescher Institute [163]. Later the name 'western blot' was given to the technique by W Neal Burnette [164]. Blotting of electrophoresis protein bands from an SDS-polyacrylamide gel onto nylon or nitrocellulose membrane and their recognition with antibody probes is known as western blotting. It is a technique by which proteins that have been substantially separated and then immobilized on the surface of a membrane are probed for reactivity with different types of affinity reagents, e.g. antibodies and receptors, and are verified for the presence of interacting proteins in pure preparations or complex mixtures. Western blot can examine any protein sample whether

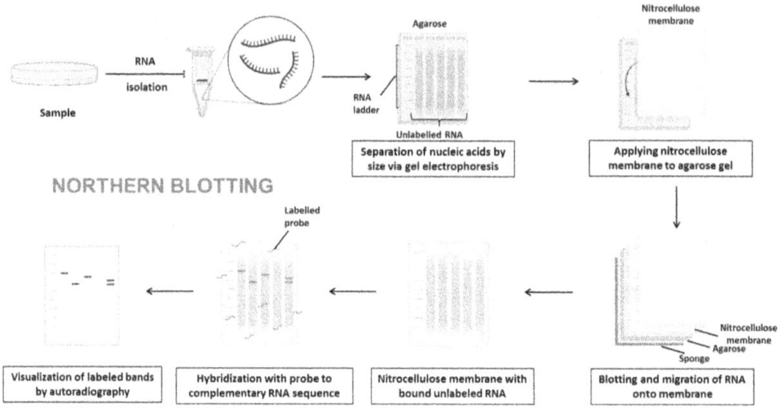

Figure 2.14. Diagrammatic representation of northern blotting.

from cells or tissues, including recombinant proteins produced *in vitro*. Western blot is reliant on the quality of the affinity reagents used to probe the protein of interest, and how specific they are to this protein. Such reagents are commercially available according to the protein of interest. Accessibility of an antibody or affinity reagent is compulsory for new proteins. For this procedure, a lesser quantity of protein (either purified from cell extracts or made as a recombinant) and its relevant antibody or affinity reagent are essential. These vigorous antibodies precisely bind to the protein of interest as an alternative to the thousands of proteins on the western blot. In the first step (electrophoresis), proteins are separated according to their variation in size, which results in the development of a series of bands. Owing to the bulky size of antibodies, a gel matrix does not permit them to enter, therefore the sample proteins are transported to a solid support. Superimposition of gel with nitrocellulose in the presence of an electric field results in the migration of proteins from the gel to the sheet where they become bound. This step provides membranes of nitrocellulose with a similar pattern of proteins as in the gel. This procedure has vast applications in the immune recognition of proteins.

2.13.6.1 Principle

Western blotting (also known as immunoblotting) is a widely used molecular biology technique for the detection and characterization of specific proteins within a complex mixture [165]. The technique derives its name from its similarity to the Southern and northern blotting techniques used for DNA and RNA analysis, respectively. Here's an overview of the principle of western blotting:

1. Protein separation: The first step in western blotting is to separate proteins from a biological sample by size using a technique called polyacrylamide gel electrophoresis (PAGE). The proteins are denatured and loaded into wells in a gel matrix, and an electric current is applied to separate them based on their molecular weight. Proteins are typically reduced and denatured before loading to ensure uniform mobility.

2. Transfer to membrane: After separation, the proteins are transferred (blotted) from the gel onto a solid support membrane, which is typically made of nitrocellulose or polyvinylidene difluoride (PVDF). This transfer can be achieved through a technique known as electroblotting, which uses an electrical current to move the proteins from the gel to the membrane.
3. Blocking: To prevent non-specific binding, the membrane is soaked in a blocking solution, often containing a protein (e.g., bovine serum albumin or non-fat dry milk). This step saturates any remaining protein-binding sites on the membrane.
4. Primary antibody incubation: The membrane is then incubated with a primary antibody that is specific to the protein of interest. The primary antibody recognizes and binds to the target protein on the membrane.
5. Washing: After the primary antibody incubation, the membrane is washed to remove any unbound primary antibody.
6. Secondary antibody incubation: A secondary antibody is applied to the membrane. This secondary antibody is conjugated with an enzyme or a fluorophore. The secondary antibody specifically binds to the primary antibody, creating a 'sandwich' with the target protein.
7. Washing: The membrane is again washed to remove any unbound secondary antibody.
8. Detection: The presence of the target protein is visualized by adding a substrate for the enzyme linked to the secondary antibody or by detecting the fluorescence signal if a fluorophore-conjugated secondary antibody was used. This results in the appearance of bands on the membrane, with each band corresponding to a specific protein.
9. Analysis: The bands on the membrane are analyzed to determine the presence, size, and relative abundance of the target protein. This analysis can be qualitative or quantitative, depending on the specific purpose of the experiment.

The western blotting technique is widely used in molecular biology and biochemistry for a variety of applications, including protein detection, protein quantification, and the study of post-translational modifications. It is a powerful tool for characterizing and confirming the presence of specific proteins in complex biological samples [165]. A diagrammatic representation of western blotting is given in figure 2.15. A comparative analysis of northern blotting, Southern blotting and western blotting is given in table 2.3.

2.13.7 Dot blot technique

This procedure is usually employed to detect, examine and identify proteins. It is a basic form of blotting procedure in which the biomolecule to be examined is not initially separated by electrophoresis. This procedure indicates the presence or absence of biomolecules that can be examined by the DNA probes or the antibody. Nevertheless, it presents no information on the size of the target biomolecules. This

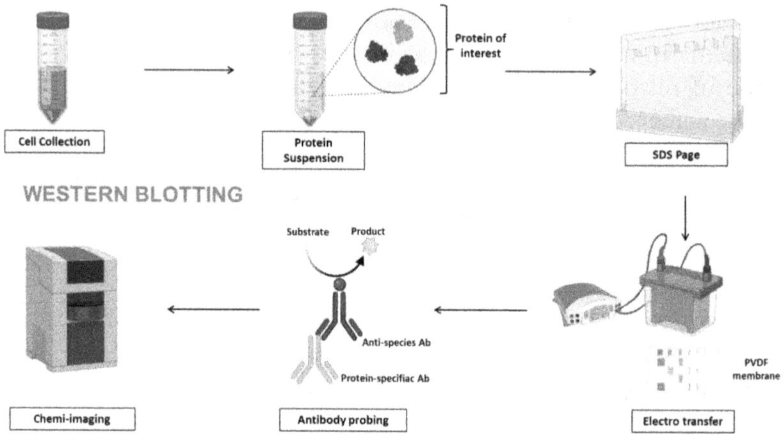

Figure 2.15. Diagrammatic representation of western blotting.

Table 2.3. Comparative study between northern blotting, Southern blotting and western blotting.

Factors	Northern blotting	Southern blotting	Western blotting
Molecule targeted	RNA	DNA	Protein
Probe used	RNA, DNA, Oligonucleotides	A nucleic acid probe which have similar sequence with the target molecule	Primary antibody
Membrane utilized	Diazobenzoxymethyl (DBM)/nylon membrane)	Nitrocellulose/nylon membrane	Nitrocellulose/PVDF membrane
Technique of separation	Agarose gel electrophoresis	Agarose gel electrophoresis/ polyacrylamide gel electrophoresis	Polyacrylamide gel electrophoresis
Techniques of blotting	Capillary transfer	Capillary transfer	Electroblotting
Methods of detection	Chemilluminescence/ colorimetry/x-ray film	Chemilluminescence/ colorimetry/x-ray film	Cooled CCD, infrared imaging
Applications	Used in gene expression studies and in diagnosis of diseases	Used in DNA mutation study and forensic	Used in identifying specific antigen present in biologicals

procedure includes application of dot and consequently hybridization and identification of proteins. DNA does not attach well to the filters; therefore it is crucial to denature the proteins. This method is both easier to apply and considerably less time-consuming than other procedures. One of the currently reported applications of this method is the detection of potato viruses and viroids, which is one of the main constraints for the development of potato (*Solanum tuberosum* L.) production globally [166]. By means of applying the dot blot procedure, spindle tuber viroids were recently discovered in potato leaf tissue.

2.13.8 Techniques for the detection of specific proteins

2.13.8.1 Hybrid-arrested translation (HART)

The procedure of recognition of rDNA clones by their capability to hybridize and avoid the translation of a specific messenger RNA in a cell-free system is called HART [167]. In this procedure, the mRNA molecule is incubated with recombinant plasmid DNA, which comprises a sequence complementary to mRNA. Consequently DNA/RNA hybrids are formed. Attraction of the mRNA acts as a probe which will pick up the clones. After positive selection, a negative selection can be executed by using mRNA from the same organisms but from a cell that does not symbolize the preferred sequence. Any positively chosen colonies that hybridize with negative probes are rejected. Even hybrids formed by positive selection could not be translated. The plasmids thus found by the probe are missing from the translation product.

Hybrid-arrested translation (HART) is a molecular biology technique used to study the translation of mRNA (messenger RNA) by ribosomes. It is a variation of the traditional translation assay that allows researchers to analyze the translational activity of specific mRNA molecules or specific regions of mRNA. HART was developed as a tool for studying the interactions between RNA and ribosomes [168].

2.13.8.2 Working principle

1. mRNA Isolation and preparation: The first step in HART involves isolating and preparing the mRNA of interest. This can be a full-length mRNA or a specific mRNA region, such as the 5′ untranslated region (UTR) or the coding region. The mRNA is typically isolated from cells or tissues.
2. RNA labeling: In HART, the mRNA is labeled with a radioactive or fluorescent marker. This label can be incorporated into the mRNA during *in vitro* transcription or added to the mRNA after isolation.
3. Translation extract preparation: A cell-free translation extract, which contains all the necessary components for protein synthesis, is prepared. This extract includes ribosomes, tRNAs, and other translation factors.
4. Hybrid formation: The labeled mRNA is mixed with the translation extract. If the labeled mRNA region has a complementary sequence to a specific antisense oligonucleotide, this oligonucleotide can be added to the mixture to form a stable RNA–DNA hybrid. The antisense oligonucleotide can be designed to target a specific region of the mRNA.

5. Translation assay: Translation of the labeled mRNA is initiated in the presence of the translation extract. The ribosomes bind to the mRNA, and translation proceeds as they move along the mRNA template. If the mRNA–DNA hybrid is formed, translation is 'arrested' at the specific location corresponding to the hybridization site.
6. Analysis: The translation products are then analyzed. Researchers can use techniques like gel electrophoresis, autoradiography (for radioactive labeling), or fluorescence detection (for fluorescent labeling) to visualize and quantify the translated products. By observing where translation was arrested, researchers can gain insights into the dynamics of translation and the interactions between ribosomes and the mRNA of interest.

HART is a valuable tool for studying various aspects of translation, including ribosome binding, translation initiation, and translation elongation. It allows researchers to investigate the roles of specific mRNA regions and their interactions with ribosomes, providing insights into the regulation of gene expression and translation [168].

2.13.8.3 Hybrid-released translation (HRT)

Many situations arise in rDNA research in which it is necessary to identify the mRNA encoded by a particular cloned DNA sequence. Cloned DNA fragments can be characterized by hybridization to mRNA, which is further identified by translation *in vitro*. There are two different approaches to this procedure: (i) hybrid-arrest translation and (ii) hybrid-release translation. In the former, hybridization of cloned DNA to an mRNA population in solution can be used to identify the complementary mRNA, since the mRNA/DNA hybrid will not be translated *in vitro*. In the latter, cloned DNA bound to a solid support is used to isolate the complementary mRNA, which can then be eluted and translated *in vitro*. This technique is more sensitive than hybrid-arrested translation. The plasmid is fixed on a filter and incubated with mRNA, which is used as a probe. Washing is done to remove unbound probes. The bound mRNA is eluted and translated. This procedure utilizes the presence of a specific protein encoded by it [167].

2.13.9 Electrophoresis techniques

2.13.9.1 Agarose gel electrophoresis

Agarose gel electrophoresis is one of numerous physical methods for evaluating the size of DNA. In this methodology, DNA is allowed to run through (elute) a highly cross-linked agarose matrix under the influence of an electric current. In the solution, the phosphates of the DNA are negatively charged, and the molecule will thus migrate to the positive (red) end. There are three issues that disturb the migration rate through a gel: conformation of the DNA, size of the DNA and ionic strength of the running buffer [169]. Assembly of agarose electrophoresis is shown in figure 2.16.

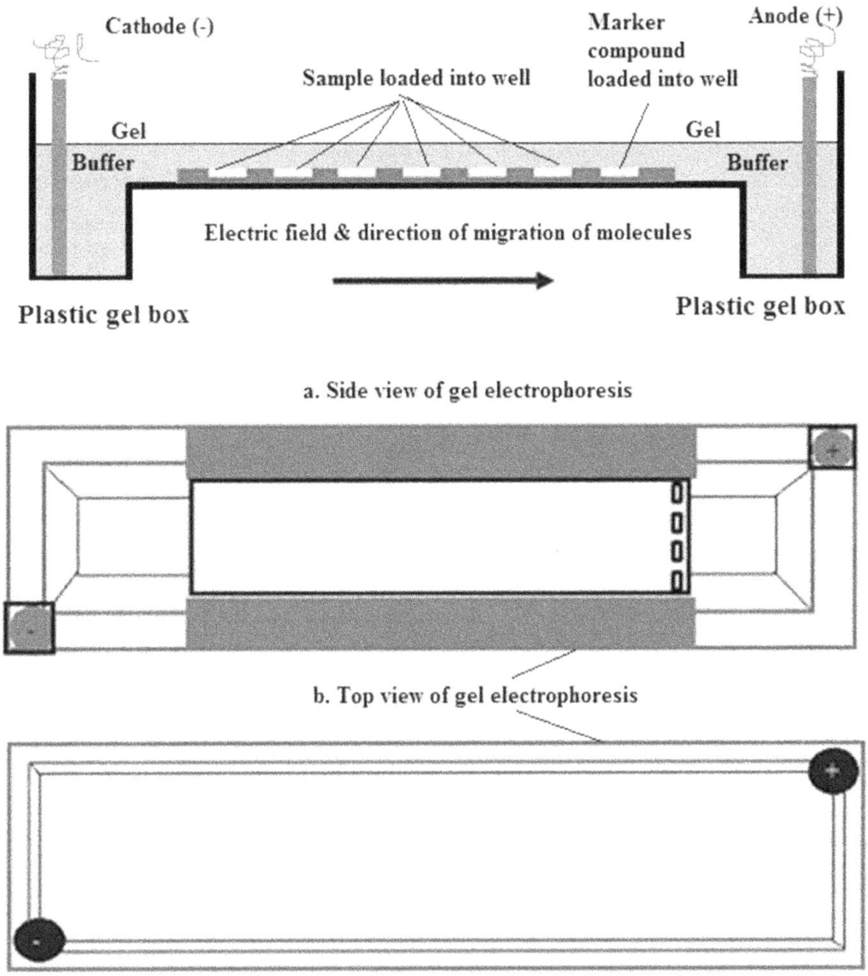

Figure 2.16. Construction of agarose electrophoresis.

Agarose gel electrophoresis is a widely used laboratory technique for separating and analyzing macromolecules, particularly DNA and RNA, based on their size [170]. It is a fundamental tool in molecular biology and biochemistry for a variety of applications, including DNA and RNA fragment analysis, DNA purification, and DNA quantification. There follows an overview of how agarose gel electrophoresis works.

2.13.9.1.1 Principle of agarose gel electrophoresis:

1. Preparation of the gel: Agarose powder is mixed with a buffer (commonly Tris-acetate-EDTA, TAE, or Tris-borate-EDTA, TBE) to create a gel matrix. The concentration of agarose can be adjusted to control the size range of molecules that can be separated. The gel is typically cast in a gel tray with wells to hold the sample.

2. Sample loading: The DNA or RNA sample is mixed with a loading buffer (often containing glycerol and a tracking dye) and then carefully loaded into the wells of the agarose gel. The tracking dye helps monitor the progress of electrophoresis.
3. Electrophoresis: An electrical field is applied across the gel by placing it in an electrophoresis chamber. DNA and RNA molecules are negatively charged due to their phosphate groups, and they move through the agarose matrix toward the positive electrode (anode) when an electric current is applied. Smaller molecules move more quickly through the gel than larger ones, leading to separation based on size.
4. Visualization: After electrophoresis is complete, the gel is removed from the chamber, and the separated DNA or RNA molecules are visualized. This is typically done by staining the gel with a fluorescent dye (e.g., ethidium bromide or SYBR Safe) that binds to DNA or RNA and fluoresces under ultraviolet (UV) light. The DNA or RNA bands appear as distinct, well-separated regions on the gel.
5. Analysis: The size of the DNA or RNA fragments is determined by comparing their migration distance on the gel to that of known molecular weight markers (also known as DNA ladders or DNA size standards). The concentration of nucleic acids can also be estimated based on the intensity of the bands.

Agarose gel electrophoresis is used in a wide range of applications, including DNA fragment analysis, checking the quality and quantity of isolated DNA or RNA, verifying PCR products, and preparing DNA fragments for downstream applications such as DNA sequencing or cloning. It is an essential technique for researchers in genetics, molecular biology, and related fields [170].

2.13.9.2 Pulsed field electrophoresis

In recent times, there has been huge demand for methods that can easily examine complete genomes. Apart from *Arabidopsis* and rice genome examination, growth in evaluating the complete genome in plants has been slow. Among the most successful practices, pulsed-field gel electrophoresis (PFGE) is currently used. Schwartz and Cantor presented PFGE for the determination of separation of several megabase-sized DNA molecules [171]. This technology is based on standard agarose gel electrophoresis, employed for separation of nucleic acids. This conventional agarose-based separation cannot resolve fragments greater than 20 kb. Owing to the inability of bulky DNA to migrate through the agarose gel matrix like smaller DNA, simple agar electrophoresis fails to separate the bulky or long DNA molecules. A constant electric field stretches them out so that they travel in a snake-like manner. This mode of movement is known as reputation. Agarose gel with low concentrations of agarose (0.1%–0.2%) is proficient in resolving particularly large DNA. Even after that it is unable to resolve some large DNA. In the PFGE process, using pulsed irregular orthogonal electric fields, DNA molecules are forced to reorient before continuing in a snake-like fashion through the gel. Through this reorientation period larger DNA molecules take longer to pass gradually through the gel. Bulky DNA molecules become entrapped in their repatation tubes and the electric field is changed every time. The bigger the DNA molecule, the longer the time required for this alignment. Nevertheless, in conventional electrophoresis a single electric field is compulsory, which restricts the separation range to kilobases. Segregation in PFGE is accomplished by applying twin perpendicularly oriented electric fields in an irregular mode to separate chromosomes up to 2000 kb.

PFGE is a specialized and powerful technique used in molecular biology to separate and analyze large DNA fragments, typically those ranging from tens of kilobases to megabases (hundreds of thousands to millions of base pairs) in size. Unlike traditional agarose gel electrophoresis, which is limited by the size of the DNA fragments that can be resolved, PFGE allows for the separation of very large DNA molecules. PFGE is particularly useful in various applications, including genomic mapping, fingerprinting, and analyzing large DNA structures [172]. Below is a description of how PFGE works.

2.13.9.2.1 Principle of pulsed-field gel electrophoresis (PFGE)

1. Preparation of the gel: A gel is cast using agarose or other specialized gel-forming substances. The key feature of this gel is that it is oriented in a way that allows the electrophoresis field to be applied alternately in different directions, hence the term 'pulsed-field.' The gel may be oriented horizontally, vertically, or even as a 'CHEF' (contour-clamped homogeneous electric field) gel, depending on the specific experimental setup.
2. Sample preparation: Large DNA molecules are isolated, typically from genomic DNA or large DNA fragments, and are treated with specific enzymes or restriction enzymes that cut the DNA into smaller fragments. These fragments, however, remain quite large compared to what can be resolved using conventional gel electrophoresis.
3. Electrophoresis with pulsed fields: In PFGE, the electrophoresis field is not applied continuously as in conventional gel electrophoresis. Instead, it is pulsed on and off in a controlled manner. The direction of the field is also alternated during different pulse periods. This allows the large DNA fragments to reorient themselves during the off periods.
4. Separation of large fragments: The pulsed-field electrophoresis system is designed to exert forces on the DNA molecules that help overcome the limitations of traditional gel electrophoresis. This results in the separation of very large DNA fragments according to their size.
5. Visualization: After the electrophoresis is complete, the gel is stained with a DNA-specific dye, and the separated DNA fragments are visualized using methods such as ethidium bromide staining, SYBR staining, or other DNA-specific dyes. The bands on the gel represent different-sized DNA fragments.

2.13.9.2.2 PFGE has various applications, including

1. Genomic mapping: PFGE is used to create a physical map of an organism's genome, revealing the arrangement and sizes of large DNA fragments.

2. Fingerprinting: It is employed in DNA fingerprinting for epidemiological studies, forensic investigations, and microbial strain typing.
3. Genomic analysis: PFGE is useful for the study of large DNA structures, such as plasmids, bacterial chromosomes, and viral genomes.
4. Genomic DNA isolation: In some cases, PFGE is used to isolate large DNA fragments or perform large DNA fragment purification.

Overall, PFGE is a valuable technique for resolving and analyzing large DNA fragments and is especially useful in studies requiring a high degree of resolution for such large genetic materials [172].

2.13.9.3 Field inversion gel electrophoresis

This method was presented by Carle *et al* [173] using a device in which there was the facility for intermittent inversion of a single electric field. The applied field is constant in both directions. The onward pulse is somewhat longer than the reverse pulse, resulting in the migration of the DNA along a perfectly straight path. This method determines DNA fragments up to 2000 kb in length.

Field inversion gel electrophoresis (FIGE) is a variation of PFGE that is used to separate and analyze DNA fragments, particularly large fragments, in a gel matrix. FIGE is a powerful technique often employed in molecular biology and genomics to study DNA molecules with sizes ranging from tens of kilobases to several megabases (millions of base pairs). It allows for the precise separation and analysis of very large DNA fragments by applying electric fields in a controlled and alternating manner [174]. Below is a description of how FIGE works.

2.13.9.3.1 Principle of field inversion gel electrophoresis (FIGE)

1. Preparation of the gel: A gel is prepared using agarose or other suitable gel-forming materials. The gel can be cast in various orientations, such as horizontal or vertical, depending on the specific experimental setup. The key feature of FIGE is the ability to apply electric fields in alternating directions within the gel.
2. Sample preparation: Large DNA molecules, such as genomic DNA, are isolated and treated with restriction enzymes to generate DNA fragments. These fragments are quite large compared to what can be resolved using conventional gel electrophoresis.
3. Electrophoresis with field inversion: FIGE applies electric fields to the gel in an alternating fashion. This means that the direction of the electric field periodically changes, which results in the reorientation of DNA fragments during the field inversion phases. This prevents the large DNA molecules from migrating too far and becoming tangled in the gel.
4. Separation of large fragments: The controlled application of electric fields in alternating directions during electrophoresis allows for the precise separation of very large DNA fragments. This separation is based on the size of the DNA fragments, and it prevents smearing and entanglement.
5. Visualization: After electrophoresis is complete, the gel is typically stained with a DNA-specific dye and visualized using methods like ethidium bromide

staining, SYBR staining, or other DNA-specific dyes. The resulting gel displays separated DNA fragments as distinct bands.

2.13.9.3.2 Applications

1. Genomic mapping: FIGE is used to create physical maps of an organism's genome, enabling the investigation of the arrangement and sizes of large DNA fragments.
2. Fingerprinting: Similar to PFGE, FIGE can be employed in DNA fingerprinting for epidemiological studies, forensic investigations, and microbial strain typing.
3. Genomic analysis: FIGE is useful for the study of large DNA structures, such as bacterial chromosomes, viral genomes, and plasmids.
4. Large DNA fragment isolation: In some cases, FIGE can be used to isolate and purify large DNA fragments for further analysis.

Field inversion gel electrophoresis is a valuable technique when studying very large DNA molecules and is particularly well-suited for applications that require high resolution and precise separation of these large genetic materials [174].

2.13.9.4 Vertical pulse field gradient electrophoresis

This method was designed and developed by Gardiner *et al* [175], using two oppositely positioned electrodes in such a manner that when the electric field is switched DNA moves towards another set of electrodes, which results in a zigzag movement of DNA from the traveling point to the bottom of the gel. There is no horizontal distortion of the DNA because the entire DNA is exposed to an equivalent electric field.

Vertical pulse field gradient electrophoresis (VPFGE) is a specialized form of PFGE that is used to separate and analyze DNA molecules, particularly large fragments, in a vertical gel setup. It is a powerful technique in molecular biology and genomics for the precise separation of DNA fragments based on their size. VPFGE, like conventional PFGE, is particularly useful when studying large DNA molecules, such as genomic DNA, by applying pulsed electric fields in a controlled and alternating manner [174]. There follows an overview of how VPFGE works.

2.13.9.4.1 Principle

1. Gel preparation: A vertical agarose gel is cast in a gel box, with wells formed at the top to allow the loading of DNA samples. The gel is positioned in a vertical orientation.
2. Sample preparation: Large DNA molecules, typically genomic DNA, are isolated and treated with restriction enzymes to generate DNA fragments. These fragments are often quite large.
3. Electrophoresis with pulsed fields: VPFGE applies pulsed electric fields to the vertical gel in a controlled and alternating manner. The key feature is that the field is applied both horizontally and vertically, creating a gradient of electric fields that runs perpendicular to the direction of electrophoresis. This

controlled pulsing allows for the reorientation of DNA fragments during field inversion phases, preventing the large DNA molecules from migrating too far and becoming entangled.

4. Separation of large fragments: The alternating and controlled application of electric fields in both horizontal and vertical directions during electrophoresis results in the precise separation of very large DNA fragments based on their size. The gel gradient allows for high resolution in both dimensions, preventing smearing and entanglement.
5. Visualization: After electrophoresis is complete, the vertical gel is stained with a DNA-specific dye and visualized using methods like ethidium bromide staining, SYBR staining, or other DNA-specific dyes. The separated DNA fragments appear as distinct bands in the vertical gel.

2.13.9.4.2 Applications

1. Genomic mapping: VPFGE is used to create physical maps of an organism's genome, revealing the arrangement and sizes of large DNA fragments.
2. Fingerprinting: It is employed in DNA fingerprinting for epidemiological studies, forensic investigations, and microbial strain typing.
3. Genomic analysis: VPFGE is useful for the study of large DNA structures, such as bacterial chromosomes, viral genomes, and plasmids.
4. Large DNA fragment isolation: In some cases, VPFGE can be used to isolate and purify large DNA fragments for further analysis.

Vertical pulse field gradient electrophoresis is a valuable technique when studying very large DNA molecules and is particularly well-suited for applications that require high resolution and precise separation of these large genetic materials in both the horizontal and vertical dimensions.

2.13.9.5 Contour-clamped homogeneous electric field gel electrophoresis

In this procedure the electric field is produced from various electrodes that are arranged in a square or hexagonal shape around the horizontal gel and are held to a fixed potential [176]. This results in the development of a homogeneous electric field, which makes it possible to determine DNA molecules up to 5000 kb in length.

2.13.9.6 Polyacrylamide gel electrophoresis

Chemically inactive polyacrylamide gel (porous gel) is made by the polymerization of acrylamide at a specific concentration in the presence of a cross-linking agent (methylene bisacrylamide), which can further govern the pore size of the gel. In this procedure proteins are applied to porous polyacrylamide gel and segregated in an electric field. When proteins are placed in an electric field they are segregated on the basis of their size and net electric charge. As the entire procedure is performed in a gel, this sort of segregation acts as a molecular sieve, which means smaller molecules travel faster through the pores in comparison to larger molecules.

Polyacrylamide gel electrophoresis (PAGE) is a widely used laboratory technique for separating and analyzing macromolecules, particularly proteins and nucleic acids (DNA and RNA), based on their size, charge, or conformation [177]. It is a fundamental tool in molecular biology, biochemistry, and other fields for various applications, including protein and nucleic acid analysis, purification, and quantification. There follows an overview of how polyacrylamide gel electrophoresis works.

2.13.9.6.1 Principle

1. Gel preparation: Polyacrylamide gels are prepared by polymerizing acrylamide and bisacrylamide in the presence of a chemical initiator. The concentration of acrylamide in the gel can be adjusted to create gels with different porosities, allowing for the separation of molecules of different sizes.
2. Sample loading: The sample, which may contain proteins or nucleic acids, is mixed with a loading buffer that contains tracking dyes and, in the case of protein samples, a reducing agent to denature proteins. The mixture is then loaded into wells or slots at one end of the gel.
3. Electrophoresis: An electric field is applied across the polyacrylamide gel by placing it in an electrophoresis chamber. The molecules in the sample become negatively charged and move through the gel toward the opposite electrode. The rate of migration is determined by the size, charge, and conformation of the molecules, with smaller and more negatively charged molecules moving faster.
4. Visualization: After electrophoresis, the separated molecules are visualized. For proteins, this is typically done by staining the gel with Coomassie Brilliant Blue or silver stain. For nucleic acids, ethidium bromide or other DNA-specific dyes are often used. Stained bands or spots on the gel represent the separated molecules.
5. Analysis: The size and quantity of the separated molecules are determined by comparing their migration distances on the gel to that of known molecular weight markers. The concentration of proteins or nucleic acids can be estimated based on the intensity of the stained bands or spots.

2.13.9.6.2 Applications

Protein electrophoresis:

1. SDS–PAGE: Sodium dodecyl sulfate-polyacrylamide gel electrophoresis is used for protein separation based on size and is a standard method for protein analysis.
2. Native PAGE: Used to analyze native (non-denatured) proteins and study protein conformation and activity.
3. Isoelectric focusing (IEF: Separates proteins by their isoelectric point, allowing for the separation of proteins with different charges.

Nucleic acid electrophoresis:

1. DNA and RNA Electrophoresis: Used for separating DNA or RNA fragments based on size, often to verify PCR products, isolate specific fragments, or analyze DNA ladders.

2. Denaturing polyacrylamide gel electrophoresis (dPAGE): Used to separate single-stranded nucleic acids, such as DNA sequencing products.

Polyacrylamide gel electrophoresis is a versatile and essential technique for molecular biologists, biochemists, and researchers in various fields. It provides a means to analyze and quantify macromolecules, contributing to a better understanding of their properties and functions [178].

2.13.9.7 Isoelectric focusing

The isoelectric point is defined as the point at which the overall charge of the protein becomes zero, i.e. a neutral charge. Segregation of proteins at the isoelectric point is called isoelectric focusing. During isoelectric focusing a gradient of pH and an electric potential are applied across the gel, making one end more positive than the other. Segregation takes place on the basis of the positive or negative groups present on the molecule. If they are positively charged, they will be dragged towards the more negative end of the gel, and if they are negatively charged they will be dragged to the more positive end of the gel. The proteins tested in the first dimension will move through the gel and will accumulate at their isoelectric point. At this phase the protein's complete charge is zero and thus it does not migrate in an electric field.

2.13.9.8 2D gel electrophoresis

In 2D gel electrophoresis a specimen is initially exposed to isoelectric focusing and then sodium dodecyl sulfate-polyacrylamide gel electrophoresis (SDS–PAGE) is used to attain much higher solution separations. Specimen proteins are initially transferred onto the strip of gel containing polyampholytes where proteins are segregated on the basis of isoelectric focusing. This procedure initiates with 1D electrophoresis when the specimen proteins/molecules lie along a lane, followed by the 2D electrophoresis when the specimen is spread out across a 2D gel, and separation of the molecules occurs in a direction 90 °C from the first. Usually, electrophoresis segregation is based on the properties of the protein molecules that are intended for separation, e.g. mass and charge, while the segregation of a single band/spot is formed if either the mass (SDS–PAGE) or charge (isoelectric focusing) of two dissimilar proteins is alike. Thus, a blend of these methods offers 2D separation of the proteins, which is more effective than 1D electrophoresis.

2.13.9.9 Polymerase chain reaction (PCR)

PCR is an amplification tool for cloning the specific or targeted parts of a DNA sequence to produce multiple copies of DNA of interest. It is based on cell-free *in vitro* fast cloning and replication of both strands of DNA in the test tube rather than in living cells like *E. coli*. This technique was developed by Kary Mullis of Cetus Corporation in 1983 and was awarded the Nobel Prize in 1993 [179]. The main feature of the PCR technique is the exponential nature of amplification. This rapid amplification and generation of pure DNA of interest is accomplished by a repetitive series of thermal cycling, which includes three main steps: denaturation of DNA duplex at 94 °C, annealing of oligonucleotide primers to the target sequences of separated DNA strands and DNA synthesis from the 3-OH end of each primer by DNA polymerase at 72 °C. With the purpose of executing PCR we must be familiar with the portion of DNA sequence that we wish to replicate. Later, short DNA fragments or primers (short oligonucleotides) are produced from the nucleotides' base pairs. These primers are opposite to the sequence of the DNA that is also amplified. Four types of deoxyribonucleotides and primers, which comprise a complementary sequence of the target sequence, are supplemented to the solution. This procedure is performed in an Eppendorf tube and afterward transferred in an automated piece of equipment called a thermocycler in which thermal cycling, comprising of cycles of recurrent heating and cooling for DNA melting and enzymatic replication of the DNA, takes place. Primers allow selective and repeated amplification of the targeted sequence. As PCR progresses, the DNA generated is itself used as a template for replication, setting in motion a chain reaction in which the DNA template is exponentially amplified. PCR can be extensively modified to perform a wide array of genetic manipulations. This technique has become a beneficial technique to amplify a selected DNA sequence in a multifold genome without including the bacterial cells. It is completely performed *in vitro*. PCR is a much quicker technique than gene cloning. This process can only be started when the opposite sequence of the targeted sequence is known. A heat stable enzyme DNA polymerase, which is active at 50 °C–70 °C, catalyzes these reactions. DNA polymerase is derived from a species of bacteria existing in hot springs at a temperature of 90 °C. It is supplemented to the solution of Tris–HCl buffer containing the dsDNA with a targeted nucleotide sequence.

The whole method is described in figure 2.17. The polymerase reaction involves the following steps:

1. The DNA is heated for 30 s to detach its strands at 94 °C.
2. The detached strands of DNA are allowed to cool for 1.5 min at 52 °C, which allows binding of primers by hydrogen bonds at the ends of the target sequences.
3. DNA polymerase or Taq DNA polymerase catalyzes the supplementation of nucleotides to the primers by taking the longer DNA sequence as templates. This procedure ends in 1 min at 72 °C. This reaction cycles for more than 20 min. The products of the first cycle of replication are denatured, annealed to oligonucleotide primers, and replicated with DNA polymerase. This reaction is recycled until adequate amplification of the targeted sequence is accomplished.
4. This whole process is repeated, which results in four copies. The procedure is repeated at least 20 times or more depending upon the desired amount of targeted sequences of DNA, resulting in eight after three cycles, 16 after four cycles, 1024 after ten cycles and so on.

The aims of gene cloning and PCR are quite similar. PCR is very fast and takes less time (1 day) in isolating the gene than gene cloning (which usually takes 2–3 months). However, PCR has some drawbacks, e.g. for designing primers the nucleotide sequences of the targeted part of the DNA should be familiar, minor

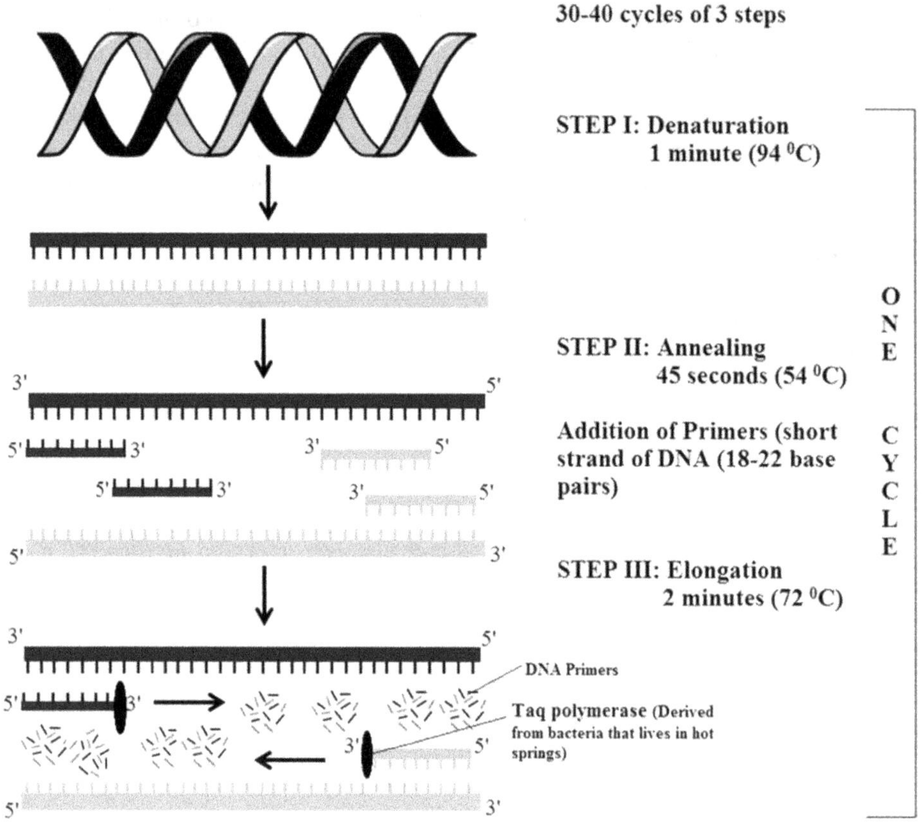

Figure 2.17. Polymerase chain reaction.

contamination of the DNA specimen can provide incorrect results and it is challenging to amplify long stretches through PCR.

2.13.9.10 Microarray

A DNA microarray, also called a DNA chip, biochip gene or chip, is a collection of high-density microscopic single-stranded DNA attached to a solid surface by biochemical analysis. The microarray was proposed by Chang [180]. It is made from either cDNA (cDNA microarray) or synthesized short oligonucleotides (oligonucleotide microarray). In this case cDNA or RNA (molecules of recognized sequences or probes, reporters, oligos or antisense RNA) are covalently linked on the solid surface. Each DNA spot encompasses picomoles (10−12 moles) of a particular DNA sequence. The experimental DNA or RNA (unknown sequence or test, target or sample DNA or RNA) are tagged with fluorescent dye and poured over the probe area for hybridization. Probe-target hybridization is typically examined and enumerated by procedures such as autoradiography, fluorescence, laser scanning and enzyme detection devices. Such practices can be employed to read the chip surface and hybridization pattern. The framework of a microarray is

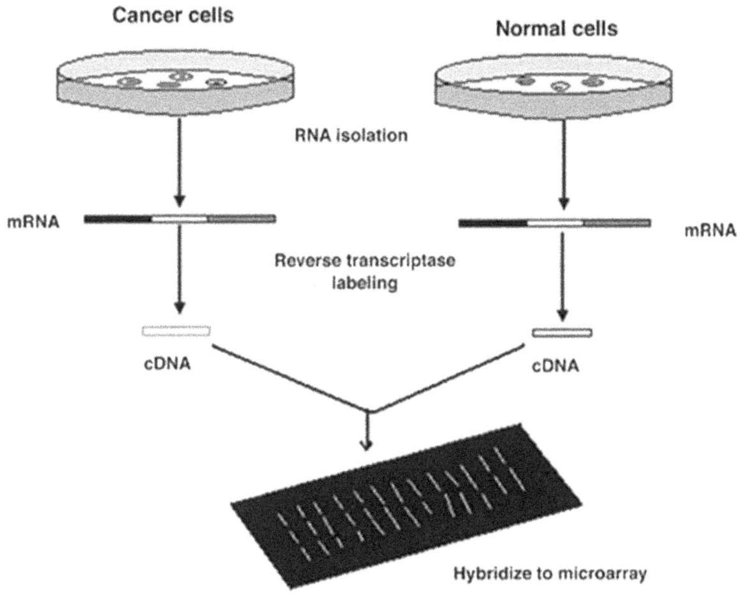

Figure 2.18. Outline of a microarray.

highlighted in figure 2.18. Researchers use DNA microarrays to determine the expression levels of large numbers of genes or their multiple regions simultaneously. Several strategies (photolithography, mechanical microspotting and ink jetting) are employed to manufacture microarrays for exploring their diverse applications in gene expression investigation, DNA sequencing, description of mutants, diagnostics and genetic mapping, proteomics and agricultural biotechnology.

2.14 Triplex DNA, TFOS, PNAs, RNA–DNA hybrids and DSRNA/RNAI

Utilization of DNA probes for the recognition of homologous nucleic acid sequences is a current hot topic in molecular biology. These DNA probes should possess optimal characteristic's including, stability, ease of preparation, rapid hybridization, specificity, sensitivity, specific activity, stringency and should be compatible with different hybridization formats and detection systems [181]. These DNA probes have been found to be valuable tools in molecular biology investigations involving:

- In-gel hybridization (particularly for oligonucleotide fingerprinting using synthetic SSRs).
- Southern blots (particularly for RFLPs).
- Northern blots (for mRNA investigation).

These practices comprising nucleic acid hybridization have also been exploited for different purposes containing inhibition of the expression of different genes (by means of antisense technology). The DNA probe is a versatile tool that can be used for recognition of complementary sequence in DNA or RNA samples, to identify a specific allele or mutations associated with diseases, to measure expression level of thousands of genes, and to study spatial organization of genes within cells with the help of fluorescence *in situ* hybridization technique [182]. They have also been employed for fundamental investigation such as investigation of expression and regulation of gene as well as for crop technology. Various inputs are made to advance the affinity, rate and specificity of nucleic acid identification technology. Nevertheless, major progress has been made through minor modifications in the nucleotide bases or in the phosphate backbone of the nucleic acid molecules. Triplex DNA, triplex establishing oligonucleotides, peptide nucleic acid, chimeric RNA–DNA molecules and double-stranded RNA are some of these modified forms of nucleic acids which have shown substantial growth in biotechnology (table 2.4). More specifically, a new strategy demonstrating a dramatic departure from standard oligonucleotide chemistry involves the use of peptide nucleic acids, which vary from DNA and RNA in having a pseudo-peptide backbone instead of a sugar phosphate backbone.

Table 2.4. Modern DNA probes and descriptions.

DNA probes	Description
Triplex DNA [183]	It was reported that RNA or DNA encompassing purines in one strand and pyrimidines in the other strand form triple-stranded structures comprising one polypurine strand and two polypyrimidine strands. In these helices, the triple DNA remains connected to duplex DNA via non-Watson–Crick interactions, now called Hoogstein pairing. Triplexes are also representative of supercoiled H = DNA. Some homopyrimidines and some purine-rich oligonucleotides can also form stable triplexes at homopurine–homopyrimidine sites of a duplex DNA
TFOs [184]	The oligonucleotides that enter duplex DNA and form triplexes are known as triplex-forming oligonucleotides (TFOs). TFO-DNA identification also results in the development of an antisense strategy so that TFO can be employed to yield universal drugs or targeted gene knockouts, in both plants and animals.
PNAs [185]	Peptide nucleic acids (PNAs) with a peptide-like backbone in place of a sugar phosphate backbone also form triplexes and can be employed for different purposes. PNAs are principally DNA correspondents, in which 2-aminoethylglycine linkages substitute the normal phosphodiester bonds. Specifically, they are oligonucleotide equivalent containing normal DNA bases with a polyamide uncharged backbone, where a methylene carbonyl linker links standard nucleotide bases to this backbone.
PNAs–RNA–DNA hybrids	PNAs lack 3′ to 5′ polarity and can connect DNA or RNA strands in either parallel or anti-parallel fashion, even though the anti-parallel mode is favored.

DsRNA/RNAi [185]	It has been found that small-stranded RNA molecules can encourage a potent and specific gene silencing both in animal and plant systems. This process was defined as RNA interference. The silencing of genes is attained at the post-transcriptional level and the process thus is also defined as post-transcriptional gene silencing.
Chimeraplasty [186]	In the past several methods have been employed for targeted gene modifications both for the investigation of gene function and for the assembly of better transgenic animals and plants. Moreover, the methodology of transposon mutagenesis is widely used for the destructive gene function with a view to allotting function to a DNA sequence. There are also strategies such as the use of TFOs and chimeraplasty (use of RNA–DNA hybrids) for gene modifications.

2.15 Isolation, sequencing, and synthesis of genes

In the last three decades considerable developments have been made in the techniques for the isolation of different genes, comprising those for

- Ribosomal RNA.
- Specific protein products.
- Phenotypic traits with unknown products.
- Regulatory functions, e.g. promoter genes.

2.15.1 Isolation of ribosomal RNA

Ribosomes consist of ribosomal RNA and proteins [187]. This ribosomal RNA makes up 80% of cellular RNA and is synthesized from ribosomal genes, which could be isolated. The rRNA consists of simple nucleotide sequence due to base pairing where it is folded into secondary structure such as internal loops, stems, bulges. These conserved secondary structures form domains in small subunits and interwoven in large subunits of ribosome. The structure of rRNA has been established and confirmed by various methods including chemical and x-ray crystallography method. Ribosomal RNA has a fundamental role in protein synthesis, and it can also be used to identify and understand evolutionary relationships among bacterial species [188]. Isolation of ribosomal genes has been considered due to the following reasons:

- Accessibility of homogeneous rRNA.
- Variances between ribosomal RNA genes and other genes, owing to their comparatively high G + C content.
- Ribosomal genes are present in multiple copies.

For the above reasons, ribosomal RNA genes were initially isolated in 1966 in an amphibian called *Xenopus*, by H Wallace and M L Birnstiel in 1966, while working at the University of Edinburgh in the UK [189]. The different steps involved are stated in figure 2.19. Isolation of ribosomal DNA permitted the first description of ribosomal genes which was enabled by the isolation of 5S DNA genes from *Xenopus laevis* by D Brown in 1977 [190].

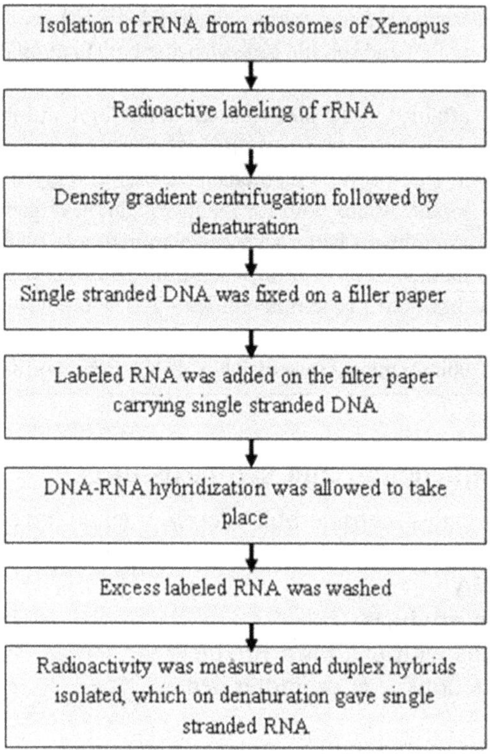

Isolation of rRNA from ribosomes of Xenopus
Radioactive labeling of rRNA
Density gradient centrifugation followed by denaturation
Single stranded DNA was fixed on a filler paper
Labeled RNA was added on the filter paper carrying single stranded DNA
DNA-RNA hybridization was allowed to take place
Excess labeled RNA was washed
Radioactivity was measured and duplex hybrids isolated, which on denaturation gave single stranded RNA

Figure 2.19. Isolation of ribosomal DNA [189].

2.15.2 Isolation of genes coding for specific proteins

Isolation of genes for particular proteins became promising only after the detection of the reverse transcriptase enzyme in 1970 [186]. The enzyme can be used for the production of copy DNA or complementary DNA from mRNA. This complementary DNA can be employed for the isolation of analogous genes from genomic DNA. It is thus noticeable that the isolation of a specific gene should first be available for the isolation of specific mRNA [191]. For this reason, antibodies are formed against a particular protein for the gene to be isolated. Thus, it precipitates the cluster of ribosomes which is bound to mRNA for translation. After extraction and purification of mRNA it can be utilized to synthesize cDNA. This derived cDNA is cloned with expression vectors to prepare a cDNA library. For identification of a specific cDNA clone, different electrophoretic and immunological techniques are used. For a known proteins gene sequence, the genomic DNA of an organism is isolated and cleaved with restriction of the endonuclease followed by gel electrophoresis and Southern blotting techniques using DNA probes. One can utilizing the specific cDNA probes to isolate the gene from genomic DNA by screening a complete or partial genomic library [192]. The isolation of a gene coding for a specific protein contains the steps illustrated in figure 2.20.

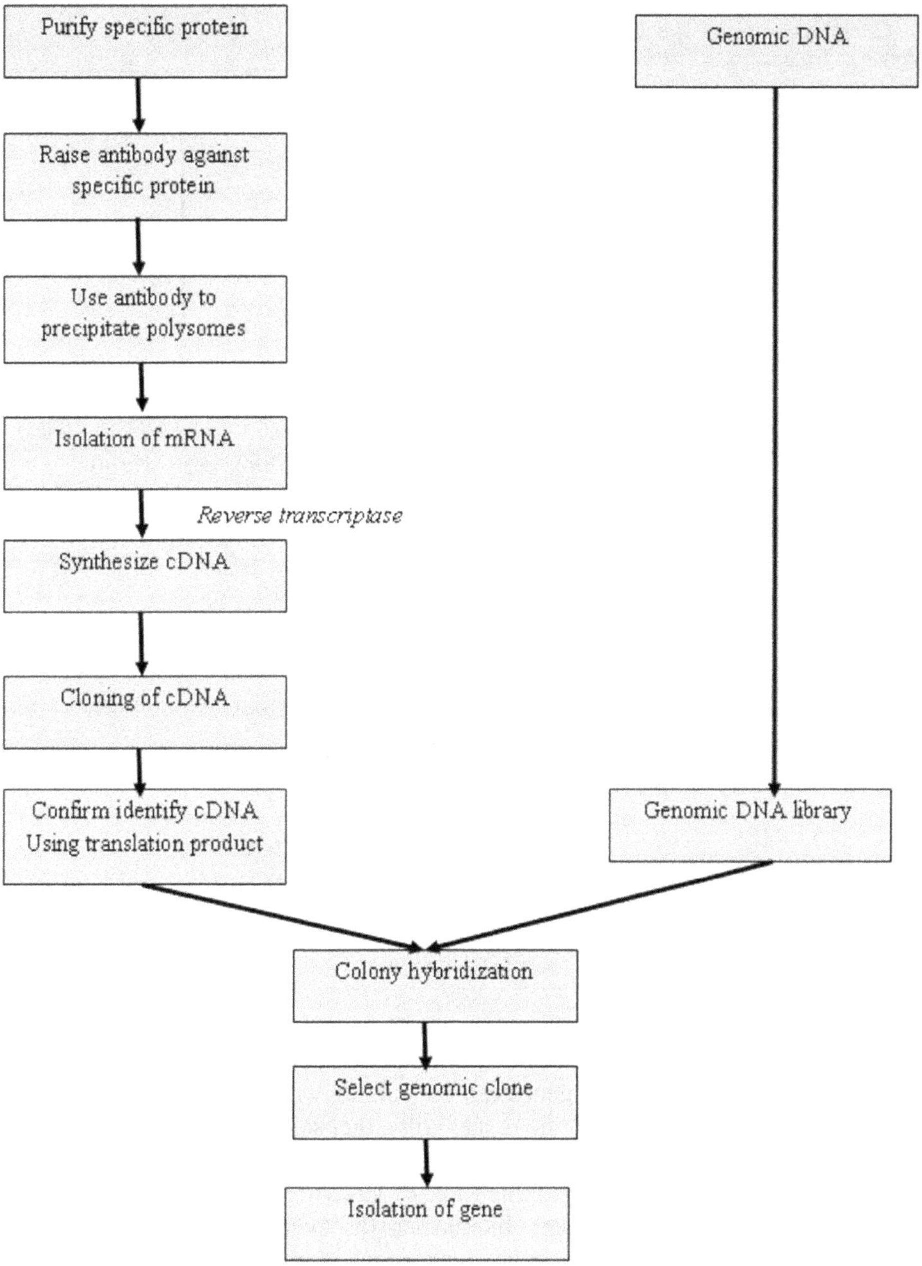

Figure 2.20. Isolation of genes for a specific protein [191].

2.15.2.1 Isolation of genes (with known or unknown products) using tissue-specific expression

It is very straightforward to isolate genes that are expressed in specific tissues. For example, genes for storage proteins are expressed in oviducts, or globin genes are

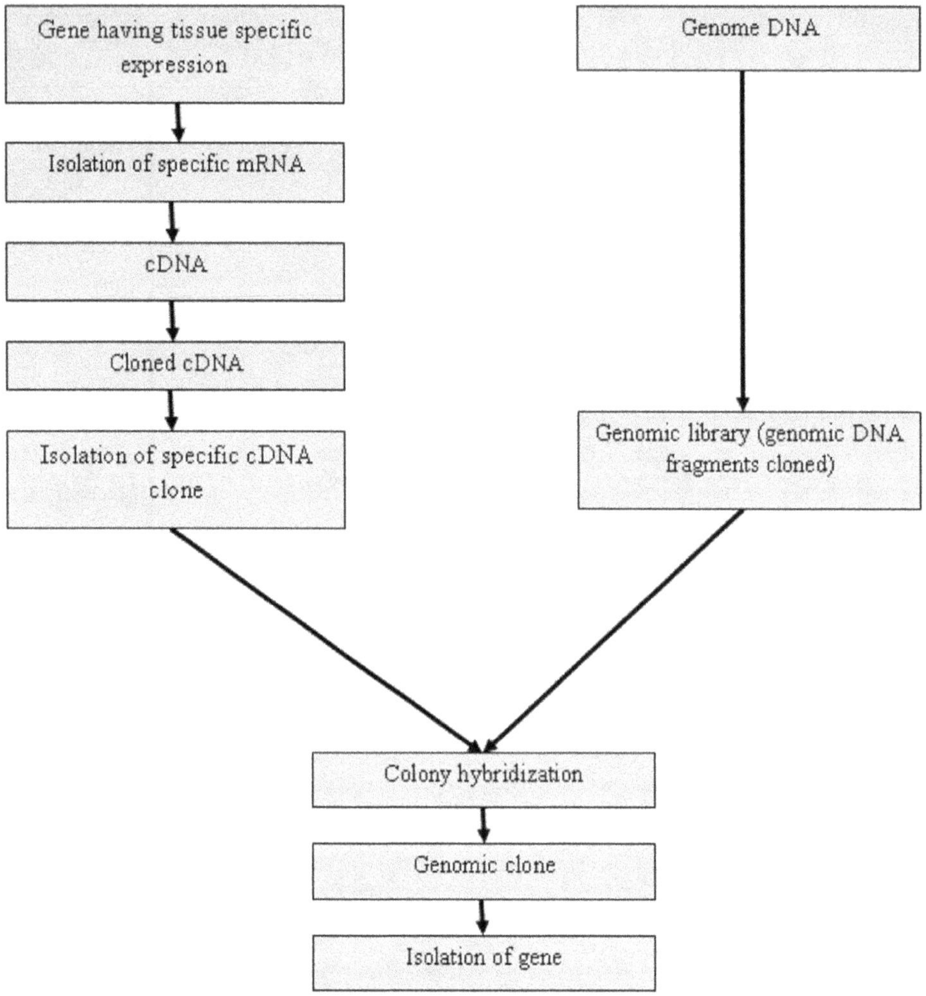

Figure 2.21. Isolation of a gene with tissue-specific expression using its mRNA [193].

expressed in erythrocytes. Such genes can be isolated without any problem because mRNA extracted from these specific tissues will either solely belong to the GOI, or it will be rich in species of mRNA from tissues where this gene is silent [193]. This method of genes isolation is a valuable tool for studying disease-related regulatory information, functional genomics, biomarker discovery and in developmental biology, because tissue-specific gene expression is mainly regulated by gene regulatory networks. It consists of specific interaction between transcription factors and gene followed by gene product [194]. This approach is described in figure 2.21.

2.15.3 Isolation of genes (with known or unknown products) using DNA or RNA probes

Particular molecular probes (whether DNA or RNA probes), if accessible, can be employed for the isolation of specific genes [195]. These probes may be accessible from another species for the same gene or may be artificially synthesized using a part of the amino acid sequence of the protein product of the gene in question. (figure 2.22). To use a DNA probe for gene isolation from bacteria, the first step is to isolate the target DNA from the bacterial chromosome, plasmid, or plasmid fragment. This can be done by denaturing the target DNA and transferring it to appropriate blotting paper. The DNA probe can be prepared by nick translation, which involves labeling the DNA with a radioactive isotope (such as 32P) or a biotin molecule. The DNA probe, which can be labeled with biotin or 32P, is mixed with the target DNA and allowed to anneal at points of genetic complementarity. This forms duplexes between the probe and the target DNA, allowing for the detection of specific gene sequences in bacterial species. In order to isolate the gene for a particular unknown protein, the protein of interest is identified by peptide

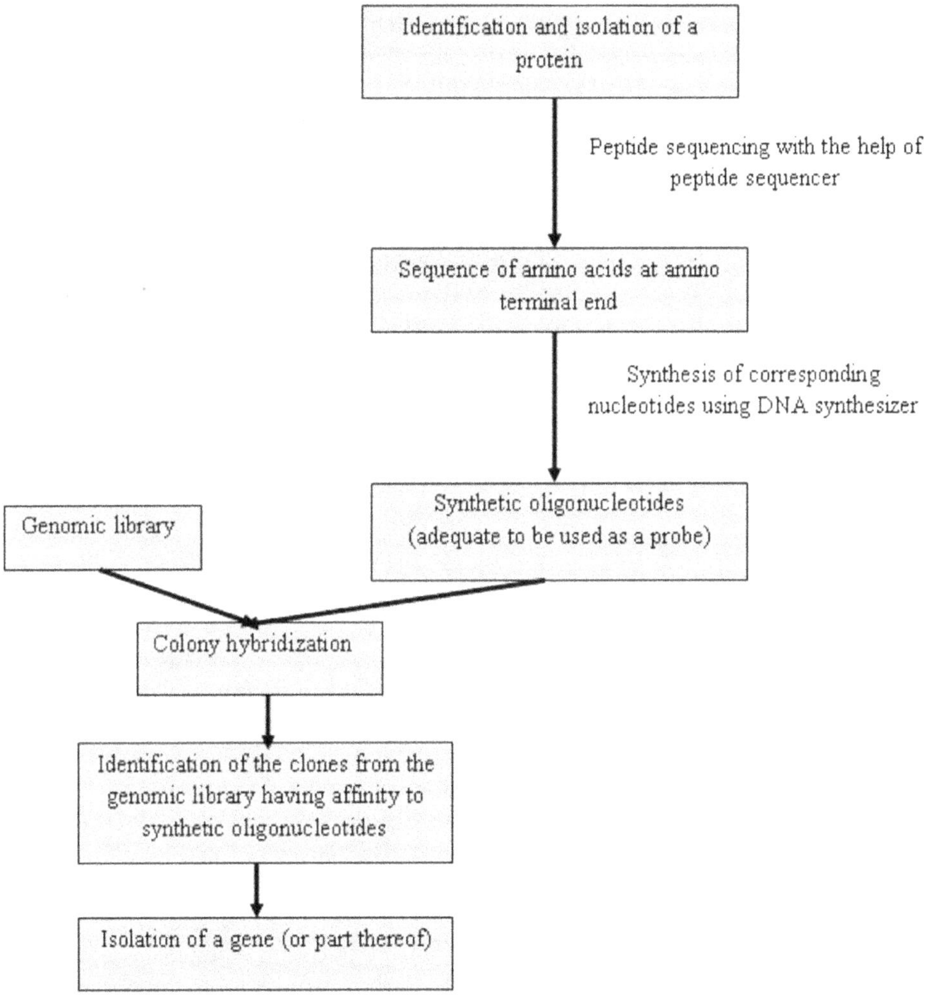

Figure 2.22. Isolation of a gene using the probe, artificially synthesized on the basis of the amino acid sequence of a part of the protein [195].

sequencing with the help of peptide sequencer followed by isolation of the identified protein. The identified protein peptide is then used to construct the sequence of corresponding oligonucleotides using DNA synthesizer. Synthetic DNA is used as a probe for the advancement to colony hybridization. A positive clone that has the affinity to this synthetic oligonucleotide probe is identified and is used further for the isolation of the gene of interest [196].

2.15.3.1 Use of heterologous probes

Probes obtained from one species and used for another species are known as heterologous probes. These probes have been reported to be effective in detecting gene clones during colony hybridization or plaque hybridization, or on Southern blots. For example, the gene for *Chalcone synthase* was isolated from *Antirrhinum majus* and *Petunia hybrida* using heterologous cDNA probes from parsley [197]. Heterologous DNA can be used as a probe for genes on which evolutionary constraints have been exercised. This approach may be useful in systems lacking easily isolatable messenger RNA or other direct selection procedures. The method used with heterologous DNA probes involved using cloned fragments of known genes from one species as probes in DNA–DNA hybridizations with restriction endonuclease fragments of another species gene. This technique allowed the identification and cloning of unknown genes, demonstrating the feasibility of using heterologous probes to identify genes for which no traditional genetic selection exists. The patterns of hybridization observed revealed the DNA sequence [198]. These probes give accurate detection and diagnosis of disease-causing bacterial species, such as *Borrelia* species, particularly in cases of Lyme disease and relapsing fever, and for identification of *Borrelia burgdorferi* and *Borrelia hermsii*. The researchers purified the DNA from the bacterial strains and labeled it with radioactive isotopes. The labeled probes were then hybridized with specific DNA fragments of the target bacteria. The hybridization was performed on GeneScreen Plus membranes using specific hybridization conditions. The membranes were then washed and exposed to x-ray film for detection. The researchers also performed Southern blot analysis to further confirm the specificity of the probes [199].

2.15.3.2 Use of synthetic probes

If proteins (purified using the technique of 2D gel electrophoresis) are used for microsequencing of 5–15 consecutive amino acids, this data can be used for the production of oligonucleotides (using automated DNA synthesizers). These oligonucleotides can be directly employed for the screening of cDNA or genomic libraries for isolation of specific genes [200]. Synthetic probes have revolutionized the detection of genes. These probes, which act as biosensors, offer improved performance compared to natural nucleic acid probes. They are more stable, efficient, and specific, making them ideal for various applications in clinical diagnostics and research. Synthetic nucleic acid analogues like locked nucleic acids (LNAs) and peptide nucleic acids (PNAs) have replaced traditional nucleic acids due to their enhanced properties. Additionally, the development of tools for probe designing and quality assessment has further facilitated the use of synthetic probes in gene detection. various tools are available for probe designing and quality evaluation in the field of omics research, such as OMICtools, OligoWiz, Teolenn, and MathFISH [201].

2.15.4 Isolation of genes coding for unknown products, when probes are not available

In certain cases we are involved in the isolation of a gene whose phenotypic effect is unidentified, but the gene product has not been known or cannot be isolated, and no probe exists. Such genes comprise those for morphological traits such as dominancy, photoperiodicity, disease resistance, etc [200]. This area of study, in which genetics is considered by isolating the gene first without knowing the gene product, is frequently defined as reverse genetics. The approaches used for the isolation of these genes are different from those used for gene coding for identified proteins. Some of these methods are mentioned below.

2.15.5 Use of transposable elements (transposon tagging) for isolation of gene

Transposons are DNA fragments that can move within the genome. By inserting these transposons randomly into the genome, researchers can disrupt specific genes and study the resulting phenotypic changes. This approach allows for large-scale mutagenesis and the identification of genes associated with specific traits or functions. Transposon tagging has been successfully used in various organisms to study gene function and genetic interactions such as *Caenorhabditis elegans* and *Drosophila*. In the process of transposon tagging, the transposon is inserted into the genome of the organism using various methods such as transposase-mediated excision or Agrobacterium T-DNA-mediated insertion. Once inserted, the transposon can disrupt the function of the gene it has inserted into, it is helpful for studying the effects of gene inactivation. Transposon tagging can be used to generate large collections of mutants in organisms such as *Arabidopsis thaliana*, *Caenorhabditis elegans*, *Drosophila*, and zebrafish. These mutants can then be analyzed to identify genes involved in specific biological processes or pathways. Transposon tagging, while a powerful tool for studying gene function, has one limitation, that of transposon excision [202]. The transposable elements in certain cases have been efficiently employed for the isolation of genes when the gene product is unknown. In this case the transposon works as a gene tag. The sequential steps are described in figure 2.23.

2.15.6 T-DNA insertion mutagenesis for isolation of plant genes

T-DNA insertion mutagenesis is a technique used to isolate and study plant genes. T-DNA, or transfer DNA, is a piece of exogenous DNA that is randomly inserted into the plant genome. This insertion can result in mutagenesis of the gene, leading to altered gene function. The technique involves analyzing pools of DNA from plants and identifying positive pools that contain T-DNA insertions. Individual members of these positive pools are then analyzed to identify specific genes that have been mutated [202]. The whole mechanism of insertional mutagenesis is described in figure 2.24. A method similar to transposon tagging is T-DNA insertion for isolation

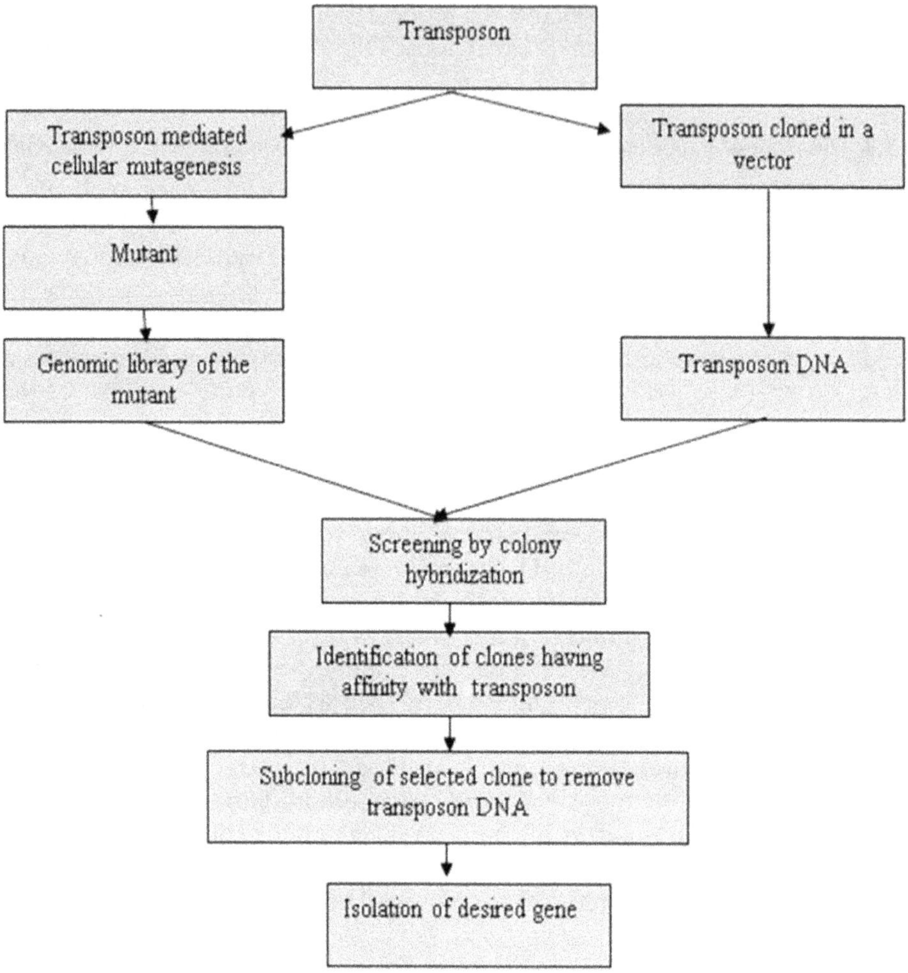

Figure 2.23. The use of transposon mutagenesis (or tagging) for identification and isolation of a gene [203].

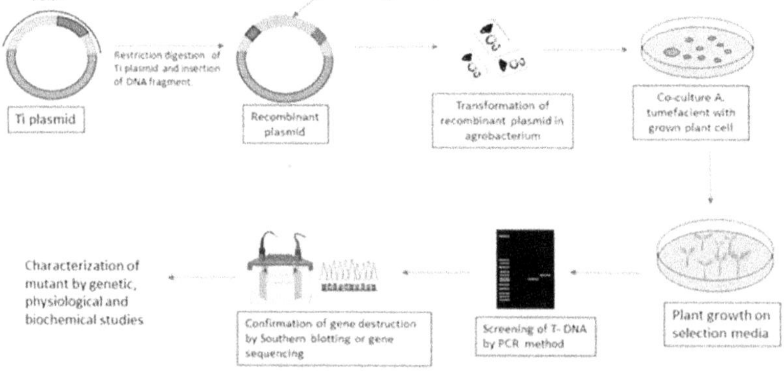

Figure 2.24. Schematic representation of T-DNA insertion mutagenesis for isolation of plant genes.

of genes. T-DNA insertion comprises the random insertion of T-DNA into the genome when *Agrobacterium tumefaciens* mediated transformation has been exploited, because it shows mutation of more than two-thirds of the genes [204]. T-DNA insertion mutagenesis is a widely used method for generating mutants in plants. However, there are several limitations to this approach. T-DNA insertions often result in hypomorphic alleles, meaning that the gene function is only partially disrupted. This can make it challenging to obtain mutants with the desired characteristics, as screening a large number of individuals may be required. Another is non-random insertion profiles, i.e. they have a preference for certain integration sites in the genome. This can result in some loci being targeted for insertions, while others may be refractory [202].

2.15.7 Promoter, enhancer and gene trap for isolation of genes

Although transformants for a large number of traits have now become accessible, all genes are not tagged in these transformants. Therefore, a major effort is essential to isolate any new gene that is not tagged in any of the available transformants. One such approach encompasses the insertion of a reporter gene with or without a Tata box or a splice acceptor. Such an approach comprises an enhancer trap, promoter trap and gene trap. In each circumstance, the reporter gene will be expressed under the influence of the enhancer/promoter sequence of a gene of unknown function and can be used as a tag for the isolation of the gene involved [205]. A promoter is a region of DNA that initiates the transcription of a particular gene. It plays a crucial role in regulating gene expression by binding to RNA polymerase and other transcription factors. In the context of gene isolation, the promoter is important for identifying and characterizing the expression patterns of specific genes. By inserting a gene-trap construct containing a minimal promoter with limited basal activity into the genome, it can be utilized for study the expression patterns of the trapped gene [206].

An enhancer is a DNA sequence that can increase the transcriptional activity of a gene. It acts by binding to specific transcription factors and promoting the recruitment of RNA polymerase to the gene's promoter region. In the context of gene isolation, enhancers are particularly useful for identifying genes that are regulated by specific enhancer elements. When an enhancer-trap construct is inserted near an enhancer, the minimal promoter in the construct is stimulated, leading to the expression of a reporter gene. This allows researchers to identify and study genes that are regulated by the enhancer [207].

Gene trapping is a technique used to identify and isolate genes based on their expression patterns. It entails inserting a gene-trap construct, usually made up of a reporter gene and a splice acceptor site into the genome. The construct is spliced with the gene's upstream exon(s) when it is placed into an intron of an expressed gene. As a result, the cellular protein that the enslaved gene encodes is expressed in a shortened and usually non-functional form. it can identify and investigate genes based on their expression patterns because the reporter gene encoded by the gene-trap device reflects the expression pattern of the trapped gene [208].

2.15.8 Mutation complementation

A genetic process known as 'mutation complementation' happens when two distinct mutations in unrelated genes can fix a single mutation-damaged gene's functionality. This suggests that both genes collaborate or interact to fulfill a certain biological function. Genes with related functions or those operating in the exact same pathway can be distinguished via complementation. Complementation studies can be used in reverse genetics to investigate synthetic-lethal relations among genes, in which cells carrying one of the two single mutations are surviving but not those carrying both. Synthetic-lethal mutation combinations can reveal information about the products required to complete a biological function [202, 209]. In this method DNA clones from the wild type are chosen which should be able to complement mutant strains, which are then transformed into the wild type by the production of transgenic plants using protoplasts obtained from the mutant plant [210].

2.15.9 Differential screening and differential display technique for isolation of genes

A variety of genes with unidentified gene products are expressed in specialized tissues. Mutations in these genes may also not result in easily detectable phenotypic changes. Such gene isolation can be attained via differential screening. In this method mRNA is prepared from contrasting tissues of plants [211]. The differential display technique is a molecular biology method used to compare gene expression patterns between different samples. It involves the amplification of cDNA fragments using random primers and PCR, followed by the separation of the amplified fragments on a gel gene. Differential expression between samples is identified by analyzing the banding patterns on the gel [212].

2.15.10 Subtractive hybridization for gene isolation

Subtractive hybridization methods offer a medium to isolate genes that are explicitly expressed in a cell type or tissue, genes that are differentially controlled during activation or differentiation of cells, or genes that are involved in pathological disorders such as cancer. Such approaches are appropriate for the isolation of low-expression genes [213, 214]. The aim of these methods is to eliminate the mRNA species shared by different cell types or tissues by subtraction, leaving the cell type/tissue-specific mRNAs for further manipulation and examination. Otherwise, mRNA from both the subtracted and/or target population can be reverse transcribed and amplified by PCR followed by subtractive hybridization and isolation of specific sequences. Preparing the driver and tester DNA is the initial stage in the subtractive hybridization process. The DNA of the tester is the sample of interest, while the DNA of the driver represents the control sample. Both DNA samples are fragmented into smaller pieces. The fragmented driver DNA is mixed with an excess of tester DNA and allowed to hybridize. This step allows for the binding of complementary sequences between the driver and tester DNA. After hybridization, the unbound tester DNA is separated from the hybridized DNA. This can be done using techniques such as column chromatography or magnetic bead separation. The unbound tester DNA represents the sequences that are unique to the tester sample. The subtracted tester DNA is then amplified using techniques such as PCR. This step increases the amount of the unique sequences present in the tester sample. This amplified tester DNA can be analyzed using various methods, such as DNA sequencing or microarray analysis, to identify the specific genes or sequences of interest that were present in the tester sample but not in the driver sample. Overall, subtractive hybridization is a technique used to isolate and identify genes or sequences that are differentially expressed or unique to a specific sample of interest. It involves the hybridization of driver and tester DNA, subtraction of unbound tester DNA, amplification of the unique sequences, and analysis of the amplified DNA to identify the genes or sequences of interest [215].

In the previous 20 years, numerous subtractive approaches have been demonstrated, but subtraction hybridization/cloning remains a technically demanding, time-consuming and labor-intensive process, including the requirement for huge amounts of mRNA or highly purified single-stranded DNA. Numerous subtractive hybridization approaches based on solid-phase hybridization on magnetic Dynabeads have previously been described.

2.15.11 Map-based cloning for gene isolation

Map-based cloning is a technique used to isolate and identify specific genes based on their physical location on a genetic map. This approach involves the identification and analysis of genetic markers that are closely linked to the gene of interest. By mapping the location of these markers, it can narrow down the region of the genome where the gene is located. Once the region of interest is identified, further analysis can be done to identify candidate genes within that region. This can involve sequencing the DNA in the region, comparing it to known gene sequences, and analyzing gene expression patterns. Map-based cloning has been successfully used in various model organisms, including yeast, zebrafish, *Drosophila*, mice, and *Xenopus*. In these organisms, collections of mutants have been generated using techniques such as gene deletion, gene trap, and insertional mutagenesis. These collections provide valuable resources for identifying and studying genes of interest. The cost of map-based cloning can vary depending on the organism and the specific techniques used also depending on the complexity of the procedure and the resources required. It is important to note that map-based cloning is dependent on the species and the specific biological question being studied. Although it has limitations when interpreting phenotypes, different approaches may have off-target effects. To avoid this problem, one should confirm results obtained with one approach by using another method [216].

Map-based cloning can be employed for the isolation of a gene for which a mutation can be identified in a crop for which a saturated molecular map is available. In the past decade various resistance genes have been isolated from model plant species, e.g. *Arabidopsis thaliana* and rice, or from diploid crop plants such as tomatoes and barley [217]. In numerous cases, gene isolation was conducted via map-based cloning. This process needs the growth of high-density genetic maps and the possibility to perform chromosome walking on large genomic fragments. Until now, such positional cloning has been restricted to small genomes, and it has remained very problematic in large (5000 Mb) and repetitive (80%) genomes, e.g. those of barley and wheat. Mlo, the first barley disease resistance gene isolated by map-based cloning was identified by the use of a yeast artificial chromosome (YAC) library and the subsequent construction of a bacterial artificial chromosome (BAC) library from the YAC clone spanning the resistance locus.

2.15.12 Isolation of novel genes

Novel genes such as oxalate decarboxylase and genes for specific proteins with a nutritionally balanced composition of amino acids were isolated by A Raina and A Datta at JNU in New Delhi in 1992. The work was selected for the Birla Award for science and technology for cloning and characterization of these two novel genes [190].

2.15.13 Sequencing of a gene or a DNA fragment

Once a gene or a DNA fragment has been cloned, its further study includes DNA sequencing. The practice of DNA sequencing was very lengthy until 1975, when a discovery was made in DNA sequencing methods [218] (table 2.5). The first two of the different techniques explained below are now often used for determination of DNA sequences, although numerous other methods have been proposed for this purpose [218]. Maxam and Gilbert's chemical sequencing method is based on chemical sequencing of an unknown sample to determine its sequence by chemical termination process. During this process sample DNA of unknown sequences is treated with certain chemicals to cleave the DNA sample at certain sites such as G, A, T, C. which allows the identification of the actual sequence of the DNA sample, as shown in figure 2.25. One common approach is Sanger sequencing, also known as chain termination sequencing. In this method, the DNA fragment is first amplified using PCR. Then, the DNA is mixed with a primer, DNA polymerase, and a mixture of normal deoxynucleotides (dNTPs) and dideoxy nucleotides (ddNTPs), which lack a 3′ hydroxyl group. As the DNA polymerase incorporates the nucleotides into the growing DNA strand, the incorporation of a ddNTP terminates the chain elongation. The resulting mixture of DNA fragments is separated by size using gel electrophoresis, and the sequence is determined by reading the order of the terminated fragments. Another method is next-generation sequencing (NGS), which allows for high-throughput sequencing of multiple DNA fragments simultaneously. NGS technologies, such as Illumina sequencing, involve fragmenting the DNA into smaller pieces, attaching adapters to the fragments, and amplifying them using PCR. The fragments are then loaded onto a sequencing platform, where they undergo cycles of DNA synthesis and imaging. The sequence of each fragment is determined by the incorporation of fluorescently labeled nucleotides and detected by the imaging system. The resulting sequences are then aligned and assembled to reconstruct the original gene or DNA fragment sequence. Overall, sequencing a gene or a DNA fragment involves amplifying the target DNA, incorporating labeled nucleotides, and determining the sequence either through chain termination sequencing or next-generation sequencing technologies [219].

Table 2.5. Gene sequencing methods and their functions.

Gene sequencing method	Function
Maxam and Gilbert's chemical degradation method	The sequential steps are shown in figure 2.25. This process involves cleavage of the specific nucleobase-specific partial in DNA by using certain chemicals such as DMSO, which is followed by the successive cleavage of the DNA backbone at locations next to the modified nucleotides.
Sanger's dideoxynucleotide synthetic method	Frederick Sanger had initially developed a method for DNA sequencing that utilized DNA polymerase to extend DNA chain length. Subsequently he developed a more powerful method utilizing single-stranded DNA as a template for DNA synthesis.
Automatic DNA sequencers	A variant of the above method was later developed which allowed the production of automatic sequencers. In this new approach different fluorescent dyes are tagged to the oligonucleotide primer in each of the reaction tubes.
Slab gel sequencing systems	These systems make use of ultrathin slab gels and involve running of at least 96 lanes per gel, the runs being completed twice daily.
Capillary gel sequencing systems	In these systems slab gel electrophoresis is replaced by capillary gel electrophoresis to analyze DNA samples.
Direct DNA sequencing using PCR	PCR has also been used for sequencing the amplified DNA product. This method of DNA sequencing is faster and more reliable and can utilize either the whole genomic DNA or cloned fragments for sequencing a particular DNA segment.
DNA sequencing through transcription	Recently, DNA sequencing was successfully achieved using RNA polymerase enzyme for transcription instead of using the sequenase or thermosequenase used in Sanger's didedoxynucleotide method of chain termination. This method of sequencing is described as transcriptional sequencing.
DNA sequencing by hybridization using microarrays on DNA chips	The main objective of several genome projects is the large-scale analysis of genomes and its application to individual case studies in medicine and research. Sequencing by hybridization for the detection of SNPs using DNA microchips was developed to meet this objective.
DNA sequencing by DE MALDI-TOF mass spectrometry	Matrix-assisted laser desorption mass spectrometry has the potential to rapidly acquire DNA sequence information and is widely used for confirmation of the sequences of short synthetic oligonucleotides. For the purpose of DNA sequencing, MALDI-TOF mass spectrometry can also be used in combination with Sanger's termination reactions.

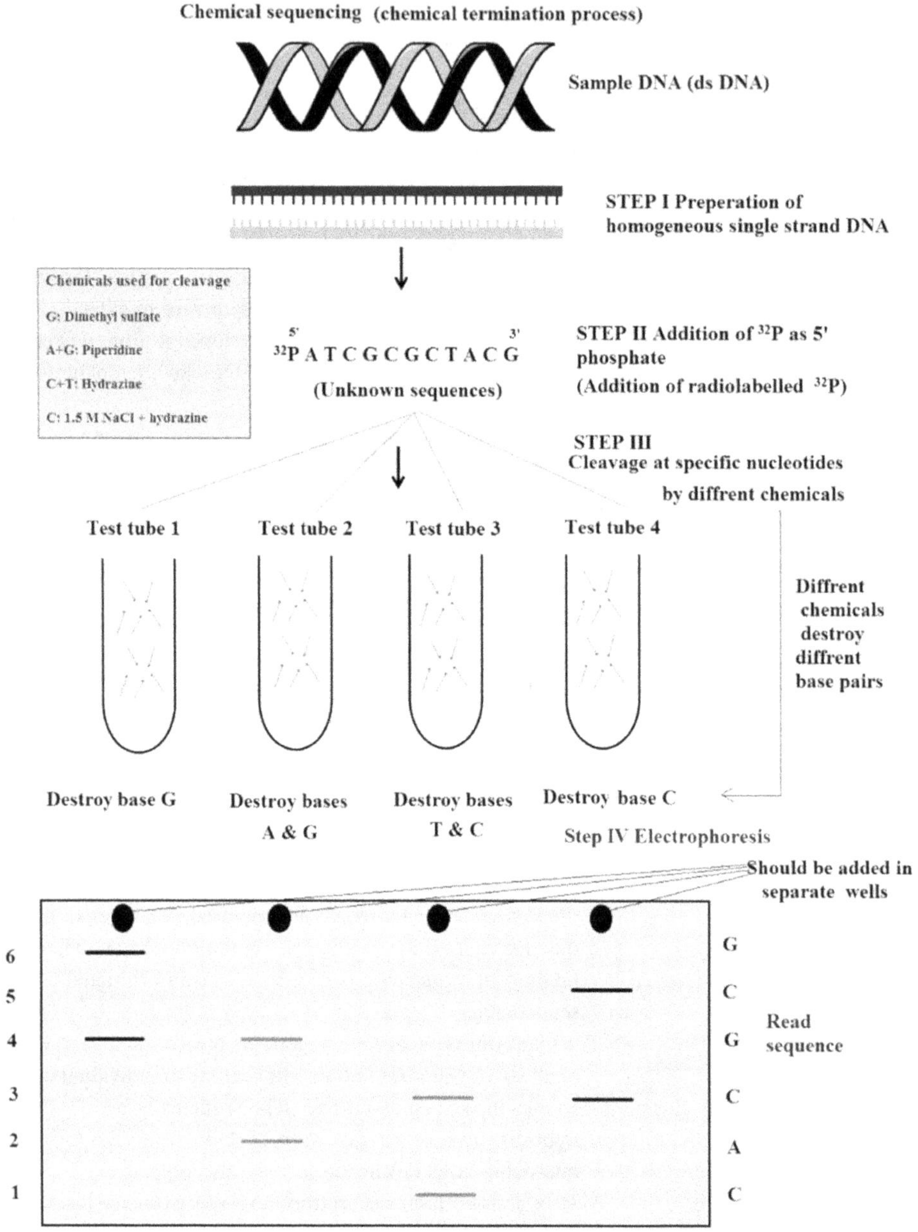

Figure 2.25. Step by step description of the Maxam–Gilbert DNA sequencing method.

2.16 Synthesis of genes

There are two approaches available for the synthesis of genes:

- When the complete structure of the gene is accessible, this gene can be produced by a purely chemical method as synthesized by H G Khorana in his work on the synthesis of genes for a tRNA (described for the first time in 1970) [220].

- If the comprehensive nucleotide sequence is not accessible, one may use the RNA directed DNA polymerase (reverse transcriptase) enzyme for the production of the gene in question in the form of complementary DNA from the mRNA of the gene isolated in its pure form. This cDNA gene nevertheless would lack intron sequences and other sequences that are transcribed but are eliminated during RNA processing. As mentioned above, cDNA is therefore often used for the isolation of a gene either from: (a) DNA extracted from living cells utilizing restriction digestion, electrophoresis and the technique of Southern blot hybridization, or (b) the genomic library.

2.16.1 Chemical synthesis of tRNA genes

As mentioned above, before one can start the chemical-based production of a gene, the structure of the gene needs to be familiar. The structure of a gene cannot not be figured out by direct chemical examination, because there is no means for isolating the gene. The structure of a gene can therefore be inferred only from its product [221]. For example, if a gene is responsible for giving rise to a polypeptide chain and the structure of this chain is identified, then from the genetic code database, the structure of the gene can be easily concluded. Such genes are primarily considered to be too long to manufacture, as an average gene contains about 1500 bp. In contrast, since tRNA molecules are fairly small in size, a gene responsible for giving rise to a tRNA molecule is within reach of synthesis. The total synthesis of the gene for an alanine transfer ribonucleic acid (tRNA) from yeast was achieved in 1970. This was a significant milestone in the field of DNA and RNA chemical synthesis. The synthesis of tRNA genes involves the chemical assembly of nucleotides to create a functional tRNA molecule. The process of chemical gene synthesis allows for the creation of custom-designed tRNA genes with specific sequences and properties. This technology has been used to study the structure and function of tRNA molecules and to engineer new tRNA variants with desired characteristics [222].

2.16.2 Synthesis of the gene for yeast alanyl tRNA

As researchers may be aware, the structure of a large number of tRNAs has now been identified. The first tRNA whose structure was known was yeast alanyl tRNA. R W Holley and co-workers provided the complete structure of yeast alanyl tRNA [223]. This information was instantly used by Khorana and co-workers to infer that the structure of the gene would noticeably be such that one of the two strands of DNA would be complimentary to the base sequence of yeast alanyl tRNA. The other strand would then automatically have the same sequence as in tRNA except that in place of the uracil of tRNA there would be thymine in DNA. Different approaches for the synthesis of the gene are as follows:

- Synthesis of the gene from three duplex fragments: three fragments a, b and c are joined to give a complete gene.

- Synthesis of oligonucleotides: 15 oligonucleotides ranging from pentanucleotide to an icosanucleotide are synthesized.
- Synthesis of three duplex fragments: with the help of 15 oligonucleotides three duplex fragments (a, b and c), each with a single-stranded end, are prepared.

2.16.3 Synthesis of a gene from true precursor tRNA

Before Khorana could complete the synthesis protocol of the gene for yeast alanyly tRNA in 1970, it became clear that tRNA was not the first direct product of transcription. In its place a precursor molecule is first produced which, then losing segments of RNA by cleavage, gives rise to tRNA. Thus the authentic gene for yeast alanyl tRNA will be longer than the DNA duplex synthesized by Khorana. In view of this Khorana later started the synthesis of a gene for the *E. coli* tyrosine suppressor tRNA precursor [224]. They chemically synthesized and ligated together 17 oligonucleotides to encode the gene for a 77-nucleotide alanine tRNA. This early work laid the foundation for modern *de novo* gene synthesis techniques. Improvements in oligonucleotide synthesis chemistries and techniques in the early 1980s led to the development of solid-phase synthesis, which allowed for the efficient production of longer DNA sequences. This advancement paved the way for the synthesis of larger genes, such as the 14-amino-acid hormone somatostatin, which was expressed in recombinant *E. coli* [225]. A DNA duplex which would result in this tRNA precursor was synthesized in the form of 26 small oligonucleotide segments. These were then settled into six DNA duplex fragments with single-stranded ends. These six single-stranded fragments resulted in the presumed gene for *E. coli* tyrosine suppressor tRNA precursor [224].

In recent years, advancements in gene synthesis methods have enabled the synthesis of even larger and more complex genes. For example, the synthesis of the first minimal bacterial genome, which consists of 473 genes, was achieved using a combination of *de novo* gene synthesis and whole-genome assembly techniques. This breakthrough has provided valuable insights into the complexities and challenges of engineering biology [226].

The synthesis of a gene from a true precursor tRNA involves several steps. First, the nucleotide sequence of the gene is designed based on the desired amino acid sequence. Then, the oligonucleotides corresponding to the gene sequence are chemically synthesized using solid-phase synthesis. These oligonucleotides are then assembled using various methods, such as enzymatic joining or DNA assembly techniques, to form the complete gene sequence. One of the challenges in gene synthesis is the fidelity of the synthetic DNA. Errors can occur during the synthesis process, leading to mutations in the final gene sequence. To address this issue, several error correction methods have been developed, including consensus shuffling and protein-mediated error correction. Another challenge is the cost of gene synthesis, which is primarily driven by the reagents needed for oligonucleotide synthesis. To reduce costs, approaches that reduce reagent consumption improve the robustness and accuracy of the gene assembly process and enable increased throughput, have been developed. These advancements have made synthetic DNA more accessible and affordable for researchers. In conclusion, the synthesis of a gene from a true precursor tRNA has come a long way since its inception in the mid-1960s. Advances in oligonucleotide synthesis chemistries, gene assembly techniques, and error correction methods have enabled the synthesis of larger and more complex genes. These advancements have not only expanded our understanding of biology but also have the potential to revolutionize various fields, including medicine, agriculture, and biotechnology [227].

2.16.4 Mass spectrometry for genomics and proteomics

Mass spectrometry encompasses segregation of charged atoms or molecules according to their mass-to-charge (*M*/*E*) ratio and thus supports the determination of the relative molecular masses of organic compounds and biomolecules with very high precision and sensitivity. Application of mass spectrometry (MS) for the investigation of biomolecules took a long time to achieve, as it requires charged gaseous molecules for analysis, and the polymeric biomolecules, being large and polar, cannot be easily transformed into the gaseous phase and ionized. Nevertheless, the accessibility of ionization techniques, e.g. MALDI, electrospray and other major developments made in sample preparation for MS [228], this made it possible to obtain polymeric biomolecules in a gaseous state and in an ionized form, so that MS has been explored widely for the investigation of biomolecules. In the early and mid-1990s, software algorithms also became accessible which permitted the investigation of the connections between the information collected from MS with the data available in massive databases/databanks. Therefore, in the last decade of the 20th century MS became a significant tool for genomics and proteomics research [228].

2.16.4.1 Applications of MS for genome/proteome analysis

Mass spectrometry in the form of MALDI-TOF has been broadly exploited for the investigation of nucleic acids, proteins and peptides, although initially the tool was more frequently used for the investigation of peptides. For biotechnology applications we need to investigate both nucleic acids and proteins and thus the use of MS for the investigation of both nucleic acids and proteins will be briefly discussed [229].

2.16.4.1.1 Genome analysis using MS

DNA sequencing by DE MALDI-TOF MS We are familiar with Sanger's dideoxy termination method of DNA sequencing which depends on a high level of resolution to permit sequential distribution of the termination fragments of lengths n and $n + 1$. The termination products of Sanger's termination reactions nevertheless can also be investigated by delayed extraction (DE) MALDI-TOF MS In this strategy mass spectra of each of the four specific dideoxy termination reactions generated from Sanger's chemistry are covered and each sized product is connected to one of the four base termination reactions, as the mass of each base is known. A major plus point of this strategy is the fast procurement of information by MALDI-TOF MS, which requires only minutes per sample. A further merit is that there is no requirement for gel electrophoresis or for any radioactive or fluorescence labeling [229].

2.16.4.1.2 SNP detection using MS

A variety of methods have been developed for the analysis of point mutations that are due to SNPs. Several methods that require neither gel electrophoresis nor labeling utilize MALDI-TOF MS. The study of DNA polymorphism using MS depends largely on the determination of relative masses of individual DNA fragments with sufficient accuracy, so that even a single base replacement can be identified due to the unique mass of each base. However, the methods have been applied only to relatively short oligonucleotides because the resolution and sensitivity of MALDI-MS generally falls off dramatically with the increase in size of oligonucleotides. Analysis of nucleic acid by MALDI-TOF MS has several advantages:

- In contrast with electrophoretic separation, ionization takes milliseconds to separate by size.
- The results are more accurate than for electrophoretic and hybridization-based techniques which are influenced by secondary structures formed by nucleic acids.
- Complete automation involving both sample preparation and processing of data is possible.

2.16.4.1.3 Pinpoint assay for SNP detection using MALDI-TOF MS of PCR products

One of the methods that is defined as pinpoint is based on using a primer directly upstream of a known point mutation or SNP, so that in PCR the primer is extended by a single deoxynucleotide triphosphates (ddNTP). In other cases a primer may anneal several bases away from SNP and extend more than one base before incorporating specific ddNTP, which terminates the reaction. The PCR products are solid-phase purified and examined by mass/charge (*m/z*) ratio values specific to the nucleotide added in the extension reaction. The method is described as minisequencing, since it includes sequencing of a segment a few bases long.

2.16.4.1.4 SNP detection using PNA probes

PNAs are being used for a variety of purposes, including as hybridization probes. They are much preferred over DNA/RNA probes due to:

- Their ability to hybridize under low ionic strength.
- The increased hybridization specificity for complementary DNA.
- The increased thermal stability they provide to the hybrid duplexes formed.

PNAs can also be more easily investigated by MALDI-TOF MS, as the peptide backbone does not fragment during MALDI.

2.16.4.1.5 SNP detection using invader cleavage

Invader cleavage is a technique that allows SNP direction without PCR. SNP detection involves minisequencing using MALDI on a chip technology. In this technology nanoliter amounts of sample from minisequencing SNP analysis reactions are piezoelectrically pipetted onto a silicon chip. This silicon chip is directly inserted into a mass spectrometer and each separate sample spot is automatically analyzed using the MALDI-TOF MS approach.

2.16.4.2 Proteome investigation using MS

In the post-genomic era, proteome investigation will be crucial for understanding different biological processes. To attain this objective, MS has been extensively utilized for:

- Peptide sequencing.
- Identification of proteins.
- Investigation of protein expression in different tissues and under different conditions.
- Identification of post-translational modification of proteins in response to different stimuli.
- Characterization of protein interactions that comprise protein ligand, protein–protein and protein–DNA interactions. Recent developments in MS have led to its increased use for protein structure and function.

2.16.4.3 Peptide sequencing

The sequence of a peptide can be evaluated by understanding MS data resulting from any of the following techniques:

- Tandem MS of trypsinized peptide fragments ionized using electrospray from a mixture.
- TOF-MS of a mixture of fragments resulting from sequential chemical degradation of a peptide from the N-terminus or C-terminus, a technique described as ladder sequencing.
- RETOF-MS of the post-source decay fragmentation of metastable peptide ions that are produced with MALDI. The basic principle involved in the approach, where MS is used for peptide sequencing, is described above.

2.16.4.4 Determination of molecular weights of intact proteins

Mass spectra of intact protein fragments allow the identification of precise molecular weights of major and minor proteins; however, larger proteins, being heterogeneous, make determination of their precise molecular weights difficult. Nevertheless, high-resolution Fourier transform ion cyclotron resonance MS has been employed for precise determination of the masses of small intact proteins. However, the molecular weight only may not be adequate for protein identification and peptide sequencing by tandem MS as mentioned above.

2.16.4.5 Protein identification by combining MS with database search

Mass spectrometry has been combined with database search to create a valuable and automatic protein identification tool. Three main types of databases are examined by mass spectrometric data. Non-redundant protein databases encompass known sets of full-length protein sequences, devoid of duplicates. In this application intact proteins are degraded into pools of peptides whose masses are determined by MS and then examined against genomic DNA, cDNA/EST and non-redundant

Table 2.6. Three main programs for protein identification using database mining.

Program	Website	Basis
Mascot	www.matrixscience.com	Includes probability-based implementations of the MOWSE[a] algorithm.
Profound	http://prowl.rockefeller.edu/	Analyzes the probability that a protein in a database is the protein under analysis and uses the Z-score as an indicator of the quality of the search result.
Protein prospector (Ms-Fit)	www.prospector.urcsf.edu	Uses the MOWSE score to assess a hit in protein identification.

[a] MOWSE: molecular weight search algorithm.

database (NRDB) entries (table 2.6). These databases can be searched both by mass fingerprints and tandem mass spectrometric data.

2.16.4.6 Searching with tandem mass spectrometric data

Databases can also be inspected for similarities with tandem mass spectrometric data obtained on peptides from the protein of interest. Since the tandem mass spectra encompass structural data related to the sequence of the peptide, rather than only its mass, these searches are more consistent and specific. Several methods exist, one of the most significant being the peptide sequence tag method. It makes use of the information that approximately every tandem mass spectrum contains at least a short run of fragment ions that clearly specify a short amino acid sequence.

2.16.4.7 Searching for protein modifications

Protein modifications can also be explored by database searching. For example, a phosphopeptide can be related to a peptide sequence in the database with an additional mass increment due to the phosphogroup. The algorithm used for the peptide sequence tag permits detection of mass difference on either side of the tag sequence.

2.16.4.8 Searching with peptide mass fingerprints

In this process, first a mixture of protein is exposed to 2D gel electrophoresis. A particular protein is then used for in-gel digestion with sequence-specific protease, e.g. trypsin and a mass spectrum designated as a mass fingerprint is obtained by MALDI-TOF. The mass data are matched to the theoretically predictable tryptic peptide masses for each entry in the database. The protein in the database may vary according to the number of peptide matches.

2.16.4.9 Investigation of post-translational modifications

Mass spectrometry is also employed for the investigation of post-translational modifications in proteins. For example, protein phosphorylation, which is so common within the cell, can be identified by MS However, it involves more time and additional preparative steps. When tryptic peptides are frequently examined in mass spectrometer, the phosphorylated peptides may need to be separated from the non-phosphorylated peptides, the presence of which may obscure the signal from the phosphorylated peptides.

2.17 Genomics and proteomics research

In the last quarter of the 20th century (1975–2000), significant development was observed in the area of genetics and biotechnology. This was possible primarily due to the growth of a variety of techniques such as rDNA, PCR, DNA chips, MALDI-TOF MS and automated DNA synthesis and sequencing machines. However, in the majority of these cases the growth was made through investigation involving individual genes or individual DNA fragments/sequences, rather than whole genomes. This was a serious drawback and did not permit the investigation of many sequences for which polymorphism did not exist. Likewise, at the phenotypic level, the roles of most of the genes could not be determined owing to non-availability of mutant alleles. This was mainly true of housekeeping genes, for which mutants would be lethal and would never be available for investigation. Such an investigation of individual genes or DNA fragments was essential in the early stages of the growth in biotechnology, since techniques for the investigation of complete genome sequences were not available. Nevertheless, starting in the mid-1990s, due to the progressing high-throughput approaches, it became possible to examine an entire genome at a time. This involved the examination of DNA sequences of the complete genome of an organism and assigning function to all these sequences. This investigation of all the genes of an organism was possible either at the level of DNA/mRNA or at the level of proteins, the former designated as genomics and latter designated as proteomics. Starting in 1995, substantial growth was rapidly made in the field, which was also designated as reverse genetics, as it involved the examination of the DNA sequence first and then finding out its effect on the phenotype, rather than starting from the phenotype and recognizing its gene, as is done in the Mendelian forward genetics method. Significant methods used in genomic research are:

- Building of clone counting (overlapping series of cloned DNA fragments).
- Construction of whole-genome BAC map: BAC-by-BAC approach.
- Electronic PCR: bridging the gaps between mapping and sequencing of genomes.
- Map first, sequence later or clone-by-clone strategy, also called hierarchical shotgun sequencing.
- Methods for annotation of genome sequences (annotation by sequence search and loss of function by mutation approach).
- Proteomics research (2D-PAGE, MS, differential display comparative 2D gel approach, protein chip approach).
- Whole-genome sequence data.
- Whole-genome shotgun sequencing.

Current accomplishments demonstrate the role of MS-based proteomics as a crucial technique for molecular and cellular biology and for the developing field of systems biology. These include the investigation of protein–protein interactions via affinity-based isolations on a small and proteome-wide scale, the simultaneous description of the malaria parasite genome and proteome, the mapping of numerous organelles, and the production of quantitative protein profiles from diverse species. The capability of MS to detect and, progressively, to accurately measure multiple proteins from complex samples is likely to impact widely on biology and medicine [56].

Genomics and proteomics research are two transformative disciplines within the field of molecular biology, offering profound insights into the genetic and protein components of living organisms. Over the past few decades, these fields have witnessed exponential growth, driven by advancements in technology, which has allowed scientists to explore the complete genetic and proteomic make-up of various species. For a comprehensive overview see reference [230].

2.17.1 Genomics

Genomics, derived from 'genetic' and 'informatics,' is the comprehensive study of an organism's entire genetic material, including its DNA, genes, and the sequences that regulate gene expression. The genomic information within an organism's DNA contains the instructions for building and maintaining the organism. Genomics involves the analysis of these instructions to unravel the genetic basis of traits, diseases, and evolutionary relationships [231]. One of the cornerstones of genomics is the sequencing of an organism's genome. Genome sequencing involves determining the order of nucleotide bases (adenine, thymine, cytosine, and guanine) in the DNA. This sequence, often represented as a linear string of letters, provides a complete 'instruction manual' for the organism. Genome sequencing has been significantly facilitated by the development of high-throughput sequencing technologies, such as next-generation sequencing (NGS) and third-generation sequencing. These technologies enable the rapid and cost-effective determination of DNA sequences, making it feasible to sequence entire genomes. The Human Genome Project, completed in 2003, was a watershed moment in genomics, as it provided the first comprehensive sequence of the human genome [232]. Beyond genome sequencing, genomics encompasses gene mapping, functional genomics, comparative genomics, and structural genomics. Gene mapping involves locating individual genes on chromosomes, while functional genomics investigates the roles and functions of genes and their products, such as proteins and non-coding RNAs. Comparative genomics explores the similarities and differences in the genomes of different species to gain insights into evolution and genetic relationships. Structural genomics focuses on the three-dimensional structures of genes and their products, particularly proteins [233]. One of the key applications of genomics is personalized medicine. Genomic information is used to identify genetic variations associated with diseases, drug responses, and other medical conditions. By understanding an individual's genetic make-up, healthcare professionals can tailor treatments and medications to optimize their effectiveness while minimizing potential side effects [234]. In agriculture, genomics research plays a vital role in crop improvement and breeding programs. By identifying genes related to desirable traits like drought resistance, disease resistance, and higher yields, scientists and breeders can develop more resilient and productive crops. Genomic information can also be used to address global challenges such as food security [235]. Genomics research has applications beyond medicine and agriculture. In evolutionary biology, comparative genomics helps trace the evolutionary history of species and understand the genetic changes that have occurred over time. In biotechnology, genomics is instrumental in the development of genetically modified organisms (GMOs) and the field of synthetic biology, where new biological systems are designed and constructed [236]. The list of different methods used for genomic research is summarized in table 2.7.

Table 2.7. Pros and cons of different methods of study essential for various types of genomic research.

Genomics method of study	Pros	Cons
Fluorescent *in situ* hybridization (FISH)	It provides high-resolution mapping of specific DNA sequences on chromosomes. direct visualization of the location of genes or DNA sequences within cells.	It performed on a small number of chromosomes or cells at a time, labor-intensive, especially for large-scale studies.
Single nucleotide polymorphism (SNP) arrays:	SNP arrays can genotype thousands to millions of SNPs across the genome, provide quantitative information about allele frequencies.	It focuses on single nucleotide variations, not on other types of genetic variations. Genome Coverage depending on the array design.
Microarray techniques	Analyze the expression levels of thousands of genes simultaneously, provide quantitative information on gene expression.	Can detect highly or lowly expressed genes. Cross-hybridization can lead to inaccurate results.
Gene expression profiling (GEP)	Used in comprehensive genomics of a given sample. Detect potential biomarkers associated with diseases.	Costly, and expression data alone may not provide a complete understanding of protein function or post-translational modifications.

(*Continued*)

Table 2.7. (*Continued*)

Genomics method of study	Pros	Cons
RNA sequencing (RNAseq)	It can detect low-abundance transcripts with high sensitivity, provides both quantitative and qualitative expression level information such as alternative splicing.	Analysis of RNA-Seq data, more expensive than microarrays, especially for large-scale studies.
ChIP-Seq (chromatin immuno precipitation sequencing)	It allows genome-wide mapping of protein–DNA interactions. Provides quantitative information on the enrichment of specific DNA sequences.	Involves complex experimental procedures, analysis of ChIP-Seq data requires bioinformatics expertise.
Whole-genome sequencing (WGS)	Provides a complete sequence of an organism's genome for detailed comparative analysis. Identification of structural variations: Enables the identification of structural variations such as insertions, deletions, and rearrangements.	Whole-genome sequencing can be expensive, especially for large genomes. Analyzing and interpreting large genomic datasets require substantial computational resources.
Phylogenetic tree construction tools	Represent evolutionary relationships. Provide a visual representation of the relatedness among species.	Accuracy depends on the quality and choice of input sequences.
Gene ontology (GO) analysis tools	Functional annotation provides understanding of biological processes associated with the gene.	Results are influenced by the completeness and accuracy of gene annotations. Interpreting results may require biological knowledge.

2.17.2 Application of human genome sequencing

These applications highlight the wide range of uses for human genome sequencing, from understanding genetic variations and disease mechanisms to unraveling the complexities of human evolution and diversity.

2.17.2.1 Assembly of genomes and discovery of variants

In order to enhance the assembly of genomes, it is noteworthy that the current read lengths have reached a sufficient extent to effectively traverse the majority of repetitive structures inside the genome. In the case of diploid genomes, such as those found in humans, the current objective is to attain precise haplotype resolution over the entirety of the genome, without relying on a reference as a guide [237]. Various methods for genome assembly exist, including *de novo* genome assembly and telomere-to-telomere chromosome assemblies. *De novo* genome assembly refers to the procedure wherein a collection of arbitrarily chosen sequence fragments is rebuilt in order to ascertain the precise arrangement of each nucleotide inside a genome [238]. Contigs are designated as stitched-together sequencing fragments, and in an optimal scenario, each chromosome is represented by a single contig. As an illustration, Shafin and colleagues successfully produced eleven human genome assemblies of high contiguity (with a median NG50 of 18.5 Mb) using long-read Oxford Nanopore Technologies (ONT) data. This achievement was accomplished utilizing a mere three PromethION flow cells and 6 h of computational work on a 28-core system equipped with over 1 TB of RAM per genome [239]. In a comparable manner, Chin and Khalak successfully constructed human genomes within a time frame of less than 100 min (equivalent to 30 CPU hours), excluding the computational expense incurred during the generation of PacBio HiFi reads. Notably, their approach yielded a contig N50 surpassing 20 Mb, solely utilizing PacBio HiFi data [240]. In the context of alternative methodologies, the optimal genome assembly entails an independent contig for each chromosome, whereby the arrangement and orientation of the entire chromosome sequence are determined from one telomere to the other. A majority of the existent inadequacies in long-read genome assemblies are found in regions that are characterized by segmental duplications [241–244]. Furthermore, these variants can be easily distinguished by the use of higher read depth. The occurrence of these collapses is attributed to the inability to effectively resolve sequences that possess a high degree of similarity. Nevertheless, it is possible to achieve assembly of these regions with an accuracy over 99.9% by employing methodologies that include partitioning the lengthy reads based on a graph of paralogous sequence variants. One such strategy is the utilization of segmental duplication assembler [242].

2.17.2.2 Structural variant detection

The utilization of long-read genome sequencing has significantly advanced our insight of the comprehensive range of genetic variation within the human population [245–247]. The research comparing individuals sequenced using the Illumina short-read and PacBio long-read platforms revealed that Illumina whole-genome sequencing missed 47% of deletions and nearly 78% of insertions, even after utilizing 11 different variant callers specifically designed to detect genomic insertions, deletions, inversions, and duplications [248]. In addition, a study was conducted to analyze challenging sequences derived from 748 human genes. These sequences were difficult to assay due to low mapping quality of certain protein-coding exons when using Illumina-based exome sequencing. The results of this analysis revealed significant improvements in sensitivity when employing long-read sequencing. Notably, this approach led to the identification of potentially pathogenic variants linked to Alzheimer's disease [249]. The greater specificity has promptly led to various practical applications, such as the identification and sequencing of more intricate forms of disease-causing variations [250–253]. These include the detection of novel

GGC repeat expansions linked to neuronal intranuclear inclusion disease and adults with leukoencephalopathy [254–256], the identification of founder SVA retrotransposon insertions responsible for X-linked dystonia-parkinsonism in the Philippines [257], the discovery of new candidate mutations associated with schizophrenia and bipolar disorder [258], and the detection of large complex triplications and regions of segmental uniparental disomy associated with Temple syndrome [259]. However, it is worth noting that prior to these breakthroughs, the successful assembly of the gene model or locus of interest was typically achieved by laborious and rigorous approaches. These crucial components were absent from the original human genome, but can now be effectively assembled using comprehensive whole-genome assembly techniques [242].

2.17.2.3 Beyond DNA sequencing

Long-read sequencing techniques have been utilized for purposes beyond genome assembly and variant discovery. This has enabled the identification of whole RNA isoforms [260–262] and the detection of alterations in native RNA and DNA [263–266]. One notable advantage of long-read sequencing technology lies in its capacity to accurately ascertain the complete sequence of RNA transcripts originating from genes. Both PacBio sequencing technology and ONT sequencing technology have the capability to accurately determine the sequence of complete RNA molecules. This can be achieved either by cDNA sequencing using PacBio and ONT platforms [267, 268], or through native RNA sequencing using ONT technology [260–262]. Sequence data of such kind enhances gene annotation and facilitates subsequent analysis by eliminated the necessity to recreate isoforms through the error-prone assembly of abbreviated RNA sequencing reads. The utilization of native RNA sequencing has facilitated the identification of previously unknown isoforms originating from disease-associated genes linked to psychiatric illnesses [269] and chronic lymphoid leukemia [270]. These findings hold promise for the identification of novel targets for early disease detection in clinical contexts and the development of pharmaceutical interventions. Prior to the advancement of these methods, the prevalent kind of base modification that could be identified was methylated cytosine, employing an indirect methodology referred to as bisulfite sequencing. Bisulfite sequencing involves the treatment of DNA with bisulfite, a chemical agent that induces the conversion of cytosine to uracil while preserving the integrity of modified cytosines. The identification of changed cytosines can be achieved through the analysis of the ensuing DNA sequencing, in conjunction with an untreated control. Nevertheless, the current method fails to differentiate between various forms of cytosine modifications [271] and lacks the capability to identify additional types of changed bases. The utilization of long-read sequencing technology significantly enhances the ability to identify changed RNA bases by obviating the need for highly specific techniques that are often employed for the detection of various sorts of modifications [272, 273]. The utilization of direct sequencing techniques on native DNA and RNA molecules is significantly contributing to the advancement of epigenomics and epitranscriptomics. This approach enables the identification of formerly unidentified modifications on DNA and RNA, which may be detected simultaneously with the sequencing process. A wide range of computer algorithms have been devised for the identification of DNA and RNA modifications, leveraging distinctive disruptions. These tools include Nanopolish [274], DeepSignal [275], mCaller [276], DeepMod [277], and Tombo [278]. The utilization of these methodologies has facilitated the exploration of methylation patterns in genomic and transcriptomic regions that were previously unexplored. Notably, these techniques have been essential in investigating the methylation states of the X chromosome centromere [279] and cancer-associated genes [280], hence contributing to the generation of novel biological knowledge.

2.17.2.4 Human genetic diversity and evolution

The implicit nature of sequencing and assembling novel human genomes, as well as the heightened presence of structural variation, is evident. The discovery pertains to an enhanced comprehension of human genetic diversity and the mutational mechanisms that have influenced the composition of our genomes [245–247, 268, 279]. As an illustration, the application of long-read sequencing on a limited diversity panel consisting of 15 human genomes revealed the presence of about 100 000 structural variants, a significant proportion of which had not been previously found. Among them, it was demonstrated that a variable number tandem repeats (VNTRs) exhibited a significant departure from random distribution, as nearly half of them were found to be located within the last 5 megabases (Mb) of subtelomeric areas. This observation may be attributed to higher frequencies of double-strand breaks occurring in these specific genomic regions [281]. The recent application of sequencing and assembly techniques has facilitated the identification of substantial copy number polymorphisms. These structural variants have been found to be linked to positive selection and introgression, exhibiting a notable specificity towards particular human populations [282]. An instance of a duplication polymorphism of 386 kilobases was comprehensively sequenced and assembled, demonstrating a notable specificity towards persons of Melanesian ancestry. The phenomenon of gene duplication, including the presence of duplicated genes, originated within the ancient Denisovan lineage and was subsequently introduced into the ancestral human population through interbreeding. The observed duplication exhibits several indications of positive selection and is currently prevalent in 79% of individuals of Melanesian descent, while being very rare in other ethnic groups. The identification and arrangement of intricate structural variations not only facilitate the process of genotyping, but also enable the improvement of association studies, particularly in datasets consisting of short-read sequences [247, 281].

2.17.2.5 Proteomics

Proteomics, a term derived from 'protein' and 'genomics,' is the scientific study of the complete set of proteins in an organism, collectively known as the proteome. Proteins are the workhorses of biology, responsible for a wide range of functions, from catalysing biochemical reactions to forming the structure of cells and tissues [283]. This research aims to understand the structure, function, and interactions of proteins. Unlike genomics, which focuses on the static genetic information, proteomics delves into the dynamic aspects of cellular processes. This involves studying how proteins are produced, modified, interact with one another, and function within living organisms [284]. Protein identification, protein expression, protein–protein interactions, and post-translational modifications are key concepts one can use study proteomics-based research. Protein identification is the process of determining the identity of proteins in a given sample, which can be complex due to the vast number of proteins in the proteome. Understanding protein expression involves quantifying the levels of specific proteins under different physiological conditions, which can provide insights into the regulation of cellular processes [284] in protein–protein interactions, as these interactions form the basis of many biological functions. Investigating how proteins bind to each other and form complexes is crucial for understanding cellular signaling pathways, metabolic networks, and disease mechanisms [285]. Post-translational modifications (PTMs) are chemical changes that occur on proteins after they are synthesized. PTMs can influence a protein's activity, stability, localization, and interactions with other molecules. Common PTMs include phosphorylation, glycosylation, acetylation, and ubiquitination [286].

Techniques used in proteomics are diverse and continually evolving such as two-dimensional electrophoresis (2D-PAGE), which is a classic method that separates proteins based on their isoelectric point and molecular weight, allowing for the visualization of individual proteins in a complex mixture. However, mass spectrometry (MS) has become the central technique in proteomics [287]. Mass spectrometry is a versatile tool that can identify, quantify, and analyze PTMs of proteins. It involves ionizing proteins, separating them based on their mass-to-charge ratio, and measuring their abundance. Modern mass spectrometers are highly sensitive and capable of analyzing complex mixtures of proteins [287, 288]. Protein chips, also known as microarrays for proteins, enable high-throughput analysis of protein interactions, PTMs, and expression. Affinity-based isolations, such as immunoprecipitation and pull-down assays, allow researchers to study protein–protein interactions and identify binding partners [289]. There are several different advantages and disadvantages that are present for performing proteomics research, which are listed here in table 2.8.

2.17.2.6 Applications of proteomics are vast and encompass multiple fields

Disease biomarkers: Proteomics is instrumental in the discovery of biomarkers for various diseases, including cancer, neurodegenerative diseases, and cardiovascular disorders. Biomarkers are proteins that can be detected in bodily fluids and tissues and can serve as indicators of disease presence or progression [290].

Drug development: Proteomics is essential for drug discovery and development. By identifying and validating drug targets, understanding the mechanisms of action of drugs, and evaluating drug efficacy and safety, proteomics accelerates the development of new pharmaceuticals [291].

Systems biology: Proteomics contributes to systems biology, which aims to understand the complex network of interactions between genes, proteins, and

Table 2.8. Different methods for conducting proteomics studies along with their respective pros and cons.

Proteomics	Pros	Cons
Two-dimensional gel electrophoresis (2D-GE)	Separates proteins based on charge and size. Visual separation of proteins, quantitative analysis.	Limited dynamic range, challenges in reproducibility.
Protein microarray	Identifies proteins by digesting them into peptides and analyzing the peptide mixture. Comprehensive identification, suitable for complex mixtures	data analysis complexity, potential for missing low-abundance proteins.
MALDI-TOF MS	Generates ions for analysis. High sensitivity, specificity, large-scale protein identification.	Complex data analysis, potential for sample degradation during ionization.
LC-MS-MS	Separates and analyzes peptides. High sensitivity, specificity, and large-scale protein identidication.	Complex data analysis, potential for sample degradation during ionization.

metabolites in living organisms [292]. It helps to model and predict cellular processes.

Functional analysis: Proteomics enables researchers to study the functions of specific proteins in cellular processes. By perturbing proteins and observing the resulting effects on cell function, scientists gain insights into the roles of individual proteins [284].

Proteome mapping: Mapping the proteome of specific organelles or cellular compartments provides detailed information about the functions and composition of these structures [293].

The integration of genomics and proteomics is particularly powerful in systems biology, as it allows researchers to bridge the gap between genetic information and protein function. By combining genomic data with proteomic analyses, scientists can gain a comprehensive view of how genes are transcribed, translated, and regulated to perform specific cellular functions [294].

2.17.2.7 Integration and synergy: genomics and proteomics

Genomics and proteomics are inherently intertwined, with the former providing the genetic blueprint, and the latter revealing how that blueprint is executed [295]. The synergy between these two disciplines is crucial for understanding the complexities of biology. Below are some examples of how they complement each other.

Functional genomics: While genomics provides information about the presence of genes and their regulatory elements, proteomics reveals which of these genes are actively transcribed and translated into proteins [296]. This insight into the functional roles of proteins is a vital link in understanding how genes contribute to cellular processes.

Protein expression profiling: Genomic data can guide proteomic experiments. For instance, genomics can identify genes of interest (e.g., potential drug targets or disease-related genes), which can then be investigated at the protein level through proteomics [231].

Post-translational modifications: Genomics cannot capture post-translational modifications, which are critical for protein function. Proteomics provides information on PTMs, shedding light on how proteins are modified to perform specific functions [286].

Protein–protein interactions: Genomic data can suggest potential interactions between genes, but proteomics can confirm and characterize these interactions. Understanding protein–protein interactions is essential for deciphering complex cellular pathways and signaling networks [297].

Network analysis: The integration of genomics and proteomics data enables researchers to construct comprehensive biological networks. These networks depict how genes, proteins, and other molecules interact and cooperate to drive cellular processes [298].

Functional validation: Proteomics can validate the functional roles of genes identified through genomics. By perturbing the expression or activity of specific genes and monitoring the resulting changes in the proteome, researchers can confirm the functions of these genes [299].

Disease mechanisms: Integrating genomics and proteomics data aids in unraveling the molecular mechanisms underlying diseases. Genomic variants associated with diseases can be explored at the proteomic level to understand how they disrupt protein function and contribute to pathology [155].

The synergy between genomics and proteomics has broad implications, from basic research to clinical applications. This integration has led to the emergence of systems biology, an interdisciplinary field that seeks to understand the complex interplay between genes, proteins, and other cellular components in the context of living organisms.

2.17.2.8 Challenges and future directions

While genomics and proteomics have made significant strides, they are not without challenges. Some of these challenges, including integrating and analyzing vast amounts of genomic and proteomic data, can be complex [290]. Developing robust bioinformatics tools and databases to handle these data is an ongoing challenge [300]. Also, to understand the functional implications of genomic and proteomic data is a multifaceted task. Researchers must bridge the gap between genetic information and its consequences at the protein level. Keeping pace with rapidly evolving sequencing and mass spectrometry technologies is essential.

Precise quantification of protein abundance in complex mixtures remains a challenge. Improvements in quantification techniques are vital for accurately assessing protein expression changes. Many PTMs remain poorly characterized. Identifying and understanding the functions of these modifications represent significant challenges [290].

Personalized medicine: Realizing the full potential of genomics and proteomics in personalized medicine requires addressing ethical, privacy, and regulatory issues [301].

The future of genomics and proteomics research promises continued growth and innovation. Some of the directions in which these fields are advancing include single-cell genomics. Researchers are increasingly focusing on analyzing the genomes and proteomes of individual cells, providing insights into cellular heterogeneity and developmental processes [302].

Long-read sequencing: Third-generation sequencing technologies, such as nanopore sequencing, enable the sequencing of long DNA fragments and have the potential to reveal complex genomic structures and reduce assembly errors [303].

Multi-omics integration: Combining genomics, proteomics, metabolomics, and other 'omics' data allows for a more comprehensive understanding of biological systems. Multi-omics approaches are instrumental in systems biology and personalized medicine [304].

Functional genomics and CRISPR-Cas9: Advances in genome editing technologies, such as CRISPR-Cas9, have revolutionized functional genomics by enabling precise gene manipulation and the study of gene function in various organisms [305].

Pharmacoproteomics: The application of proteomics in pharmacology and drug development is growing. Proteomics helps identify drug targets, predict drug responses, and assess drug safety [284].

Environmental genomics and proteomics: These fields explore the genomic and proteomic adaptations of organisms to their environments and have applications in environmental monitoring and bioremediation [306].

References

[1] Watson J D and Crick F H C 1953 Molecular structure of nucleic acids: a structure for deoxyribose nucleic acid *Nature* **171** 737–8

[2] Dawkins R 1989 *The Selfish Gene* 2nd edn (Oxford: Oxford University Press) pp 142–5

[3] Hoffman R E 1996 The gene wars: science, politics, and the human genome *Am. J. Psychiatry* **153** 959

[4] Garrod A E 1908 The Croonian lectures on inborn errors of metabolism, lecture IV *Lancet* **2** 214–20

[5] Beadle G W and Tatum E L 1941 Genetic control of biochemical reactions in *Neurospora* *Proc. Natl Acad. Sci. USA* **27** 499–506

[6] Horowitz N H 1948 The one gene-one enzyme hypothesis *Genetics* **33** 612

[7] Roy B, Haupt L M and Griffiths L R 2013 Review: alternative splicing (AS) of genes as an approach for generating protein complexity *Curr. Genomics* **14** 182–94

[8] Brem R B, Yvert G, Clinton R and Kruglyak L 2002 Genetic dissection of transcriptional regulation in budding yeast *Science (1979)* **296** 752–5

[9] Sandberg R, Yasuda R, Pankratz D G, Carter T A, Del Rio J A, Wodicka L *et al* 2000 Regional and strain-specific gene expression mapping in the adult mouse brain *Proc. Natl Acad. Sci. USA* **97** 11038–43

[10] Primig M, Williams R M, Winzeler E A, Tevzadze G G, Conway A R, Hwang S Y *et al* 2000 The core meiotic transcriptome in budding yeasts *Nat. Genet.* **26** 415–23

[11] Cavalieri D, Townsend J P and Hartl D L 2000 Manifold anomalies in gene expression in a vineyard isolate of *Saccharomyces cerevisiae* revealed by DNA microarray analysis *Proc. Natl Acad. Sci. USA* **97** 12369–74
[12] Karp C L, Grupe A, Schadt E, Ewart S L, Keane-Moore M, Cuomo P J *et al* 2000 Identification of complement factor 5 as a susceptibility locus for experimental allergic asthma *Nat. Immunol.* **1** 221–6
[13] Jin W, Riley R M, Wolfinger R D, White K P, Passador-Gurgell G and Gibson G 2001 The contributions of sex, genotype and age to transcriptional variance in Drosophila melanogaster *Nat. Genet.* **29** 389–95
[14] Oleksiak M F, Churchill G A and Crawford D L 2002 Variation in gene expression within and among natural populations *Nat. Genet.* **32** 261–6
[15] Jansen R C and Nap J P 2001 Genetical genomics: the added value from segregation *Trends Genet.* **17** 388–91
[16] Watson J D and Crick F H 1953 Genetical implications of the structure of deoxyribonucleic acid *Nature* **171** 964–7
[17] Watson J D and Crick F H 1953 Molecular structure of nucleic acids; a structure for deoxyribose nucleic acid *Nature* **171** 737–8
[18] Shampo M A and Kyle R A 2002 Kary B Mullis—Nobel Laureate for procedure to replicate DNA *Mayo Clin. Proc.* **77** 606
[19] Champoux J 2001 DNA topoisomerases: structure, function, and mechanism *Annu. Rev. Biochem.* **70** 369–413
[20] Lodish H 2000 *DNA Replication, Repair, and Recombination* (New York: Freeman) ch 12 pp 85–92
[21] Lodish H 2004 *Molecular Biology of the Cell* 5th edn (New York: Freeman)
[22] Lindahl T and Barnes D E 2000 Repair of endogenous DNA damage *Cold Spring Harb. Symp. Quant. Biol.* **65** 127–33
[23] Mathews L A, Cabarcas S M and Hurt E M 2013 *DNA Repair of Cancer Stem Cells: DNA Repair Pathways and Mechanisms* (Berlin: Springer) pp 19–32
[24] Lindahl T 1993 Instability and decay of the primary structure of DNA *Nature* **362** 709–15
[25] Apel K and Hirt H 2004 Reactive oxygen species: metabolism, oxidative stress, and signal transduction *Annu. Rev. Plant Biol.* **55** 373–99
[26] Marnett L J 2000 Oxyradicals and DNA damage *Carcinogenesis* **21** 361–70
[27] Cadet J, Berger M, Douki T and Ravanat J L 1997 Oxidative damage to DNA: formation, measurement, and biological significance *Rev. Physiol., Biochem. Pharmacol.* **131** 1–87
[28] Burney S, Caulfield J L, Niles J C, Wishnok J S and Tannenbaum S R 1999 The chemistry of DNA damage from nitric oxide and peroxynitrite *Mutat. Res.* **424** 37–49
[29] McCulloch S D and Kunkel T A 2008 The fidelity of DNA synthesis by eukaryotic replicative and translesion synthesis polymerases *Cell Res.* **18** 148–61
[30] Ravanat J L, Douki T and Cadet J 2001 Direct and indirect effects of UV radiation on DNA and its components *J. Photochem. Photobiol.,* B **63** 88–102
[31] Ward J F 1988 DNA damage produced by ionizing radiation in mammalian cells: identities, mechanisms of formation, and reparability *Prog. Nucleic Acid Res. Mol. Biol.* **35** 95–125
[32] Wogan G N, Hecht S S, Felton J S, Conney A H and Loeb L A 2004 Environmental and chemical carcinogenesis *Semin. Cancer Biol.* **14** 473–86

[33] Irigaray P and Belpomme D 2010 Basic properties and molecular mechanisms of exogenous chemical carcinogens *Carcinogenesis* **31** 135–48

[34] Noll D M, Mason T M and Miller P S 2006 Formation and repair of inter strand cross-links in DNA *Chem. Rev.* **106** 277–301

[35] Sinha B K 1995 Topoisomerase inhibitors. A review of their therapeutic potential in cancer *Drugs* **49** 11–19

[36] Bedard L L and Massey T E 2006 Aflatoxin B1-induced DNA damage and its repair *Cancer Lett.* **241** 174–83

[37] Altieri F, Grillo C, Maceroni M and Chichiarelli S 2008 DNA damage and repair: from molecular mechanisms to health implications *Antioxid. Redox Signal* **10** 891–937

[38] Lindahl T 1993 Instability and decay of the primary structure of DNA *Nature* **362** 709–15

[39] Zharkov D O 2008 Base excision DNA repair *Cell. Mol. Life Sci.* **65** 1544–65

[40] Li G M 2008 Mechanisms and functions of DNA mismatch repair *Cell Res.* **18** 85–98

[41] Costa R M, Chigancas V, Galhardo Rda S, Carvalho H and Menck C F 2003 The eukaryotic nucleotide excision repair pathway *Biochimie* **85** 1083–99

[42] Nouspikel T 2008 Nucleotide excision repair and neurological diseases *DNA Repair (Amst.)* **7** 1155–67

[43] Alberts B 2002 *Molecular Biology of the Cell* 4th edn (New York: Garland Science)

[44] Alberts B 2002 Site-specific recombination *Molecular Biology of the Cell* 4th edn (New York: Garland Science)

[45] Alberts B 2002 DNA replication, repair, and recombination *Molecular Biology of the Cell* 4th edn (New York: Garland Science) ch 5

[46] Dorado G, Unver T, Budak H and Molina P H 2017 *Molecular Markers* (Amsterdam: Elsevier)

[47] Amiteye S 2021 Basic concepts and methodologies of DNA marker systems in plant molecular breeding *Heliyon* **7** e08093

[48] Clancy J A, Jitkov V A, Han F and Ullrich S E 1996 Barley tissue as direct template for PCR: a practical breeding tool *Mol. Breed.* **2** 81–3

[49] Ikeda N, Bautista N S, Yamada T, Kamijima O and Ishii T 2001 Ultrasimple DNA extraction method for marker-assisted selection using microsatellite markers in rice *Plant Mol. Biol. Rep.* **19** 27–32

[50] Dayteg C, Vos Post L, Lund R and Tuvesson S 1998 Quick DNA extraction method for practical plant breeding programmes *Plant and Animal Genome VI (San Diego, CA, Jan. 18–22))* p 39

[51] Murray M G and Thompson W F 1980 Rapid isolation of high molecular weight plant DNA *Nucleic Acids Res.* **8** 4321–5

[52] Dellaporta S L, Wood J and Hicks J B 1983 A plant DNA minipreparation: version II *Plant Mol. Biol. Rep.* **1** 19–21

[53] Shetty P 2020 The evolution of DNA extraction methods *Am. J. Biomed. Sci. Res.* **8** 39–45

[54] Paterson A H, Brubaker C L and Wendel J F 1993 A rapid method for extraction of cotton (*Gossypium* spp.) genomic DNA suitable for RFLP or PCR analysis *Plant Mol. Biol. Rep.* **11** 122–7

[55] Thompson D and Henry R J 1995 Single step protocol for preparation of plant tissue for analysis by PCR *Biotechniques* **19** 394–7

[56] Gu W K, Weeden N F, Yu J and Wallace D H 1995 Large-scale, cost effective screening of PCR products in marker-assisted selection applications *Theor. Appl. Genet.* **91** 465–70

[57] Beckmann J S 1988 Oligonucleotide polymorphisms: a new tool for genomic genetics *Biotechnology* **6** 161–4

[58] Landegren U, Kaiser R, Sanders J and Hood L 1988 DNA diagnostics. molecular techniques and automation *Science* **241** 1077–80

[59] Wang G, Mahalingan R and Knap H T 1998 (C-A) and (GA) anchored simple sequence repeats (ASSRs) generated polymorphism in soybean, *Glycine max* (L.) *Merr. Theor. Appl. Genet.* **96** 1086–96

[60] Zietkiewicz E, Rafalski A and Labuda D 1994 Genome fingerprinting by simple sequence repeats (SSR)-anchored PCR amplification *Genomics* **20** 176–83

[61] Welsh J and McClelland M 1990 Fingerprinting genomes using PCR with arbitrary primers *Nucleic Acids Res.* **18** 7213–8

[62] Akopyanz N, Bukanov N O, Westblom T U and Berg D E 1992 PCR-based RFLP analysis of DNA sequence diversity in the gastric pathogen *Helicobacter pylori Nucleic Acid Res.* **20** 6221–5

[63] Konieczny A and Ausubel F M 1993 A procedure for mapping *Arabidopsis* mutations using co-dominant ecotype-specific PCR-based markers *Plant* J **4** 403–10

[64] Telenius H, Carter N P, Bebb C E, Nordenskjold M, Ponder B A J and Tunnacliffe A 1992 Degenerate oligonucleotide-primed PCR: general amplification of target DNA by a single degenerate primer *Genomics* **13** 718–25

[65] Jaccoud D, Peng K, Feinstein D and Kilian A 2001 Diversity arrays: a solid state technology for sequence information independent genotyping *Nucleic Acids Res.* **29** e25

[66] Caetano-Anolles G, Bassam B J and Gresshoff P M 1991 DNA amplification fingerprinting using very short arbitrary oligonucleotide primers *Biotechnology* **9** 553–7

[67] Adams M D 1991 Complementary DNA sequencing: expressed sequence tags and human genome project *Science* **252** 1651–6

[68] Triglia T, Peterson M G and Kemp D J 1988 A procedure for *in vitro* amplification of DNA segments that lie outside the boundaries of known sequences *Nucleic Acids Res.* **16** 8180–6

[69] Rohde W 1996 Inverse sequence-tagged repeat (ISTR) analysis, a novel and universal PCR-based technique for genome analysis in the plant and animal kingdom *J. Genet. Breed.* **50** 249–61

[70] Meyer W, Mitchell T G, Freedman E Z and Vilgalys R 1993 Hybridization probes for conventional DNA fingerprinting used as single primers in the polymerase chain reaction to distinguish strains of *Cryptococcus neoformans J. Clin. Microbiol.* **31** 2274–80

[71] Shuber A P, Michalowsky L A, Nass G S, Skoletsky J, Hire L M, Kotsopoulos S K, Phipps M F, Barberio D M and Klinger K W 1997 High throughput parallel analysis of hundreds of patient samples for more than 100 mutations in multiple disease genes *Hum. Mol. Genet.* **6** 337–47

[72] Wu K, Jones R, Dannaeberger L and Scolnik P A 1994 Detection of microsatellite polymorphisms without cloning *Nucleic Acids Res.* **22** 3257–8

[73] Hantula J, Dusabenygasani M and Hamelin R C 1996 Random amplified microsatellites (RAMS)—a novel method for characterizing genetic variation within fungi *Eur. J. For. Path.* **26** 15–166

[74] Williams J G K, Kublelik A R, Livak K J, Rafalski J A and Tingey S V 1990 DNA polymorphism's amplified by arbitrary primers are useful as genetic markers *Nucleic Acids Res.* **18** 6531–5

[75] Morgante M and Vogel J 1994 Compound microsatellite primers for the detection of genetic polymorphisms *US Patent Application* no. 08/326 456
[76] Botstein D, White R L, Skolnick M and Davis R W 1980 Construction of a genetic linkage map in man using restriction fragment length polymorphisms *Am. J. Hum. Genet.* **32** 314–31
[77] Paran I and Michelmore R W 1993 Development of reliable PCR-based markers linked to downy mildew resistance genes in lettuce *Theor. Appl. Genet.* **85** 985–93
[78] Waugh R, Bonar N, Baird E, Thomas B, Graner A, Hayes P and Powell W 1997 Homology of AFLP products in three mapping populations of barley *Mol. General Genet.* **255** 311–21
[79] Beckmann J S and Soller M 1990 Toward a unified approach to genetic mapping of eukaryotes based on sequence tagged microsatellite sites *Biotechnology* **8** 930–2
[80] Olsen M, Hood L, Cantor C and Botstein D 1989 A common language for physical mapping of the human genome *Science* **245** 1434–5
[81] Hamada H, Petrino M G and Kakunaga T 1982 A novel repeat element with Z-DNA-forming potential is widely found in evolutionarily diverse eukaryotic genomes *Proc. Natl Acad. Sci. USA* **79** 6465–9
[82] Dietrich W, Katz H, Lincoln S E, Shin H S, Friedman J, Dracopoli N C and Lander E S 1992 A genetic map of the mouse suitable for typing intraspecific crosses *Genetics* **131** 423–47
[83] Akkaya M S, Bhagwat A A and Cregan P B 1992 Length polymorphisms of simple sequence repeat DNA in soybean *Genetics* **132** 1131–9
[84] Jordan S A and Humphries P 1994 Single nucleotide polymorphism in exon 2 of the BCP gene on 7q31-q35 *Hum. Mol. Genet.* **3** 1915
[85] Gupta M, Chyi Y S, Romero-Severson J and Owen J L 1994 Amplification of DNA markers from evolutionarily diverse genomes using single primers of simple-sequence repeats *Theor. Appl. Genet.* **89** 998–1006
[86] Orita M, Suzuki Y, Sekiya T and Hayashi K 1989 Rapid and sensitive detection of point mutations and DNA polymorphisms using polymerase chain reaction *Genomics* **5** 874–9
[87] Koes R 1995 Targeted gene inactivation in petunia by PCR-based selection of transposon insertion mutants *Proc. Natl Acad. Sci.* **92** 8149–53
[88] Walker G T, Little M C, Nadeau J G and Shank D D 1992 Isothermal *in vitro* amplification of DNA by a restriction enzyme/DNA polymerase system *Proc. Natl Acad. Sci.* **89** 392–6
[89] Nakamura Y 1987 Variable number tandem repeat (VNTR) markers for human gene mapping *Science* **235** 1616–22
[90] Wallace H and Birnstiel M L 1966 Ribosomal cistrons and the nucleolar organizer *Biochem. Biophys. Acta* **114** 296–310
[91] Reddy M P, Sarla N and Siddiq E A 2002 Inter simple sequence repeat (ISSR) polymorphism and its application in plant breeding *Euphytica* **128** 9179–17
[92] Grodzicker T, Williams J, Sharp P and Sambrook J 1975 Physical mapping of temperature sensitive mutants of adenovirus *Cold Spring Harb. Symp. Quant. Biol.* **39** 439–46
[93] Helentjaris T, Slocum M, Wright S, Schaefer A and Nienhuis J 1986 Construction of genetic linkage maps in maize and tomato using restriction fragment length polymorphisms *Theor. Appl. Genet.* **61** 650–8
[94] Terachi T 1993 The progress of DNA analyzing techniques and its impact on plant molecular systematics *J. Plant Res.* **106** 75975–9

[95] Arrigo A-P and Landry J 1994 Expression and function of the low-molecular-weight heat shock proteins *The Biology of Heat Shock Proteins and Molecular Chaperones* ed R Morimoto, A Tissieres and C Georgopoulus Cold Spring Harbor Monograph Series 26th edn (Cold Spring Harbor, NY: Cold Spring Harbor Laboratory Press) pp 335–73

[96] Holtke H J, Ankenbauer W, Muhlegger K, Rein R, Sagner G, Seibl R and Walter T 1995 The digoxigenin (DIG) system for non-radioactive labelling and detection of nucleic acids —an overview *Cell. Mol. Biol.* **41** 883–905

[97] Potter R H and Jones M G K 1991 Molecular analysis of genetic stability *In Vitro Methods for Conservation of Plant Genetic Resources* ed J H Dodds (London: Chapman and Hall) pp 71–91

[98] Southern E M 1975 Detection of specific sequences among DNA fragments separated by gel electrophoresis *J. Mol. Biol.* **98** 503–17

[99] Staub J E and Serquen F C 1996 Genetic markers, map construction, and their application in plant breeding *HortScience* **31** 729–40

[100] Mansfield E S, Worley J M, McKenzie S E, Surrey S, Rappaport E and Fortina P 1995 Nucleic acid detection using non-radioactive labeling methods *Mol. Cell. Probes* **9** 145–56

[101] Perez de la Vega M P 1993 Biochemical characterization of populations *Plant Breeding: Principles and Prospects* ed M D Hayward, N O Bosemark and I Romagosa (London: Chapman and Hall) pp 182–201

[102] Yu K F, Deynze A V and Pauls K P 1993 Random amplified polymorphic DNA (RAPD) analysis *Methods in Plant Molecular Biology and Biotechnology* ed B R Glick and J E Thompson (Boca Raton, FL: CRC Press)

[103] Roy A, Frascaria N, Mackay J and Bonsquet J 1992 Segregating random amplified polymorphic DNA (RAPDs) in *Betula alleghaniensis Theor. Appl. Genet.* **85** 173–80

[104] Wolfe A D and Liston A 1998 Contribution of PCR-based methods to plant systematics and evolutionary biology *Molecular Systematics of Plants II: DNA Sequencing* ed D E Soltis, P S Soltis, J J Doyle and Kluwer pp 43–86

105Caetano-Anolles GWelsh J and McClelland M 1991 Genomic fingerprinting using arbitrarily primed PCR and a matrix of pairwise combinations of primers *Nucleic Acids Res.* **19** 5275–9

[107] Bassam B J, Caetano-Anolles G and Gresshoff P M 1992 DNA amplification fingerprinting of bacteria *Appl. Microbiol. Biotechnol.* **38** 70–6

[108] Williams J G K, Kublelik A R, Livak K J, Rafalski J A and Tingey S V 1990 DNA polymorphisms amplified by arbitrary primers are useful as genetic markers *Nucleic Acids Res.* **18** 6531–5

[109] Huff D R, Peakall R and Smouse P E 1993 RAPD variation within and among natural populations of outcrossing buffalograss [*Buchloe dactyloides* (Nutt.) Engelm] *Theor. Appl. Genet.* **86** 927–34

[110] Pammi S, Schertz K, Xu G, Hart G and Mullet J E 1994 Randomamplified-polymorphic DNA markers in Sorghum *Theor. Appl. Genet.* **89** 80–8

[111] Corley-Smith G E, Lim C J, Kalmar G B and Brandhorst B P 1997 Efficient detection of DNA polymorphisms by fluorescent RAPD analysis *BioTechniques* **22** 690–2

[112] Devos K M and Gale M D 1992 The use of random amplified polymorphic DNA markers in wheat *Theor. Appl. Genet.* **84** 567–72

[113] Heun M and Helentjaris T 1993 Inheritance of RAPDs in F1 hybrids of corn *Theor. Appl. Genet.* **85** 9618961

[114] Wolff K, Schoen E D and Peters-Van Rijn J 1993 Optimizing the generation of random amplified polymorphic DNA in chrysanthemum *Theor. Appl. Genet.* **86** 1033–7
[115] Micheli M R, Bova R, Pascale E and D'Ambrosio E 1994 Reproducible DNA fingerprinting with the random amplified polymorphic DNA (RAPD) method *Nucleic Acids Res.* **22** 1921–2
[116] Skroch P and Nienhuis J 1995 Impact of scoring error and reproducibility of RAPD data on RAPD based estimates of genetic distance *Theor. Appl. Genet.* **91** 1086–91
[117] Kresovich S, Williams J G K, McFerson J R, Routman E J and Schaal B A 1992 Characterization of genetic identities and relationships of *Brassica oleracea* L. via a random amplified polymorphic DNA assay *Theor. Appl. Genet.* **85** 190–6
[118] Schierwater B, Metzler D, Kruger K and Strit B 1996 The effect of nested primer binding sites on the reproducibility of PCR: mathematical modeling and computer simulation studies *J. Computational Biol.* **3** 235–51
[119] Thormann C E, Ferreira M E, Camargo L E A, Tivang J G and Osborn T C 1994 Comparison of RFLP and RAPD markers to estimating genetic relationships within and among cruciferous species *Theor. Appl. Genet.* **88** 973–80
[120] Weising K, Nybom H, Wolff K and Meyer W 1995 *DNA Fingerprinting in Plants and Fungi* (Boca Raton, FL: CRC Press)
[121] Ridout C and Donini P 1999 Use of AFLP in cereals research *Trends Plant Sci.* **4** 76–9
[122] Vos P 1995 AFLP: a new technique for DNA fingerprinting *Nucleic Acids Res.* **23** 44074414
[123] Mueller U G and Wolfenbarger L L 1999 AFLP genotyping and fingerprinting *Trends Ecol. Evol.* **14** 389–94
[124] Rouppe van der Voort J N, van Zandvoort P, van Eck H J, Folkertsma R T, Hutten R C B, Draaistra J, Gommers F J, Jacobsen E, Helder J and Bakker J 1997 Use of allele specificity of co-migrating AFLP markers to align genetic maps from different potato genotypes *Mol. General Genet.* **255** 438–47
[125] Jones C J 1997 Reproducibility testing of RAPD, AFLP, and SSR markers in plants by a network of European laboratories *Mol. Breed.* **3** 381–90
[126] Powell W, Morgante M, Andre C, Hanafey M, Vogel J, Tingey S and Rafalski A 1996 The comparison of RFLP, RAPD, AFLP and SSR (microsatellite) markers for germplasm analysis *Mol. Breed.* **2** 225238
[127] Joshi S P, Gupta V S, Aggarwal R K, Ranjekar P K and Brar D S 2000 Genetic diversity and phylogenetic relationship as revealed by intersimple sequence repeat (ISSR) polymorphism in the genus *Oryza Theor. Appl. Genet.* **100** 1311–20
[128] Kojima T, Nagaoka T, Noda N and Ogihara Y 1998 Genetic linkage map of ISSR and RAPD markers in Einkorn wheat in relation to that of RFLP markers *Theor. Appl. Genet.* **96** 37–45
[129] Fang D Q and Roose M L 1997 Identification of closely related citrus cultivars with inter-simple sequence repeat markers *Theor. Appl. Genet.* **95** 408–17
[130] Moreno S, Martin J P and Ortiz J M 1998 Inter simple sequence repeats PCR for characterization of closely related grapevine germplasm *Euphytica* **101** 117–25
[131] Tsumura Y, Ohba K and Strauss S H 1996 Diversity and inheritance of inter-simple sequence repeat polymorphisms in Douglas-fir (*Pseudotsuga menziesii*) and sugi (*Cryptomeria japonica*) *Theor. Appl. Genet.* **92** 40–5
[132] Sankar A A and Moore G A 2001 Evaluation of inter-simple sequence repeat analysis for mapping in Citrus and extension of genetic linkage map *Theor. Appl. Genet.* **102** 206–14

[133] Sanchez M P, Davila J A, Loarce Y and Ferrer E 1996 Simple sequence repeat primers used in polymerase chain reaction amplifications to study genetic diversity in barley *Genome* **39** 112–17
[134] Hancock J M 1999 Microsatellites and other simple sequences: genomic context and mutational mechanisms *Microsatellites: Evolution and Applications* ed D B Goldstein and C Schlotterer (Oxford: Oxford University Press) pp 191–9
[135] McDonald D B and Potts W K 1997 DNA microsatellites as genetic markers for several scales *Avian Molecular Evolution and Systematics* ed D P Mindell (San Diego, CA: Academic) pp 29–49
[136] Goldstein D B and Pollock D D 1997 Launching microsatellites: a review of mutation processes and methods of phylogenetic inference *J. Hered.* **88** 335–42
[137] Schlotterer C 1998 Microsatellites *Molecular Genetic Analysis of Populations: A Practical Approach* ed A R Hoelzel (Oxford: IRL) pp 237–61
[138] Armour J A L, Alegre S A, Miles S, Williams L J and Badge R M 1999 Minisatellites and mutation processes in tandemly repetitive DNA *Microsatellites: Evolution and Applications* ed D B Goldstein and C C Schlotterer (Oxford: Oxford University Press) pp 24–33
[139] Chambers G K and MacAvoy E S 2000 Microsatellites: consensus and controversy *Comparative Biochem. Physiol.* B **126** 455–76
[140] Tautz D, Trick M and Dover G A 1986 Cryptic simplicity in DNA is a major source of genetic variation *Nature* **322** 652–6
[141] Levinson G and Gutman G A 1987 Slipped-strand mispairing: a major mechanism for DNA sequence evolution *Mol. Biol. Evol.* **4** 203–21
[142] Eisen J A 1999 Mechanistic basis for microsatellite instability *Microsatellites: Evolution and Applications* ed D B Goldstein and C Schlotterer (Oxford: Oxford University Press) pp 34–48
[143] Freudenreich C H, Stavenhagen J B and Zakian V A 1997 Stability of a CTG:CAG trinucleotide repeat in yeast is dependent on its orientation in the genome *Mol. Cell. Biol.* **4** 2090–8
[144] Queller D C, Strassman J E and Hughes C R 1993 Microsatellites and kinship *Trends Ecol. Evol.* **8** 2858285
[145] Vieira M L, Santini L, Diniz A L and Munhoz Cde F 2016 Microsatellite markers: what they mean and why they are so useful *Genet. Mol. Biol.* **39** 312–28
[146] Rudd S 2003 Expressed sequence tags: alternative or complement to whole genome sequences? *Trends Plant Sci.* **8** 321–9
[147] Maeda M, Uryu N, Murayama N, Ishii H, Ota M, Tsuji K and Inoko H 1990 A simple and rapid method for HLA-DP genotyping by digestion of PCR-amplified DNA with allele specific restriction endonucleases *Hum. Immunol.* **27** 111–21
[148] Michaels S D and Amasino R M 1998 A robust method for detecting single-nucleotide changes as polymorphic markers by PCR *Plant* J. **14** 381–5
[149] Iwata H, Ujino-Ihara T, Yoshimura K, Nagasaka K, Mukai Y and Tsumura Y 2001 Cleaved amplified polymorphic sequence markers in sugi, *Cryptomeria japonica* D. Don, and their locations on a linkage map *Theor. Appl. Genet.* **103** 881–95
[150] Matsumoto A and Tsumura Y 2004 Evaluation of cleaved amplified polymorphic sequence markers *Theor. Appl. Genet.* **110** 80–91
[151] Neff M M, Neff J D, Chory J and Pepper A E 1998 dCAPS, a simple technique for the genetic analysis of single-nucleotide polymorphisms: experimental applications in *Arabidopsis thaliana* genetics *Plant* J. **14** 387–92

[152] Kiran U, Khan S, Mirza K J, Ram M and Abdin M Z 2010 SCAR markers: a potential tool for authentication of herbal drugs *Fitoterapia* **81** 969–76
[153] Romano I, Ventorino V and Pepe O 2020 Effectiveness of plant beneficial microbes: overview of the methodological approaches for the assessment of root colonization and persistence *Front. Plant Sci.* **11** 6
[154] Marwal A, Sahu A K and Gaur R K 2014 Molecular markers: tool for genetic analysis *Animal Biotechnology* ed A S Verma and A Singh (San Diego, CA: Academic) pp 289–305
[155] Gupta P K, Roy J K and Prasad M 2001 Single nucleotide polymorphisms: a new paradigm for molecular marker technology and DNA polymorphism detection with emphasis on their use in plants *Curr. Sci.* **80** 524–35
[156] Campbell T N and Choy F Y M 2002 Approaches to library screening *J. Mol. Microbiol. Biotechnol.* **4** 551–4
[157] Arencibia A 2000 *Plant Genetic Engineering: Towards the Third Millennium* (Amsterdam: Elsevier) p 65
[158] Brown T 1993 Hybridization analysis of DNA blots *Curr. Protoc. Mol. Biol.* **21** 2.10.1–16
[159] Brown T A 2001 *Southern Blotting and Related DNA Detection Techniques* www.els.net
[160] Tofano D, Wiechers I R and Cook-Deegan R 2006 Edwin Southern, DNA blotting, and microarray technology: a case study of the shifting role of patents in academic molecular biology *Genomics, Society and Policy* **2** 1–12
[161] Alwine J C, Kemp D J and Stark G R 1977 Method for detection of specific RNAs in agarose gels by transfer to diazobenzyloxymethyl-paper and hybridization with DNA probes *Proc. Natl Acad. Sci. USA* **74** 5350–4
[162] Lovatt D and Eberwine J 2013 Northern blotting *Brenner's Encyclopedia of Genetics* (Academic Press) 2ndedn pp 105–7
[163] Towbin H, Staehelin T and Gordon J 1979 Electrophoretic transfer of proteins from polyacrylamide gels to nitrocellulose sheets: procedure and some applications *Proc. Natl Acad. Sci. USA* **76** 4350–4
[164] Burnette W N 1981 Western blotting: electrophoretic transfer of proteins from sodium dodecyl sulfate–polyacrylamide gels to unmodified nitrocellulose and radiographic detection with antibody and radioiodinated protein A *Analyt. Biochem.* **112** 195–203
[165] Towbin H 1998 Western blotting *Encyclopedia of Immunology* (Elsevier) pp 2503–7
[166] Bernardy M G, Jacoli G G and Ragetli H W J 1987 Rapid detection of potato spindle tuber viroid (PSTV) by dot blot hybridization *J. Phytopathol.* **118** 171–80
[167] Dudley K 1988 Hybrid-arrested translation *Methods Mol. Biol.* **4** 39–45
[168] Dudley K 1988 Hybrid-arrested translation *New Nucleic Acid Techniques* (Humana Press) pp 39–45
[169] Perrimon N, Ni J Q and Perkins L 2010 *In vivo* RNAi: today and tomorrow *Cold Spring Harb. Perspect. Biol.* **2** a003640
[170] Masoodi K Z, Lone S M and Rasool R S 2021 Agarose gel electrophoresis *Advanced Methods in Molecular Biology and Biotechnology* (Elsevier) pp 7–12
[171] Schwartz D C and Cantor C R 1984 Separation of yeast chromosome sized DNA by pulse field gradient gel electrophoresis *Cell* **37** 67–75
[172] Perrett D 2000 Electrophoresis *Encyclopedia of Separation Science* (Elsevier) pp 103–18
[173] Carle G F, Frank M and Olson M V 1986 Electrophoretic separation of large DNA molecules by periodic inversion of large DNA molecules by periodic inversion of electric field *Science* **232** 65

[174] Carle G F and Carle G F 1992 Field-inversion gel electrophoresis *Pulsed-Field Gel Electrophoresis* (Humana Press) pp 3–18

[175] Gardiner A, Lass R W and Patterson D 1986 Function of large mammalian DNA restriction fragments using vertical pulse field gradient gel electrophoresis *Somat. Cell Mol. Gene* **12** 185

[176] Chu G, Vollrath D and Davis R W 1986 Separation of large DNA molecule by contour clamped homogeneous electric fields *Science* **234** 582–5

[177] Bhattacharya T K 2020 Application of genomics tools in meat quality evaluation *Meat Quality Analysis: Advanced Evaluation Methods, Techniques, and Technologies* (Academic Press) pp 369–89

[178] Petrov A, Tsa A and Puglisi J D 2013 Analysis of RNA by analytical polyacrylamide gel electrophoresis *Methods Enzymol.* **530** 301–13

[179] Bartlett J M S and Stirling D 2003 A short history of the polymerase chain reaction *PCR Protocols* **226** 363–6

[180] Chang T W 1983 Binding of cells to matrixes of distinct antibodies coated on solid surface *J. Immunol. Meth.* **65** 217–23

[181] Tyagi S DNA probes *Encyclopedia of Analytical Chemistry* (Wiley)

[182] Vizzini P, Iacumin L, Comi G and Manzano M 2017 Development and application of DNA molecular probes *AIMS Bioeng* **4** 113–32

[183] Chan P P and Glazer P M 1997 Triplex DNA: fundamentals, advances, and potential applications for gene therapy *J. Mol. Med. (Berl.)* **75** 267–82

[184] Besch R, Giovannangeli C and Degitz K 2004 Triplex-forming oligonucleotides—sequence-specific DNA ligands as tools for gene inhibition and for modulation of DNA-associated functions *Curr. Drug Targets* **5** 691–703

[185] Almarsson O and Bruice T C 1993 Peptide nucleic acid (PNA) conformation and polymorphism in PNA–DNA and PNA–RNA hybrids *Proc. Natl Acad. Sci. USA* **90** 9542–6

[186] Graham I R and Dickson G 2002 Gene repair and mutagenesis mediated by chimeric RNA–DNA oligonucleotides: chimeraplasty for gene therapy and conversion of single nucleotide polymorphisms (SNPs) *Biochim. Biophys. Acta* **1587** 161–6

[187] Felske A, Engelen B, Nübel U and Backhaus H 1996 Direct ribosome isolation from soil to extract bacterial rRNA for community analysis *Appl. Environ. Microbiol.* **62** 4162–7

[188] Liljas A 2013 Ribosomal RNA *Brenner's Encyclopedia of Genetics* (Elsevier) pp 244–6

[189] Brown D D, Carroll D and Brown R D 1977 The isolation and characterization of a second oocyte 5S DNA from xenopus laevis *Cell* **12** 1045–56

[190] Raina A and Datta A 1992 Molecular cloning of a gene encoding a seed-specific protein with nutritionally balanced amino acid composition from Amaranthus *Proc. Natl Acad. Sci. USA* **89** 11774–8

[191] Luo Y, Gong X, Xu L and Li S 2007 Isolation of RNA and RT-PCR, cloning, and sequencing of noncoding RNAs from Fungi *Biochem. Mol. Biol. Educ.* **35** 355–8

[192] Kerovuo J, Lauraeus M, Nurminen P, Kalkkinen N and Apajalahti J 1998 Isolation, characterization, molecular gene cloning, and sequencing of a novel phytase from *Bacillus subtilis Appl. Environ. Microbiol.* **64** 2079–85

[193] Griffiths A J F 1999 *Modern Genetic Analysis* (New York: Freeman)

[194] Sonawane A R, Platig J, Fagny M, Chen C Y, Paulson J N, Lopes-Ramos C M *et al* 2017 Understanding tissue-specific gene regulation *Cell Rep.* **21** 1077–88

[195] Griffiths A J F 1999 *Cloning a Specific Gene* (New York: Freeman)
[196] Trevors J T 1985 DNA probes for the detection of specific genes in bacteria isolated from the environment *Trends Biotechnol.* **3** 291–3
[197] Purdy D I and Park S F 1993 Heterologous gene expression in *Campylobacter coli*: the use of bacterial luciferase in a promoter probe vector *FEMS Microbiol. Lett.* **111** 233–7
[198] Mazur B J, Rice D and Haselkorn R 1980 Identification of blue-green algal nitrogen fixation genes by using heterologous DNA hybridization probes *Proc. Natl Acad. Sci. USA* **77** 186–90
[199] Schwan T G, Simpson W J, Schrumpf M E and Karstens R H 1989 Identification of Borrelia burgdorferi and B. hermsii using DNA hybridization probes *J. Clin. Microbiol.* **27** 1734–8
[200] Suggs S V, Wallace R B, Hirose T, Kawashima E H and Itakura K 1981 Use of synthetic oligonucleotides as hybridization probes: isolation of cloned cDNA sequences for human beta 2-microglobulin *Proc. Natl Acad. Sci. USA* **78** 6613–7
[201] Zahra S, Singh A and Kumar S 2018 Synthetic probes, their applications and designing *Synthetic Biology: Omics Tools and Their Applications* ed S Singh (Singapore: Springer Singapore) pp 207–26
[202] Hardy S, Legagneux V, Audic Y and Paillard L 2010 Reverse genetics in eukaryotes *Biol. Cell.* **102** 561–80
[203] Muñoz-López M and García-Pérez J L 2010 DNA transposons: nature and applications in genomics *Curr. Genomics.* **11** 115–28
[204] Krysan P J, Young J C and Sussman M R 1999 T-DNA as an insertional mutagen in *Arabidopsis Plant Cell* **11** 2283–90
[205] Springer P S 2000 Gene traps: tools for plant development and genomics *Plant Cell* **12** 1007–20
[206] Villao-Uzho L, Chávez-Navarrete T, Pacheco-Coello R, Sánchez-Timm E and Santos-Ordóñez E 2023 Plant promoters: their identification, characterization, and role in gene regulation *Genes* **14** 1226
[207] Kawakami K, Largaespada D A and Ivics Z 2017 Transposons as tools for functional genomics in vertebrate models *Trends Genet.* **33** 784–801
[208] Springer P S 2000 Gene traps: tools for plant development and genomics *Plant Cell* **12** 1007–20
[209] Ramsey M E, Hackett K T, Kotha C and Dillard J P 2012 New complementation constructs for inducible and constitutive gene expression in Neisseria gonorrhoeae and Neisseria meningitidis *Appl. Environ. Microbiol.* **78** 3068–78
[210] Griffiths A J F 2000 *Complementation, an Introduction to Genetic Analysis* 7th edn (New York: Freeman)
[211] Lievens S, Goormachtig S and Holstersa M 2001 A critical evaluation of differential display as a tool to identify genes involved in legume nodulation: looking back and looking forward *Nucleic Acids Res.* **29** 3459–68
[212] Crawford D R, Kochheiser J C, Schools G P, Salmon S L and Davies K J 2002 Differential display: a critical analysis *Gene Expr.* **10** 101–7
[213] Choi J H, Lee M Y, Kim Y, Shim J Y, Han S M, Lee K A, Choi Y K, Jeon H M and Baek K H 2010 Isolation of genes involved in pancreas regeneration by subtractive hybridization *Biol. Chem.* **391** 1019–29

[214] Aasheim H C, Logtenberg T and Larsen F 1997 Subtractive hybridization for the isolation of differentially expressed genes using magnetic beads *cDNA Library Protocols* ed I G Cowell and C A Austin (New York: Humana) (Methods in Molecular Biology vol 69) pp 115–28

[215] Clark D and Pazdernik N 2013 *Cloning Genes for Analysis* pp 194–226

[216] He J P 2010 The application and evaluation of map-based gene isolation in crops *Yi Chuan* **32** 903–13

[217] Tanksley S D, Ganal M W and Martin G B 1995 Chromosome landing: a paradigm for map-based gene cloning in plants with large genomes *Trends Genet.* **11** 63–8

[218] Gupta P K 2008 *Molecular Biology and Genetic Engineering* (Rastogi Publications) pp 355–400

[219] Wolf S F, Mareni C E and Migeon B R 1980 Isolation and characterization of cloned DNA sequences that hybridize to the human X chromosome *Cell* **21** 95–102

[220] Agarwal K L 1970 Total synthesis of the gene for an alanine transfer ribonucleic acid from yeast *Nature* **227** 27–34

[221] Brown E L, Belagaje R, Ryan M J and Khorana H G 1979 Chemical synthesis and cloning of a tyrosine tRNA gene *Methods Enzymol.* **68** 109–51

[222] Hughes R A and Ellington A D 2017 Synthetic DNA synthesis and assembly: putting the synthetic in synthetic biology *Cold Spring Harb. Perspect. Biol.* **9** a023812

[223] Khorana H G 1976 Total synthesis of the structural gene for the precursor of a tyrosine suppressor transfer RNA from *Escherichia coli*. 1. General introduction *J. Biol. Chem.* **251** 565–70

[224] Kresge N, Simoni R D and Hill R L 2009 Total synthesis of a tyrosine suppressor TRNA: the work of H Gobind Khorana *J. Biol. Chem.* **284** e5

[225] Agarwal K L, Büchi H, Caruthers M H, Gupta N, Khorana H G, Kleppe K *et al* 1970 Total synthesis of the gene for an alanine transfer ribonucleic acid from yeast *Nature* **227** 27–34

[226] Itakura K, Hirose T, Crea R, Riggs A D, Heyneker H L, Bolivar F *et al* 1977 Expression in *Escherichia coli* of a chemically synthesized gene for the hormone somatostatin *Science (1979)* **198** 1056–63

[227] Ma S, Saaem I and Tian J 2012 Error correction in gene synthesis technology *Trends Biotechnol.* **30** 147–54

[228] Gstaiger M and Aebersold R 2009 Applying mass spectrometry-based proteomics to genetics, genomics and network biology *Nat. Rev. Genet.* **10** 617–27

[229] Aebersold R and Mann M 2003 Mass spectrometry-based proteomics *Nature* **422** 198–207

[230] Tyers M and Mann M 2003 From genomics to proteomics *Nature* **422** 193–7

[231] Manzoni C, Kia D A, Vandrovcova J, Hardy J, Wood N W, Lewis P A *et al* 2018 Genome, transcriptome and proteome: the rise of omics data and their integration in biomedical sciences *Brief Bioinform.* **19** 286–302

[232] Slatko B E, Gardner A F and Ausubel F M 2018 Overview of next-generation sequencing technologies *Curr. Protoc. Mol. Biol.* **122** e59

[233] Gonzaga-Jauregui C, Lupski J R and Gibbs R A 2012 Human genome sequencing in health and disease *Annu. Rev. Med.* **63** 35–61

[234] Ginsburg G S and Willard H F 2009 Genomic and personalized medicine: foundations and applications *Transl Res.* 277–87

[235] Gao C 2021 Genome engineering for crop improvement and future agriculture *Cell* **184** 1621–35

[236] Sivashankari S and Shanmughavel P 2007 Comparative genomics—a perspective *Bioinformation* **1** 376–8

[237] Logsdon G A, Vollger M R and Eichler E E 2020 Long-read human genome sequencing and its applications *Nat. Rev. Genet.* **21** 597–614

[238] Lander E S, Linton L M, Birren B, Nusbaum C, Zody M C, Baldwin J *et al* 2001 Initial sequencing and analysis of the human genome *Nature* **409** 860–921

[239] Shafin K, Pesout T, Lorig-Roach R, Haukness M, Olsen H E, Bosworth C *et al* 2020 Nanopore sequencing and the Shasta toolkit enable efficient de novo assembly of eleven human genomes *Nat. Biotechnol.* **38** 1044–53

[240] Chen-Shan Chin A K 2019 Human genome assembly in 100 min bioRxiv: https://www.biorxiv.org/content/10.1101/705616v1

[241] Porubsky D, Ebert P, Audano P A, Vollger M R, Harvey W T, Marijon P *et al* 2021 Fully phased human genome assembly without parental data using single-cell strand sequencing and long reads *Nat. Biotechnol.* **39** 302–8

[242] Vollger M R, Dishuck P C, Sorensen M, Welch A E, Dang V, Dougherty M L *et al* 2019 Long-read sequence and assembly of segmental duplications *Nat. Methods* **16** 88–94

[243] Vollger M R, Logsdon G A, Audano P A, Sulovari A, Porubsky D, Peluso P *et al* 2020 Improved assembly and variant detection of a haploid human genome using single-molecule, high-fidelity long reads *Ann Hum Genet* **84** 125–40

[244] Chaisson M J P, Wilson R K and Eichler E E 2015 Genetic variation and the de novo assembly of human genomes *Nat. Rev. Genet.* **16** 627–40

[245] Pendleton M, Sebra R, Pang A W C, Ummat A, Franzen O, Rausch T *et al* 2015 Assembly and diploid architecture of an individual human genome via single-molecule technologies *Nat. Methods* **12** 780–6

[246] Chaisson M J P, Huddleston J, Dennis M Y, Sudmant P H, Malig M, Hormozdiari F *et al* 2015 Resolving the complexity of the human genome using single-molecule sequencing *Nature* **517** 608–11

[247] Huddleston J, Chaisson M J P, Steinberg K M, Warren W, Hoekzema K, Gordon D *et al* 2017 Discovery and genotyping of structural variation from long-read haploid genome sequence data *Genome Res.* **27** 677–85

[248] Zheng G X Y, Lau B T, Schnall-Levin M, Jarosz M, Bell J M, Hindson C M *et al* 2016 Haplotyping germline and cancer genomes with high-throughput linked-read sequencing *Nat. Biotechnol.* **34** 303–11

[249] Ebbert M T W, Jensen T D, Jansen-West K, Sens J P, Reddy J S, Ridge P G *et al* 2019 Systematic analysis of dark and camouflaged genes reveals disease-relevant genes hiding in plain sight *Genome Biol.* **20** 20 97

[250] Wenzel A, Altmueller J, Ekici A B, Popp B, Stueber K, Thiele H *et al* 2018 Single molecule real time sequencing in ADTKD-MUC1 allows complete assembly of the VNTR and exact positioning of causative mutations *Sci Rep.* **8** 4170

[251] Zeng S, Zhang M Y, Wang X J, Hu Z M, Li J C, Li N *et al* 2019 Long-read sequencing identified intronic repeat expansions in *SAMD12* from Chinese pedigrees affected with familial cortical myoclonic tremor with epilepsy *J. Med. Genet* **56** 265–70

[252] Mizuguchi T, Suzuki T, Abe C, Umemura A, Tokunaga K, Kawai Y *et al* 2019 A 12-kb structural variation in progressive myoclonic epilepsy was newly identified by long-read whole-genome sequencing *J. Hum. Genet* **64** 359–68

[253] Miao H, Zhou J, Yang Q, Liang F, Wang D, Ma N *et al* 2018 Long-read sequencing identified a causal structural variant in an exome-negative case and enabled preimplantation genetic diagnosis *Hereditas* **155** 32

[254] Dutta U R, Rao S N, Pidugu V K, V.S V, Bhattacherjee A, Bhowmik A D *et al* 2019 Breakpoint mapping of a novel de novo translocation t(X;20)(q11.1;p13) by positional cloning and long read sequencing *Genomics* **111** 1108–14

[255] Sone J, Mitsuhashi S, Fujita A, Mizuguchi T, Hamanaka K, Mori K *et al* 2019 Long-read sequencing identifies GGC repeat expansions in NOTCH2NLC associated with neuronal intranuclear inclusion disease *Nat. Genet.* **51** 1215–21

[256] Okubo M, Doi H, Fukai R, Fujita A, Mitsuhashi S and Hashiguchi S 2019 GGC repeat expansion of *NOTCH2NLC* in adult patients with leukoencephalopathy *Ann. Neurol.* **86** 962–8

[257] Aneichyk T, Hendriks W T, Yadav R, Shin D, Gao D, Vaine C A *et al* 2018 Dissecting the causal mechanism of X-linked dystonia-Parkinsonism by integrating genome and transcriptome assembly *Cell* **172** 897–909.e21

[258] Song J H T, Lowe C B and Kingsley D M 2018 Characterization of a human-specific tandem repeat associated with bipolar disorder and schizophrenia *Am. J. Human Genet.* **103** 421–30

[259] Carvalho C M B, Coban-Akdemir Z, Hijazi H, Yuan B, Pendleton M, Harrington E *et al* 2019 Interchromosomal template-switching as a novel molecular mechanism for imprinting perturbations associated with temple syndrome *Genome Med.* **11** 25

[260] Soneson C, Yao Y, Bratus-Neuenschwander A, Patrignani A, Robinson M D and Hussain S 2019 A comprehensive examination of Nanopore native RNA sequencing for characterization of complex transcriptomes *Nat. Commun.* **10** 3359

[261] Workman R E, Tang A D, Tang P S, Jain M, Tyson J R, Razaghi R *et al* 2019 Nanopore native RNA sequencing of a human poly(A) transcriptome *Nat. Methods* **16** 1297–305

[262] Garalde D R, Snell E A, Jachimowicz D, Sipos B, Lloyd J H, Bruce M *et al* 2018 Highly parallel direct RNA sequencing on an array of nanopores *Nat. Methods* **15** 201–6

[263] Rand A C, Jain M, Eizenga J M, Musselman-Brown A, Olsen H E, Akeson M *et al* 2017 Mapping DNA methylation with high-throughput nanopore sequencing *Nat. Methods* **14** 411–3

[264] Vilfan I D, Tsai Y C, Clark T A, Wegener J, Dai Q, Yi C *et al* 2013 Analysis of RNA base modification and structural rearrangement by single-molecule real-time detection of reverse transcription *J. Nanobiotechnol.* **11** 8

[265] Flusberg B A, Webster D R, Lee J H, Travers K J, Olivares E C, Clark T A *et al* 2010 Direct detection of DNA methylation during single-molecule, real-time sequencing *Nat. Methods* **7** 461–5

[266] Feng Z, Fang G, Korlach J, Clark T, Luong K, Zhang X *et al* 2013 Detecting DNA modifications from SMRT sequencing data by modeling sequence context dependence of polymerase kinetic *PLoS Comput. Biol.* **9** e1002935

[267] Au K F, Sebastiano V, Afshar P T, Durruthy J D, Lee L, Williams B A *et al* 2013 Characterization of the human ESC transcriptome by hybrid sequencing *Proc. Nat. Acad. Sci.* **110** E4821–30

[268] Sharon D, Tilgner H, Grubert F and Snyder M 2013 A single-molecule long-read survey of the human transcriptome *Nat. Biotechnol.* **31** 1009–14

[269] Clark M B, Wrzesinski T, Garcia A B, Hall N A L, Kleinman J E, Hyde T *et al* 2020 Long-read sequencing reveals the complex splicing profile of the psychiatric risk gene CACNA1C in human brain *Mol. Psychiatry* **25** 37–47
[270] Tang A D, Soulette C M, van Baren M J, Hart K, Hrabeta-Robinson E, Wu C J *et al* 2020 Full-length transcript characterization of SF3B1 mutation in chronic lymphocytic leukemia reveals downregulation of retained introns *Nat. Commun.* **11** 1438
[271] Huang Y, Pastor W A, Shen Y, Tahiliani M, Liu D R and Rao A 2010 The behaviour of 5-hydroxymethylcytosine in bisulfite sequencing *PLoS One* **5** e8888
[272] Bakin A V and Ofengand J Mapping of pseudouridine residues in RNA to nucleotide resolution *Protein Synthesis* (New Jersey: Humana Press) pp 297–310
[273] Incarnato D, Anselmi F, Morandi E, Neri F, Maldotti M, Rapelli S *et al* 2017 High-throughput single-base resolution mapping of RNA 2′-O-methylated residues *Nucleic Acids Res.* **45** 1433–41
[274] Simpson J T, Workman R E, Zuzarte P C, David M, Dursi L J and Timp W 2017 Detecting DNA cytosine methylation using nanopore sequencing *Nat. Methods* **14** 407–10
[275] Ni P, Huang N, Zhang Z, Wang D P, Liang F, Miao Y *et al* 2019 DeepSignal: detecting DNA methylation state from nanopore sequencing reads using deep-learning *Bioinformatics* **35** 4586–95
[276] McIntyre A B R, Alexander N, Grigorev K, Bezdan D, Sichtig H, Chiu C Y *et al* 2019 Single-molecule sequencing detection of N6-methyladenine in microbial reference materials *Nat. Commun.* **10** 579
[277] Liu Q, Fang L, Yu G, Wang D, Xiao C L and Wang K 2019 Detection of DNA base modifications by deep recurrent neural network on Oxford nanopore sequencing data *Nat. Commun.* **10** 2449
[278] Hiroki U 2020 nanoDoc: RNA modification detection using nanopore raw reads with deep One2 class classification bioRxiv https://www.biorxiv.org/content/10.1101/2020.09.13.295089v2
[279] Miga K H, Koren S, Rhie A, Vollger M R, Gershman A, Bzikadze A *et al* 2020 Telomere-to-telomere assembly of a complete human X chromosome *Nature* **585** 79–84
[280] Gilpatrick T, Lee I, Graham J E, Raimondeau E, Bowen R, Heron A, Sedlazeck F J and Timp W 2019 Targeted nanopore sequencing with Cas9 for studies of methylation, structural variants, and mutations bioRxiv https://www.biorxiv.org/content/10.1101/604173v2
[281] Audano P A, Sulovari A, Graves-Lindsay T A, Cantsilieris S, Sorensen M, Welch A E *et al* 2019 Characterizing the major structural variant Alleles of the human genome *Cell* **176** 663–675.e19
[282] Hsieh P, Vollger M R, Dang V, Porubsky D, Baker C, Cantsilieris S *et al* 2019 Adaptive archaic introgression of copy number variants and the discovery of previously unknown human genes *Science (1979)* **366** 6463
[283] Mesri M 2014 Advances in proteomic technologies and its contribution to the field of cancer *Adv. Med.* **2014** 238045
[284] Al-Amrani S, Al-Jabri Z, Al-Zaabi A, Alshekaili J and Al-Khabori M 2021 Proteomics: concepts and applications in human medicine *World J. Biol. Chem.* **12** 57–69
[285] Rao V S, Srinivas K, Sujini G N and Kumar G N S 2014 Protein-protein interaction detection: methods and analysis *Int. J. Proteomics* **2014** 147648

[286] Uversky V N 2013 Posttranslational modification *Brenner's Encyclopedia of Genetics (Second Edition)* ed S Maloy and K Hughes (San Diego, CA: Academic) pp 425–30
[287] Büyükköroğlu G, Dora D D, Özdemir F and Hızel C 2018 Techniques for protein analysis *Omics Technologies and Bio-Engineering* ed D Barh and V Azevedo (New York: Academic) ch 15 pp 317–51
[288] Han X, Aslanian A and Yates 3rd J R 2008 Mass spectrometry for proteomics *Curr. Opin. Chem. Biol.* **12** 483–90
[289] Hall D A, Ptacek J and Snyder M 2007 Protein microarray technology *Mech. Ageing Dev.* **128** 161–7
[290] Chandramouli K and Qian P Y 2009 Proteomics: challenges, techniques and possibilities to overcome biological sample complexity *Hum. Genomics Proteomics* **2009** 239204
[291] Amiri-Dashatan N, Koushki M, Abbaszadeh H A, Rostami-Nejad M and Rezaei-Tavirani M 2018 Proteomics applications in health: biomarker and drug discovery and food industry *Iran. J. Pharm. Res.* **17** 1523–36
[292] Moore J B and Weeks M E 2011 Proteomics and systems biology: current and future applications in the nutritional sciences *Adv. Nutr.* **2** 355–64
[293] Borner G H H 2020 Organellar maps through proteomic profiling 2013; a conceptual guide *Mol. Cell. Proteom.* **19** 1076–87
[294] Chase Huizar C, Raphael I and Forsthuber T G 2020 Genomic, proteomic, and systems biology approaches in biomarker discovery for multiple sclerosis *Cell Immunol.* **358** 104219
[295] Franklin S and Vondriska T M 2011 Genomes, proteomes, and the central dogma *Circ. Cardiovasc. Genet* **4** 576
[296] Chatterjee S and Ahituv N 2017 Gene regulatory elements, major drivers of human disease *Annu. Rev. Genomics Hum. Genet* **18** 45–63
[297] Kaake R M, Wang X and Huang L 2010 Profiling of protein interaction networks of protein complexes using affinity purification and quantitative mass spectrometry *Mol. Cell Proteom.* **9** 1650–65
[298] Cline M S, Smoot M, Cerami E, Kuchinsky A, Landys N, Workman C *et al* 2007 Integration of biological networks and gene expression data using Cytoscape *Nat. Protoc.* **2** 2366–82
[299] Graves P R and Haystead T A 2002 Molecular biologist's guide to proteomics *Microbiol. Mol. Biol. Rev.* **66** 39–63
[300] Hu, Canon B, Eloe-Fadrosh S, Anubhav E A, Babinski M, Corilo Y *et al* 2022 Challenges in bioinformatics workflows for processing microbiome omics data at scale *Front. Bioinform.* **1** 826370
[301] Goetz L H and Schork N J 2018 Personalized medicine: motivation, challenges, and progress *Fertil. Steril.* **109** 952–63
[302] Shao X, Weng L, Gao M and Zhang X 2019 Single-cell analysis for proteome and related researches *TrAC, Trends Anal. Chem.* **120** 115666
[303] Wang Y, Zhao Y, Bollas A, Wang Y and Au K F 2021 Nanopore sequencing technology, bioinformatics and applications *Nat. Biotechnol.* **39** 1348–65
[304] Pinu F R, Beale D J, Paten A M, Kouremenos K, Swarup S, Schirra H J *et al* 2019 Systems biology and Multi-Omics integration: viewpoints from the metabolomics research community *Metabolites* **9** 76

[305] Li H, Yang Y, Hong W, Huang M, Wu M and Zhao X 2020 Applications of genome editing technology in the targeted therapy of human diseases: mechanisms, advances and prospects *Signal Transduct Target Ther.* **5** 1

[306] Lacerda C M R and Reardon K F 2009 Environmental proteomics: applications of proteome profiling in environmental microbiology and biotechnology *Brief. Funct. Genom.* **8** 75–87

IOP Publishing

Introduction to Pharmaceutical Biotechnology, Volume 1
(Second Edition)
Basic techniques and concepts
Ahmed Al-Harrasi, Saif Hameed, Zeeshan Fatima and Saurabh Bhatia

Chapter 3

Introduction to genetic engineering

Sarika Bano, Isha Bansal, R Joshma, Aanvi Goel, Tanuja Sarkar and Munindra Ruwali

3.1 Introduction

Genetic engineering, also known as genetic modification or genetic manipulation has emerged as a revolutionary and rapidly advancing field of science and technology. This multidisciplinary discipline involves the deliberate alteration of an organism's genetic material to achieve specific outcomes, such as the introduction of desirable traits or the correction of genetic disorders. It is an assembly of techniques employed for direct genetic modification of organisms or populations of organisms by means of recombination of DNA. These techniques are used to identify, replicate, modify and transfer the genetic material of cells, tissues or whole organisms [1, 2]. Most procedures are associated to the direct manipulation of DNA concerned with the expression of particular genes. In a wider sense, genetic engineering encompasses the introduction of DNA markers for selection (marker-assisted selection, or MAS) to increase the efficiency of the so-called 'traditional' approaches of breeding based on phenotypic material. The most well-known purpose of genetic engineering is the direct manipulation of DNA sequences. These methods include the ability to isolate, cut and transfer particular DNA fragments, analogous to particular genes [3, 4]. The mammalian genome has a bigger size and has multifaceted associations with viruses, bacteria and plants. Therefore, genetic modification of animals, by means of molecular genetics and rDNA technology, is more challenging and expensive than that of simpler organisms. In mammals, methods for reproductive manipulation of gametes and embryos, e.g. procurement of a complete new organism from adult differentiated cells (cloning), and measures for artificial reproduction, e.g. *in vitro* fertilization, embryo transfer (ET) and artificial insemination, are normally a significant part of these procedures [5, 6]. The application of genetic engineering techniques has provided unprecedented insights into the genetic basis of life, enabling

doi:10.1088/978-0-7503-5382-3ch3

scientists to modify genes with precision. Recent research into genetic engineering of animals is focused on different possible medical, pharmaceutical and agricultural uses. Moreover, there is great interest in enhancing our basic knowledge about mammalian genetics and physiology, including complex traits controlled by many genes, e.g. many human and animal disorders [7–11]. Table 3.1 lists the different branches of biotechnology.

Table 3.1. Different types of biotechnology and their characteristic features.

S. No.	Type of biotechnology	Areas covers
1.	Red biotechnology	This is the health branch and responsible, according to the Biotechnology Innovation Organization (BIO), for the development of more than 250 vaccines and medications such as antibiotics, regenerative therapies and the production of artificial organs [23].
2.	Green biotechnology	It is used by more than 13 million farmers worldwide to fight pests and nourish crops and strengthen them against microorganisms and extreme weather events, such as droughts and frosts [21].
3.	White biotechnology	The industrial branch works to improve manufacturing processes, the development of biofuels and other technologies to make industry more efficient and sustainable [8].
4.	Yellow biotechnology	This branch is focused on food production and, for example, it carries out research to reduce the levels of saturated fats in cooking oils. Its main function is to genetically improve products so that there is a higher quantity or quality of food [52].
5.	Blue biotechnology	This exploits marine resources to obtain aquaculture, cosmetics and healthcare products. At the environmental level, the aim is to preserve marine species and ecosystems. In addition, it is the branch most widely used to obtain biofuels from certain microalgae [182].
6.	Grey biotechnology	Its purpose is the conservation and restoration of contaminated natural ecosystems through, as mentioned above, bioremediation processes.
7.	Gold biotechnology	Also known as bioinformatics it is responsible for obtaining, storing, analyzing and separating biological information, especially that related to DNA and amino acid sequences [11].
8.	Brown biotechnology	This comes from green biotechnology with the aim of taking advantage of arid and desert soils to include highly resistant plant species that increase the flora and biodiversity of these environments [21].
9.	Purple biotechnology	It deals with the legal study of the very aspects of this science. They are closely related to intellectual property, patents and the biosafety of processes involving living organisms [24].

10.	Orange biotechnology	This includes the dissemination of information of interest to the other branches. It is carried out both in the fields of education and scientific dissemination with new advances in biotechnologies.
11.	Black biotechnology	This includes all research work on microorganisms that can be manipulated to attack human health. Its main activities are related to biological warfare and bioterrorism.

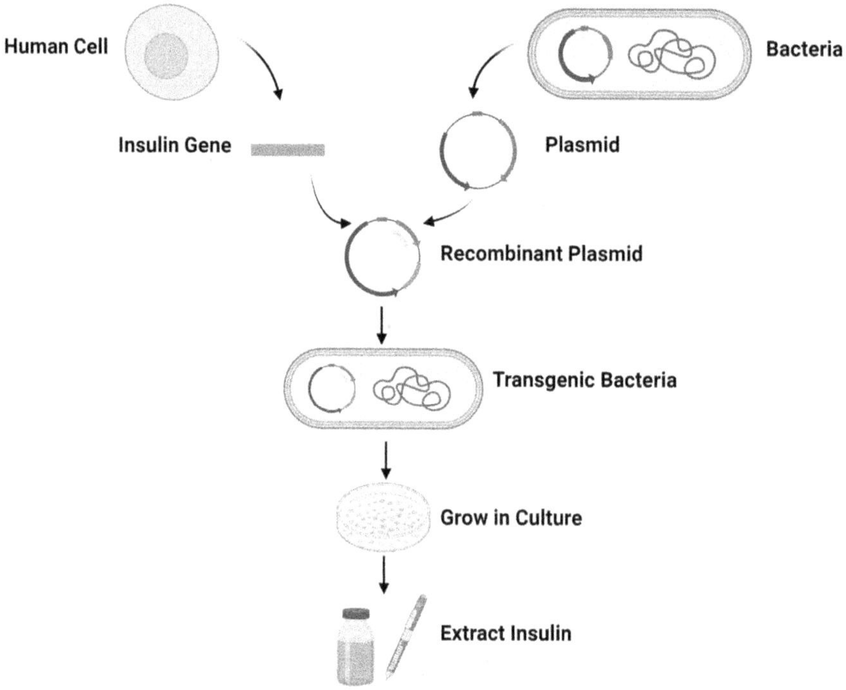

Figure 3.1. Application of genetic engineering in production of insulin.

The importance in genetic engineering of mammalian cells is based on knowledge of, for instance, the use of gene therapy to treat genetic disorders such as cystic fibrosis by substituting the injured copies of the gene for normal ones in fetuses or infants (gene therapy) [12, 13]. Genetically engineered animals, e.g. the 'knockout mouse', in which one particular gene is 'turned off', are used to model genetic disorders in humans and to determine the role of particular sites of the genome [14]. Genetically engineered animals, e.g. pigs, will perhaps be employed to produce organs for transplant to humans (xenotransplantation) [5–15]. Additional applications include production of particular therapeutic human proteins, e.g. insulin in the mammary glands of genetically engineered milking animals such as goats (transgenic animals, bioreactors) (figure 3.1) [16]. These practices may be employed to enhance disease resistance and output in agriculturally important animals by enhancing the frequency of the desired alleles in the populations used in food production. This can be attained by transferring alleles or allele mixtures, over-expressing or eliminating the expression of particular genes (the use of genetic engineering in animal breeding) [17–20]. Moreover, these procedures expose the prospect of using artificially modified genes to enhance the biological competence of proteins. In agriculture, genetically modified (GM) crops have been developed to enhance crop yields, improve resistance to pests and diseases, and reduce the need for chemical pesticides and fertilizers [21]. In medicine, gene therapy offers new avenues for treating genetic diseases and disorders, including cystic fibrosis and muscular dystrophy [22]. Moreover, genetic engineering is playing a pivotal role in the development of advanced pharmaceuticals and vaccines, such as the mRNA-based COVID-19 vaccines [23].

The progress in genetic engineering has also raised important ethical, social, and environmental considerations. Questions about the potential risks, unintended consequences, and equitable access to genetic engineering technologies are subjects of ongoing debate. Regulatory frameworks and ethical guidelines continue to evolve to address these concerns [24].

3.2 Gene transfer technologies

Genetic engineering has revolutionized the field of biology, offering scientists the ability to manipulate and modify the genetic material of organisms. A fundamental aspect of genetic engineering is the transfer of specific genes or genetic material from one organism to another. This process, known as gene transfer, is instrumental in creating genetically modified organisms (GMOs), gene therapies, and various biotechnological applications. Gene transfer tools offer the capability to genetically manipulate the cells of higher animals. In the 1970s it became possible to incorporate exogenous DNA constructs into higher eukaryotic cells *in vitro*. Mammalian (germline) transgenesis was first attained in the early 1980s. The model used in this work was mice. The transport of genes *in vitro* can be achieved by treating the cells with viruses using, e.g. calcium phosphate, liposomes, retrovirus or adenovirus, particle bombardment, fine needle naked DNA injection, electroporation or any combination of these methods. These are the potential techniques for research and have possible applications in gene therapy. Certain valuable techniques used to transfer genes in animals and plants cells and their application and contributions are described below.

3.2.1 Electroporation

Transient pores in the plasma membrane are produced by electroporation to allow macromolecules entry into the cells. Electroporation is an effective method to transfer DNA into cells. In biological membranes microscopic pores are induced by the application of an electric field. These pores are called electropores and permit the molecules, ions and water to pass from one side of the membrane to another. These pores can only be recovered if an appropriate electric pulse is applied. Application of an electric field allows impulsive resealing of electropores and the cell can recover. During electroporation, cells are exposed to short, high-voltage electrical pulses. This causes the formation of nanoscale pores in the lipid bilayer of the cell membrane, enabling the passage of molecules that would otherwise be impermeable, such as DNA, RNA, or proteins. Following electroporation, the pores reseal, and the foreign genetic material can enter the cell [25]. The development of electropores depends upon the type of cells considered and the intensity and interval of the electric pulse that is applied to them. These electric currents can result in intense heating of the cells which can lead to cell death. Heating effects are reduced by using a comparatively high amplitude, a short duration pulse. Otherwise, utilization of two very short duration pulses can also be considered as an alternative to the former procedure. This method has gained widespread use in various fields, from molecular biology and biotechnology to gene therapy. Recent advances have improved the precision, safety, and efficiency of electroporation. For mammalian transgenesis, electroporation is an efficient process of introducing exogenous DNA into embryonic stem (ES) cells. This practice has recently been utilized to deliver genes into cultured mammalian embryos at particular stages of development [26–32]. It was reported [26–32] that there is an escalation from 12% to 19% of transgenic bovine blastocysts when electroporation was involved in an otherwise passive sperm-DNA uptake procedure. Related results were described [26–32], again with transgenic bovine blastocysts. Fish species were also shown to be genetically manipulated in this method [26–32]. Electroporation has been described as increasing the level of gene expression and considerably developing immune responses elicited to DNA vaccines in both large [26–32] and small [26–32] animals. The procedure of electroporation is depicted in figure 4.16 (section 4.6.2.5).

Recent research has focused on optimizing pulse parameters, such as pulse duration, frequency, and amplitude, to enhance electroporation efficiency and minimize cell damage. These developments have led to gentler yet more effective electroporation protocols [33]. Microfluidic systems have been integrated with electroporation, enabling precise control and manipulation of cells during the process. This advancement allows for high-throughput and single-cell electroporation, which is valuable for research and therapeutic applications [34].

Electroporation techniques have evolved to accommodate three-dimensional (3D) cell cultures and tissues. Researchers have developed strategies for gene transfer into complex, multicellular structures, offering new possibilities in regenerative medicine and tissue engineering [35].

Electroporation is used in the delivery of therapeutic genes, including those for cancer treatment and DNA vaccines. Recent advancements in electroporation have improved the efficiency of gene delivery for therapeutic purposes [36]. It is an efficient method for delivering CRISPR-Cas9 components into target cells, facilitating gene editing and knockout experiments. Ongoing research aims to refine electroporation for precise genome editing [37]. It is a valuable tool in molecular biology for introducing plasmid DNA, siRNA, and other molecules into cells. Recent improvements have enhanced the transfection efficiency, reducing cell toxicity [38]. Electroporation remains a versatile and indispensable method for introducing genetic material into cells, and ongoing developments continue to refine its precision and applications in research, biotechnology, and medicine.

3.2.2 Microinjection

Microinjection is a sophisticated technique employed for introducing genetic material, such as DNA, RNA, or proteins, directly into individual cells or embryos. Microinjection involves the use of a fine, hollow needle to physically puncture the cell or embryo membrane and deliver genetic material directly into the nucleus or cytoplasm. The microinjection process offers precise control over the delivery of genetic material, allowing for the manipulation of specific cells or organelles [39]. In the microinjection technique DNA can be incorporated into cells or protoplast with the assistance of very fine needles or glass micropipettes with diameters of 0.5–10 μm. Certain inserted DNA may be taken up by the nucleus. Computerized regulation of the holding pipette, needle, microscope stage and video technology has advanced the effectiveness of this technique. Microinjection is possibly a valuable method for simultaneous transfer of multiple bioactive compounds such as antibodies, peptides, RNAs, plasmids, diffusion markers, elicitors and Ca^{2+}, as well as the nucleus and artificial micro- or nanoparticles containing those chemicals, into the same target single cells [40–45]. Macroinjection is the technique reported for artificial DNA transfer to cereal plants that show an inability to regenerate and develop into whole plants from cultured cells. The needles used in this process for delivering DNA have diameters greater than the cell diameter. DNA is introduced with a conventional syringe into the region of the plant that will further develop into floral tillers. About 0.3 ml of DNA solution is injected at a point above the tiller node until several drops of the solution come out from the top of the young inflorescence [40–45]. Injection timing is always important and should be 14 days before meiosis. A schematic representation of this technique is presented in chapter 4, figure 4.13 (section 4.6.2.2). It is renowned for its precision and is commonly used in various research fields and applications.

Recent advances have seen the integration of robotics and automation with microinjection, enhancing the accuracy and throughput of the technique. Robotic systems are capable of high-throughput microinjection, making them more applicable in large-scale genetic screening and drug discovery [46]. Innovations have allowed for the microinjection of single cells, which is particularly valuable for applications such as single-cell genomics and the generation of transgenic animals or stem cell lines [47]. Microinjection is a preferred method for delivering CRISPR-Cas9 components into zygotes or embryonic stem cells for precise genome editing. Refinements in this process aim to improve the efficiency and specificity of gene editing [48].

Microinjection is instrumental in creating transgenic animals by introducing foreign genes into embryos. This technique is used in biomedical research to study gene function and disease modeling [49]. Microinjection is employed to modify the genetic make-up of stem cells for regenerative medicine. It allows for the generation of patient-specific induced pluripotent stem cells (iPSCs) and the correction of genetic disorders [50]. In assisted reproduction, microinjection is used for *in vitro* fertilization (IVF) procedures, such as intracytoplasmic sperm injection (ICSI), where a single sperm is injected into an egg to overcome infertility issues [51]. Microinjection remains an indispensable tool for precise genetic manipulation, particularly in the development of transgenic organisms, stem cell research, and gene editing applications.

3.2.3 Biolistics or microprojectiles for DNA transfer

Biolistics, or the microprojectile method, is a gene transfer technology that allows for the direct delivery of DNA or other genetic material into cells or tissues using microscopic particles, typically gold or tungsten microcarriers. This technique offers unique advantages in terms of precision and can be used in various applications. Biolistics or particle bombardment for DNA transfer is a physical technique that uses faster microprojectiles to deliver DNA or other molecules into intact tissues and cells. The method was established by Sanford *et al* primarily to deliver genes into plants [52–55]. Biolistics transformation is a comparatively new and unique method among the physical methods for artificial delivery of exogenous DNA. This procedure avoids the requirement for protoplast and is superior in efficiency. The procedure can be used for any plant cells, root sections, embryos, seeds and pollen. The gene gun is a method that accurately fires DNA into target cells [31]. Initially DNA is coated onto microscopic beads made of either gold or tungsten to be transformed into the cells. The beads are carefully coated with DNA and these beads are then fixed to the end of a plastic bullet. Afterwards these beads are loaded into the firing chamber of the gene gun. With high force the gene gun fires the bullet down the barrel of the gun in the direction of the target cells that lie just beyond the end of the barrel. When the bullet arrives at the end point of the barrel it is caught and stopped. The DNA coated beads continue to move toward the target cells. Certain beads pass via the cell wall into the cytoplasm of the target cells. Now the beads and the DNA become separated and the cells are transformed. After gaining entry inside the target cells, the DNA is solubilized and may be expressed. This strategy, occasionally called 'biolistics', was originally developed for plant transgenesis but has been shown to be effective for transferring transgenes into mammalian cells *in vivo* [52–55]. The gene gun is mainly suitable for transforming cells that are difficult to transform by other methods. This approach can also be used for transferring DNA constructs into whole animals. The procedure of particle bombardment is depicted in chapter 4, figure 4.14 (section 4.6.2.3).

Recent advancements in biolistics have focused on improving control over particle size and velocity. This optimization allows for better penetration and increased transfection efficiency while minimizing damage to target cells [56]. Researchers have developed strategies for the simultaneous delivery of multiple genes using biolistics. This is crucial for genetic studies and applications requiring the expression of multiple genes [57]. Innovations in microcarrier design have led to the use of biodegradable materials. This reduces the risk of potential toxicity associated with non-biodegradable materials like gold or tungsten [58].

Biolistics is commonly used to introduce foreign DNA into plant cells. It has contributed to the development of genetically modified crops with traits such as herbicide resistance, pest resistance, and improved nutritional content [57]. It has been explored for gene therapy and vaccine delivery, particularly for diseases such as cancer and infectious diseases. Recent studies focus on optimizing delivery techniques for therapeutic applications [59]. It is utilized in neuroscience to deliver genetic material into neuronal tissues, enabling the study of neural development and function. Recent advancements enhance precision in this context [60]. Biolistics remains a valuable gene transfer method with diverse applications, particularly in plant biotechnology, gene therapy, and neuroscience research. Ongoing developments aim to enhance its efficiency and broaden its utility.

3.2.4 Liposome-mediated gene transfer

Liposome-mediated gene transfer, also known as lipofection, is a widely employed technique for introducing genetic material into cells. Liposomes are artificially constructed vesicles made of lipid bilayers that can encapsulate and protect DNA, RNA, or other molecules and facilitate their entry into target cells. Lipid vesicles can be used to deliver molecules into cells. These are lipid-based artificial spherical vesicles that can act as transporting agents for exogenous materials including transgenes [61]. They are defined as a sphere of lipid bilayers surrounding the molecule to be delivered and encourage delivery after interacting with the cell membrane. For the delivery of nucleic acid positive charged cationic lipids are used. These liposomes are proficient in interacting with the negatively charged cell membrane more quickly than uncharged liposomes. This type of interaction between cationic liposomes and the cell surface allows the delivery of the DNA directly across the plasma membrane. The process involves forming liposome-DNA complexes (lipoplexes) and exposing cells to these complexes. The liposomes fuse with the cell membrane, allowing the genetic material to be taken up into the cell through endocytosis or fusion. Once inside, the genetic material can exert its effects [62]. Different types of lipid bases are usually used for the preparation of cationic liposomes and can be produced from a number of cationic lipids, e.g. DOTAP (*N*-1 (-(2,3-dioleoyloxy)propyl)-*N*,*N*,*N*-trimethylammonium ethyl sulfate) and DOTMA (*N*-(1-(2,3-dioleoyloxy)propyl)-*N*,*N*,*N*-trimethylammonium chloride) [61]. These lipids are usually available, in particular some that are commercially available as *in vitro* transfecting agents, e.g. lipofectin. Specifically for gene transfer, liposome vehicles are fabricated by supplementing an appropriate mix of bilayer constituents to an aqueous solution of DNA molecules. This aqueous environment allows self-association of hydrophobic tails to exclude water from within the lipid bilayer while phospholipid hydrophilic heads associate with water. This self-association produces separate spheres of a continuous lipid bilayer membrane enveloping a small amount of DNA solution. These lipid-based vesicles are then ready to be added to target cells. Some of the commonest examples of this type of delivery are germline transgenesis with liposome-mediated gene transfer, and ES cells have also been effectively transfected by liposomes [61]. The procedure of liposome-mediated delivery is demonstrated in chapter 4, figure 4.14 (section 4.6.2.4).

Researchers have developed stimuli-responsive liposomes that release their cargo in response to specific cues, such as changes in pH, temperature, or enzymatic activity. This innovation enhances control over the release of genetic material within target cells [63]. Lipid nanoparticles have emerged as a promising alternative to traditional liposomes. They are better suited for the delivery of mRNA, especially for vaccines, due to their improved stability and efficiency [64]. Recent research has explored hybrid nanoparticles composed of both lipids and polymers. These nanoparticles combine the advantages of both liposomes and polymeric nanoparticles, resulting in improved transfection efficiency [65].

Liposome-based delivery systems have been employed in vaccine development, particularly for mRNA vaccines and subunit vaccines. Recent advancements in liposome design enhance vaccine efficacy and stability [66]. In molecular biology and research, liposome-mediated gene transfer is used to introduce genes for the purpose of studying gene function or gene regulation. Ongoing developments focus on improving transfection efficiency and minimizing cytotoxicity [67]. Liposome-mediated gene transfer remains a versatile and widely-used technique for delivering genetic material into cells. Advances in liposome design and applications continue to expand its utility in gene therapy, vaccines, and research.

3.2.5 Calcium phosphate-mediated DNA transfer

Calcium phosphate-mediated DNA transfer, often referred to as calcium phosphate transfection, is a method used to introduce DNA into cells. This technique relies on the precipitation of calcium and phosphate ions with DNA to form DNA-loaded calcium phosphate precipitates, which are then taken up by the target cells. The entire process of transfection entails the amalgamation of isolated DNA (10–100 μg) with a solution of calcium chloride and potassium phosphate. This is achieved under conditions that allow the precipitation of calcium phosphate. Subsequently cells are incubated with precipitated DNA either in solution or in a tissue culture dish. A small part of the cells will take up the calcium phosphate DNA precipitate by a process called endocytosis. The transfection efficiencies of this method can be quite low, somewhere in the range of 1%–2%. However, it can be increased if very high purity DNA is used which allows the precipitate to form slowly [68]. Various protocols have been developed where cell take up of exogenous DNA could be up to 20%. This method is used for introducing DNA into mammalian cells. ES cells can also be transfected by co-precipitation [68]. A schematic representation of calcium phosphate-mediated DNA transfer is demonstrated in figure 3.2.

Recent research has focused on optimizing co-precipitants or additives used in calcium phosphate transfection. This optimization aims to improve the efficiency of the transfection process, minimize cell toxicity, and enhance transgene expression [69]. Innovations have sought to enhance the stability and delivery efficiency of calcium phosphate-DNA precipitates. This includes modifying the precipitates to

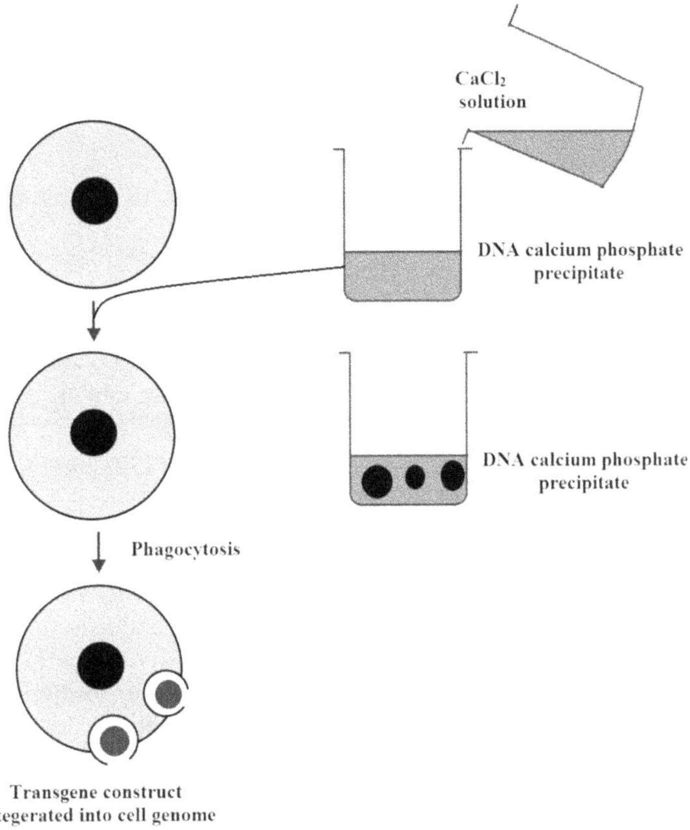

Figure 3.2. Schematic representation of calcium phosphate-mediated DNA transfer.

make them more biocompatible and improve their transfection ability [70]. Efforts have been made to develop strategies for cell-specific targeting using calcium phosphate-mediated DNA transfer. Recent studies have explored modifications to the precipitates and the use of targeting ligands to improve specificity [71]. It is widely used for transfecting cells in basic research to study gene function and regulation. Recent advancements aim to improve transfection efficiency, which is particularly valuable for experiments requiring high gene expression [72]. Calcium phosphate transfection is employed to produce viral vectors for gene therapy and gene delivery applications. It plays a crucial role in the production of lentiviral and retroviral vectors [73]. The technique is used for protein production in mammalian cells, making it useful in biotechnology and the pharmaceutical industry. Recent developments seek to enhance the production of recombinant proteins [74]. Calcium phosphate-mediated DNA transfer remains a cost-effective and widely used method for transfecting a variety of cell types. Ongoing research focuses on optimizing this classic technique for modern applications in gene therapy, biotechnology, and research.

3.2.6 DNA transfer by DEAE-dextran method

The DEAE-dextran method is a gene transfer technique that relies on a cationic polymer, diethylaminoethyl-dextran, to enhance the uptake of DNA by cells. DEAE-dextran forms a complex with DNA and promotes its internalization through cell membranes. DNA can also be transferred by diethylaminoethyl (DEAE)-dextran (a derivative of carbohydrate polymer dextran) method. DEAE-dextran may be used in the transfection medium in which DNA is present. DEAE-dextran is a polycationic, high molecular weight derivative and suitable for transient assays in COS cells (fibroblast-like cell lines derived from monkey kidney tissue). It does not appear to be efficient for the production of stable transfectants. If DEAE-dextran treatment is coupled with dimethyl sulfoxide (DMSO) shock, then up to 80% of transformed cells can express the transferred gene. It is well known that serum inhibits this transfection, so cells are washed well to make them serum free [75]. Stable expression is very difficult to obtain by this method. Treatment with chloroquinine enhances the transient expression of DNA. The main benefit of this technique is that it is cheap, simple and can be used for transient cells which cannot survive even after short exposure to calcium phosphate, while its disadvantages include cytotoxicity and low transfection efficiency for a variety of cells (typically less than 10% in primary cells), as well as the requirement for reduced serum media during the transfection procedure. In this method the cationic DEAE-dextran molecule tightly associates with the negatively charged backbone of the nucleic acid and the net positive charge of the resulting nucleic acid–DEAE-dextran complex allows it to adhere to the cell membrane and enter into the cytoplasm via endocytosis or osmic shock induced by DMSO or glycerol. A schematic representation of cDNA transfer by the DEAE-dextran method is depicted in figure 3.3.

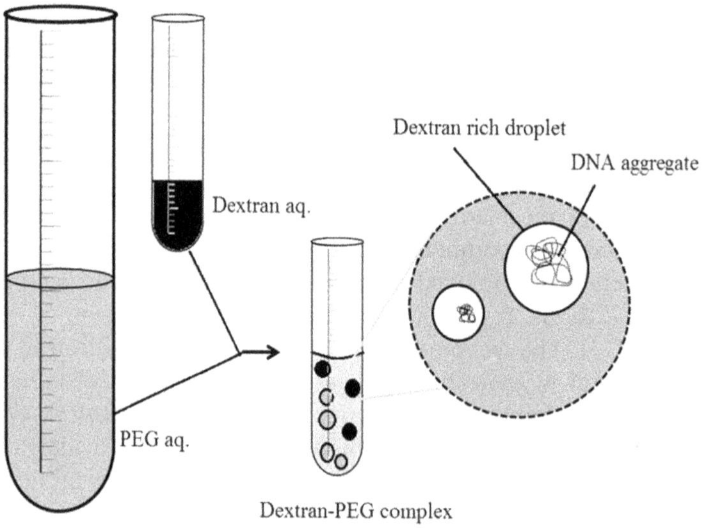

Figure 3.3. Schematic representation of cDNA transfer by the DEAE-dextran method.

Recent research has focused on optimizing DEAE-dextran parameters such as concentration, molecular weight, and polymer modifications to enhance transfection efficiency. This is especially relevant for applications requiring high levels of gene expression [76]. Efforts have been made to achieve cell-specific targeting with the DEAE-dextran method. Modifications to the DEAE-dextran complex or the inclusion of targeting ligands have been explored to improve the selectivity of gene delivery [77]. Researchers are working to reduce the cytotoxic effects associated with DEAE-dextran transfection. Strategies such as optimizing the ratio of DEAE-dextran to DNA and using lower molecular weight DEAE-dextran aim to enhance safety [78].

The DEAE-dextran method is used in the production of recombinant viruses, such as retroviruses and lentiviruses, which are essential in gene therapy, vaccine development, and functional genomics studies [79]. The DEAE-dextran method is widely employed for transient transfection of cultured cells in basic research. Recent developments aim to improve transfection efficiency and reduce cytotoxicity in these experiments [38]. This method has been explored for delivering therapeutic genes in cancer gene therapy. Efforts are ongoing to enhance the selectivity and safety of the DEAE-dextran method for this application [80]. The DEAE-dextran method remains a valuable technique for gene transfer into a wide range of cell types. Ongoing research seeks to optimize and expand its applications in various fields, including virology, molecular biology, and gene therapy.

3.2.7 Transfer of DNA by polycation-DMSO

Although the calcium phosphate method of DNA transfer is reproducible and efficient, there are a narrow range of optimum conditions. This is a new protocol for DNA transfection in a system of chicken embryo fibroblast cells and cloned *Rous sarcoma virus* DNA. In this method polycation reagent is used as a mediator to adsorb DNA to the cell surface and dimethyl sulfoxide as an agent to allow the uptake of adsorbed DNA by the cells. This is a simple and convenient polycation-dimethyl sulfoxide transfection method, which requires no carrier DNA even with small amounts of DNA, and the number of transformed cell foci induced by *Rous sarcoma virus* DNA was proportional to the dose of the transfecting DNA. In addition, chicken embryo fibroblast cells were positively transformed by v-Src (gene present in *Rous sarcoma virus* that encodes a *tyrosine kinase*) containing subgenomic DNA. DNA transfer by polycation (Polybrene) is used to enhance the adsorption of DNA to the cell surface followed by a brief treatment with 25%–30% DMSO to enhance membrane permeability and increase uptake of DNA. In this technique no carrier DNA is required and stable transformants are produced. This procedure works with mouse fibroblasts and chick embryos [81].

Researchers have focused on optimizing the formation of DNA-polycation complexes to improve transfection efficiency. Adjusting the ratio of DNA to polycations and fine-tuning the preparation process have been explored [82]. Efforts have been made to minimize the cytotoxic effects of DMSO, which can be harmful to cells. Strategies include reducing the concentration of DMSO or seeking alternative permeabilization agents [83]. Recent studies have investigated combining polycation-DMSO transfection with other techniques, such as electroporation or lipid-based transfection, to further enhance transfection efficiency [38]. The DNA transfer by polycation-DMSO method is commonly used for transient gene expression in mammalian cells. This is useful for studying gene function, protein production, and various other molecular biology applications [84]. This method has been employed to deliver CRISPR-Cas9 components for gene knockout and functional genomics studies. It enables the editing of specific genes and the study of their functions [85]. The DNA transfer by polycation-DMSO method remains a valuable tool for delivering genetic material into mammalian cells. Recent developments aim to improve transfection efficiency, minimize cytotoxicity, and expand its applications in areas such as gene editing and drug discovery.

3.2.8 Polyethylene-glycol-mediated transfection

Polyethylene glycol (PEG)-mediated transfection is a gene transfer technique that utilizes PEG to enhance the uptake of genetic material into cells. PEG is a hydrophilic polymer that helps facilitate the fusion of cell membranes and the internalization of DNA or RNA. Direct introduction of DNA into plant protoplasts allows a quick analysis of transient gene expression, along with the production of stably transformed transgenic plants. Transient gene expression assays achieved after DNA transformation allow a reasonable analysis of cis-acting regulatory sequences and their function in transcriptional control of plant genes. There are various methods for introducing DNA into plant protoplasts, but the most frequently used technique is polyethylene glycol (PEG) facilitated DNA uptake. The PEG-mediated transformation is very simple and effective, allowing a concurrent processing of various samples, and yields a transformed cell population with high survival and division rates. This method utilizes reasonable supplies and equipment and helps to overcome the hurdle of the host range limitations of *Agrobacterium*-mediated transformation. PEG-mediated DNA transfer can be readily adapted to a broad range of plant species and tissue sources. This technique is utilized for protoplasts only. PEG encourages endocytosis and thus DNA uptake occurs. In this method protoplasts are placed in a solution containing PEG. The molecular weight of PEG used is 8000 Da at concentration of 15%. Calcium salt in the form of calcium chloride is added and sucrose and glucose act as osmotic buffering agents. To minimize the effects of the nuclease present, carrier DNA from salmon or herring sperm may also be added. Once the protoplast is exposed to exogenous DNA in the presence of PEG and other chemicals, PEG can be removed. Subsequently, intact surviving protoplasts are cultured to form cells with walls and colonies in turn. After some development in selectable medium, the occurrence of transformation is calculated [86]. PEG-based vehicles are less toxic and more resistant to non-specific protein adsorption, making them an attractive alternative for non-viral gene delivery [86]. For oral squamous cell carcinoma, PEG p-lactoglobulin (BLG) nanoparticle-mediated herpes simplex virus–thymidine kinase (HSV-TK)/ganciclovir (GCV) gene therapy has also been reported [86].

Recent research has focused on optimizing the concentration of PEG to achieve the most efficient transfection while minimizing cytotoxicity. The ideal PEG concentration can vary depending on the cell type and application. PEG is often used in combination with lipid-based delivery systems to improve transfection efficiency. Recent developments have sought to enhance the design and performance of these lipid-PEG complexes [87]. Efforts have been made to achieve cell-specific targeting using PEG-mediated transfection. Modifications to the PEG complexes, such as adding targeting ligands, aim to improve the selectivity of gene delivery [88]. PEG-mediated transfection is widely used for transfection in basic research to study gene function, regulation, and cellular pathways. Researchers aim to enhance transfection efficiency for these studies [38]. PEG-mediated transfection has been applied in gene therapy to deliver therapeutic genes or RNA-based therapeutics. Recent advancements aim to improve the safety and efficacy of this method [89]. The technique is utilized in drug screening and development to assess the effects of potential drug candidates on specific genes or pathways in cell-based assays [90]. PEG-mediated transfection remains a versatile and widely-used method for delivering genetic material into cells. Ongoing research focuses on optimizing this method for various applications in molecular biology, gene therapy, and drug discovery.

3.2.9 Gene transfer through peptides

Gene transfer through peptides is a relatively newer approach that utilizes short peptide sequences to facilitate the delivery of genetic material into cells. This method has gained attention due to its potential for enhancing transfection efficiency and minimizing cytotoxicity. Peptides are designated as tools for development of the system because of their biodegradability, reduced size, diverse and tunable features, as well as their potential to gain intracellular/organellar access. A range of peptide sequences exist which can potentially bind to, and condense, DNA to make it more suitable for entry into cells, e.g. the tetrapeptide serine-proline-lysine-lysine (present on the C-terminus of the histone H1 protein) helps in DNA transfer [91]. Lysine, a positively charged amino acid, helps to counteract the negatively charged phosphate DNA backbone and permits the DNA molecules to pack tightly to each other. Coherent design of peptide sequences has also been used to develop synthetic DNA-binding peptides. Tyrosine-lysine-alanine-(Lysine)s-tryptophan-lysine is another example of a peptide which is very effective at forming complexes with DNA [91]. DNA-binding peptides that can be coupled to cell-specific ligands can also be synthesized. It facilitates receptor-mediated targeting of the peptide/DNA complexes to specific cell types.

Researchers have been actively working on the design and modification of peptides to improve their transfection efficiency and specificity. This includes altering peptide sequences, introducing cell-targeting motifs, and optimizing charge and structure [92]. Recent studies have explored the development of multifunctional peptides that can both condense the genetic material and enhance endosomal escape. This improves the overall transfection process [93]. Peptide-mediated transfection is sometimes combined with nanoparticles or lipids to form more complex delivery systems. These systems aim to increase the stability and efficiency of gene transfer [94]. This method holds promise for gene therapy applications, where it can be used to deliver therapeutic genes or RNA-based therapeutics for the treatment of genetic diseases and acquired disorders [89].

Gene transfer through peptides is employed in functional genomics studies, including gene knockout and gene overexpression experiments to understand gene function and regulation [95]. Peptide-based transfection is utilized in cancer research for delivering genetic material for studying cancer-related genes and developing potential gene therapies [96]. The method is also applied in drug development for assessing the effects of compounds on specific genes or pathways in cell-based assays [97]. Gene transfer through peptides continues to be an active area of research with the potential to address the challenges associated with traditional transfection methods. Ongoing developments aim to optimize this approach for diverse applications in the fields of gene therapy, molecular biology, and drug discovery.

3.2.10 Gene transfer by retroviruses

The comparatively low efficiency of foreign DNA integration into animal cells, combined with the absence of naturally occurring plasmids, results in the manipulation of viruses as potential vectors for gene transfer. Retrovirus-mediated expression cloning was discovered in the mid-1990s. Retrovirus-mediated gene transfer is a potential technique that can be used to understand gene functions. Retroviruses are present in many species including most mammals [98]. Retroviruses are a family of enveloped RNA viruses that include various genera, such as lentiviruses and gamma-retroviruses, commonly used for gene transfer. The genome of retroviruses can be manipulated to carry exogenous DNA. The merits of using retrovirus-based vectors arise from the stability of the integration of the viral genome into the host. The integration of a single copy of the viral DNA at a random location within the host's genome allows for the long-term expression of the integrated foreign gene. Moreover, retroviruses signify a highly efficient mechanism for the transfer of DNA into cells. Virus uptake is effective for many somatic cell lines, but germline cells are infected at low frequency, owing to a high level of mosaicism [98]. The retrovirus-mediated expression cloning method is effective because the number of provirus integrations in each cell is limited. Consequently, it is not essential to recover and reintroduce the plasmid from, and into, the cells repeatedly, as in the conventional method using COS7 cells (fibroblast-like cell lines obtained from monkey kidney tissue). During the retrovirus-mediated expression cloning procedure, the infection efficiencies should be controlled between 10% and 30% to circumvent multiple integration in a cell as much as possible. Otherwise, one can recover the integrated retroviruses by transfecting a helper construct harboring gag-pol and env genes into the isolated clone that has acquired a phenotype of interest after transduction of the cDNA library. In this case, the recovered retroviruses are infected to the target cells to decide which integration was responsible for the phenotype. The most significant advantage over the conventional method is that any functional assay can be applied to recognize cDNAs by their

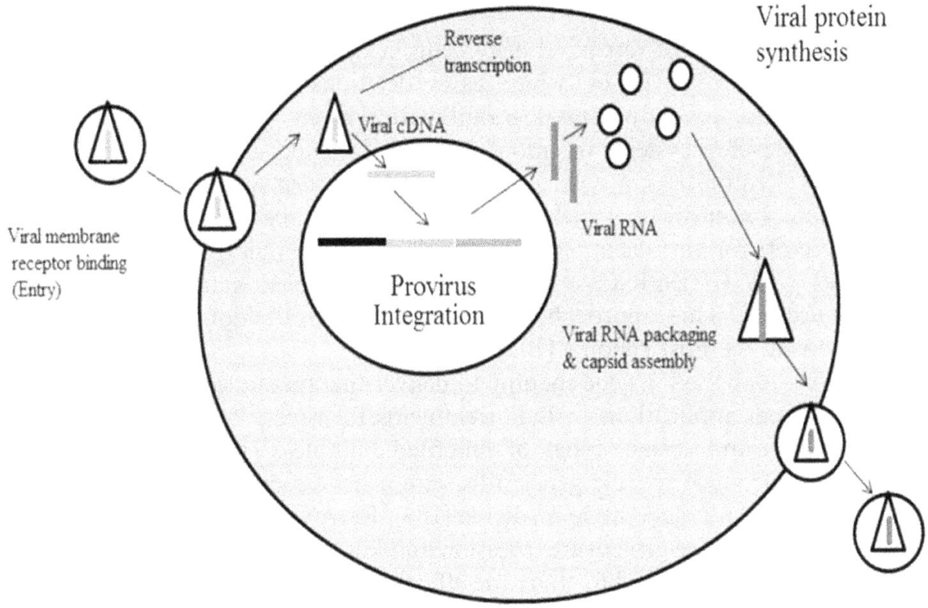

Figure 3.4. Schematic representation of gene transfer by retroviruses.

functions because, once integrated, the expression of the retrovirally transduced cDNA is usually stable. The virus can be used for highly developed tissues, e.g. those of fetuses, juveniles or adults [98]. This holds great promise in the context of somatic gene therapy. Retroviral vectors have also been used to introduce transgenes into the ES cell genome [98]. However, retroviral vectors are limited or problematic in a number of respects. They show the random nature of the integration process, which may have harmful effects on the host cell, and the overall requirement that retroviruses have to infect only dividing cells. A schematic representation of gene transfer by retroviruses is depicted in figure 3.4.

The process of gene transfer by retroviruses involves several steps [99]:

1. **Attachment and entry**: The retrovirus attaches to the host cell membrane via viral envelope proteins and enters the cell through receptor-mediated endocytosis.
2. **Reverse transcription**: Once inside the cell, the retroviral RNA genome is reverse transcribed into DNA by the enzyme reverse transcriptase. This newly synthesized DNA, known as cDNA, is then transported to the cell nucleus.
3. **Integration**: The cDNA is integrated into the host cell's genome by the viral enzyme integrase, becoming a provirus. The provirus remains stably integrated and is replicated along with the host cell's DNA during cell division.
4. **Transcription and expression**: The integrated provirus is transcribed by the host cell's machinery, leading to the expression of the introduced gene. This expression is generally stable over time.

To improve the safety of retroviral gene transfer, researchers have developed self-inactivating (SIN) retroviruses, which carry deletions in the viral long terminal repeats (LTRs) to prevent potential recombination events. Additionally, efforts are underway to develop systems for more precisely targeted integration of retroviral vectors [100]. Lentiviruses, a type of retrovirus, have been widely used due to their ability to infect non-dividing cells. Recent advances have focused on optimizing lentiviral vectors for various applications, including gene therapy [101]. Combining retroviruses with CRISPR-Cas9 technology has enabled gene editing through retroviral vectors. This approach allows for the introduction of targeted gene modifications in the host genome [102].

Retroviruses are used in gene therapy to deliver therapeutic genes to treat genetic disorders. Recent applications include treatments for severe combined immunodeficiency (SCID) and certain types of inherited blindness [103]. Retroviruses are employed to introduce specific genes into stem cells, directing their differentiation and potential use in regenerative medicine [104]. Retroviruses are valuable tools in functional genomics for gene overexpression and knockout studies to elucidate gene function [105]. They are used to study the effects of specific genes in cancer cell lines and animal models, facilitating cancer research and drug development [106]. Gene transfer by retroviruses remains a significant method for stable and long-term gene expression and has continued to evolve with advancements in safety, specificity, and a growing range of applications.

3.2.11 CRISPR-Cas9-mediated gene editing

CRISPR-Cas9-mediated gene editing is a revolutionary and highly precise technology for introducing targeted modifications into the genome of an organism. It has gained immense popularity and is widely used in both basic research and potential therapeutic applications [107]. CRISPR-Cas9 (Clustered Regularly Interspaced Short Palindromic Repeats and CRISPR-associated protein 9) is a genome editing system that allows scientists to make precise modifications to DNA. It functions by using a guide RNA (gRNA) to target a specific DNA sequence and the Cas9 enzyme to introduce modifications to that sequence. This technology enables the addition, deletion, or replacement of DNA sequences with a high degree of accuracy.

3.2.12 Mechanism of CRISPR-Cas9-mediated gene editing [108]

1. **Designing gRNA**: The process begins with designing a gRNA that is complementary to the target DNA sequence. The gRNA directs the Cas9 protein to the specific location in the genome.
2. **Cas9 cleavage**: The Cas9 protein acts as molecular scissors and binds to the DNA at the target site guided by the gRNA. It then creates a double-strand break (DSB) at that location.
3. **DNA repair mechanisms**: The cell's DNA repair machinery comes into play to repair the DSB. There are two main repair pathways:

- **Non-homologous end joining (NHEJ)**: Often results in small insertions or deletions (indels) at the site of the break. These indels can disrupt the target gene's function.
- **Homology-directed repair (HDR)**: Involves using a repair template to precisely introduce or replace a specific DNA sequence.

Recent developments in CRISPR-Cas9-mediated gene editing include base editing, which allows for precise changes of single DNA bases without introducing DSBs [109]. Another breakthrough is prime editing, which enables highly precise edits without DSBs and allows for the introduction of insertions, deletions, or substitutions at specific sites [110]. High-throughput CRISPR-Cas9 screens are being used to systematically investigate the functions of genes and regulatory elements [111]. *In vivo* gene editing approaches are being advanced to target and modify genes directly within living organisms. Enhanced delivery methods, such as viral vectors and nanoparticles, are being developed for more efficient and specific delivery of CRISPR components.

Applications of CRISPR-Cas9-mediated gene editing include functional genomics, where it is used to study gene function by knocking out (gene disruption) or modifying specific genes in a controlled manner. It also has the potential to treat genetic diseases through gene therapy by correcting or replacing faulty genes [112]. In agriculture, CRISPR-Cas9 is used to develop genetically modified crops with desired traits, such as disease resistance and improved yields [113]. In biotechnology, it is employed for engineering microbial strains for the production of biofuels, pharmaceuticals, and chemicals. The technology is also used in drug discovery to create cellular models for drug screening and development, as well as in cancer research to study the genetics of cancer and develop potential therapies [114].

3.2.13 Viral-like particles (VLPs) for transfection

Viral-like particles (VLPs) have become a promising approach for transfection and gene delivery due to their structural similarity to viruses and their potential for efficient and safe genetic material delivery. VLPs are engineered structures that mimic the outer shell or capsid of viruses. VLPs do not contain the viral genome, making them safe vehicles for delivering genetic material into target cells. Their structural resemblance to viruses enhances their ability to interact with cellular receptors and efficiently enter cells [115].

3.2.14 Mechanism of VLP-mediated transfection [116]

1. **VLP design**: VLPs are designed to encapsulate genetic material, such as plasmid DNA or RNA. The genetic cargo can be incorporated within the VLP structure.
2. **Cellular uptake**: VLPs efficiently interact with cellular receptors, which can trigger endocytosis or direct fusion with the cell membrane. Once inside the cell, the genetic cargo is released into the cytoplasm.

3. **Release of genetic material**: The genetic material can be released from the VLP and transported to the cell nucleus for gene expression.

Researchers are developing customized VLPs that can be engineered to carry specific cargo and target particular cell types or tissues. This allows for precise and efficient transfection [117]. Efforts are being made to improve the stability of VLPs, ensuring that they protect the genetic cargo during delivery [118]. Surface modifications are being explored to enhance the specificity of VLPs for target cells. This can include the addition of ligands or antibodies that interact with receptors on the cell surface [119]. VLPs have been widely used in vaccine development, particularly for viruses like human papillomavirus (HPV) and hepatitis B. They can be engineered to present viral antigens, inducing an immune response [115]. VLPs have the potential to be used in gene therapy for the delivery of therapeutic genes to treat genetic disorders. Their safety profile makes them attractive for clinical applications [120]. VLPs can be employed for drug delivery, especially in the field of targeted therapies. They can encapsulate and deliver drug payloads to specific cells or tissues [121]. VLPs are used in basic research to study cellular processes, gene function, and regulatory mechanisms. They offer a versatile tool for transfection in a wide range of cell types [119]. VLPs have the potential to revolutionize gene delivery, vaccine development, and targeted drug delivery due to their safety, efficiency, and ability to be tailored for specific applications. Continued research and development in this area is expected to expand their utility.

3.3 Plasmids

A plasmid is a tiny circular DNA molecule that lives in a cell separate and apart from its chromosomal DNA. Plasmids, which are primarily found in bacteria and certain other microorganisms, are responsible for carrying genetic information apart from the necessary genomic material. These DNA structures have the ability to replicate on their own and frequently contain genes that confer extra characteristics to the host cell, like resistance to antibiotics or the capacity to metabolize particular drugs. In molecular biology and genetic engineering, plasmids are frequently employed as vectors to introduce foreign genes into host cells. This allows scientists to control the expression of genes, generate proteins, and modify organisms for a variety of biotechnological uses. Genetic engineering, a field at the forefront of modern biotechnology, has revolutionized our ability to manipulate and modify the genetic material of organisms. One essential tool in genetic engineering is the plasmid, a small, circular piece of DNA that plays a pivotal role in the transfer of genetic information [122]. Plasmids are widely used in recombinant DNA technology, enabling the introduction of specific genes into host organisms, the production of valuable proteins, and the study of gene function.

Plasmids are extrachromosomal, circular, dsDNA molecules that are separate from a cell's chromosomal DNA and replicate independently [123]. Plasmids occur naturally in bacteria, yeast, and some higher eukaryotic cells. They exist in a parasitic or symbiotic relationship with their host cell. Plasmid sizes vary from a few thousand base pairs to more than 100 kb. Similarly to the host cell's chromosomal DNA, plasmid DNA is duplicated before every cell division. Through cell division, at least one copy of the plasmid DNA is separated to each daughter cell. This assures the continued propagation of the plasmid through consecutive generations of the host cell. Various naturally occurring plasmids contain genes that offer various benefits to the host cell. This may satisfy the plasmid's portion of the symbiotic relationship, e.g. certain bacterial plasmids encode enzymes that inactivate antibiotics. Such drug-resistance plasmids have now become a major problem in the treatment of various bacterial pathogens. As antibiotic use became common, plasmids containing several drug-resistance genes developed, making their host cells resistant to a range of different antibiotics simultaneously [123]. Most of these plasmids also comprise 'transfer genes' encoding proteins that can form a macromolecular tube, or pilus, by which a copy of the plasmid can be transferred to other host cells of similar or related bacterial species. This type of transfer can lead to the rapid spread of drug-resistance plasmids, expanding the number of antibiotic-resistant bacteria in an environment such as a hospital. Handling the spread of drug-resistance plasmids is a key challenge for modern medicine. A schematic representation of a cloning vector derived from a plasmid is shown in figure 3.5.

The versatility of plasmids in genetic engineering is evident in their numerous applications. Recent advancements have expanded their use in various fields, including medicine, agriculture, and biotechnology [124]. For instance, plasmids are used in the development of recombinant DNA vaccines, gene therapies, and the production of biopharmaceuticals like insulin and monoclonal antibodies [125]. Additionally, they play a critical role in the creation of GMOs with improved agricultural traits and in synthetic biology projects to design and construct novel genetic circuits [126]. Recent developments in plasmid design and engineering have enhanced their efficiency and safety in genetic modification processes. The use of CRISPR-Cas9 technology in combination with plasmids has revolutionized genome editing, allowing for precise and targeted modifications in a variety of organisms [127].

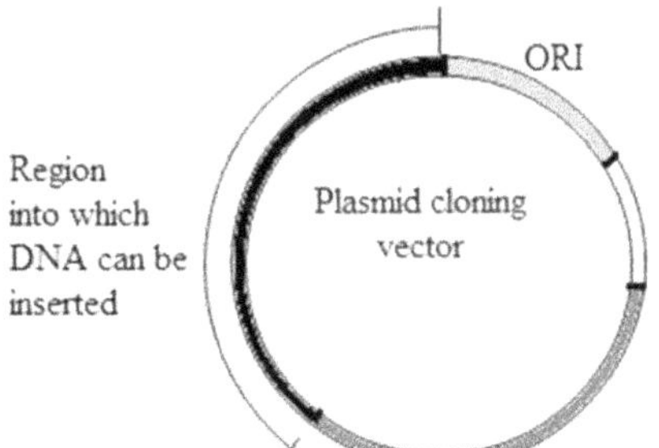

Figure 3.5. Illustration of a simple cloning vector derived from a plasmid, a circular dsDNA molecule that can replicate within *E. coli*.

3.4 Different hosts and protein expression technologies

Genetic engineering is a dynamic field that has transformed our ability to produce specific proteins of interest, ranging from therapeutic enzymes to industrial enzymes, by harnessing various host organisms and protein expression technologies. Host organisms, ranging from bacteria to eukaryotes, serve as factories for protein production in genetic engineering. Bacteria, such as *Escherichia coli* (*E. coli*), have long been favored for their rapid growth and well-characterized genetic systems. *E. coli*-based systems are still heavily utilized, especially in research and small-scale applications [128]. Beyond bacteria, yeasts like *Saccharomyces cerevisiae* and *Pichia pastoris* have gained prominence due to their capacity for eukaryotic post-translational modifications and ease of genetic manipulation [129]. Filamentous fungi, like *Aspergillus niger*, are advantageous for the secretion of complex proteins and enzymes [130]. In recent years, mammalian cell lines, including Chinese hamster ovary (CHO) cells, have become essential for the production of biopharmaceuticals. Their ability to perform intricate post-translational modifications is critical for the production of therapeutic proteins [131].

Protein expression uses rDNA technology to copy a protein coding DNA (cDNA) into a plasmid vector and express the protein in a host cell. However, a number of problems related to protein expression in *E. coli* have been found. The first problem is DNA cloning. Certain protein coding cDNAs seem difficult to clone. Several can only be cloned in a vector with incorrect orientation. Several others contain mutations. Still others cannot be cloned in a certain vector at all. Once a cDNA is cloned into a vector, the second issue is that the protein may not be expressed, or the expression is unpredictable. Occasionally it is expressed at a low level, other times it is just not expressed [132]. Even after a fruitful protein expression, there might be issues related to protein yield, solubility, stability and activity. Thus, various researchers have claimed that protein expression is an art rather than a science [132].

In a living system, a specific protein is expressed only at a particular subcellular location in a cell type of a tissue, in defined time period and at a particular level. This is so-called spatial, temporal and quantitative expression. In an animal system, there are various organs, tissues and cell types. There are diverse cell types at different developmental stages in a human. Each protein in these cell types appears to be correctly expressed. Incorrect expressions often cause developmental defects or severe diseases. A number of the proteins are expressed at reasonably high levels, e.g. antibodies in plasma cells and insulin in β cells in the islets of Langerhans in a pancreas. The only reasons that these cell types can correctly express these proteins are that these cells and their environment offer essential and suitable materials and tools for protein expressions.

There are several different types of expression host systems (table 3.2). Each host system has its own advantages and disadvantages. In a particular recombinant system, basic materials and techniques for protein transcription and translation are provided for protein expression. Therefore, various recombinant proteins are effectively expressed in different host cells. However, no host cell can offer all the

Table 3.2. Evaluation of frequently used host cells for protein expression.

Host cell	Advantages	Disadvantages
E. coli	• Convenient expression control. • Easy operations, rapid growth rate, low cost. • High yield, 5%–20% of total cellular proteins; some can reach 40% and up to 80% has been reported. • Inclusion bodies facilitate purification. • Large vector and fusion choices.	• Endotoxin. • Lacks post-translational modi fication. • Overexpression of proteins may be insoluble (inclusion bodies) and may not be refolded.
Yeast	• Disulfide bond formation and some glycosylation. • Low cost fermentation. • No endotoxin or human pathogens, considered to be safe. • Secretion facilitates purification. • Well-developed large-scale system.	• Different glycosylation from mammals. • Difficult to break cell wall for protein purification. • Less understanding of genetics and more difficult expression control than *E. coli*. • Fewer vector choices and more difficult vector manipulation than *E. coli*.
Insect (baculovirus)	• Clinical trials approved by the FDA using proteins produced by baculovirus. • High yield facilitates protein purification. • Post-translational modifications similar to mammals.	• High mannose glycosylation and over-phosphorylation. • Overexpression may result in insoluble inclusion bodies. • Recombinant proteins may not be 100% active.
Mammal	• Large-scale mammalian cell culture feasible. • Recombinant protein activity same as natural protein.	• Cell culture involves expensive labor, facilities and consumables. • Low cell growth rate, high cost. • Low yield, can compare with microbe yield at large scale.

materials and tools essential and appropriate for all protein expressions. Therefore, other proteins cannot be expressed in a specific tested host cell. Nearly all cDNAs are first cloned in *E. coli* [132]. *E. coli* is by far the most universally used host for protein expression in research, diagnostic and pharmaceutical investigations. It is the most studied organism in nature. *E. coli*'s comparatively simple operations, low cost, high protein yield, short growth time, convenient expression control, and large selection of vectors and strains make it the number one choice in protein expression [132].

Protein expression using transgenic animals and cell-free systems is not included here. There is no single system fulfilling all protein expression requirements. Various systems may be selected for an expression (table 3.3). However, this also increases time, labor and costs significantly.

3.4.1 rDNA technology

Recombinant DNA technology, often referred to as genetic engineering, is a revolutionary technique that allows the creation of novel DNA molecules by combining genetic material from different sources. This technology has opened up exciting possibilities for manipulating and modifying genes to produce valuable proteins, develop new medical treatments, and engineer organisms for various applications [125]. This is a protocol used in genetic engineering that includes the identification, isolation and insertion of a GOI into a vector such as a plasmid or bacteriophage to form an rDNA molecule, and the production of a large amount of the gene fragment or product encoded by that gene. Humulin is insulin developed using rDNA technology which is currently used to treat diabetes [133, 134]. Here insulin is produced inside the bacterium where we introduced the human insulin gene. The bacterial system just works as a biofactory for the production of insulin. The procedure involved in rDNA technology is demonstrated in figures 3.6(a) and (b).

Step 1. Identification and isolation of GOI.

From where do we obtain the desired gene?

From one of the following:

- Genomic library.
- cDNA library.
- Chemical synthesis of the gene if we know the sequence.
- If the number of copies of the desired gene is not enough for gene cloning, we can opt for a gene amplification technique.

Step 2. Joining of this gene to a suitable vector (construction of rDNA).

A gene cloning vector is any DNA molecule which is capable of multiplying inside the host and into which the GOI can be integrated easily for cloning. The selection of the vector depends on the size of fragments to be cloned. Most common vectors include plasmids and phage vectors. In this procedure, a restriction enzyme functions as scissors for cutting the DNA molecule. The ligase enzyme is the joining enzyme that joins the vector DNA with the GOI. The final DNA is known as the rDNA, chimera or recombinant vector.

Step 3. Incorporation of this vector into suitable organism.

Introduction of the recombinant vector into a host cell is accomplished by various gene transfer methods:

Physical gene transfer methods

- DNA transfer via pollen.
- Electroporation.
- Liposome-mediated gene transfer.

Table 3.3. Expression problems and host systems.

Host cells	Difficult cloning	No or variable expression	Low yield	Insoluble	Unstable	Dysfunctional
E. coli	Detoxification media, cell strains and vectors.	tRNA supplement cell strains. Detoxification media, cell strains and vectors.	Special media. tRNA supplement cell strains. Detoxification media, cell strains and vectors.	Special media. Co-express with chaperones. Lower temperature.	Special media. Co-express with chaperones.	Special media. Co-express with chaperones.
Yeast	*E. coli* is normally used for DNA cloning.	May express because of different codon usage.	Secretion may get good yield.	Successful secretion should be soluble.	No much help.	Some glycosylation may not help much.
Insect (baculovirus)	*E. coli* is normally used for DNA cloning.	May express because of different codon usage.	Baculovirus vector can have high yield.	High yield may result in insoluble inclusion bodies.	Not much help.	Glycosylation and
phosphorylation may not be same as mammal.						
Mammal	*E. coli* is normally used for DNA cloning.	May express because of different codon usage.	Generally lower yield than other systems.	Mostly soluble proteins.	May be stable in right cell lines.	May be functional with right modifications.

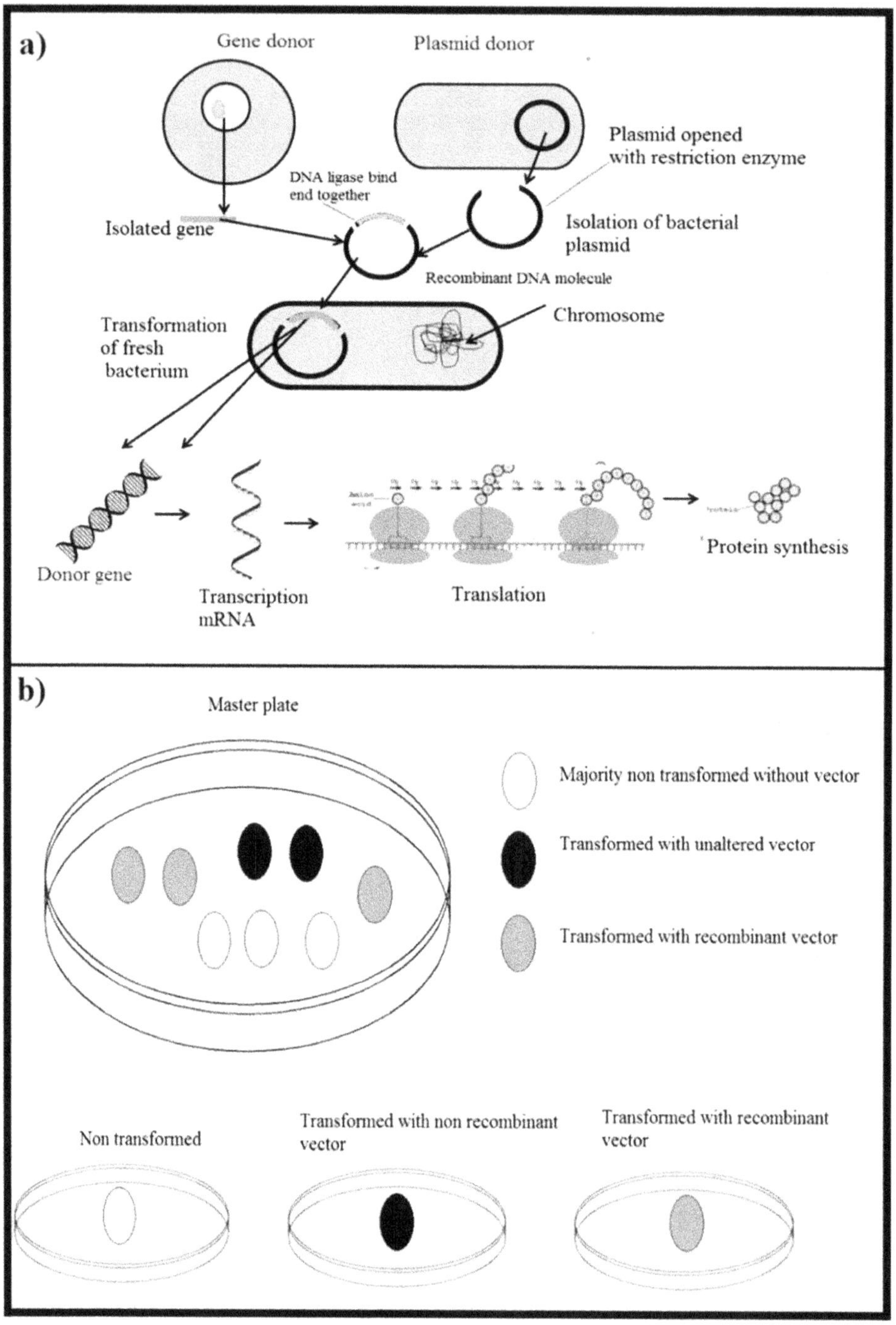

Figure 3.6. (a) Steps involved in rDNA technology. (b) Steps involved in rDNA technology.

- Microinjection.
- Silicon-carbide-fiber-mediated gene transfer.
- Ultrasound-mediated gene transfer.

Chemical gene transfer methods
- Calcium chloride-mediated.
- DEAE-dextran-mediated gene transfer.
- DNA inhibitors by cells, tissues or organs: transformation.
- PEG method.
- Virus-mediated gene transfer: transduction.

Step 4. Selection of transformed recombinant cells with GOI.

The total number of cells with the recombinant vector will be far fewer. So the next step is to select the transformed cells with our GOI from non-transformed cells. Numerous methods are used for selection of transformed cells:
- Antibiotic resistance.
- Assay for biological activity.
- Blotting test.
- Colony hybridization.
- The selected cells are cultured on a large scale.
- Visible characteristics.

Step 5. Multiplication or expression of GOI.

The main aim of gene cloning is either to make various copies of the desired gene or to produce a protein using the desired genes. The inserted gene along with the vector will replicate inside the host so that various copies of the anticipated gene will be produced. For expression of the desired gene, an expression vector is used (a vector with control elements such as promoter or operator). The product is produced in mass cultures in large amounts. This is how insulin is synthesized in large amounts in cell cultures.

3.5 Gene cloning

Gene cloning is defined as the method of copying fragments of DNA which can then be used for various purposes, e.g. creating GM crops or finding a cure for disease. Broadly, there are two types of gene cloning: one is *in vivo*, which includes the use of restriction enzymes and ligases using vectors and cloning the fragments into host cells (as can be seen in figure 3.7). The other type is *in vitro*, which entails using the PCR method to produce copies of fragments of DNA.

The concept of gene cloning dates back to the 1970s when researchers developed the first methods for cloning genes. Since then, the field has witnessed significant advancements, with numerous recent developments showcasing its growing importance in the biotechnology landscape. An exciting development in gene cloning is the synthesis of artificial genes. With advancements in DNA synthesis techniques, scientists can now design and construct genes from scratch. This capability has

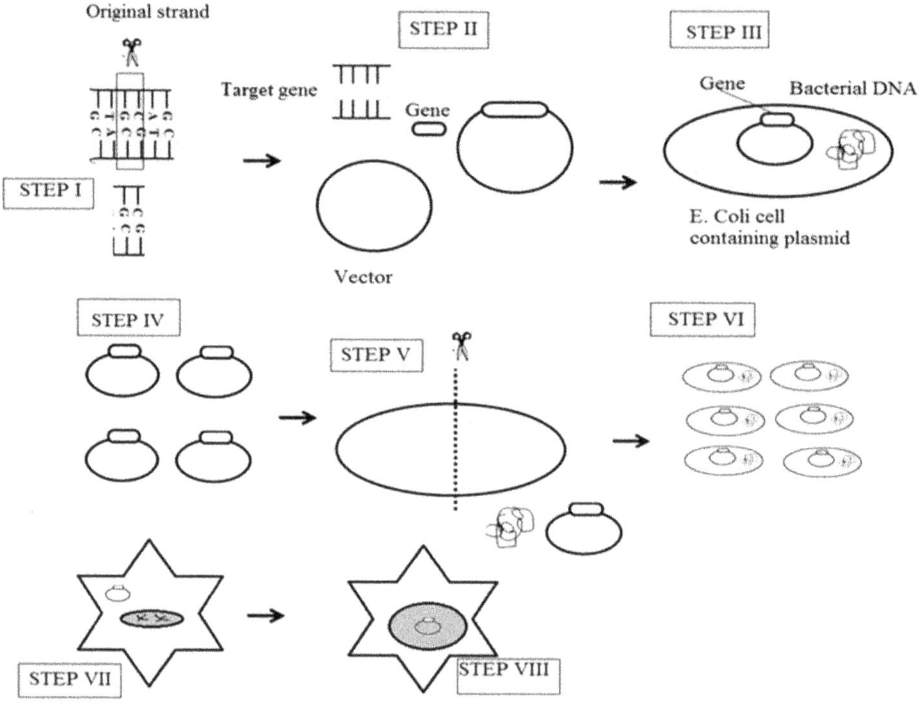

Figure 3.7. Molecular cloning is one way of studying the specific proteins involved in cell division. A gene contains the instructions for how to make a protein. By mutating a gene, the protein's shape, size and function could all be affected. Mutating a gene changes its instructions. Once a mutated gene is created and incorporated into a cell's DNA, the cell replicates, creating many cells containing the mutant gene. The cells with the changed gene can then be compared to normal cells. Shown are the steps involved in both making a mutant gene and incorporating it into the DNA of a human cell: (1). Chemically 'cut' the gene you want to study from the DNA strand. (2). Attach target gene to a small, circular piece of DNA. Together, this is called a plasmid, which serves as the vehicle for transporting the gene. (3). Put the plasmid into an *E. coli* cell (or another type of bacteria). As each *E. coli* cell divides, each new cell contains a copy of the plasmid containing the gene. (4). Grow a lot of *E. coli* cells. (5). Once the *E. coli* population has reached your desired number of cells, break apart the *E. coli* cells using a chemical that dissolves the cell wall. (6). Filter the mixture of broken *E. coli* cells and collect only the plasmids containing the gene. (7). Put the plasmids into human cells. The type of cell varies depending on the research. (8). Over time, the plasmid will be incorporated into the host cell DNA and the new gene will change the proteins produced. (9). Observe physical changes between the cells with the plasmid and those without.

far-reaching implications, including the creation of novel proteins and enzymes for industrial and medical applications [122]. Additionally, recent progress in synthetic biology has expanded the possibilities of gene cloning. By combining genetic elements from different organisms, researchers can engineer entirely new genetic circuits, enabling the development of biosensors, biocomputers, and biofuel production systems [135].

For *in vivo* cloning of a DNA fragment, containing a single gene or a number of genes, is inserted into a vector that can be amplified within another host cell [136].

A vector is a fragment of DNA that can incorporate another DNA fragment without losing the capacity for self-replication, and a vector containing an extra DNA fragment is known as a hybrid vector. If the segment of DNA includes one or more genes the process is known as gene cloning.

There are four different types of vectors:

- Cosmids.
- Expression vectors.
- Lambda (λ) phage vectors.
- Plasmid vectors.

The host cell copies the cloned DNA using its own replication mechanisms. A variety of cell types are used as hosts, including bacteria, yeast cells and mammalian cells.

One significant recent development in vector technology is the emergence of synthetic biology-derived vectors. These vectors are designed using standardized genetic parts and assemblies, making them highly modular and customizable. Researchers can now construct vectors tailored to specific applications, whether it is gene expression, protein production, or gene editing [137]. Furthermore, the rise of CRISPR-Cas technology has transformed vectors used in gene cloning. CRISPR-based vectors are engineered to carry the necessary components for precise gene editing, allowing for the targeted modification of the host organism's genome. These vectors have revolutionized the field, making gene editing faster and more accurate [138]. Recent advancements in viral vectors, particularly adeno-associated viruses (AAVs), have improved their efficiency in delivering genes to target cells. AAVs have gained prominence in gene therapy, as they can be used to deliver therapeutic genes to treat various genetic disorders. Their enhanced safety and efficacy profiles have made them a valuable tool in clinical applications [139]. Additionally, advances in nanotechnology have given rise to nanoscale vectors for gene delivery. Nanoparticles, liposomes, and other nanocarriers have shown promise in efficiently transporting genetic material to specific cells or tissues, providing potential solutions for targeted gene therapy and drug delivery [140].

3.6 Transfection methods and transgenic animals

There are various applications of animal cell and tissue culture; one of its significant applications involves the transfer of foreign genes into livestock. In organisms such as bacteria and other microbes, or even in higher plants, the uptake of genes by cells is frequently known by the term 'transformation'. However, in animals this term has been substituted by the term 'transfection', since the term 'transformation' in animal cell culture is used to describe phenotypic alteration of cells. The usage of the term 'transformation' for 'cell modification' has been unfortunate and discontinuation of its usage for this purpose is suggested. Transfection or gene transfer in animals may be done at the cellular level to obtain transfected cells, which may be used for multiple purposes, e.g. for the production of chemicals and pharmaceutical drugs. It may also be undertaken for basic investigations involving the examination of the structure and function of genes [141]. While many mammalian cell lines have often been utilized for these purposes, transfection has also been accomplished effectively for the production of transgenic animals. The development in livestock through transgenesis has already led to the following positive results:

- Enhanced milk production in cattle.
- Enhanced growth rate of livestock and fish.
- Large-scale production of valuable proteins in the milk, urine and blood of livestock, enabling the use of transgenic animals as 'bioreactors' for 'molecular farming'.
- Improvement of wool production through production of transgenic sheep. These positive results have made transfection and the production of transgenic animals an attractive growth area of research.

3.6.1 Gene transfer or transfection

In an earlier section we have already discussed the procedure involved in somatic cell fusion as a means of transfer of the whole genome from one organism to another. However, fusion can also be exercised between isolated nuclei, or between a nucleus and an enucleated whole cell. Likewise, the transfer of genetic material to whole cells can be used at the level of (i) individual chromosomes or fragments or (ii) isolated genes or gene fragments. Two related ideas in molecular biology that deal with introducing genetic material into cells are transfection and gene transfer. These methods are frequently applied in biotechnology and research to understand gene function, control cellular functions, and create gene therapies [142].

3.6.1.1 Gene transfer

Gene transfer refers to the process of introducing genetic material (such as DNA or RNA) into cells. There are several methods for gene transfer, each with its own advantages and limitations. Gene transfer can be achieved in both eukaryotic and prokaryotic cells, and it can be used for various purposes, including the expression of foreign genes, genetic modification, and gene therapy.

3.6.1.2 Transfection

Transfection is a specific method of gene transfer that involves the introduction of foreign genetic material into eukaryotic cells. The term 'transfection' is often used when the introduced material is DNA. Transfection can be accomplished using various techniques, and the choice of method depends on the type of cells being used and the specific goals of the experiment [145].

3.6.2 Transfection of fertilized eggs or embryos

The process of transfection involves introducing foreign nucleic acids into a eukaryotic cell in order to alter the genetic composition of the host cell. Because transfection has been widely used to study cellular processes and the molecular mechanisms underlying diseases, it has become more and more popular over the past thirty years. The identification of particular biomarkers that may be used to diagnose and prognose diseases is made possible by an understanding of the molecular pathways underlying disease. Additionally, transfection is a tactic used in gene therapy to treat hereditary diseases that are incurable. Many nucleic acids, including ribonucleic acids (RNAs), deoxyribonucleic acids (DNAs), and small, non-coding RNAs like siRNA, shRNA, and miRNA, can now be transfected into mammalian cells thanks to advances in life sciences technology [143]. Production of a transgenic animal requires the transfection of specialized cells or embryos, as only eggs or embryos can develop into whole animals. In contrast, in plants any cell or protoplast may be transformed, as undifferentiated plant cells, being totipotent, can develop into whole plants through differentiation and growth. The eggs can be modified by transfer of whole nuclei, whole chromosomes or parts thereof, or DNA fragments [144].

3.6.3 Transfer of whole nuclei (or split embryos)

Transfer of a whole nucleus from a somatic cell of the superior donor to the enucleated egg can be achieved using the following steps (see figure 3.8):

(i) Enucleation of the unfertilized egg is accomplished by centrifuging cytochalasin-B-treated cells, such that the nuclei detach from the eggs and pellet at the bottom of the tube, leaving enucleated eggs in the supernatant.

(ii) Karyoplasts (nuclei with only some residual plasma membrane) are similarly derived from the blastula stage of the developing embryos of the donor.

(iii) Karyoplasts obtained from the donor are incubated with enucleated eggs in the presence of PEG, and fusion is carried out.

(iv) The manipulated egg is transferred to the uterus of a surrogate mother for subsequent growth and development. Protocols have also been developed where a superior developing embryo may be bisected into two parts using a surgical blade. Each bisected part of the embryo may be separately transferred to an enucleated unfertilized egg (figure 3.9). Such a manipulated egg may then be transferred to the uterus of a surrogate mother for subsequent development. Transfer of whole individual chromosomes or fragments is possible. Chromosomes can be isolated from metaphase cells by hypotonic lysis. Incubation of these isolated chromosomes with whole cells after co-precipitation with the chromosomes once isolated can also be subjected to fractionation using density centrifugation or flow cytophotometry and individual chromosome pairs may be incorporated into recipient cells.

3.6.4 DNA microinjection into the egg

Transfer of separate cloned genes is usually accomplished by incorporating them into a fertilized egg, with a large number of copies of recombinant plasmid carrying the GOI, using the method of DNA microinjection. The DNA is microinjected into a fertilized egg before the fusion of male and female nuclei [53] (figure 3.10). The egg is first immobilized by applying mild suction to the large, blunt holding pipette and

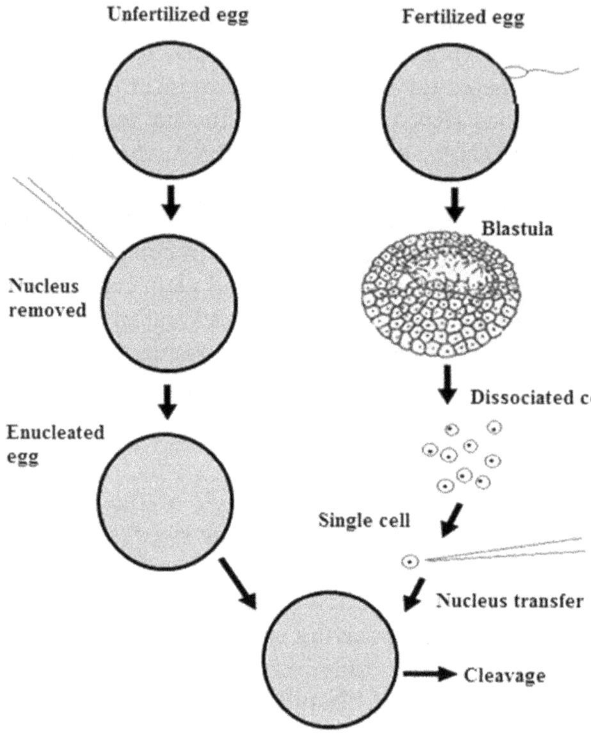

Figure 3.8. Fusion of karyoplasts with enucleated cells in the presence of PEG.

DNA is then incorporated via the sharp end of a narrow glass microneedle. Through recombination at the DNA level, the incorporated gene can be integrated into the host genome and inherited in a Mendelian manner. Transgenic mice have been produced in various laboratories utilizing this technique. The scheme has also been effectively utilized for the production of transgenic chicken, cows, fish, pigs, rabbits and sheep. In *Drosophila*, the P elements (transposons) are used as vectors, so that a recombinant P element carrying the foreign gene is used for microinjection. However, microinjected flies may not carry the inserted gene in all cells, while a number of their progeny may carry the gene in all the cells.

3.6.5 Virus-mediated gene transfer to embryo

Retrovirus infection of embryos has also been used for the production of transgenic mice. This virus has been found to be an effective vector system for animals. The virus carrying the GOI transfers it into the genome of embryonic cells leading to its integration and the production of transgenic animals.

3.6.6 Transfection of cultured mammalian cells

Transfection of cultured mammalian cells is a fundamental technique in molecular biology and biotechnology, involving the introduction of foreign genetic material,

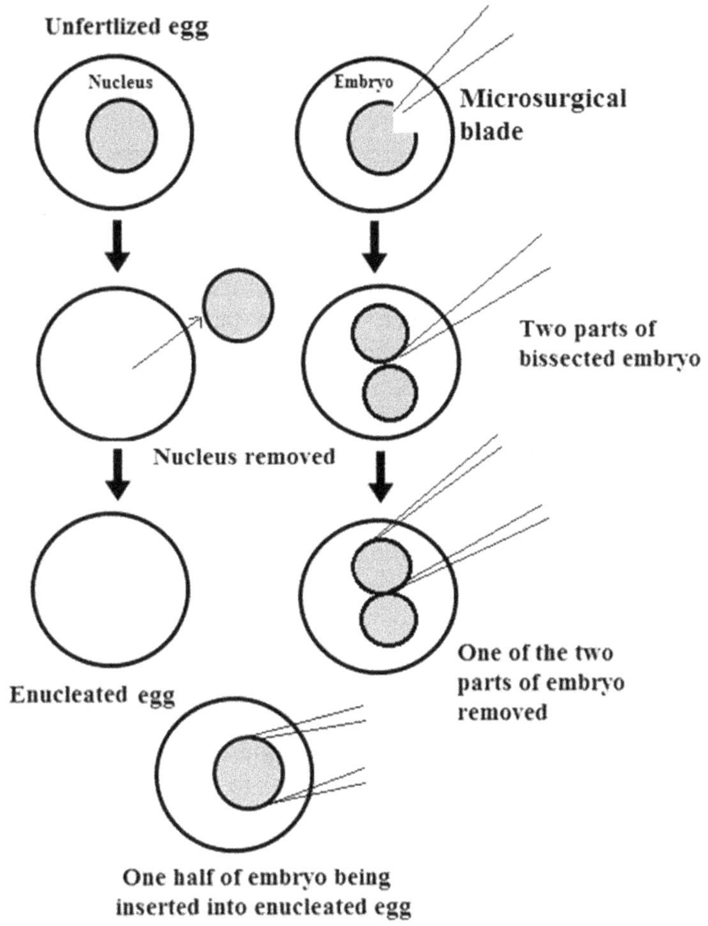

Figure 3.9. Splitting of an embryo, followed by transfer of one half of the embryo to an unfertilized egg whose contents were removed.

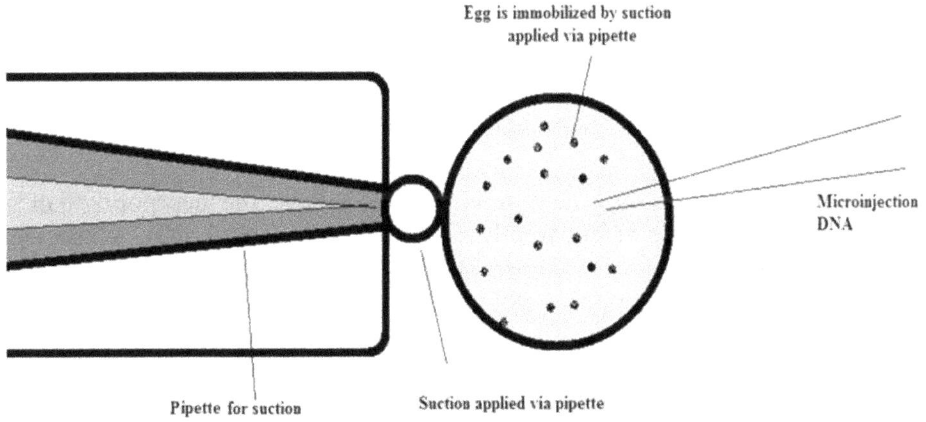

Figure 3.10. Microinjection of foreign DNA into a fertilized egg for production of transgenic animals. Calcium phosphate results in their introduction into the nuclei.

such as DNA or RNA, into cultured cells. This process enables the manipulation of gene expression, the study of cellular functions, and the production of specific proteins. Transfection methods vary and include chemical-based approaches, electroporation, and viral vectors. Researchers use transfection to elucidate gene function, model diseases, and develop therapeutic proteins. The technique is essential for advancing our understanding of cellular processes and holds significant implications for biopharmaceutical production and gene therapy research [145].

Various types of cells, from bacterial to animal cells, can be transfected through the transfer of genes, either using viruses as vectors or by physical or chemical methods. The viruses that have been found to be suitable as vectors include retroviruses, vaccinia virus, adeno-associated virus (AAV), herpes viruses and bovine papillomavirus. In animal cells, transfection frequency also rises dramatically if DNA is co-precipitated with calcium phosphate in the recipient cells [145]. In all these procedures, some of the transferred DNA may integrate with the chromosomes of the cultured cells, therefore causing stable transfection. If the donor DNA encodes a genetic trait, the recipient cells will express this trait. Transfection of cultured mammalian cells has been utilized extensively for the detection of cancer genes (oncogenes) and for gene therapy experiments. For detection of a cancer gene, DNA derived from human tumor cell lines is purified, trimmed into fragments (30–50 kb pairs in length), dissolved in phosphate buffer and finally precipitated by the addition of calcium chloride [146]. The solution is poured onto a layer of mouse 3T3 cells, which develop foci of transformed cells. These transformed cells can later be used for identification of cancer-causing genes (mouse 3T3 cell lines are efficient for DNA uptake and have been used for decades to assay cancer-causing genes). Transfection of cultured cells has also been used for gene therapy, in which the genes are incorporated into cultured cells, which are then placed into the body of a patient for gene therapy. A range of virus vectors are used for this purpose. Retroviruses were used in most of the early clinical trials (in 1990–91) including on two young girls suffering from adenosine deaminase (ADA) deficiency. A modified adenovirus and adeno-associated virus are also used. 'Naked DNA' is also utilized for gene therapy, using particle guns, liposomes or electroporation devices. Future research will categorize the most harmless and most efficient delivery methods for gene therapy [147].

3.6.7 Targeted gene transfer

In most of the procedures for gene transfer discussed above, the incorporation of the foreign gene takes place at apparently random chromosomal sites. While these 'misplaced' genes are subject to correct regulation under the control of regulatory sequences, random integration does not result in precise replacement of the defective gene at a homologous site. Gene transfer at homologous sites in the host genome is commonly defined as targeted gene transfer. Initially, such targeted gene transfer by HR for substitution of a resident wild or mutant gene was possible only in bacteria and yeast. Later, for the first time in 1985, such targeted gene transfer was effectively accomplished in human cells when Oliver Smithies at UW-Madison transferred a human eglobin gene into the eglobin gene of recipient cells by recombination [148]. The targeted gene transfer was possible because of the presence of homologous DNA sequences at the targeted site and in the vector carrying the foreign gene. Marker genes are also used for screening cells transfected with transferred gene at the targeted site. Such a selection can be achieved by several methods:

- By assaying the activity of an enzyme, as in the hypoxanthine phosphoribosyltransferase (HPRT) enzyme.
- By using a marker gene for antibiotic resistance that would enable cells to grow in a medium containing the antibiotic that would otherwise kill the cells.
- By PCR, if the sequence of the gene is available for making PCR primers. Chimeric mice have actually been prepared by targeted gene transfer, where HPRT genes or a homeobox containing genes have been modified in some embryonic cells.

If these cells contribute to the production of egg or sperm, transgenic mice will be produced. Accomplishment of targeted gene transfer has also been achieved in many other cases.

3.6.7.1 Gene targeting using ES cells

In this procedure, embryo-derived stem cells are cultured. These stem cells are transfected with a vector containing the desirable gene.

This facilitates targeting of the gene to a specific site by HR. The rare targeted cells are isolated, multiplied and used for injection of expanded blastocysts, which are then implanted into surrogate mothers to allow the development to be completed. The developed animals can be tested for transgenesis. The various steps of this technique are demonstrated in figure 3.11.

3.6.8 Transgenic animals in biotechnology

Transgenic animals play a pivotal role in biotechnology as genetically modified organisms with introduced foreign genes. These animals, often mice, rats, or livestock, are engineered to express specific traits beneficial for research, agriculture, or therapeutic purposes. In biomedicine, transgenic animals serve as invaluable models for studying human diseases, testing potential treatments, and understanding gene function. In agriculture, transgenic livestock may be designed for enhanced productivity, disease resistance, or improved nutritional content. While their applications offer substantial benefits, the development and use of transgenic animals also raise ethical considerations and require careful regulation to ensure responsible and ethical use of this biotechnological tool [149].

3.6.8.1 Transgenic mice technology

One of the first proofs of transgenic animals, reported in December 1982, involved the transfer of a GH gene (from rat) fused to the promoter for the mouse metallothionein 1 (MT) gene [151]. Since then various transgenic animals, including

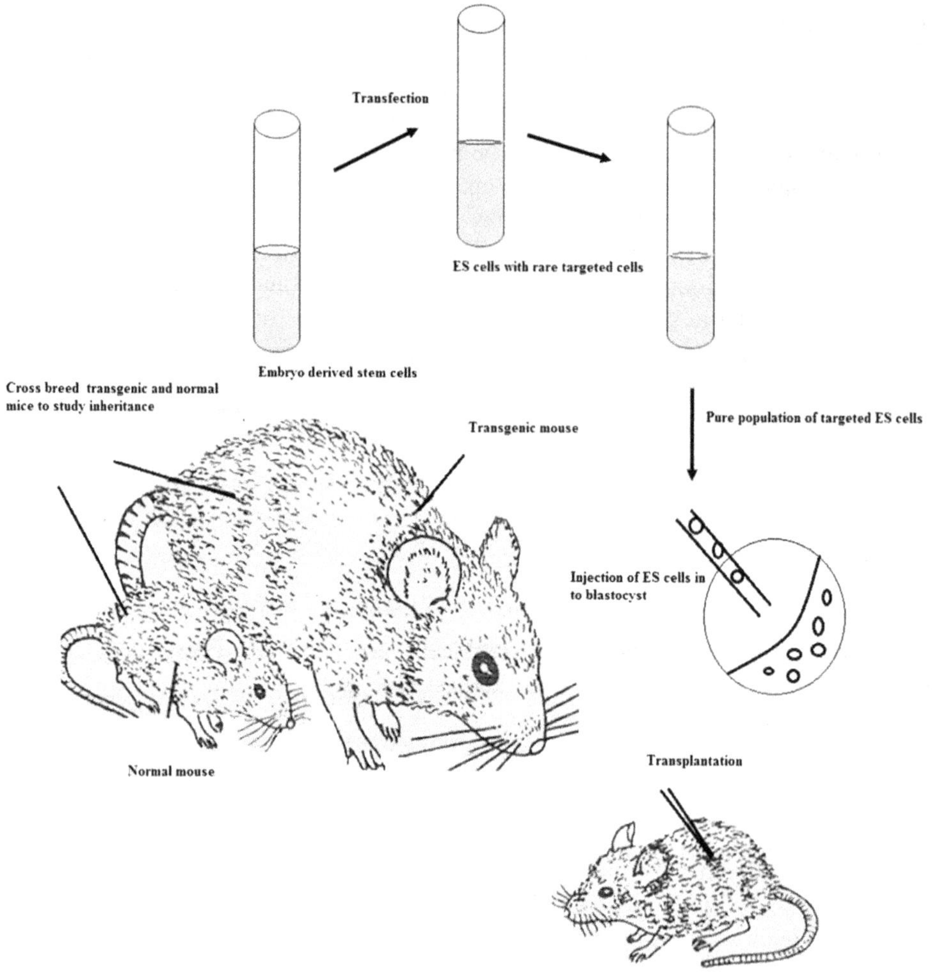

Figure 3.11. Transfection of stem cells with a vector carrying the GOI followed by microinjection of transfected stem cells into a blastocyst leading to the production of transgenic mice.

cattle, sheep, goats, pigs, rabbits, chickens and fish, have been produced and will be utilized in future for a range of purposes taking advantage of their:

- Efficiency in utilizing feed.
- Ability to provide leaner meat.
- Ability to grow to marketable size sooner.
- Resistance to certain diseases.

In addition to this, currently various attempts are being made to use transgenic animals as living bioreactors. Transgenic animals produced for this purpose will secrete valuable recombinant proteins and pharmaceuticals into their milk, blood and urine, which can be utilized for extraction of these drugs. This new prospect of manufacturing drugs via transgenic animals is frequently described as 'molecular farming' or 'molecular pharming'. Although initially many experiments leading to the production of transgenic animals did not give commercially attractive results, success has been achieved in some recent cases. Some of these cases will be discussed below.

3.6.8.2 Production of transgenic sheep

As per earlier reports, transgenic sheep production has proven difficult in comparison to the mouse and lower animals [147]. Nevertheless, due to the large benefits for human and animal health and also to improve agricultural productivity, researchers have successfully developed transgenic sheep [147]. In transgenic sheep production certain difficulties need to be addressed, such as regulation of expression of the transgenes, their phenotypic effects and optimization of the fusion gene constructs. In 1985, Hammer *et al* for the first time evidenced transgenic investigation on large animals by microinjecting the fusion gene (MT–hGH13) into the pronuclei or nuclei of eggs from superovulated rabbits, sheep and pigs [148].

The rate of transgenesis, which is very low (0.1%–0.2%), can be improved by the implantation of viable embryos into surrogate ewes. For production, embryos (8–16 cell stage) can be divided into two parts. One part of the embryo is for culture and the other is for detection of integrated genes using the gene amplification technique, PCR [149]. Previously, microinjection was the most common method for DNA delivery, but due to the considerable disadvantages of this technique gene targeting is now being utilized for the development of transgenic sheep. Before the report by McCreath *et al* in 2000, gene targeting had not yet been succeeded in mammals other than mice. This was because of the unavailability of functional embryonic stem cells [150]. As per the investigation by McCreath *et al* nuclear transfer from cultured somatic cells offers a more reliable approach for cell-mediated transgenesis [150]. Thus, they described the efficient and reproducible gene targeting in fetal fibroblasts to place a therapeutic transgene at the ovine $\alpha 1(I)$ procollagen (COL1A1) locus and the production of live sheep by nuclear transfer [150].

In this approach, transfection of the embryonic stem cells takes place with a vector that carries the GOI and HR (as discussed above) and helps in targeting the gene at specific site. Initially this approach was used in mice. The first evidence of transgenic sheep was reported by JP Simons in 1988 [151]. This process resulted in the production of two transgenic ewes. Each ewe carries around ten copies of the human anti-hemophilic factor IX gene (cDNA). Before transfection, this anti-hemophilic factor IX gene fused with the 10.5 kb BLG gene, which will ultimately help in expression of genes to produce desirable proteins in mammary glands, as shown in figure 3.12.

Expression of these genes helps in the production of milk with desirable proteins. Consequently, the gene will have tissue-specific expression. The transgenic ewes ultimately secrete human factor IX (or alpha-1 antitrypsin) into their milk. This human factor IX remains active even when the expression of the transgene is low [56]. In another approach reported by Schnieke *et al* in 1997, ovine primary fetal fibroblasts (cells that synthesize the extracellular matrix and collagen) were co-transfected (simultaneous transfection with two separate nucleic acid molecules)

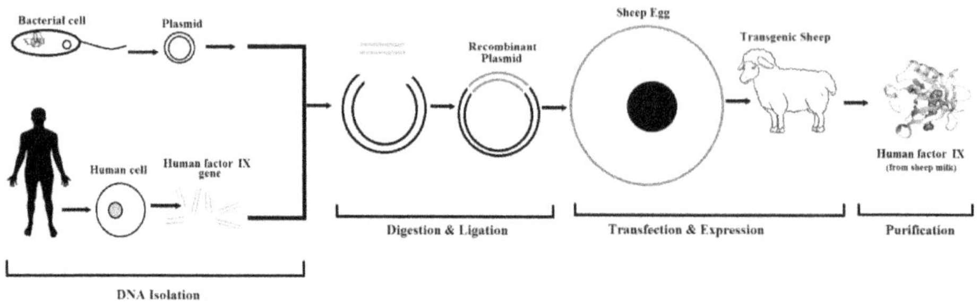

Figure 3.12. Human factor IX transgenic sheep.

with a neomycin resistance marker gene and a human coagulation factor IX genomic construct. This was prepared for expression of the encoded protein in sheep milk [152].

In 1986 transgenic ewes were born and in the same year they were successfully mated. Later in 1987, each ewe gave birth to a lamb carrying the BLG-F IX transgene and secreting factor IX in its milk. Owing to its commercial significance, this whole procedure was supported by Pharmaceutical Proteins Ltd (Cambridge, UK). Subsequently Colman *et al* produced five transgenic sheep by the fusion of ovine β-lactoglobulin gene promoter with the human antitrypsin (ha1AT) gene [153]. Out of five, four of the animals were female and one was male. In one female, a significant amount of haIAT protein (35 g) was found per liter of the milk [154]. Later, desirable protein was purified from the milk. Deficiency of ha1AT in the European population, especially among adults, resulted in a lethal disease known as emphysema (a common hereditary disorder among European population). Thus, there is a high demand for any safe and economic approach that increases the yield of the protein in milk or in any other natural consumable secretion derived from plants and animals. In this respect, production of transgenic sheep with the ha1AT gene is considered as a reliable approach. The production of therapeutic proteins in milk using transgenesis is a commercially significant approach, and similarly encouraging wool growth by means of rDNA technology can also be considered as reliable strategy. To achieve this objective, researchers discovered the genes that are responsible for the production of vital amino acids present in proteins of wool. These genes have been cloned and introduced into embryos to further produce transgenic sheep. The genes cysE and cysM for the respective enzymes serine O-acetyltransferase and O-acetylserine sulfydrylase involved in the biosynthesis of cysteine were identified and further isolated from bacteria, and ultimately cloned in a vector. These genes responsible for wool production were introduced into sheep cells and ultimately resulted in the production of transgenic sheep, where these genes are expressed to increase the wool growth. Similarly, growth hormone genes have also been introduced and can be used to promote body weight to further increase meat production. Several other genes responsible for wool production, growth hormone production and production of desirable proteins were discovered recently, which can be further used for transgenesis.

In recent research by Cornetta *et al* in 2013, the safety of HIV-1 based vectors was evaluated during the production of transgenic sheep [154]. In this procedure HIV-1 based vectors were introduced into (one-cell stage) sheep embryos by microinjection, then further transferred into recipient females [154]. This study supported the safety of this procedure for human gene therapy, as the transgenic animals and their surrogates showed no evidence of replication competent lentivirus (RCL) or transfer of inadvertent vector sequences [154]. The outcome of this research supports the safety of HIV-1 based vectors in animal and human applications.

3.6.8.3 Genetically modified pigs

In contrast to transgenic mice (2.5%–6%), the rate of the transgenesis in transgenic pigs is still very low. In the case of pigs, the efficiency for the production of transgenic pigs is 0.6%, even when as many as 7000 eggs were injected. To improve the production efficiency of large transgenic animals, researchers studied a linker-based sperm-mediated gene transfer method [155]. This approach is effective for the generation of transgenic pigs and mice by linker-based sperm-mediated gene transfer [155]. Even with a low frequency, several transgenic studies have been successfully performed on pigs for the production of desirable proteins and for other applications. Isolation of the gene responsible for growth hormone production and their expression in transgenic pigs was one of the most welcomed approaches for the production of GH. At the Agriculture Research Service in Beltsville, USA, V G Purse isolated GH genes of bovine or human origin and produced the sheep globin gene. Expression of hGH gene in transgenic pigs allowed varied levels of expression [155]. It has been observed that a mere 66% of these animals showed noticeable levels of hGH and bGH in their plasma. Comparatively, these hGH carrying animals showed significant growth, however, did not increase in size. Likewise, bGH carrying pigs did not show any noticeable changes expression of the transgene, for unknown reasons. However, these reports proved that these transgenic pigs showed a 10%–15% increase in daily weight and also a 16%–18% increase in feed consumption efficiency. Of course, these results were lower than those observed in mice, however, it was still comparable to those receiving injections of GH. More importantly, a marked reduction in subcutaneous fat was observed, signifying the prospect of producing meat with a lower fat content [156]. These reports have had a considerable influence on the livestock industry, in particular the pig industry in the USA. Additionally, it was observed that continuous production of GH is generally harmful for the health of pigs, which may result in gastric ulcers, arthritis and several other diseases. Thus, various tools have now been developed to efficiently manipulate the transgene expression by a number of procedures (e.g. modifying the genetic background or changing the husbandry regime) [157]. Therefore, techniques will have to be developed to better manipulate the transgene expression using a variety of methods (e.g. changing the genetic background or modifying the husbandry system) [157]. Several other studies have been reported, such as expression of the plant gene in a complex mammalian system to improve the PUFA concentrations in pork [158]. Recently, a PRKAG3 gene based dominant mutation has been identified, which may lead to glycogen accumulation in skeletal muscles, especially in Hampshire pigs. This type of mutation helps in the improvement of pork taste, but deceptively makes automated processing more difficult [159]. Furthermore, two quantitative-trait loci have been identified that have substantial effects on muscle mass and fat deposition [160]. The myxovirus resistance gene is responsible for broad spectrum antiviral properties and also acts as an interesting candidate gene to improve disease resistance in farm animals [161]. More recently researchers have explored the Mx1 transgene which can protect against viral infection in cells of transgenic pigs and indicate that the Mx1 transgene can be harnessed to develop disease-resistant pigs [161].

The overall draft of the pig genome is based on the most recent assembly (Sus scrofa genome build 10 (Sscrofa10), currently being annotated), which signifies around 98% of the porcine genome [162]. The utilization of organs derived from transgenic pigs for xenotransplantation into humans [163] and the production of pharmaceuticals [164] are also being explored. In medical science pigs are accepted as an excellent model for surgical testing. This study was based on their respective organs' similarity to the human kidney, lung, heart, coronary vasculature, liver, and uterine histology [165]. Pigs also act as an ideal model for genetic research, as the size and composition of the porcine genome is similar to that of humans [166].

As far as the xenotransplantation is concerned, transgenic pigs are favorable donor organisms since they have several identical anatomical and physiological characteristics to human beings. However, the most important obstacle to pig-to-primate xenotransplantation is the rejection of the grafted organ. This rejection is mediated by the number of immune mechanisms usually called hyperacute rejection, acute humoral xenograft rejection, immune cell-mediated rejection and chronic rejection. Different approaches that are based on genetic modification of pigs can be utilized to allow them to be donors for organ transplantation [165]. As per the current investigation, transgenic pigs lacking alpha-1,3-Gal epitopes, considered as the major xenoantigens triggering hyperacute rejection of pig-to-primate xenografts, are considered to be the basis for further genetic modifications that can address other rejection mechanisms and incompatibilities between the porcine and primate blood coagulation systems. Moreover, transgenic approaches have been developed to prevent the possible risk of infections by endogenous porcine retroviruses.

3.6.8.4 Production of transgenic goats

John McPherson and Karl Ebert, in the USA, successfully produced transgenic goats that expressed a heterologous protein (a variant of human tissue-type plasminogen activator, LAtPA) in their milk. This protein is usually employed for dissolving blood clots, i.e. for management of coronary thrombosis [167].

In an expression vector a complementary DNA representing LAtPA was linked with either the murine whey acid promoter or a kappa-casein promoter. Vectors carrying the GOI were injected in early embryos derived by surgical procedures from the oviducts of superovulated dairy goats [168]. These vectors carrying embryos were either directly transferred to the oviducts of recipient females or alternatively cultured for 72 h (blocked at the 8–16 cell stage), before transfer to the uterus of surrogate or recipient mothers. Out of 29 offspring from 36 recipients, one male and one female carries the transgene [168]. The transgenic female carried five offspring, out of which one was transgenic, presenting expression of LAtPA at a low level of a few milligrams per liter of milk. In another case of a transgenic goat, a few grams of LAtPA per liter of milk could be obtained. At this concentration, the dairy goat may become an economically viable bioreactor for human pharmaceuticals [168]. In recent research, several researchers have improved the nutrient content of goat milk by constructing a vector (pBLAC) containing a hybrid goat β-lactoglobulin (BLG) promoter/cytomegalovirus (CMV) enhancer. Through this approach the mammary-gland-specific expression of vector pBLAC with hybrid BLG/CMV can drive the hLA gene to expression under *in vitro* and *in vivo* environmental conditions [169].

Several approaches have been used for the production of transgenic goats. Of these, production via pronuclear microinjection of DNA expression vectors is considered as the most traditional approach, however, results in low efficiencies. The laparoscopic ovum pick-up technique with pronuclear microinjection can also be successfully utilized to produce transgenic goats. Alternative approaches, such as somatic cell nuclear transfer, has considerably improved the productivity in rates of transgenesis. This approach guarantees that kids born are transgenic and of predetermined gender [169]. Production of transgenic goats expressing human coagulation factor IX in the mammary glands using transfected fetal fibroblast cells is an excellent example of the nuclear transfer technique, which may allow the large-scale production and therapeutic application of hFIX expressed in transgenic goats [168].

At the end of 2000, several scientists from Genzyme Transgenics Corporation, Framingham, MA, investigated hormonally induced lactation in prepubertal, nulliparous and male goats (both transgenic and non-transgenic). They observed that hormonal induction of lactation in the caprine species is a feasible alternative to pregnancy for initiating lactation and milk production [169]. This procedure does not adversely influence reproductive performance long-term and can benefit the early assessment of recombinant proteins produced in a transgenic founder program [169].

Lysozyme, an antimicrobial protein, is extremely expressed in human milk, buy is not present in ruminant milk. This therapeutic protein offers protection to infants, in particular breastfeeding children, against diarrheal diseases. Several researchers have reported that consumption of milk from transgenic goats which produce human lysozyme (hLZ-milk) in their milk could accelerate recovery from diarrhea [169, 170]. In this study they have used pigs as a model for children and infected with enterotoxigenic *E. coli*. The results demonstrated that with consumption of hLZ-milk pigs recover from infection faster. This makes hLZ-milk a real treatment for *E. coli*-induced diarrhea. Similarly, several other researchers engineered transgenic goats expressing human lysozyme in the mammary gland [169, 170]. Milk from engineered animals had a shorter rennet clotting time and improved curd strength. Moreover, milk of such nature may be of value to the producer through altering udder health and milk processing [169, 170].

For the large-scale production of functional human lysozyme in transgenic cloned goats, several researchers have utilized a somatic cell-mediated transgenic cloning method by further utilizing two optimized lysozyme expression cassettes (β-casein/hLZ and β-lactoglobulin/hLZ) and introduced into goat somatic cells by cell transfection [171]. As discussed above, lysozyme is a significant non-specific immune protein in human milk, controlling the immune response against bacterial infections. In 2018, several researchers from Brazil engineered transgenic goat secreting milk expressing human lysozyme for the recovery and treatment of gastrointestinal pathogens [172]. This research demonstrated valid evidence for its potential use as a nutraceutical for the improvement of health and nutrition quality for humans [172].

Several safety issues need to be considered during the development of genetically engineered animals. One of the safety concerns for the expression of the human GH gene in transgenic goats has attracted the attention of several researchers [172]. Recently, several researchers assessed the risks of growth hormone from transgenic goats, covering the possibility of horizontal gene transfer and the influence on the microbial community of the goat's gastrointestinal tracts, feces and the surrounding soil. The outcome of this research demonstrated that expression of goat GH in the mammary glands of GH transgenic goats does not affect the microflora of the intestine, feces and surrounding soil [173]. In 2006, scientists developed a two-step membrane isolation and purification process using ultrafiltration to recover heterologous immunoglobulin from transgenic goat milk, with an 80% yield and 80% purity [174].

3.6.8.5 Genetically modified cows

The purpose of genetically modified cows is to produce cows with particular characteristics that will increase agricultural productivity, better animal welfare, and address environmental issues. These changes frequently go after characteristics like improved nutritional value, greater milk production, and disease resistance. Scientists are working to breed cows that can yield more milk by introducing genes linked to desirable traits. This could lead to increased food security and financial gains for farmers. Genetically engineered animals act as active source the production of several useful compounds with high therapeutic value, and are often called biofactories, e.g. the production of therapeutic proteins by transgenic cows in their milk. Transgenic cows are produced by introducing a desirable gene into their DNA to further assess their expression in the form of production of protein in their secretions such as milk. Thus, transgenic cows always carry an additional gene that may come from the same species or from a different species. This newly inserted gene, called an additional gene or transgene, is present in every cell in the transgenic cow, nevertheless, its expression is restricted to the mammary glands. Therefore, the transgenic cow acts as a biofactory for the production of a transgenic or recombinant protein which can be secreted in the cow's milk and can be further extracted and purified from there. In the beginning, the GOI is identified and sequenced, which is followed by DNA cloning. This allows insertion of the chosen gene in gene construct. Ultimately, the designed gene construct is introduced into female bovine (cow) cells by transfection. Afterwards, selection of transgenic bovine cells is done to fuse them with bovine oocytes, after eliminating their chromosomes.

After oocyte fusion, transgenic cell's chromosomes are re-engineered to direct development into an embryo. To achieve this the cells are implanted into a recipient cow. After 9 months of pregnancy, a female calf is born. After the delivery of her first calf she will express the transgene in the form of production of proteins in her milk during lactation. Mammary-gland-specific expression of the transgene in lactating mammary cells is regulated by a promoter specific region which allows the synthesis of desirable proteins in milk [175].

Previously, embryos or fertilized oocytes produced *in vivo* were utilized for the production of transgenic cows. In this process proembryos or fertilized oocytes are recovered by surgical procedures from superovulated and artificially inseminated cows. Via surgery zygotes are directly transferred using a microneedle into the oviduct of recipient cows or into temporary hosts such as sheep or rabbits. As this approach involves many surgical procedures it is labor intensive and expensive. During 1991, a new approach was developed for *in vitro* production of embryos. This approach allows the fertilization of oocytes derived from the ovaries of slaughter house cows under *in vitro* conditions. Microinjection of pronuclei was achieved by preparing a construct that contains a bovine alpha-S1-casein promoter driving a cDNA encoding the antibacterial human iron-binding protein lactoferrin. Developed embryos were cultured to the morula/blastula stage and then non-surgically transferred to recipient females. Out of 19 newly born calves, 10^3 transferred zygotes were transgenic (one male and the other female). This method may allow the use of cows as bioreactors at a large-scale [175].

Several researchers have also reported a disadvantage of transgenic cows in the form of experimental mastitis, which is an infection caused by *E. coli.* According to this research, transgenic cows that produce recombinant human lactoferrin in milk are not protected from experimental *E. coli* intramammary infection [176]. They have concluded that thelactoferrin transgenesis model did not provide protection against *E. coli* mastitis in dairy cows, in contrast to the findings for the experimental *S. aureus* problem in lysostaphin-transgenic cows [177].

Different approaches have been utilized for the production of transgenic cows, such as manipulating transgenic animals using transposable elements or transposons (they can be used for germline transgenesis, somatic cell transgenesis/gene therapy and random germline insertional mutagenesis) [178]. In a recent study, researchers successfully developed transgenic cattle using a two-transposon system and the cattle genomes were analyzed using next-generation sequencing. It has been observed that all these animals could be a valuable resource for agriculture and veterinary science [179].

In addition, researchers also produced transgenic cattle using reverse-transcribed gene transfer. During this procedure reverse-transcribed gene transfer can take place in an oocyte in metaphase II arrest of meiosis, resulting in generation of offspring, the majority of which are transgenic [180]. Researchers have also discussed the consequences of this mechanism both as a means of generation of transgenic livestock and as a model for naturally occurring recursive transgenesis

Additionally, genetic modifications may offer solutions to environmental challenges associated with livestock farming, such as reduced methane emissions and improved feed efficiency. However, the development and commercialization of genetically modified cows also spark ethical debates regarding animal welfare, potential environmental impacts, and the long-term consequences of altering the genetic makeup of livestock. Striking a balance between innovation and ethical considerations is crucial as researchers and society navigate the evolving landscape of genetically modified organisms in agriculture [102].

3.6.8.6 Genetically modified fish

Fish that have had their genetic makeup changed through genetic engineering are referred to as genetically modified (GM) fish. Often, the purpose of genetically modifying fish is to introduce particular traits that can enhance their growth rate, disease resistance, environmental tolerance, or other desired qualities. These are some important points to remember about genetically modified fish. Examples of GM fish include:

AquAdvantage Salmon—This genetically modified Atlantic salmon has been engineered to grow faster than conventional salmon.

Tilapia with Enhanced Omega-3—Some researchers have worked on genetically modifying tilapia to produce higher levels of omega-3 fatty acids. It is important to note that public opinion, regulatory environments, and scientific research on genetically modified organisms, including fish, continue to evolve. Public discourse often involves discussions about the potential benefits and risks associated with genetic modification, and regulatory bodies work to establish guidelines that balance innovation with safety and environmental concerns [182].

Transgenic fish are produced by the artificial transfer of rearranged genes into newly fertilized eggs. Currently microinjection is the most suitable technique, while the integration rates of transgenes are generally low [181]. Efforts to produce transgenic fish began in 1985 and some hopeful findings have been obtained. The genes that have been incorporated by microinjection into fish include the following:

- Human or rat genes for GH.
- Chicken genes for delta-crystalline protein.
- *E. coli* genes for fi-galactosidase.
- *E. coli* genes for neomycin resistance.
- Winter flounder (flat fish) gene for antifreeze protein.
- Trout genes for GH.

The procedure of microinjection has been effectively used to produce transgenic fish in various species, e.g. common carp, catfish, goldfish, loach medaka, salmon, tilapia, rainbow trout and zebrafish. In other animals (e.g. mice, cows, pigs, sheep and rabbits), typically direct microinjection of cloned DNA into male pronuclei of fertilized eggs has proved fruitful, but in most fish species investigated so far, pronuclei cannot be easily visualized (except in medaka), so the DNA needs to be inserted into the cytoplasm. Eggs and sperm from mature individuals are collected and placed into separate dry containers [181]. Fertilization is initiated by adding water and sperm to eggs, with mild stirring to facilitate the fertilization process. The egg shells are hardened in water. Around 10^6–10^8 molecules of linearized DNA in a volume of 20 ml or less are microinjected into each egg (1–4 cells stage) within the first few hours after fertilization. Following microinjection, eggs are incubated in suitable hatching trays and dead embryos are removed daily [181]. As in fish fertilization is external, for the *in vitro* culturing of embryos the subsequent transfer into foster mothers (as required in mammals) is not required. Further, the injection into the cytoplasm is not as harmful as that into the nucleus, so the survival rate in fish is higher (35%–80%). Human GH gene transferred to transgenic fish allowed growth to twice the size of their corresponding non-transgenic fish goldfish, rainbow trout and salmon. Likewise, the antifreeze protein (AFP) gene has been transferred in a number of cases and its expression was investigated in transgenic goldfish (*Carassius auratus*) for its implications to cold adaptation [182]. It was reported that the level of AFP gene expression is still too low to provide protection against freezing. There was also an investigation in 1991 based on the production of transgenic zebrafish from an Indian laboratory at Madurai Kamaraj University [183]. In this effort, a plasmid-containing rat GH was microinjected into fertilized zebrafish eggs, and its presence was confirmed in adult fish.

3.7 Applications of genetic engineering in biotechnology

Most of the genes derived from the higher eukaryotes are quite large, extending over hundreds and thousands of base pairs. Coding of the eukaryotic genome is not continuous, however; it is always interrupted by introns that are spliced from primary mRNA. From this it is clear that among higher eukaryotes, very little of the genome codes for protein. Then question raised for *Homo sapiens* what is in the remaining genome, is that can be called 'junk' DNA, covering almost 97% of the genome? If a region is gene-poor; is that because there are massive deserts of intergenic DNA between adjacent genes, or is it because the few genes that are there are large, with vast introns? Much of the length is made up of introns which are excised from the mRNA in processing [184].

The structure of eukaryotic genes is more complex and includes several distinct components such as:

Promoter: The promoter is a region at the beginning of a gene where RNA polymerase (an enzyme responsible for transcription) binds to initiate the transcription process. Promoters contain specific DNA sequences, such as the TATA box, which help recruit the transcription machinery.

Transcription start site (TSS): This is the specific point on the DNA strand where transcription begins. It is typically located just downstream of the promoter.

Coding region (Exons): The coding region of a gene, also known as exons, contains the actual genetic information that codes for a protein or functional RNA molecule. Exons are interrupted by introns.

Introns: Introns are non-coding regions within a gene that interrupt the coding sequence. During the process of transcription, introns are transcribed into pre-mRNA but are later spliced out during RNA processing to create mature mRNA. This splicing step allows for the removal of non-coding regions, ensuring that only the coding sequence is retained in the final mRNA.

Polyadenylation signal (Poly-A Signal): At the end of the gene, there is a sequence called the polyadenylation signal. This signal indicates where the polyadenylation machinery should add a poly-A tail to the mRNA molecule. The poly-A tail is important for mRNA stability and translation.

Terminator: The terminator is a sequence that marks the end of the gene and signals the RNA polymerase to stop transcription. It is located downstream of the coding region.

Enhancers and silencers: These are regulatory elements that can be located either upstream or downstream of the gene. They control the level of gene expression by binding transcription factors that enhance (activate) or suppress (silence) transcription.

Splicing signals: These signals are found at the boundaries between exons and introns and help guide the splicing machinery during the removal of introns from pre-mRNA.

3' and 5' untranslated regions (UTRs): These regions are found on either side of the coding region in mRNA. They play a role in regulating translation and mRNA stability.

After the discovery in 1977 that genes present in eukaryotes are comprised of 'extra' pieces of DNA that do not appear in the mRNA that the gene encoded, these sequences became known as intervening sequences or introns [185]. This is one of the most amazing discoveries regarding eukaryotic genes. These sequences are always present with the sequences that will make up the mRNA, known as exons [185]. In numerous cases, number and total length of the introns are greater than that of the exons, e.g. as in the case of the chicken ovalbumin gene (has total of seven introns making up more than 75% of the gene) [186]. After more research and the development of a better understanding of eukaryotic genes, it was concluded that eukaryotic genes are extremely complex, and perhaps very large indeed [186].

This demonstrates the wonderful range of sizes for human genes, the smallest of which may be only a few hundred base pairs in length [186]. At the other end of the scale, the dystrophin gene is spread over 2.4 Mb of DNA on the X chromosome, with the 79 exons representing only 0.6% of this length of DNA. In eukaryotes the existence of introns clearly has significant effects for the expression of genetic information [186]. The introns must be removed before the mRNA can be translated. This event takes place in the nucleus, where the introns are spliced out of the primary transcript.

It is essential to understand the molecular biology behind genetic engineering to further understand the structure and function of DNA and its organization within the genome (the total genetic complement of an organism) [186]. In modern biotechnology, the understanding of molecular biology has allowed genetic engineering to explore several applications, as follows:

- As microorganisms have a higher metabolic rate, the genes coding for anticipated enzymes could be inserted into the plasmids of bacteria. For example, a gene responsible for amylase synthesis can be obtained from yeast and can be introduced into the plasmids of microbes to further encourage beer fermentation. A similar example is found in the case of genes responsible for cellulose synthesis; the introduction of such genes encourages cellulose degradation. Both applications have demonstrated commercial significance [187].

- Chimeric monoclonal antibodies (made by fusion of the antigen-binding region from one species, e.g. mouse, with the effector region from another species, e.g. rabbit) in the human Fc (fragment of crystallization) region can be made [187].
- Genetic engineering has also been used to treat a number of the genetic diseases by means of gene therapy.
- Several products, such as alpha-1 antitrypsin, antithrombin, factor VIII, tissue plasminogen activator, erythropoeitin, etc, are produced using this technology.
- Additionally, some more therapeutic protein-based products such as subunit vaccines can be produced by rDNA technology. For the production of subunit vaccines, instead of producing antibodies against all the antigens in the pathogen, a specific antigen is used in such a manner that once the antibody produced by a B cell binds to it, infection is prevented. Thus an effective subunit vaccine is produced by identifying the particular antigen or combination of antigens to trigger specific immune reactions. The most common examples of subunit vaccines are hepatitis B and haemophilus influenzae b (Hib) that use only one antigen; influenza is an example of a subunit vaccine with two antigens (haemagglutinin and neuraminidase) [188].
- Several antigenic microbial proteins are allowed to express in plant host systems in such a way that their immunogenic properties are retained. The product derived from this procedure is called an edible vaccine [189].
- By using this technology several products with high therapeutic and commercial value, such as the hormone somatostatin (growth hormone–inhibiting hormone), thymosin alpha-I (peptide fragment resulting from prothymosin alpha) and β-endorphin (hormone that is produced in certain neurons), have been produced.
- Transgenic animals with valuable features have been created using this technique.
- Weissmann and colleagues produced alpha-interferon using an rDNA technique. The enzyme urokinase, which is used to dissolve blood clots, has been produced by genetically engineered microorganisms [190].
- Plasmid technology has proven that biopharmaceuticals such as insulin, interferon, vaccines and human GH may be commercially possible. In 1984, almost 200 industries were involved in the production of these types of products by either gene splicing experiments or by exploring other applications of genetic engineering. Products such as Humulin (human insulin), interferon, a human growth hormone known as protropin (the hormone used to treat dwarfism), urokinase (a clot dissolving enzyme) and endorphin (a pain killer) have been produced through genetic engineering by inserting the desirable gene into bacterial plasmids to produce multiple copies

initially and then later on these were allowed to be expressed in a suitable host for the production of these therapeutic proteins.

Some of the key applications of genetic engineering in various domains of biotechnology include (191–194):

1. Medical biotechnology:
   (a) Production of recombinant proteins: Genetic engineering is used to produce therapeutic proteins like insulin, growth hormones, and clotting factors, which are used to treat diseases like diabetes, growth disorders, and haemophilia.
   (b) Gene therapy: It involves the introduction or correction of specific genes in a patient's cells to treat genetic disorders or diseases, such as cystic fibrosis or certain types of cancer.
   (c) Pharmacogenomics: Genetic engineering helps tailor drug treatments to an individual's genetic makeup, improving drug efficacy and reducing side effects.
2. Agricultural biotechnology:
   (a) GM crops: Genetic engineering is used to create crops with improved traits such as resistance to pests, herbicides, or harsh environmental conditions, and enhanced nutritional profiles.
   (b) Crop yield enhancement: Genetic engineering can increase crop yields by improving traits like drought tolerance, disease resistance, and nutrient uptake.
   (c) Reduced food spoilage: Genetically engineered crops can have extended shelf life and reduced susceptibility to spoilage.
3. Environmental biotechnology:
   (a) Bioremediation: Genetic engineering aids in designing microorganisms capable of breaking down or detoxifying pollutants in soil and water, helping to clean up contaminated environments.
   (b) Biofuel production: Engineered microorganisms can produce biofuels like ethanol and biodiesel, providing renewable energy sources with reduced environmental impact.
4. Industrial biotechnology:
   (a) Enzyme production: Genetic engineering is used to produce enzymes for various industrial processes, including textile manufacturing, detergent production, and biofuel processing.
   (b) Bioplastics: Microorganisms can be engineered to produce biodegradable plastics, reducing the environmental impact of plastic waste.
5. Pharmaceuticals and drug development:
   (a) Biopharmaceuticals: Genetic engineering is essential in the development of biopharmaceuticals like monoclonal antibodies and vaccines.
   (b) Drug discovery: Engineered cells and organisms are used in drug screening assays and studies of drug interactions.

6. Synthetic biology:
   (a) Creation of novel organisms: Genetic engineering allows scientists to design and create entirely new organisms with specific functions or capabilities, contributing to fields like biofuels, materials science, and medicine.
   (b) Bio-computing: Genetic circuits and engineered biological systems can be used to perform computational tasks and logic operations.
7. Diagnostics:
   (a) Genetic testing: Genetic engineering is used in DNA sequencing, PCR (polymerase chain reaction), and other diagnostic techniques to detect genetic disorders, infectious diseases, and paternity testing.
8. Vaccine development: Genetic engineering plays a critical role in the development of vaccines for infectious diseases, including mRNA-based COVID-19 vaccines.
9. Gene editing: Technologies like CRISPR-Cas9 enable precise gene editing in various organisms, offering potential therapies for genetic diseases and creating genetically modified organisms (194).

3.8 Mammalian cell line characterization

Mammalian cell lines are crucial for research and development in the areas of biology and medicine. These cell lines have to be grown in suitable media containing the required nutrients and should be provided with optimal growth condition.

Characterization of cell lines is the first essential step after each cell line is generated for evaluating its functionality, authenticity, contamination, origin, etc (tables 3.4 and 3.5). A cell line is defined as a growth that develops after a primary culture is sub-cultured or passaged. It is further divided into two parts: the normal cell line (divides a limited number of times) and the continuous cell line (the cell line with the capacity for infinite survival (immortal)) [195]. Characterization is an essential step that entails defining/outlining those many traits of the cell line, some of which may be unique. Morphology, chromosome and DNA analysis have now become the major standard procedures for cell line identification.

Mammalian cell lines are ideal for producing recombinant proteins due to their remarkable characteristics such as proper protein folding, assembly and post-translational modification. As recently as 2007, 70% of the therapeutic recombinant proteins were produced using specific mammalian cells lines called Chinese hamster ovary cell lines [196]. Initially researchers were concerned to use mammalian cells for producing recombinant therapeutic proteins as they were derived by altering the oncogenes which has the potential to cause proliferation. But, in contrast it was proved that CHO cells lines do not cause any potential risks [196]. Tissue plasminogen was the first recombinant therapeutic protein produced using CHO cell line and it was approved in the year 1987 [196].

Table 3.4. Techniques involved in cellular characterization.

Methods of characterization	
DNA fingerprinting analysis	• RFLP, AmpFLP (Amplified FLP), STR, SNP
Identity testing	• Barcode analysis • DNA fingerprinting (STR analysis) • Isoenzyme • Karyology
Virological safety testing	
Genetic stability testing	• Copy number determination • DNA and RNA sequencing • Restriction map analysis
DNA content (DNA content can be measured using DNA flourochromes)	• Propidium iodide, Hoechst 33 258, DAPI, Pico green. Analysis of DNA content is particularly useful in the characterization of transformed cells that are often aneuploid and heteroploidy. • DNA fingerprinting [197] DNA fingerprinting is a valuable approach developed by Alec Jeffrey for characterization of cell lines.

Table 3.5. Characterization of cell lines and cell strains.

Sr No.	Target of analysis	Method
1	DNA profile	PCR of microsatellite repeats
2	Karyotype	Chromosome spread with banding
3	Isozyme	Agar gel electrophoresis
4	Genome	Microarray
5	Gene expression	Microarray
6	Proteomics	Microarray
7	Cell surface antigens	Immunochemistry
8	Cytoskeleton	Immunochemistry with antibodies to specific cytoskeleton

Some of the significant application of mammalian expression system are as follows [3]:

- monoclonal antibody production;
- protein expression analysis;
- development of active viral surface antigens;
- Cloned gene product verification.

This approach can also differentiate between closely related cell lines.

DNA profiling has been used most broadly with human cell lines where the primers are most frequently accessible; the extension of this to other animal species is still fairly limited. Speciation (the formation of new and distinctive species in the course of evolution) can be achieved using the so-called 'barcode region' of the cytochrome oxidase I as well as by isoenzyme examination. DNA profiling mainly analyses STRs. STRs are repetitive DNA elements between two and six bases long that are repeated in tandem. These STR loci are targeted with sequence-specific primers and amplified using PCR. They are most widely used with human cell lines. DNA fingerprinting, DNA profiling and DNA hybridization are the main parameters for characterization of cell lines [198].

3.9 *In vitro* fertilization (IVF) and embryo transfer in humans and domestic animals

Infertility is a serious concern in the health of humans and livestock, and causes major economic losses in the livestock industry. There are numerous possible reasons for infertility, which may be infectious or non-infectious. Currently available animal cell/tissue culture techniques offer a solution to this problem. Recently these techniques have become more advanced and are often used for the manipulation of genetic material [199]. In plant research, totipotent cells can be utilized to regenerate into a whole plant. In contrast, in animal cells only the gametes (oocytes and spermatocytes) can be fertilized under *in vitro* conditions to develop a zygote, which can be developed into the embryonic stage to study the further development of an animal. In view of this fact, it is essential to establish certain procedures which will allow:

- Oocyte recovery in large numbers.
- Fertilization of these oocytes *in vitro* condition.
- Development of the zygote to the embryonic stage.
- Selection of the same or s surrogate mother (or healthy uterus).
- Transfer of the fertilized ovum or embryo in a healthy uterus.
- Monitoring regular development of the embryo.

Recently several *in vitro* fertilization based techniques and procedures have been developed to refine the previous technology, such as genetic screening, single-embryo transfer, frozen embryos, new medications, gonadotropin-releasing hormone agonist, the hormone kisspeptin, luteal phase support and improved culture media, optimal pH of embryology media, optimal oxygen (O_2) concentration in embryo incubators, *in vitro* maturation, cryopreservation, preimplantation genetic diagnosis (pgd) and preimplantation genetic screening, secretomics and metabolomics, time lapse imaging, etc Currently various researches are in progress to refine the technology in such a way as to produce elite varieties. It is believed that these advancements help in successful transformation of desirable traits in animals, which may further results in genetic improvement. This improvement imparts quality characteristics to the livestock such as increase in growth and milk production. Previously, different methods, e.g. artificial insemination and embryo transfer, have been employed to genetically manipulate livestock. Recent genetic advances such as quantitative-trait mapping will allow these conventional animal-breeding procedures to increase the quality of farm animals. With the help of genetic engineering it is possible to produce livestock with high quality traits, e.g. milk composition, wool growth, body growth and disease resistance [200]. Transgenic animals have been produced worldwide, however, the rate of producing these animals is still low and the method involved is costly. It is assumed that by 2025, the cloning and breeding of superior varieties of animals will be carried out by industries which will be equivalent to those that now involve the artificial insemination industry [200].

Louise Joy Brown (25 July 1978) was the first child born of an IVF procedure [201]. IVF is now readily available in many neonatal and other healthcare centers, in which viable oocytes are recovered and fertilized under *in vitro* conditions. This fertilization is followed by ET which is again followed by normal development of the fetus, and ultimately the delivery of a baby conceived in this way [202].

3.10 IVF in humans and embryo transfer

Different strategies have been suggested for the recovery of human oocytes, followed by *in vitro* fertilization, embryo culture, embryo transfer and monitoring embryo development [150]. An overview of these stages is shown in figure 3.13.

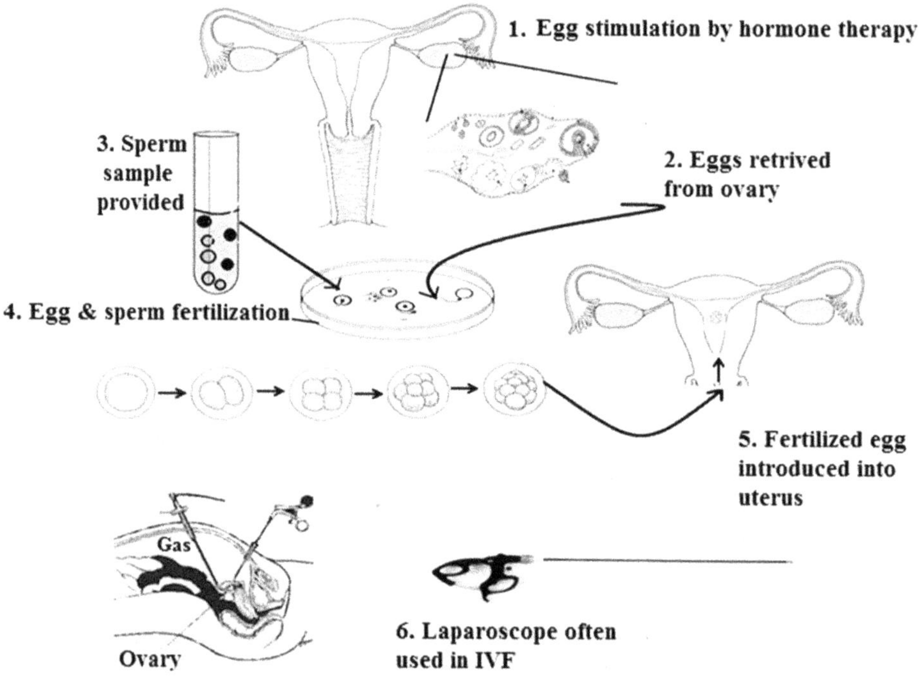

Figure 3.13. Overview of IVF.

3.10.1 Types and causes of infertility

Infertility is not accepted as a disease by most third-party payers, and medical diagnosis agents and treatment usually requires the couple to provide payment. IVF is frequently limited to couples who are unsuccessful with less aggressive treatment, but it is the first-line treatment for those with tubal factor or severe male factor infertility [203]. Ofyen infertile couples have had some earlier assessments of their infertility and this information must be carefully studied [204]. There are several reasons behind infertility and this technique is limited to couple who may have infertility for specific reasons [205]. The following section describes some common examples of infertility:

3.10.1.1 What causes female infertility?

One of the most common causes for female infertility is damage to the fallopian tubes or uterus, problems with ovulation, or problems with the cervix.

3.10.1.1.1 Tubal factor infertility

The fallopian tubes (the tubes which receive oocytes from the follicles of the ovaries to allow fertilization) or uterus can be damaged for several reasons, such as pelvic inflammatory disease, a previous infection, polyps in the uterus, endometriosis or fibroids, scar tissue or adhesions, chronic medical illness, a previous ectopic (tubal) pregnancy, and a birth defect or syndrome. Previously, a low success rate was usually achieved in the surgical treatment (repair) of damaged or non-functional fallopian tubes [206]. This traditional surgical treatment of fallopian tube obstruction (also called tuboplasty) was overtaken by the modern method IVF, since it is more cost-effective, less invasive and the results are immediate [206]. Several other strategies have also been used previously to treat tubal infertility, such as ovarian implantation, tubal transplantation or replacement of tubes by grafting. After the arrival of IVF techniques, the utilization of these approaches became limited as after fertilization has taken place under *in vitro* conditions, no fallopian tubes are required, only a functional uterus is required for embryo transfer.

3.10.1.1.2 Absent or non-functional ovaries

Sometimes the ovaries are non-functional or inaccessible. In that case a healthy oocyte will not be produced so one can be procured from a healthy donor, which can be fertilized by the chosen spermatozoa under *in vitro* conditions. Subsequently the developing embryo may then be implanted in the infertile recipient, which requires an external supply of steroid hormones (if the ovaries are non-functional).

3.10.1.1.3 Non-functional (or absent) uterus

In this case the oocytes are derived from the female and subjected to IVF; however, the developing embryo will be implanted into the uterus of a surrogate mother for pregnancy and further development [207–209]. This is done when the uterus is absent or non-functional, such as the presence of uterine leiomyomas (commonly known as fibroids, which are non-cancerous tumors), a unicornuate uterus (rudimentary horn is the rarest congenital anatomic anomaly of the female genital system), Mayer–Rokitansky–Kuster–Hauser syndrome (aplasia or hypoplasia of the uterus and vagina due to an early arrest in development of Mullerian ducts), etc [207–209].

3.10.1.1.4 Unexplained or idiopathic infertility

Worldwide almost 30% of infertile couples are diagnosed with unexplained or idiopathic infertility. Based on European Society of Human Reproduction and Embryology (ESHRE) guidelines, several examinations for unexplained infertility are:

- Semen analysis.
- Assessment of ovulation and the luteal phase.
- Assessment of tubal patency by hysterosalpingogram or laparoscopy.

Nevertheless, there are debatable views over the value of endometrial biopsy, ovarian reserve post-coital tests and serum prolactin levels [210]. One of the effective treatments available for idiopathic infertility is cycles without ovarian stimulation. Cycles without ovarian stimulation are more effective in women below 35, nevertheless cycles without ovarian stimulation increase the chances of multiple gestations. However, cycles without ovarian stimulation are not effective for couples with long duration infertility. This type of infertility, where the exact cause is not known, is called idiopathic infertility. Often, this may result in failure of fertilization or abnormal fertilization [211]. Current advancements in IVF and ET offer a useful therapeutic technique for the treatment of idiopathic infertility.

3.10.1.2 What causes male infertility?

Infertility can be explained as the incapability to conceive within 12 months of unprotected intercourse [212]. Male factor infertility is expected to contribute to two-thirds of all cases. In examining reasons for infertility in men, 13.7% of reports are related with a sperm or semen problem and 18.1% of reports are with male factor infertility. In a fertile human the total count of sperm should be 15–20 million per ml [213, 214]. As per the literature, 10–20 000 per ml of sperm should be required to pursue IVF [214]. Several conditions of male infertility, such as oligospermia (the number of sperm decreases) and azoospermia (when the amount of non-motile sperm is high), require an alternative approach such as IVF. A reduced sperm count in a male is often defined as oligospermia, whereas the absence or very low concentration of motile sperm (while non-motile sperm may be found) is defined as azoospermia. As a result of this, it is likely that a patient suffering with oligospermia may have sufficient motile spermatozoa for IVF but not for fertilization *in vivo*.

3.10.2 Evaluation and assessment of patients

The evaluation and assessment of a patient is essential for both diagnosis of infertility and the selection of patients for treatment with IVF or intracytoplasmic sperm injection (ICSI). Ideally during IVF, normal sperm fertilization function is required, meaning that sperm should bind to the zona pellucida and experience the acrosome reaction. Then it will enter the zona pellucida and fuse with the oolemma before fertilization takes place [215]. In contrast, most sperm functions are not essential for fertilization in ICSI as sperm bypass the zona pellucida and oolemma by injection of sperm directly into the cytoplasm of the oocyte. Consequently, the clinical analysis report of patients is often dependent on the results of sperm tests [215].

A number of techniques based on semen analysis are currently available which are important in preparing diagnostic and prognostic information on male infertility [215]. This information which can be assessed by using these techniques cannot be determined in conventional semen examination alone, and also it is important in deciding whether an assisted reproductive technology (ART) technique (IVF or ICSI) is to be employed or not. In addition to this, structural assessment of chromatin fibers can give an idea about the extent of structure/sperm DNA damage. DNA damage can result in infertility; this factor can be considered as the most likely cause for male infertility, as it can be inherited from paternal genes by offspring [215].

Additionally, genetic defects can be root-level cause for the several male infertility conditions such as non-obstructive azoospermia and cryptozoospermia [215–217]. These conditions may arise due to chromosome abnormalities, Y chromosome microdeletions in the AZFc region, cystic fibrosis transmembrane conductance regulator gene mutations and androgen receptor gene mutations [215–217]. Moreover, to have the most fruitful effect of treatment it is essential to evaluate the female partner, mainly a genetic and reproductive system evaluation. The female partner involved in the IVF course should meet the following criteria [152]:

- Female partner must be healthy to carry a pregnancy and it is equally important to evaluate the impact of invasive or surgical procedures on patient health. It has also been observed that health issues such as obesity and earlier abdominal operations obstruct oocyte collection.
- Advancement in technology trying to offer maximum comfort and best treatment for the patient health, e.g. retrieval of oocyte at 140 mmHg negative aspiration pressure can be a favorable approach for the flushing and aspiration in assisted reproduction, in particular for women with a low ovarian reserve [218].
- For IVF, female ovaries should be available for oocyte recovery. Due to adhesions, sometime ovaries are out of sight. In this case procedures such as initial laparotomy and ovariolysis may require.
- In patients who have suffered from cancer chemotherapy often has a harmful impact on fertility. Such patients should receive this information about the fertility risks associated with their cancer treatment and how it can be circumvented by fertility preservation. After controlled ovarian hyperstimulation, facilities such as oocyte or embryo banking are considered as an effective method for preserving female fertility. Currently various protocols are available for ovarian stimulation exclusively to allow cancer patients to submit an oocyte or embryo for cryopreservation, irrespective of the phase of

the cycle or without an exogenous follicle-stimulating hormone-related increase in serum estradiol levels [219].
- The uterus of the patient should be functional, i.e. it should support the growth of the embryo for the full term of 9 months.
- The patient should have a physiologically functional cervical canal (cervix) for embryo transfer. Alternatively, for embryo transfer, the fundus can also be used if cervical canal is not functional. The male patient should also be assessed for a suitable concentration of motile sperm. If there is an insufficient concentration, an alternative male donor with suitable semen may have to be used.

3.10.3 IVF fertility treatment

IVF has been considered as one of the medical innovations of the twentieth century. Almost 5 million children have been born by means of the procedures first established by Robert Edwards. Nevertheless, there is ongoing concern about certain outcomes of IVF treatment [220], mainly the high number of multiple births, an issue which became apparent only a few years after the birth of Louise Brown (1978).

Another concern is the high cost of this technique, which restricts the utilization of this technology to the upper classes and wealthy societies. There are various strategies to reduce the cost of IVF, such as male-factor subfertility examination through semen analysis using a light microscope [221, 222]. This examination of the semen is suggested as the ideal approach for assessing sperm [222]. The trust-worthiness over manual semen analysis should not be surpassed by the more expensive methods such as computer-aided sperm examination [223]. Examination of the pelvic anatomy and ovarian reserve using antral follicle count involves an ultrasound scan machine with satisfactory resolution; advanced digital function or 3D imaging is not essential and has not been proven to offer any additional advantage [224].

Patients who have undergone IVF are instructed to record their menstrual cycles for nearly six months. This practice may allow the health practitioner to take the necessary steps to determine [152]:

- The date of admitting the patient to hospital.
- The date of urine sampling for luteinizing hormone (LH) surge.
- The date of administration of human chorionic gonadotrophin (hCG) to control the last stages of follicular and oocyte development.

Menstruation is the cyclic shedding of the uterine lining, in concert with the interactions of hormones secreted by the hypothalamus, pituitary and ovaries. This orderly cycle can be divided into two phases: (1) the follicular or proliferative phase and (2) the luteal or secretory phase. The type of treatment recommended for an individual patient will depend on which of the following three cycles is utilized for oocyte recovery for IVF.

3.10.3.1 Roles of hormones in the menstrual cycle

To regulate the menstrual cycle, hormones are secreted in a negative and positive feedback loop. Gonadotropin-releasing hormone (GnRH) is secreted in the hypothalamus at the onset of puberty in a pulsatile, increased manner. After that, GnRH is delivered to the anterior pituitary, where it binds to the G-protein receptor on its 7-transmembrane membrane. This signals the anterior pituitary to release luteinizing hormone (LH) and stimulating follicle hormone (FSH). The ovaries receive input from FSH and LH. Theca cells and granulosa cells are the two cell types found in ovarian follicles that produce hormones. By activating the enzyme cholesterol desmolase, LH stimulates the production of progesterone and androstenedione in theca cells. Androstenedione diffuses to the surrounding granulosa cells after it is secreted [219].

Here, aromatase is activated by FSH, which prompts the granulosa cells to convert androstenedione to testosterone and subsequently 17-beta-estradiol. There is a negative feedback loop back to the anterior pituitary to lower the levels of FSH and LH being produced and, consequently, the levels of 17-beta-estradiol and progesterone produced, as levels of these hormones rise according to the phases of the menstrual cycle. During ovulation, this is not the case. In this instance, the production of 17-beta-estradiol triggers the anterior pituitary to release more FSH and LH after a critical level is reached. Furthermore, the granulosa cells within the feedback system generate activin and inhibin, which both stimulate and inhibit the anterior pituitary's release of FSH. This feedback mechanism is controlled by upregulating, to increase hormone production, or downregulating to decrease hormone production, the GnRH receptors on the anterior pituitary.

3.10.3.2 Phase 1: the follicular, or proliferative phase

The follicular or proliferative phase is the first stage of the menstrual cycle. With an average duration of 28 days, it happens from day 1 to day 14 of the menstrual cycle. Variations in the length of the follicular phase are the cause of the variability in the menstrual cycle duration. In this phase, 17-beta-estradiol, or oestrogen, is the primary hormone. The follicle's FSH receptors are upregulated at the start of the cycle, which results in an increase in this hormone. But as the follicular phase comes to an end, the anterior pituitary will receive negative feedback from the elevated levels of 17-beta-estradiol. The uterus's endometrial layer is supposed to grow during this phase. 17-beta-estradiol achieves this by increasing the growth of the endometrial layer of the uterus, stimulating increased amounts of stroma and glands, and increasing the depth of the arteries that supply the endometrium, the spiral arteries.

Since ovulation always happens 14 days before menstruation, ovulation happens on day 14 of an average 28-day cycle. 17-beta-estradiol levels are high at the end of the proliferative phase because of follicle maturation and increased hormone production. Only during this period does 17-beta-estradiol stimulate the production of FSH and LH in a positive manner. When 17-beta-estradiol reaches a critical level—at least 200 picograms per millilitre of plasma—this happens. The LH surge is the term for the elevated levels of FSH and LH that occur during this period. The mature follicle splits as a result, releasing an oocyte. The changes to the cervix as initiated during the

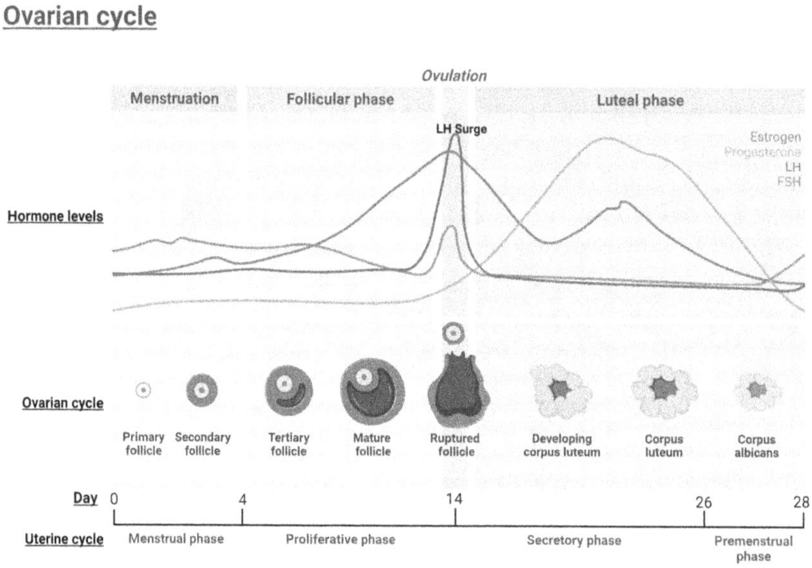

Figure 3.14. The luteal or secretory phase of the ovarian cycle.

follicular phase further increase, allowing for increased, waterier cervical mucous to better accommodate the possible sperm—the levels of 17-beta-estradiol fall at the end of ovulation.

The luteal, or secretory, phase of the menstrual cycle comes next (figure 3.14). This stage of the cycle always lasts from day 14 to day 28. During this stage, progesterone, which is stimulated by LH, is the main hormone that gets the corpus luteum and the endometrium ready for a potential implantation of fertilized eggs. Progesterone will give the anterior pituitary negative feedback as the luteal phase comes to an end, lowering FSH and LH levels and, in turn, progesterone and 17-beta-estradiol levels. The mature follicle rupture site in the ovary forms the corpus luteum, a structure that produces progesterone and 17-beta-estradiol, which is predominant at the end of the phase because of the negative feedback system. The endometrium prepares by increasing its vascular supply and stimulating more mucous secretions. This is achieved by the progesterone stimulating the endometrium to slow down endometrial proliferation, decrease lining thickness, develop more complex glands, accumulate energy sources in the form of glycogen, and provide more surface area within the spiral arteries. Contrary to the cervical mucous changes seen during the proliferative phase and ovulation, progesterone decreases and thickens the cervical mucous making it non-elastic since the fertilization period passed, and sperm entry is no longer a priority. Additionally, progesterone increases the hypothalamic temperature, so body temperature increases during the luteal phase. Near the end of the secretory phase, plasma levels of 17-beta-estradiol and progesterone are produced by the corpus luteum. If pregnancy occurs, a fertilized ovum is implanted within the endometrium, and the corpus luteum will persist and maintain the hormone levels. However, if no fertilized ovum is implanted, then the corpus luteum regresses, and the serum levels of 17-beta-estradiol and progesterone decrease rapidly [226].

3.10.4 Development of ovarian follicles in natural menstrual cycles

Natural cycle *in vitro* fertilization is a process which mimics the body's natural fertilization process. It does not involve the use of fertility drugs that induce the ovaries to produce multiple eggs as in controlled ovarian hyperstimulation [COH] approach. Natural cycle IVF alters the endometrium making it suitable for the implantation of the embryo [225]. Natural cycle IVF procedure with a spontaneous LH surge is the simplest, entirely drug-free and most 'natural' version of IVF. It was often practiced by the innovators of IVF, but later fell out of favor due to the new gonadotropin/GnRH analogue regimens. However, the natural cycle procedure was revived again when medical practitioners slowly documented the harmful effects related to high-dose ovarian stimulation [226].

To understand the natural cycle, it is important to understand the spontaneous LH surge under whose effect all completely developed follicles of both ovaries burst, ovulate and ova are collected by the fallopian tubes [226]. Therefore, it is very important to examine the LH surge at the right stage. During the natural cycle, the spontaneous LH surge is examined using urine or plasma sampling at 3–6 h intervals [226]. The spontaneous cycle has benefits in terms of early term pregnancy and of a natural hormonal environment for ET. The drawbacks include the accessibility and recovery of only one oocyte, resulting in a low success rate of IVF and ET. Although evidence supports stimulated *in vitro* fertilization, a number of patients do not respond to it well. Also, stimulated treatment could be related to reduced ovarian response. In 2008, researchers observed that mature oocyte recovery achieved through natural rather than stimulated *in vitro* fertilization could be a possible treatment for individuals of an advanced age once stimulated IVF has repeatedly failed [227]. According to a recent report, a modified natural cycle IVF (GnRH antagonist, gonadotrophin, Indocid are administered on a daily basis from detection of a dominant follicle until ovulation induction) is an adequate treatment option for individuals considering IVF, mainly for women younger than 35 and for women older than 36 with normal ovarian response [228]. MNC-IVF is a cost-effective approach as it does not not include the use of drugs and laboratory tests. This method is suitable for suboptimal responders to traditional IVF. This approach is atraumatic as it does not involve sedation whole retrieving egg from the patient [229]. NC-IVF is a patient-friendly and negligible risk approach of IVF. The disadvantage of this method is higher cancellation rate due to LH rise and premature ovulation, but these can be overcome by medication like indomethacin [GnRH antagonist] [230]. This method requires more research and apprehension to resolve the challenges associated with it [230].

3.10.4.1 Two types of natural cycle IVF [231]

Natural cycle IVF [NC-IVF]:

- Fertility drugs are not administered to induce the ovaries.

- Human chorionic gonadotrophin hormone [pregnancy hormone] induces ovulation when the folic size is around 15–20 mm.
- Focused in retrieval of one matured oocyte.
- Oocyte is retrieved under guidance of vaginal ultrasound and mild sedation.

Modified natural cycle IVF [MNC-IVF]:

- This method uses gonadotrophins to induce follicular growth, stimulation period is around 2–6 days.
- In order to prevent premature ovulation, GnRH antagonist is used to suppress LH secretion.
- Focused on retrieval of one matured oocyte.
- Oocyte is retrieved under guidance of vaginal ultrasound and mild sedation.
- Cryopreservation of embryos after NC- IVF and MNC-IVF is not possible. Therefore, these methods are preferred by couples who are contrary to cryopreservation of embryos due to cultural and religious reasons.

Merits of using NC- IVF and MNC-IVF

- Multiple pregnancy can be prevented.
- Less risk of ovarian hyperstimulation syndrome.
- Less cost.
- No requirement of resting cycle after a failed cycle.

3.10.5 Development of ovarian follicles in stimulated cycles

After the introduction of IVF technology, natural cycle IVF have been replaced by IVF with ovarian stimulation. However, natural cycle IVF has a number of benefits. It avoids multiple pregnancy and there is also zero possibility of ovarian hyperstimulation syndrome [232]. Per cycle, natural cycle IVF is less time consuming, physically and emotionally less difficult for patients, and less expensive than stimulated IVF; however, it is also less effective [232]. Growth follicles and maturation of eggs are controlled by hormones like FSH and LH [233]. Usually in a stimulated cycle, by administering clomiphene and/or human menopausal gonadotrophin (hMG), multiple follicular developments are encouraged. The LH surge remains spontaneous and must be inspected at the right stage, as mentioned above. During this protocol human chorionic gonadotrophin (hCG) is also administered to check the inhibition of the LH surge caused by hMG [232]. It was also observed that rate of growth of follicles of a woman undergoing stimulated cycles is higher than for natural menstrual cycles [234]. A major advantage of the stimulated cycle is the accessibility of multiple follicles and oocytes so that several embryos are accessible for embryo transfer, which may result in a higher success rate. This protocol also involves certain disadvantages, such as the effort to understand variable hormonal levels, the requirement for ultrasonic scanning to measure the number of maturing follicles, the recovery of oocytes at different development stages (some of these oocytes are abnormal), the abnormal environment and the high possibility of abnormal pregnancy [232]. Today, there are milder ways by which the ovaries can be stimulated, which are much safer approach. In some of the cases, treatments used in the earlier stages of IVF might affect the later stages so in such scenarios the embryos are cryopreserved [233]. A strategy for mild ovarian stimulation was developed in 1999, which involves the use of less medication and prevents the risk of ovarian hyperstimulation. This procedure has several advantages such as faster pregnancy achievement and reduced dropout rates. This approach is also cost effective and increases patience tolerance for repeated treatment [235].

3.10.6 Development of ovarian follicles during a controlled cycle

The first live birth with IVF was after a natural cycle IVF. Later, gonadotropin-releasing hormone (GnRH) analogs and gonadotropins were added to foil the luteinizing hormone (LH) surge. This is done to escalate the number of recruited follicles, which results in an increase of the number of oocytes retrieved and embryos fertilized. By this approach multiple embryos can be retrieved which can give options for selection. Thus better quality embryos can be transferred to improve the success rate. Simultaneously, the surplus better quality embryos can be vitrified for future transfers. Therefore, the main objective of controlled ovarian hyperstimulation (COH) is multi-follicular development while simultaneously inhibiting spontaneous ovulation.

Since the application of IVF has started increasing over the last few years, a number of approaches have emerged, such as controlled ovarian stimulation. In this approach, the further development of the follicles is arrested at the ideal stage of maturation by the administration of hCG. This approach offers greater comfort to the patients as in this cycle oocyte recovery can be achieved via laparoscopy at a time suitable to the doctor and the patient. The difficulty, however, is in estimating the ideal time for hCG administration, which should also differ for different preovulatory forms. Out of the three cycles discussed above, the stimulated and controlled cycles are considered to have higher success rates in oocyte recovery, embryo transfer and pregnancies achieved.

3.10.7 Ovarian stimulation protocols for IVF

To use a stimulatory cycle for IVF, the female patient needs to be administered with doses of clomiphene and hMG during the chosen time period. Gonadotropins have long been used to increase the oocyte yield [236, 237]. GnRH analogs (agonist and antagonist) have been used to prevent LH surge [238]. The clomiphene-based stimulation protocol in IVF is anticipated as a cheaper treatment because of the reduction in the dose requirement of gonadotropins. Moreover, there is no need to add GnRH analogs to avoid LH surge. The main concern with such continued use of clomiphene citrate is its antiestrogenic effect on the uterus. This can harmfully affect implantation. Nevertheless, if clomiphene-based procedures are employed in oocyte donors, its antiestrogenic effect on the uterus will no longer be a matter of concern. Once the decision has been taken that the stimulatory cycle needs to be used, as mentioned above, the female patient needs to be administered with doses of clomiphene and hMG. Clomiphene (the medicine which is used to stimulate ovulation) is given to the patient at the optimum rate of 150 mg per day from the fifth day to the ninth day of the cycle. Certain patients do not respond to a five-day course, so prolonged administration for ten days may be required. As discussed above, this prolonged treatment will, however, also extend the anti-estrogen effect so that uterus receptivity for embryo implantation may be reduced. This may finally result in an increased spontaneous abortion rate. Nevertheless, the rate of abortion is low if hMG is used instead of clomiphene. One of the limitations of using hMG is its high cost, so a combination of clomiphene and hMG is often used. hMG administration also results in hyperstimulation. This hyperstimulation may not support pregnancy and therefore it may result in a variety of complications including abdominal discomfort, ascites, pleural effusion and thromboembolic phenomena, sometimes leading to death. Another approach which is called frozen–thawed embryo transfer is employed for the storage and transfer of excess embryos derived during IVF-ICSI cycles. Recently, developments in laboratory conditions and limitations on the number of embryos to be transferred have resulted in progressive increase in frozen–thawed embryo transfer cycles. An alternative procedure to avoid multiple pregnancies in IVF cycles is to transfer a single embryo and freeze all surplus embryos [239–242]. Nevertheless, the best answer for endometrial preparation in these cycles is still a matter of discussion [239–242]. Frozen–thawed embryo transfer averts embryo waste and improves the chances of pregnancy in a single stimulated cycle.

3.10.7.1 Monitoring ovarian stimulation

In the beginning, monitoring ovarian of stimulation was achieved by observing the LH surge just before ovulation. Recently, in all assisted reproductive technology facilities, the monitoring of stimulated ovulatory cycles is achieved by conventional 2D ultrasound to measure follicle diameter [243]. Another way to monitor ovulatory cycles is by taking blood tests that examine certain hormones levels such as estradiol, progesterone and LH. Such an examination facilitates determination of the numbers and quality of growing ovarian follicles. Moreover, it also helps in evaluation of follicle maturity before selecting the suitable time for ovulation triggering. Ovulatory monitoring has become more advance with the arrival of new software known as SonoAVC [242]. This tool facilitates the utilization of 3D blocks to directly analyze the total number and volume of the follicles inside the ovary. This robust method is faster, more precise and more reliable. Additionally, it has better reproducibility than the classical 2D parameters. The, following are the factors that are considered as indicators for ovarian stimulation to facilitate the harvesting of oocytes at the perfect stage of development:

- Examination of the day of LH surge based on information available about length and dates of the menstrual cycle (while this prediction is equally perfect in normal cycles, its precision in stimulatory cycles is yet to be established).
- Basal body temperature charts for menstrual cycles of women should be evaluated. A temperature chart (showing the temperature increase at pre-ovulatory and post-ovulatory stages).

- The detection of changes in cervical mucus score indicates follicular development as initially it will increase to five days before the LH surge and reached a maximum level a day before and decreased suddenly on the day of the LH surge.
- The amount of plasma or urinary estrogen can be assessed with 24 h urine collection. This estimation can be used to determine the timing for the LH surge and hCG injection; the established method of Brown *et al* from 1968 is used [243], but more recently radioimmunoassays have been fruitfully utilized.
- Ultrasonic examination can be used to determine follicular size, as mentioned above. Sonography and ultrasound-based examinations have become a valuable tool for the examination of spontaneous and induced ovulation. This technique helps in understanding folliculogenesis and reproductive endocrinology. Practically, during ovulation induction, sonography helps in the estimation of the number and distribution of follicles. This is again essential for satisfactory interpretation of estrogen levels. While there is no ideal size at which it can be considered that a follicle is mature, assessment of follicle size is of importance as size measurement guides the suitable timing of hCG administration. In the case that the follicles are very small, there is an indication of hyperstimulation. These reports, along with the E2 levels, may be utilized to determine whether a further ultrasonic investigation is necessary for the examination of follicular growth or whether the treatment cycle should be uncontrolled. On the condition that follicular size is under normal limits, the diameter of the largest follicle can also be used in IVF procedure to assess when the individual must be admitted to the hospital. Once the patient is admitted follicular development is carefully monitored and administration of hCG is carried out [235]. Sonography is also important in individuals with one ovary accessible to laparoscopy. If the largest follicle is present inside the inaccessible ovary, the treatment cycle does not have to be abandoned, on the condition that the number of follicles is increasing in the contralateral ovary [235]. However, in the case that none of the ovary is accessible, then surgical procedures such as laparoscopy and percutaneous oocyte aspiration provide the individual an opportunity for IVF and embryo transfer [244].
- In females, ovulation of mature follicles inside the ovary is triggered by a large burst of LH secretion, which is known as the preovulatory LH surge. Residual cells within ovulated follicles multiply to yield corpora lutea, which may further release the steroid hormones progesterone and estradiol [244]. Identification of the LH surge and progesterone determination allow the most precise ovulation timing.

3.10.8 Spontaneous luteinizing hormone (LH) surge

Determination of LH surge is required for forecasting the correct ovulation time, because if laparoscopy is performed after ovulation, then no oocyte will be recovered, and if it is done more than 6 h prior, fertilization may not take place. Due to recent advancements in technology there is an immense scope for culturing oocytes under *in vitro* conditions. This may allow oocyte collection at the right stage of its development, making the time of oocyte collection less critical. It is not possible to quantitate gonadotropin in the blood of 'normal' women by utilizing bioassays, researchers have observed that the amount of LH can be estimated from urine (at three-hourly intervals) either by haemagglutination or by radioimmunoassay, to facilitate the right prediction of time for laparoscopy [245].

The level of progesterone present in plasma is determined as they begin to increase 24 h prior to the LH surge in stimulated cycles [245]. Thus, an escalation in progesterone means that a spontaneous LH surge will occur within the next 24 h. Ultimately, this will also confirm suspected ovulation [245]. LH determination is also required for the administration of hCG, since no increase in LH should be detected before administering hCG, which is used to govern the time of ovulation. If the LH amount has already risen prior to the administration of hCG, then no hCG is administered and laparoscopy is timed to 21–28 h after the midpoint of the first sample which showed an increased amount of LH [245].

3.10.9 Administration of hCG for controlled ovulation

As reported, new opportunities such as improved treatment using recombinant human LH are currently available for patients suffering from ovulatory disorders. The ovarian response to gonadotrophins varies significantly among female patients. Recently, it has been proven that in female patients administered GnRH analogues, a short-term pre-treatment with recombinant LH, prior to recombinant follicle-stimulating hormone (FSH) administration, upsurges the number of small antral follicles prior to FSH stimulation and the yield of normally fertilized embryos [246]. Moreover, rLH pre-treatment can have a significant impact on the subsequent ovarian responsiveness to FSH. hCG administration in combination with aromatase inhibitor in the early follicular phase allows androgen priming and results in a subsequent increase in the number of good quality embryos [247].

As discussed earlier, hCG is administered to control the ovulation. The choice to administer hCG is made on the basis of:

- The day of the menstrual cycle.
- The absolute amount and variations in the amount of oestrodial 17/3.
- The size and number of follicles assessed through ultrasonic examinations and cervical mucus score.

Sonography should be performed to determine the number and size of follicles (at least 1.9 cm diameter). hCG administration should be delayed if the follicles are small. This can be extended until the follicles attain preovulatory size. In addition, the amount of LH present in urine should not peak before hCG administration (as mentioned above). Laparoscopy is performed 28–36 h after hCG administration in female patients with no symptoms of spontaneous LH surge.

3.10.9.1 Oocyte recovery (laparoscopy) methods

Oocyte recovery in IVF and embryo transfer can be achieved by laparoscopy or by sonography. According to a recent survey, transvaginal ultrasound-guided follicle aspiration has become the ideal method for oocyte retrieval during ART. In contrast to laparoscopic methods, this approach improves safety and efficacy [247–251].

The potentially beneficial follicular flushing is still criticized yet continues to be a common procedure in many ART clinics. Numerous methods for oocyte recovery have been tried in the past and included the following:

- Previously, the entire follicular fluid was aspirated. Since this aspiration allows the retrieval of in-follicular aspirates, if an oocyte is present in the aspirated fluid further aspiration is not essential.
- A surgically removed ovary is minced for oocyte recovery.
- Intact follicles are dissected prior to puncture to study the developmental stage.
- Follicles are sliced under the microscope and oocytes are recovered.

3.10.10 Equipment and technique for laparoscopy

Laparoscopy is a minimally invasive surgical technique that allows for visual examination and intervention within the abdominal or pelvic cavity through small incisions. The primary equipment for laparoscopy includes a laparoscope, which is a long, thin, and illuminated tube with a camera on one end, providing high-resolution images of the internal organs. Carbon dioxide gas is used to inflate the abdominal cavity, creating a workspace for the surgeon. Phillip Bozzini has developed the first cystoscope, although it was not used in humans. P F Boesch, (a Swiss gynecologist) performed the first laparoscopic sterilization by electro-coagulation of the fallopian tubes [252]. The first surgeon to accomplish a laparoscopic cholecystectomy was Erich Muhe (a German surgeon), who used a galloscope, a 3 cm, direct-vision laparoscope to remove a gallbladder [253]. In 1987, Phillip Mouret (a French surgeon) performed the first videolaparoscopic cholecystectomy [254]. The first robot-assisted aortofemoral bypass was performed by Zimmerman and Kelley in 2000 [255]. Robotic surgery was considered by several researchers as one of the next advancements in minimally invasive surgery [256]. The first robotic system for laparoscopic surgery became available in 1994. Da Vinci became the first United States FDA-approved integrated robotic surgical system in July 2000. It is now the only commercially available robotic system for laparoscopic and thoracoscopic use [256].

Previously used methods caused extensive damage to the ovary, thus their application was restricted. Laparoscopy was a major breakthrough in techniques for oocyte recovery [153]. In this approach, follicles are initially identified in the ovary using microscopic equipment. Then the ovulating follicles are aspirated with apparatus consisting of:

- A 23 cm long stainless-steel needle with an external diameter of 2.1 mm and an internal diameter of 1.6 mm. This stainless-steel needle is lined on the inside with Teflon, which reduces the internal diameter to 1.0 mm.

- External tubing, a 52 cm long continuous tube that runs along the needle (covers the needle) and through a silicone rubber bung (the outer end maintains the gas seal when the instrument is inserted) into a 5 ml or 10 ml tissue culture tube.
- Between the needle and the tubing there is an entire fluid space of 1.2 ml.
- From the rubber bung, 18 gauge needles perforate.
- The needle is connected to a suction pump operated by foot.

The optimum adjustment of pressure and flow parameters facilitates effective tissue rinsing and effective aspiration of fluid. The optimum pressure should be within the range of 80–100 mm of mercury. The laparoscopic procedure includes insufflation of a gas (typically carbon dioxide) into the peritoneal cavity producing a pneumoperitoneum. This causes an increase in intra-abdominal pressure which allows easier access to organs during the laparoscopy. Based on recent research, during insufflation (inflation with CO_2) in the peritoneal cavity, nitrogen (non-reactive substance) and oxygen are also included (90% N_2, 5% O_2, 5% CO_2). CO_2 gas insufflation is ideal as it has a high diffusion coefficient and also is a normal metabolic end product rapidly removed from the body. Additionally, CO_2 has higher blood solubility than air, therefore decreasing the chances of problems after venous embolism. The presence of adhesive material or omentum over the ovary can cause problems, thus this can be removed by using laparoscopic scissors. To select the oocytes, the ovarian ligament is grabbed moderately and the ovulating follicles are carefully examined. Subsequently ovulating follicles are selected for aspiration. After selection, those follicles with ova and which are suitable for fertilization are further selected, provided their size is smaller than 1.5 cm. However, if case the follicles are within the ovarian tissue, it is difficult to measure their size precisely. Further, suction assembly must be examined properly by using culture medium to avoid leakage of fluid and that can also prevent the loss of oocytes because of the failure of the pump. By applying optimum suction, follicular fluid around 4–12 ml is aspirated completely from the ovulating follicle, as mentioned above. The aspirated fluid should be straw-colored, as often it is contaminated with blood. If blood appears in the aspirated fluid, heparinized culture medium must be immediately added to the aspirate to prevent clotting. Prevention of clotting is very important as a blood clot may disturb in the selection, isolation and fertilization of the ovum. Aspiration of the fluid results in the walls of the follicle collapsing.

As the fluid is aspirated, the walls of the follicle collapsed (corpus luteum). The aspirated fluid should be carefully examined. After the identification of the oocyte further aspiration is not required. However, until the oocyte is identified, flushing of the follicle with heparinized culture medium is repeated to obtain the oocytes through reaspiration of the distended follicle. This procedure can be repeated as frequently as required until an oocyte is not recovered. Mature oocytes can only be recovered by careful follicular monitoring and identification of the timing between the LH surge and hCG administration should be carefully understood. This may help in development of the oocyte culture *in vitro* for a minimum period prior to the fertilization. This will enhance the chances of fertilization and subsequent embryo development [153].

3.10.11 Oocyte culture and IVF culture of oocytes

From the earliest times of IVF, it has been well accepted that not all oocytes retrieved after COH have a similar potential for attaining pregnancy. In addition to the number of oocytes, the maturity of the retrieved oocytes is also equally important for the success of ART. Usually, about 5%–20% [154, 155] of recovered oocytes in COH are immature. Some are at metaphase I (MI absence of both a germinal vesicle and a first polar body) or some are at germinal vesicle (GV) stage [156, 157]. A number of these oocytes have the potential for spontaneous maturation in the course of *in vitro* culturation and can be used as a source of oocytes for sperm injection in ICSI cycles. For the development of oocyte culture, initially the oocyte is examined under a microscope and is handled with great care. This examination is followed by incubation for 5–10 h after oocyte recovery, which can further depend upon the expected maturity of the follicles and oocytes. Various culture media are currently available for oocyte culture and IVF:

- Earl's solution.
- Modified Ham's F10 medium.
- Modified Whitten's culture medium.
- Whittingham's T6 medium [257].

The culture medium is prepared in a week and can be examined by culturing mouse embryos from the two-cell stage to the blastocyst stage. After examination the same media can be utilized for fertilization and embryo culture.

3.10.12 Preparation of semen

Semen can be procured from healthy individual by masturbation, which should be approximately 60–90 min before insemination. At the time of ejaculation semen is collected as thick gel, however, it usually becomes liquid 20 min after ejaculation [158]. Thus liquefaction time is the time require by the fresh sample (semen) after ejaculation to liquefy. However, delayed liquefaction does not necessarily indicate infertility nor does it significantly impact fertility. Once the sample is liquefied, it can be centrifuged and the subsequent sperm pellet is finally resuspended in the culture medium. After resuspension the sample is again allowed to incubate in the culture medium at 37 °C for 30–60 min. Finally, the sample is collected from the surface so that it contains the most active spermatozoa [258]. By using recent innovations in animal tissue culture, it is possible to separate functional spermatozoa from those that are immotile, have poor morphology or are not capable of fertilizing oocytes [258]. For IVF, the initial procedure for sample preparation starts from the washing of spermatozoa, then it includes a set of separation techniques. These separation techniques are selected according to the basic principles such as migration, filtration or density gradient centrifugation. One of the most conventional and economic approaches is the swim-up procedure; however, the most sophisticated is migration–

sedimentation. Recent innovations led to the exploration of new separation methods that may offer higher numbers of motile spermatozoa: glass wool filtration and density gradient centrifugation with different media. Different media have been explored, such as Percoll® as a density medium, and later other media such as IxaPrep®, Nycodenz, SilSelect®, PureSperm® and Isolate® were developed in order to replace Percoll® because of its risk of contamination with endotoxins [258]. Thus, in 1996 it was removed from the market for clinical use in humans. Soon, it was realized that ejaculates often contain ROS, which may affect the viability and motility of the whole sample, and it was observed that conventional methods such as swim-up can trigger the production of ROS and can severely damage the spermatozoa [258]. Certain substances such as caffeine, pentoxifylline and 2-deoxyadenosine have been explored to stimulate motility, and other substances such as bicarbonate, metal chelators or platelet-activating factor can also utilized to stimulate spermatozoa [258].

3.10.13 *In vitro* fertilization

In vitro fertilization (IVF) has a transformative history since the birth of Louise Brown, the first 'test-tube baby,' in 1978. Pioneered by Drs Patrick Steptoe and Robert Edwards, IVF has undergone significant advancements, including refined ovarian stimulation protocols, the introduction of intracytoplasmic sperm injection (ICSI) to address male infertility, and the implementation of preimplantation genetic testing (PGT) for genetic screening of embryos. Innovations in culture media, embryo selection techniques, and cryopreservation methods have contributed to increased success rates [259]. IVF has become a globally accepted assisted reproductive technology, offering hope to millions facing fertility challenges and evolving continually with ongoing research and technological breakthroughs [260].

The field of IVF is rapidly progressing with several new developments in the last decade. Certain topics, such as improving oocyte quality by preventing DNA damage and defining the role of mitochondria, still require attention. Moreover, to reduce ROS production, approaches such as co-enzyme Q10 supplementation and mitochondrial transfer are now more focused, while treatment with gonadotropins and letrozole, and pre-treatment with dehydroepiandrosterone/testosterone bring more success to IVF.

Based on the above-described procedures, a total number of 10 000–50 000 motile spermatozoa are prepared. The prepared sample is subsequently added to 10 μl–1 ml of culture medium containing the healthy oocyte. Oocytes should be inseminated between 4 and 6 h after collection. Usually, there are two techniques available, conventional insemination (IVF) and ICSI. As discussed above for conventional insemination, the motile sperm concentration should be around 100 000 per oocyte which can be inseminated with a mature oocyte in a suitable culture medium, whereas ICSI involves the injection of a single sperm into each oocyte. During ICSI, before insemination but after oocyte retrieval, usually between 2 and 4 h, the follicular cells are removed from the surroundings of the oocyte so as to examine the oocyte in greater detail. Based on this, the oocytes are classified according to their maturity. Then they are stored in culture dishes in an incubator; however, only mature oocytes are microinjected. Since male infertility factors cannot be resolved with conventional IVF, ICSI is always recommended by an embryologist. However, conventional insemination is still preferred in many ART centers. During conventional insemination, the oocyte is left for 12–13 h and then inspected for its maturity in a petri dish containing the culture medium. During this stage the oocyte may contain two pronuclei and two polar bodies. Any deviation from the normal physiology of an embryo, such as the presence of multiple pronuclei, granulation or vasculature of the cytoplasm, or abnormal shape, can be carefully monitored and such embryos are not used further. After fertilization, first cleavage takes place between 24 and 30 h and each succeeding division should occur within 10–12 h thereafter. Cleavage should be carefully monitored as, if cleavage does not occur within 24 h, this also suggests an abnormal oocyte, which should not be used for transfer. Moreover, to examine cleavage, the best embryos should be selected by the advance technique called the fluorescein diacetate test, although its utilization in humans is still is uncertain, as oocytes and embryos may both appear similar morphologically. An alternative approach is to carefully collect one cell from the embryo and examine it under an electron microscope. This examination may also be evasive, as the single cell may not represent the whole embryo. There might be the presence of certain issues in the embryo and the morphological features of the single cell may not be enough to represent the biological function of the whole embryo.

3.11 Embryo transfer (ET) in humans

ARTs have become an essential part of infertility treatment. Conventional techniques like ovarian stimulation, fertilization, culture and transfer of embryos have become more advanced to ultimately enhance the efficacy of IVF/embryo transfer [261]. Despite these developments, embryo implantation is still a difficult task for the clinician as it involves multiple steps such as zona hatching, apposition and adhesion of the blastocyst, followed by an invasion of the trophoblast into the uterine endometrium. In order to achieve successful implantation of the embryo into the uterus, the uterus has to go through functional and structural changes, these changes are controlled by two major hormones, estrogen and progesterone. These hormones work by binding to the specific receptors within the uterus. The progesterone and estrogen receptors are of two types:

Progesterone receptors: PR-A and PR-B.

Estrogen receptors: ER α and ER β.

These receptors play a significant role for successful implantation of the embryo as they facilitate hormonal signals that drive necessary modification in the uterus [262].

Fertilized embryos are implanted into the uterus using a catheter under the guidance of transabdominal ultrasound. Embryos at the cleavage stage (3 days after fertilization) or blastocyst stage (5 days after fertilization) are used for the implantation [263]. Embryos may fail to implant. One of the major reasons for unsuccessful implantation is failure in developing a sticky matrix between the blastocyst and endometrium. Numbers of improvements have been made to design suitable ET media which may further improve implantation and pregnancy rates, e.g. albumin protein supplementation provides energy, hormones, vitamins, metals and optimum viscosity to the culture medium and acts as a lubricant and also averts the adherence of embryos to the culture dish [264]. Similarly, hyaluronan (HA) supplementation in the culture medium was reported to improve the implantation and pregnancy rate in IVF–ET cycles [265]. It was also observed that HA improves the developmental potential of bovine embryos and it is appropriate to use it as a supplement for *in vitro* production, specifically when the embryos are to be cryopreserved for the future use [266]. HA-based Embryo Glue is a human ET medium, which a contains high concentration of HA and a low concentration of recombinant human albumin. There are several advantages of using HA enriched medium, it enhances the attachment and positioning of embryo while performing implantation, increases the medium's viscosity and prevents expulsion of the embryo after the transfer into the uterus [267]. Embryo Glue also contains EDTA, which is required for cleavage stage embryos, but inhibits blastocyst development [268]. Various the steps involved in embryo transfer are described in the following sections.

3.11.1 Time of ET

Since fallopian tubes can easily accommodate embryos of the 8–16 cell stage under *in vivo* conditions, which then move further to the uterus, the ideal size for transfer to the uterus is a 1–16 celled embryo. The more advanced stage embryos are not preferred. As persistent culture or subculture of an embryo under *in vitro* conditions may affect its viability and also decrease the chances of pregnancy. Thus the best stage is maybe 2–4 cells; however, these early embryos may not survive for a long time in the uterus. Alternatively, multiple embryos may also be implanted to increase the chance of subsequent pregnancy; nevertheless, this again may result in multiple pregnancies, which the patient may not desire.

Progesterone supplements are given to the patient on the day of oocyte retrieval or during embryo transfer to increase the chances of successful pregnancy [263]. The American Society of Reproductive Medicine has set some guidelines for the number of embryos that can be transferred during IVF based on the age of woman [263]:

Blastocyst stage embryos [263]:

More than two blastocysts cannot be transferred to women of 37 years or younger.

More than three blastocysts cannot be transferred to women of 38–40 years.

More than three blastocysts cannot be transferred to women of 41–42 years.

Cleavage stage embryos [263]:

More than two embryos cannot be transferred to women under 35 years of age.

More than three embryos cannot be transferred to women of age 35–37 years.

More than four embryos cannot be transferred to women of age 38–40 years.

More than five embryos cannot be transferred to women of age 41–42 years.

This criterion is developed to optimize the chances of successful pregnancy.

3.11.2 ET technique

Embryo transfer is a crucial step in assisted reproductive technology (ART) procedures, such as IVF. This technique involves the placement of fertilized embryos into the uterus of a woman with the goal of establishing a successful pregnancy [269]. Embryo transfer is a serious rate-limiting step in IVF. However, the level of skill for carrying out this procedure varies widely. It is challenging to standardize a method that combines skill with know-how. There are still IVF physicians who regularly carry out ET without using ultrasound assistance to make certain that the embryo is deposited in the uterus with accuracy. ET should be performed under direct ultrasound guidance to guarantee proper placement within the uterine cavity. This practice will considerably improve embryo implantation and pregnancy rates. For embryo transfer the healthy patient can be administered 10 mg diazepam (valium) or similar muscle relaxing anti-anxiety medications orally about half an hour prior to embryo transfer. This allows the patient to relax and decreases her apprehension. No anesthesia or analgesia is required and ET is negotiated through the cervical canal. The following steps are involved in ET:

- Once the patient is suitably relaxed, she is assisted into the position familiar to women that have received a pap smear (the test for diagnosis of cancer or precancer of the uterine cervix). A sterile bivalve vaginal speculum is slowly introduced to visualize the cervix. Cusco's speculum (a bivalve instrument) is suggested to be used in all ETs as it allows the procedure to be atraumatic and gentle. Aligning the cervix with a volsellum during ET is essential to transfer the cervical canal angulation with the catheter tip. For this, patient is positioned in the knee to chest or lithotomy position with enough head down tilt to ensure that the fundus is lower than the cervical canal.
- The uterus should be manipulated gently to align the cervical canal and uterine cavity. Once it is confirmed that the patient's bladder is sufficiently full to offer clear ultrasound images, the doctor initially introduces a speculum into the vagina to expose the cervix. Then the physician may clean the cervix to take out any mucus or other secretions. This process increases the success of implantation, pregnancy and birth [270]. The abdominal ultrasound transducer is placed against the lower abdomen in order to visualize the uterus clearly.
- By means of a vaginal speculum, the physician exposes the cervix. After this a predetermined number of embryos suspended in culture medium (10 μl) are drawn into a transfer catheter, a long, thin sterile tube with a syringe on one end, with an external diameter of 1.27 mm and an internal diameter of 1.0 mm. This Teflon-made catheter passes through the vagina and cervix into the uterus. Teflon is preferred due to its low adhesiveness and it also reduces the risk of carrying cervical secretions into the uterine cavity. Additionally, during transfer the Teflon catheter is passed down an outer Teflon sheath which offers protection to the inner catheter from vaginal contamination. This allows the successful deposition of embryos from the catheter into the uterus.

- Most clinicians introduce a catheter into the uterine cavity to a depth of 5 cm from the external os of the cervix (just short of the fundus) and deposit the embryos without touching the fundus. The distance between the fundus to the external cervical os can be pre-examined by the help of ultrasound examinations, which will help in successful deposition of embryo in uterus. It has usually been believed that embryos must be implanted 5–10 mm below the surface of the uterine fundus. Nevertheless, certain researchers have recommended that placing embryos lower in the endometrial cavity may improve pregnancy rates [271].
- After successful deposition the catheter and cannula are gradually withdrawn. Finally, the catheter should be carefully examined under a microscope to ensure that the embryo has been expelled or is not present in the tube.

The above-mentioned steps should be carried out carefully since incorrect introduction of the catheter, or the use of an excessive amount of medium for transfer, may result in the expulsion of the embryo from the uterine lumen or to possible tubal pregnancy. These complications during pregnancy following ET have been reported. After ET, the patient is recommended to rest for at least 2–7 h and to avoid intercourse for at least a week. No hormonal support is required after ET.

3.11.3 Complications associated with embryo transfer

In some of the cases the embryos do not successfully attach to the uterus, even after multiple attempts of IVF, this is called repeated implantation failure [RIF]. This might be due to the concerns in the embryo, endometrium or the mother's immune system [272]. Therefore, while dealing with RIF, it is important to assess the quality of embryos and the health of the uterus and endometrium before implantation to avoid unnecessary complications [272]. A study found that for a patient with a history of recurrent IVF failure, there was 50% success rate when embryos grown in HA enriched medium were used for the implantation in the uterus [267].

3.12 Superovulation, IVF and embryo culture in farm animals

Superovulation, IVF, and embryo culture are reproductive technologies used in the field of animal husbandry and agriculture to enhance genetic progress, increase the number of offspring from superior females, and improve the overall quality of livestock. These techniques are commonly employed in farm animals, such as cattle, sheep, and pigs [273]. Superovulation is a technique usually employed to produce genetically engineered mice. It involves the administration of equine chorionic gonadotropin to encourage follicle growth and then that of human chorionic gonadotropin to promote ovulation [274]. This technique allows the artificial increase of the number of ovulated oocytes. It is carried out to derive oocytes from oocyte donors before IVF for the production of genetically engineered mice [274]. This technique allows the production of genetically improved farm animals in good numbers, which may result in the development of new industry [154]. The major steps involved in this technique are described below:

- Fertilized eggs are retrieved from genetically superior females. These females are either ovulate spontaneously or are allowed to ovulate a number of eggs (superovulation) by hormonal administration.
- Embryos derived from such females are transferred into genetically less desirable females. This may complete the objective of retrieving more progeny from superior females.

The hormone Inhibin is released into the general blood stream of the body by granulosa cells in the ovarian follicle. Inhibin hormone inhibits the anterior pituitary gland's function of producing FSH. Follicle growth is largely affected by the concentrations of both FSH and Inhibin. Some studies of superovulation technique demonstrate that when a combination of Inhibin antiserum (IAS) with Equine Chronic Gonadotrophin (eCG) and Human Chorionic Gonadotrophin (hCG) is introduced in the body of mice, it helps in increasing the number of oocytes ovulated than by the combination of eCG and hCG used [275].

Embryos can be developed in artificial media. The sexing of embryos (this technique is based on the difference between a chromosome of different embryos, i.e. different sex or the presence or absence of the Y chromosome) is done to allow the production of more female progeny if required. Sexing techniques involves identification of Y chromosome-specific DNA sequences [276]. This approach is considered as the most reliable method to date. PCR allows amplification of a target sequence from a smaller number of blastomeres. Nevertheless, it needs technical skill and is tedious [276]. An alternative approach entails the splitting of embryos into segments, which can result in development of offspring from each segment, i.e. 20–30 calves can be obtained per year from one valuable donor [277]. Embryo splitting at the 6–8 cell stage offers much higher developmental efficiency in contrast to splitting at the 2–5 cell stage. Embryo splitting may be significant for offering more embryos to be cryopreserved and also for patients undergoing IVF but with a low response to hormonal stimulation in ART. This technology is safely and well utilized for farm animals [277].

The sexing techniques of bovine embryos consists of three steps: embryo production, embryo biopsy and polymerase chain reaction (PCR). The first step includes the fertilization of oocytes with bull's spermatozoa. The fertilized oocytes are grown on a maturation medium. In the second step, biopsied embryos are taken after five days prior to a fertilization event using a micropipette. These are then transerred onto a cultivation medium. After the seventh day of fertilization, embryos are introduced non-surgically into farm animals. In the last step, a PCR reaction using the removed blastomeres is performed. After that, electrophoresis is performed on a 2% agarose gel. The bands are analyzed. One band of the bovine product corresponds to a female embryo, whereas two bands of bovine product correspond to a male embryo [278].

By means of this technology, efficient embryo splitting in the mouse can be achieved whereas in non-human primates application of this technology has resulted in several pregnancies [277]. Recently, human embryo splitting has been reported. By means of this technology it is possible to produce superior progeny, by replacing

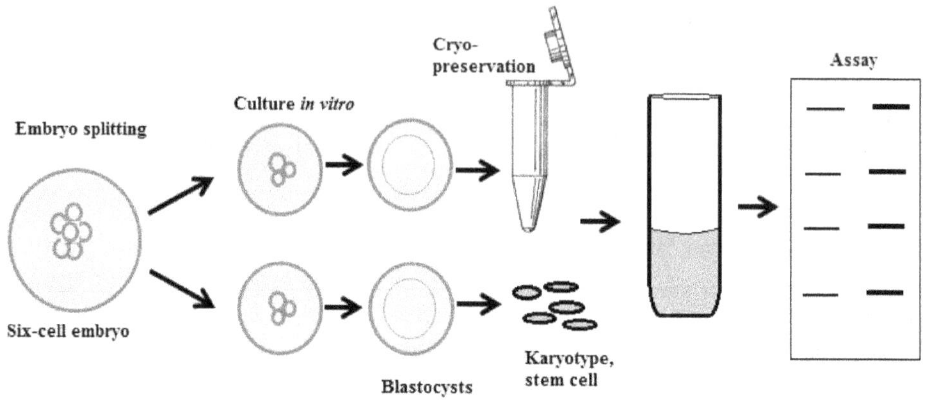

Figure 3.15. Embryo splitting.

the nucleus of an egg of a genetically less desirable female animal (i.e. it does not carry the superior characteristic) with that of a somatic cell of a superior female. The procedure involved in embryo splitting is depicted in figure 3.15.

Thus this technology offers superior eggs in large numbers. With the aid of recombinant DNA technology, it is now possible to transform the egg or embryo before embryo transfer. Several gene transfer techniques have been developed which allow the successful transformation of eggs or embryos to produce transgenic animals with desirable characteristics. Transgenic animals such as mice, cows, sheep, goats, chickens, pigs, etc, can be produce by this process.

Superovulation procedures have developed significantly after the introduction of bovine embryo transfer [278]. This was at a time when purified gonadotrophins and prostaglandin were not available. However, ovarian follicular development during the menstrual cycle has not been fully understood. Although superovulation procedures in cattle are usually introduced mid-cycle, optional control of follicular development and ovulation have great influence on the utilization of on-farm embryo transfer [278]. In farmhouse animals, more potential procedures have been developed for superovulation, *in vitro* fertilization, embryo sexing, embryo culture, transformation of embryos and ET. Furthermore, it allows the determination of gene expression, epigenetics, modifications and cytogenetic disorders during development. The nutritional requirements of culturing embryos (of farm animals) have usually been extrapolated from laboratory animals such as mice and rabbits. Nevertheless, the embryos of most mammals can be maintained under *in vitro* conditions for half a day or more with no irreversible damage [278]. A recent report underlining the antagonism between genetic advantage for milk production and the ability to produce embryos in sheep, established that high-milking sheep have a lower ovulation rate and are likely to produce fewer embryos in response to superovulation and intrauterine artificial insemination [279].

During superovulation, FSH needs to be introduced in the body of cattle daily for around 4 days, twice a day to promote growth of multiple embryos. Aluminium hydroxide (AH) gel has a unique property of taking up and releasing FSH hormone slowly with the help of protein bovine serum albumin (BSA) in the body. Now the second dose of FSH can be transferred into the body after a period of 48 h [279].

There are a number of approaches by which transgenic animals are produced. If transgenic animals produced by the above approaches are genetically superior and can be multiplied using the methods discussed above, the total cost involved will be satisfied by producing numerous superior animals via superovulation and ET in surrogate mothers. The genetic pattern of an embryo can be reproduced by dividing the embryo into groups of cells to obtain identical twins, triplets or quadruplets. An approach for freezing semen and embryos has also been developed, and will offer enormous flexibility in using these techniques for the genetic improvement of farm animals.

3.13 ET in cattle

Embryo transfer in cattle has recently gained considerable attention. Embryo transfer technology was discovered in between 1970s and1980s. During 1890, embryo transfer was first carried out and reported by Walter Heape, by transferring two Angora rabbit embryos into a gestating Belgian doe. During 1930s embryo transfer in food animals began with sheep and goats, and the first commercial embryo transfers were performed in the early 1970s. In this procedure, embryos were recovered from valuable donors and transferred to recipient animals using surgical methods.

With the help of embryonic transfer (ET), a popular reproductive technique in cattle breeding, farmers can improve the genetic potential of their herds. Superovulating a donor cow yields multiple embryos, which are then harvested and injected into recipients—surrogate cows—in the process. Through the use of this technique, it is possible to propagate superior genetics from cows that perform well, thereby improving traits like disease resistance, milk production, and overall productivity. Within a cattle herd, ET speeds up the rate of genetic improvement by facilitating the quick spread of valuable genetic material. It now forms a crucial component of contemporary cattle breeding initiatives, aiding in the long-term growth of superior livestock populations [280].

Some 40 years ago, artificial insemination emerged as a new tool to exploit the vast numbers of sperm produced by a genetically engineered livestock, although the reproductive potential of the female has been largely unutilized. Like artificial insemination in livestock, embryo transfer is a technique that can significantly increase the number of offspring. This allows significant improvement in our livestock and by using such technology semen can be stored for prolonged periods and can be transported it across distances whenever required [281]. Currently almost all commercial embryo transfer uses non-surgical recovery of the embryos rather than surgical techniques. The process includes numerous steps and considerable time as well as varied costs, as shown in figure 3.16.

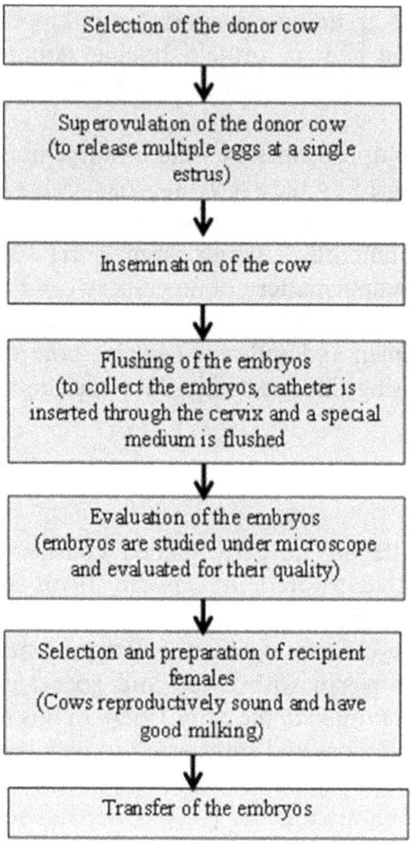

Figure 3.16. Embryo transfer technology in cattle.

3.13.1 ET technique in cattle

The reproductive biotechnology of ET in cattle entails the retrieval and transfer of embryos from a genetically superior donor cow to several recipient cows. Cattle breeders can increase the reproductive potential of elite females—those with desirable traits for producing meat or milk, for example—by using this technique. The first step in the procedure is superovulation, in which the donor cow receives hormonal therapy to encourage the release of several eggs. The embryos are transferred to synchronized recipient cows after artificial insemination, where they are recovered non-surgically and carried to term. Through the use of ET, exceptional individuals' genetic material can be quickly dispersed, improving herd genetics and advancing livestock breeding initiatives. This technology has demonstrated especially great value in in enhancing the efficiency and productivity of cattle breeding while preserving and propagating desirable genetic traits [282].

ET is a method by means of which embryos are retrieved from a donor female and then placed in the uterus of recipient females, which act as surrogate mothers for the rest of the pregnancy. ET (also called transplantation) in cattle is a more recent development, where newly formed embryos, before their implantation (after fertilization), are derived from a superior 'donor' female animal and transferred into the reproductive tract of other recipient females (often described as surrogate mothers), where they allowed to develop. Several approaches have also been developed for ET in cattle. One of the most common methods is embryo splitting in which the embryo can be divided into two or more equal parts, each part developing into an offspring giving twins, triplets, etc, after ET, as shown in figure 3.16. Thus, the ET technique can be employed for faster improvement of livestock. The developed embryo in such cases will inherit their genes partially from the donor females and partially from the males with which the donor was bred, but nothing from the surrogate mothers. The surrogate only receives the embryo from the donor for its development. The following phases are present during ET in cattle:

- After complete examination, a genetically superior high milk yielding cow should be selected as the donor. A low yielding milk cow should be considered as the recipient (surrogate mother). Estrus synchronization with prostaglandins has the potential to improve and increase artificial insemination (AI) programs with cattle. However, in 2005 it was reported that uterine secretion of PGF(2alpha) is increased after ET and administration of a PGF (2alpha) synthesis inhibitor at the time of embryo transfer enhanced pregnancy rates in cows [282].
- To achieve superovulation, follicle-stimulating hormone should be administered to the donor to further derive a higher number of ovules. Superovulation is a very inefficient approach for attaining oocytes from ovaries and is likely to be replaced by various other methods in the next decade. Nevertheless, superovulation still leads to the production ten times more embryos than single ovum recovery.
- After superovulation, the donor cow is allowed to be artificially inseminate by means of frozen semen from a genetically superior top pedigree bull. It has been also observed that the use of sexed frozen–thawed sperm cay be economically viable for commercial multiple ovulation and embryo transfer programs in Holstein heifers [283].
- After seven days of artificial insemination, the fertilized eggs (embryos) are collected (flushed) from the uterus of the donor cow, using a special nutrient medium (in a year, six flushings of embryos can be obtained from a donor cow, each flushing giving six good embryos, so 36 embryos in a year can be obtained from one donor cow).
- The embryos are isolated from the number of ovules and investigated under a stereo-microscope; good embryos are selected.
- Selected embryos are maintained in special medium at 37 °C in an incubator. To date, no chemically defined medium has been formulated to support the normal development of bovine embryos satisfactorily for longer than about 24 h. However, from 2013, medium 199, foetal bovine serum, and HEPES for buffering, has been considered as simple medium that allows bovine embryos to be held for seven days at 4 °C.

- Afterwards any one good embryo (or a part, where an embryo is split) is transferred to each surrogate mother, i.e. low milk producing cow (on an average 50% success is attained). By using this technique, eighteen superior calves from one donor cow per year can be produced, while in the natural course, merely one calf is produced by a cow per year.

3.13.2 Technique for freezing embryos in cattle

As mentioned above embryos produced *in vivo* are typically received from super-ovulated cows 7 days after estrus, and ultimately transferred to recipient cows. However, if the recipient cow is not at the anticipated stage (estrus cycle), the collected embryos can be preserved by cryopreservation using liquid nitrogen until the recipient cow is ready. However, this approach is not suitable for short-term storage since freezing by cryopreservation using liquid nitrogen unavoidably causes cryodamage to the cells. So, to freeze embryos for long-term storage, the embryos are primarily dehydrated by 'cryoprotectant' (e.g. glycerol). Once suitable osmotic pressure has been built up or equilibration is achieved, the embryos are allowed cool gradually from 25 °C to −38 °C (in a controlled manner). This cooling can be attained in a programmable controlled-rate freezer. About −38 °C embryos are plunged into liquid nitrogen (−196 °C), to be saved for posterity and used whenever required. Additionally, since the 1940s, several cell preservation media that are effective at hypothermic and cryogenic temperatures have been reported. These media are for the safe storage and transport of embryos. The latter approach of cryopreservation by means of liquid nitrogen has become dominant, particularly in the field of artificial reproductive technology. Nevertheless, the universal pregnancy rate has not been enhanced yet by means of cryopreserved mammalian embryos. This is because the freeze–thawing approach may responsible for substantial damage. Therefore, while thawing, dense cryoprotectants must be diluted very wisely to circumvent splitting of the embryo due to osmotic shock.

There exist two primary methods for cryopreservation of the embryos. The first method is referred to as controlled-rate or slow freezing. It involves the progressive combining of the embryos with the cryoprotectants, placing them in a straw, allowing them to form an ice crystal, gradually cooling at a controlled rate of 0.3 °C–0.5 °C and submerging them into liquid nitrogen when temperature (−30 °C to −65 °C) is attained. The second method is referred to as vitrification. This method is carried out in a glass-like state to prevent the ice crystal formation which can damage the cells as in the first method. Slow freezing is usually the preferred method as the embryos can be transplanted directly. Whereas in vitrification, high quantities of hazardous cryoprotectants are used, due to which embryos need to be washed properly after thawing the cells [284].

3.13.3 Benefits of ET in cattle

There are several advantages of ET:

- By preserving embryos, we can preserve superior traits of the livestock rather than preserving them in actuality, i.e., cattle embryos can be preserved, which avoids the transport of cattle from place to place, and has also become a cost effective technique. The offspring developed through this approach carry superior traits and also develop an immune system to deal with pathogens in the new environment.

- ET always improves the reproductive capability of a cow (at times their number is limited, as they are imported). Semen from one male can later be utilized for a number of females, and a single superior female can donate large number of ovules by superovulation.
- ET can be very well utilized to support breeding bull production in a cost-effective way.
- In this technique embryos can be procured by cryopreservation and can ultimately be preserved in an embryo bank. This embryo can be further utilized whenever required.
- Using this technique old superior cows that are unable to conceive can still donate ovules for ET.

3.13.4 Problems in ET in cattle

- Heat stress: When an animal is not able to strike a balance between the accumulation of heat and heat dissipated in the body is referred to as heat stress [285]. It is well known that heat stress reduces animal productivity, and climate change may make these effects worse [286].

References

[1] Marta I R 2001 *Ingeniería Genética y Transferencia Génica* 2nd edn (Madrid: Ediciones Pirámide)

[2] Gerald K 2002 *Cell and Molecular Biology: Concepts and Experiments* 3rd edn (New York: Wiley)

[3] Benjamin L 1999 *Genes VII* (Oxford: Oxford University Press)

[4] Klug W S, Cummings M R, Spencer C A and Palladino M A 2012 *Concepts of Genetics* 11th edn (Ewing, NJ: Prentice Hall)

[5] Murray J D, Oberbauer A M and McGloughlin M M 1999 *Transgenic Animals in Agriculture* (Davis, CA: CABI)

[6] Marta I R 1999 *Ingeniería Genética y Transferencia Génica* 1st edn (Madrid: Ediciones Pirámide)

[7] Louis-Marie H 1998 La transgenèse animale et ses applications *Product. Anim.* **11** 81–94

[8] Lynch M and Walsh B 1998 *Genetics and Analysis of Quantitative Traits* (Sunderland, MA: Sinauer)

[9] Montaldo H H and Meza-Herrera C A 1998 Use of molecular markers and major genes in the genetic improvement of livestock *Electron. J. Biotechnol.* **1** 12

[10] Schimenti J 1998 Global analysis of gene function in mammals: integration of physical, mutational and expression strategies *Electron. J. Biotechnol.* **1** 11

[11] Eggen A 2003 Basics and tools of genomics *Outlook Agric.* **32** 215–17

[12] Coutelle C and Rodeck C 2002 On the scientific and ethical issues of fetal somatic gene therapy *Gene Ther.* **9** 670–3

[13] NHGRI (International Human Genome Sequencing Consortium) 2001 Initial sequencing and analysis of the human genome *Nature* **409** 860–921
[14] Majzoub J A and Muglia L J 1996 Knockout mice *New England J. Med.* **334** 904–7
[15] Prather R S, Hawley R J, Carter D B, Lai L and Greenstein J L 2003 Transgenic swine for biomedicine and agriculture *Theriogenology* **59** 115–23
[16] Wall R J 1999 Biotechnology for the production of modified and innovative animal products: transgenic livestock bioreactors *Livest. Prod. Sci.* **59** 243–55
[17] Cameron E R, Harvey M J and Onions D E 1994 Transgenic science *Br. Vet. J.* **150** 9–24
[18] Kinghorn B P 1998 Future developments in animal breeding *Acta Agric. Scand.* A **28** 27–32
[19] Fries R and Ruvinsky A 1999 *The Genetics of Cattle* (Wallingford: CABI)
[20] Smidt D and Niemann H 1999 Biotechnology in genetics and reproduction *Livest. Prod. Sci.* **59** 207–21
[21] Abdul Aziz M, Brini F, Rouached H and Masmoudi K 2022 Genetically engineered crops for sustainably enhanced food production systems *Front. Plant Sci.* **13** 1027828
[22] Lu X, Zhang M, Li G, Zhang S, Zhang J, Fu X and Sun F 2023 Applications and research advances in the delivery of CRISPR/Cas9 systems for the treatment of inherited diseases *Int. J. Mol. Sci.* **24** 13202
[23] Polack F PC4591001 Clinical Trial Group 2020 Safety and efficacy of the BNT162b2 mRNA Covid-19 vaccine *New Engl. J. Med.* **383** 2603–15
[24] National Academies of Sciences, Engineering, and Medicine, National Academy of Medicine, National Academy of Sciences, and Committe on Human Gene Editing: Scientific, Medical, and Ethical Considerations. 2017 Human genome editing: science *Ethics, and Governance* (US: National Academies Press)
[25] Kotnik T, Frey W, Sack M, Haberl Meglič S, Peterka M and Miklavčič D 2015 Electroporation-based applications in biotechnology *Trends Biotechnol.* **33** 480–8
[26] Reiss M, Jastreboff M M, Bertino J R and Narayanan R 1986 DNA-mediated gene transfer into epidermal cells using electroporation *Biochem. Biophys. Res. Commun.* **137** 244–9
[27] Tur-Kaspa R, Teicher L, Levine B J, Skoultchi A and Shafritz D A 1986 Use of electroporation to introduce biologically active foreign genes into primary rat hepatocytes *Mol. Cell. Biol.* **6** 716–18
[28] Inoue K, Yamashita S, Hata J, Kabeno S, Asada S, Nagahisa E and Fujita T 1990 Electroporation as a new technique for producing transgenic fish *Cell Diff. Dev.* **29** 1238123–8
[29] Gagne M B, Pothier F and Sirad M A 1991 Electroporation of bovine spermatozoa to carry foreign DNA in oocytes *Mol. Reprod. Dev* **29** 6–15
[30] Puchalski R B and Fahl W E 1992 Gene transfer by electroporation, lipofection, and DEAE dextran transfection: compatibility with cell sorting by flow cytometry *Cytometry* **13** 23–30
[31] Whitmer K J and Calarco P G 1992 HIV-1 expression during early mammalian development *AIDS* **6** 1133–8
[32] Camper S A 1995 Implementing transgenic and embryonic stem cell technology to study gene expression, cell–cell interactions and gene function *Biol. Reprod.* **52** 246–57
[33] Potočnik T, Sachdev S, Polajžer T, Maček Lebar A and Miklavčič D 2022 Efficient gene transfection by electroporation—*In Vitro* and in silico study of pulse parameters *Appl. Sci.* **12** 8237

[34] Geng T and Lu C 2013 Microfluidic electroporation for cellular analysis and delivery *Lab Chip* **13** 3803–21
[35] Linnik D S, Tarakanchikova Y V, Zyuzin M V, Lepik K V, Aerts J L, Sukhorukov G and Timin A S 2021 Layer-by-Layer technique as a versatile tool for gene delivery applications *Expert Opin. Drug Deliv.* **18** 1047–66
[36] Rakoczy K, Kisielewska M, Sędzik M, Jonderko L, Celińska J, Sauer N, Szlasa W, Saczko J, Novickij V and Kulbacka J 2022 Electroporation in clinical applications—the potential of gene electrotransfer and electrochemotherapy *Appl. Sci.* **12** 10821
[37] Foley R A, Sims R A, Duggan E C, Olmedo J K, Ma R and Jonas S J 2022 Delivering the CRISPR/Cas9 system for engineering gene therapies: recent cargo and delivery approaches for clinical translation *Front. Bioeng. Biotechnol.* **10** 973326
[38] Fus-Kujawa A, Prus P, Bajdak-Rusinek K, Teper P, Gawron K, Kowalczuk A and Sieron A L 2021 An overview of methods and tools for transfection of eukaryotic cells *in vitro* *Front. Bioeng. Biotechnol.* **9** 701031
[39] Von Dassow G, Valley J and Robbins K 2019 Microinjection of oocytes and embryos with synthetic mRNA encoding molecular probes *Methods Cell. Biol.* **150** 189–222
[40] Gordon M F, Scangos G A, Plotkin D J, Barbosa J A and Ruddle F H 1980 Genetic transformation of mouse embryos by microinjection of purified DNA *Proc. Natl Acad. Sci. USA* **77** 7380–4
[41] Brinster R L, Chen H Y, Trumbauer M E, Senear A W, Warren R and Palmiter R D 1981 Somatic expression of herpes thymidine kinase in mice following injection of a foreign gene into eggs *Cell* **27** 223–31
[42] Costantini F and Lacy E 1981 Introduction of a rabbit-globin gene into the mouse germ line *Nature* **294** 92–4
[43] Wagner E F, Stewart T A and Mintz B 1981 The human globin gene and a functional thymidine kinase gene in developing mice *Proc. Natl Acad. Sci. USA* **78** 5016–20
[44] Wagner T E, Hoppe P C, Jollick J D, Scholl D R, Hondinka R L and Gault J B 1981 Microinjection of a rabbit globin gene in zygotes and its subsequent expression in adult mice and their offspring *Proc. Natl Acad. Sci. USA* **78** 6376–80
[45] Dunn D A, Kooyman D L C A and Pinkert 2005 Foundation review: transgenic animals and their impact on the drug discovery industry *DDT* **10** 757–67
[46] Zhang D, Gorochowski T E, Marucci L, Lee H T, Gil B, Li B, Hauert S and Yeatman E 2023 Advanced medical micro-robotics for early diagnosis and therapeutic interventions *Front. Robot. AI* **9** 1086043
[47] Volobueva A S, Orekhov A N and Deykin A V 2019 An update on the tools for creating transgenic animal models of human diseases - focus on atherosclerosis *Braz. J. Med. Biol. Res. = Rev. Bras. Pesquisas Med. Biol.* **52** e8108
[48] Menchaca A, Dos Santos-Neto P C, Mulet A P and Crispo M 2020 CRISPR in livestock: from editing to printing *Theriogenology* **150** 247–54
[49] Shakweer W M E, Krivoruchko A Y, Dessouki S M and Khattab A A 2023 A review of transgenic animal techniques and their applications *J. Genetic Eng. Biotechnol.* **21** 55
[50] Deguchi K, Zambaiti E and De Coppi P 2023 Regenerative medicine: current research and perspective in pediatric surgery *Pediatr. Surg. Int.* **39** 167
[51] Muthaiyan Shanmugam M and Manoj H 2021 Microinjection for single-cell analysis and therapy In: T S Santra and F G Tseng *Handbook of Single Cell Technologies* (Singapore: Springer)

[52] Sanford J C, DeVit M J, Russel J A, Smith F D, Harpending P R, Roy M K and Johnston S A 1991 An improved, helium-driven biolistic device *Tech. J. Meth. Cell Mol. Biol.* **3** 3163–16
[53] Sanford J C 1988 The biolistic process *TIBTECH* **6** 299–302
[54] Biewenga J E, Destre O H J and Schrama L H 1997 Plasmid-mediated gene transfer in neurons using the biolistics technique *J. Neuro. Meth.* **71** 67–75
[55] Jiao S, Cheng L, Wolff J and Yang N 1993 Particle bombardment-mediated gene transfer and expression in rat brain tissues *Nat. Biotechnol.* **11** 497–502
[56] Sharma D, Arora S, Singh J and Layek B 2021 A review of the tortuous path of nonviral gene delivery and recent progress *Int. J. Biol. Macromol.* **183** 2055–73
[57] Lacroix B and Citovsky V 2020 Biolistic approach for transient gene expression studies in plants *Methods Mol. Biol. (Clifton, N.J.)* **2124** 125–39
[58] Handral H K, Wyrobnik T A and Lam A T-L 2023 Emerging Trends in biodegradable microcarriers for therapeutic applications *Polymers* **15** 1487
[59] Shchaslyvyi A Y, Antonenko S, Tesliuk M G and Telegeev G D 2023 Current state of human gene therapy: approved products and vectors *Pharmaceuticals* **16** 1416
[60] Hamad M I K, Daoud S, Petrova P, Rabaya O, Jbara A, Melliti N, Stichmann S, Reiss G, Herz J and Förster E 2020 Biolistic transfection and expression analysis of acute cortical slices *J. Neurosci. Methods* **337** 108666
[61] Felgner P L, Gadek T R, Holm M, Roman R, Chan H W, Wenz M, Northrop J P, Ringold G M and Danielsen M 1987 Lipofection: a highly efficient, lipid-mediated DNA-transfection procedure *Proc. Natl Acad. Sci. USA* **84** 7413–17
[62] Sriwidodo , Umar A K, Wathoni N, Zothantluanga J H, Das S and Luckanagul J A 2022 Liposome-polymer complex for drug delivery system and vaccine stabilization *Heliyon* **8** e08934
[63] Nikolova M P, Kumar E M and Chavali M S 2022 Updates on responsive drug delivery based on liposome vehicles for cancer treatment *Pharmaceutics* **14** 2195
[64] Aldosari B N, Alfagih I M and Almurshedi A S 2021 Lipid nanoparticles as delivery systems for rna-based vaccines *Pharmaceutics* **13** 206
[65] Mohanty A, Uthaman S and Park I K 2020 Utilization of polymer-lipid hybrid nanoparticles for targeted Anti-cancer therapy *Molecules (Basel, Switzerland)* **25** 4377
[66] Tretiakova D S and Vodovozova E L 2022 Liposomes as adjuvants and vaccine delivery systems *Biochem. (Mosc.) Suppl. Ser. A, Membr. Cell Biol.* **16** 1–20
[67] BioMed Research International 2019 Retracted: recent trends of polymer mediated liposomal gene delivery system *Bio. Med. Res. Int.* **2019** 8195729
[68] Chen C A and Okayama H 1988 Calcium phosphate-mediated gene transfer: a highly efficient transfection system for stably transforming cells with plasmid *DNA Biotechniques* **6** 632–8
[69] Guo L *et al* 2017 Optimizing conditions for calcium phosphate mediated transient transfection *Saudi J. Biol. Sci.* **24** 622–9
[70] Levingstone T J, Herbaj S, Redmond J, McCarthy H O and Dunne N J 2020 Calcium phosphate nanoparticles-based systems for RNAi delivery: applications in bone tissue regeneration *Nanomaterials* **10** 146
[71] Levingstone T J, Herbaj S and Dunne N J 2019 Calcium phosphate nanoparticles for therapeutic applications in bone regeneration *Nanomaterials* **9** 1570

[72] Chong Z X, Yeap S K and Ho W Y 2021 Transfection types, methods and strategies: a technical review *PeerJ* **9** e11165
[73] Fiol C R, Collignon M L, Welsh J and Rafiq Q A 2023 Optimizing and developing a scalable, chemically defined, animal component-free lentiviral vector production process in a fixed-bed bioreactor. Molecular therapy *Methods Clin. Dev.* **30** 221–34
[74] Contesini F J *et al* 2020 Advances in recombinant lipases: production, engineering, immobilization and application in the pharmaceutical industry *Catalysts* **10** 1032
[75] Gulick T 2001 Transfection using DEAE-dextran *Curr. Protoc. Neurosci.* **20** 20.4
[76] Cai X, Dou R, Guo C, Tang J, Li X, Chen J and Zhang J 2023 Cationic polymers as transfection reagents for nucleic acid delivery *Pharmaceutics* **15** 1502
[77] Steffens R C and Wagner E 2023 Directing the way-receptor and chemical targeting strategies for nucleic acid delivery *Pharm. Res.* **40** 47–76
[78] Gharaati-Far N, Tohidkia M R, Dehnad A and Omidi Y 2018 Efficiency and cytotoxicity analysis of cationic lipids-mediated gene transfection into AGS gastric cancer cells *Artif. Cells, Nanomed. Biotechnol.* **46** 1001–8
[79] Lundstrom K 2019 RNA viruses as tools in gene therapy and vaccine development *Genes* **10** 189
[80] Khan M S, Gowda B H J, Nasir N, Wahab S, Pichika M R, Sahebkar A and Kesharwani P 2023 Advancements in dextran-based nanocarriers for treatment and imaging of breast cancer *Int. J. Pharm.* **643** 123276
[81] Kawai S and Nishizawa M 1984 New procedure for DNA transfection with polycation and dimethyl sulfoxide *Mol. Cell. Biol.* **4** 1172–4
[82] Loginova T P, Khotina I A, Kabachii Y A, Kochev S Y, Abramov V M, Khlebnikov V S, Kulikova N L and Mezhuev Y O 2023 Promising gene delivery properties of polycations based on 2-(*N*,*N*-dimethylamino)ethyl methacrylate and polyethylene glycol monomethyl ether methacrylate copolymers *Polymers* **15** 3036
[83] Awan M *et al* 2020 Dimethyl sulfoxide: a central player since the dawn of cryobiology, is efficacy balanced by toxicity? *Regen. Med.* **15** 1463–91
[84] Arghya Bhattacharya and Lopamudra Chakravarty 2021 'Gene transfer technologies and their applications: mitigation and curing of diseases'. acta scientific *Pharmacology* **2.4** 23–30
[85] Xu Y and Li Z 2020 CRISPR-Cas systems: overview, innovations and applications in human disease research and gene therapy *Comput. Struct. Biotechnol. J.* **18** 2401–15
[86] Hayashimoto A, Li Z and Murai N 1990 A polyethylene glycol-mediated protoplast transformation system for production of fertile transgenic rice plants *Plant Physiol.* **93** 857–63
[87] Suk J S, Xu Q, Kim N, Hanes J and Ensign L M 2016 PEGylation as a strategy for improving nanoparticle-based drug and gene delivery *Adv. Drug Deliv. Rev.* **99** 28–51
[88] Pan X, Veroniaina H, Su N, Sha K, Jiang F, Wu Z and Qi X 2021 Applications and developments of gene therapy drug delivery systems for genetic diseases *Asian J. Pharm. Sci.* **16** 687–703
[89] Qin S *et al* 2022 mRNA-based therapeutics: powerful and versatile tools to combat diseases *Signal Transduct. Target. Ther.* **7** 166
[90] Chen G G, Mao M, Qiu L Z and Liu Q M 2015 Gene transfection mediated by *Polyethyleneimine-polyethylene* glycol nanocarrier prevents cisplatin-induced spiral ganglion cell damage *Neural Regen. Res.* **10** 425–31

[91] Gottschalk S, Sparrow J T, Hauer J, Mims M P, Leland F E, Woo S L and Smith L C 1996 A novel DNA-peptide complex for efficient gene transfer and expression in mammalian cells *Gene Ther.* **3** 448–57
[92] Kalafatovic D and Giralt E 2017 Cell-Penetrating peptides: design strategies beyond primary structure and amphipathicity *Molecules (Basel, Switzerland)* **22** 1929
[93] Wickline S A, Hou K K and Pan H 2023 Peptide-based nanoparticles for systemic extrahepatic delivery of therapeutic nucleotides *Int. J. Mol. Sci.* **24** 9455
[94] Tarvirdipour S, Skowicki M, Schoenenberger C A and Palivan C G 2021 Peptide-assisted nucleic acid delivery systems on the rise *Int. J. Mol. Sci.* **22** 9092
[95] Hilton I B and Gersbach C A 2015 Enabling functional genomics with genome engineering *Genome Res.* **25** 1442–55
[96] Samec T, Boulos J, Gilmore S, Hazelton A and Alexander-Bryant A 2022 Peptide-based delivery of therapeutics in cancer treatment *Mater. Today Bio* **14** 100248
[97] Wang L, Wang N, Zhang W, Cheng X, Yan Z, Shao G, Wang X, Wang R and Fu C 2022 Therapeutic peptides: current applications and future directions *Signal Transduct. Target. Ther.* **7** 48
[98] Miller D G, Adam M A and Miller A D 1990 Gene transfer by retrovirus vectors occurs only in cells that are actively replicating at the time of infection *Mol. Cell Biol.* **10** 4239–42
[99] Nisole S and Saïb A 2004 Early steps of retrovirus replicative cycle *Retrovirology* **1** 9
[100] Vargas J E, Chicaybam L, Stein R T, Tanuri A, Delgado-Cañedo A and Bonamino M H 2016 Retroviral vectors and transposons for stable gene therapy: advances, current challenges and perspectives *J. Transl. Med.* **14** 288
[101] Mátrai J, Chuah M K and VandenDriessche T 2010 Recent advances in lentiviral vector development and applications *Mol. Ther.: J. Am. Soc. Gene Ther.* **18** 477–90
[102] Xu C L, Ruan M Z C, Mahajan V B and Tsang S H 2019 Viral delivery systems for CRISPR *Viruses* **11** 28
[103] Razi Soofiyani S, Baradaran B, Lotfipour F, Kazemi T and Mohammadnejad L 2013 Gene therapy, early promises, subsequent problems, and recent breakthroughs *Adv. Pharm. Bull.* **3** 249–55
[104] Steichen C *et al* 2014 Messenger RNA- versus retrovirus-based induced pluripotent stem cell reprogramming strategies: analysis of genomic integrity *Stem Cells Transl. Med.* **3** 686–91
[105] Gianni D and Farrow S 2020 Functional genomics for target identification *SLAS Discov.: Adv. Sci. Drug Discov.* **25** 531–4
[106] Bin Umair M *et al* 2022 Viruses as tools in gene therapy, vaccine development, and cancer treatment *Arch. Virol* **167** 1387–404
[107] Janik E, Niemcewicz M, Ceremuga M, Krzowski L, Saluk-Bijak J and Bijak M 2020 Various aspects of a gene editing system-CRISPR-Cas9 *Int. J. Mol. Sci.* **21** 9604
[108] Asmamaw M and Zawdie B 2021 Mechanism and applications of CRISPR/Cas-9-mediated genome editing *Biol.: Targets Ther.* **15** 353–61
[109] Li Y, Liang J, Deng B, Jiang Y, Zhu J, Chen L, Li M and Li J 2023 Applications and prospects of CRISPR/Cas9-mediated base editing in plant breeding *Curr. Issues Mol. Biol.* **45** 918–35
[110] Hansen S, McClements M E, Corydon T J and MacLaren R E 2023 Future perspectives of prime editing for the treatment of inherited retinal diseases *Cells* **12** 440

[111] Liu H J *et al* 2020 High-throughput CRISPR/Cas9 mutagenesis streamlines trait gene identification in maize *Plant Cell* **32** 1397–413
[112] Uddin F, Rudin C M and Sen T 2020 CRISPR gene therapy: applications, limitations, and implications for the future *Front. Oncol* **10** 1387
[113] Liu Q, Yang F, Zhang J, Liu H, Rahman S, Islam S, Ma W and She M 2021 Application of CRISPR/Cas9 in crop quality improvement *Int. J. Mol. Sci.* **22** 4206
[114] Parsaeimehr A, Ebirim R and Ozbay G 2022 CRISPR-Cas technology a new era in genomic engineering *Biotechnol. Rep. (Amsterdam, Netherlands)* **34** e00731
[115] Tariq H, Batool S, Asif S, Ali M and Abbasi B H 2022 Virus-like particles: revolutionary platforms for developing vaccines against emerging infectious diseases *Front. Microbiol.* **12** 790121
[116] He J, Yu L, Lin X, Liu X, Zhang Y, Yang F and Deng W 2022 Virus-like particles as nanocarriers for intracellular delivery of biomolecules and compounds *Viruses* **14** 1905
[117] Banskota S *et al* 2022 Engineered virus-like particles for efficient *in vivo* delivery of therapeutic proteins *Cell* **185** 250–65
[118] Mejía-Méndez J L, Vazquez-Duhalt R, Hernández L R, Sánchez-Arreola E and Bach H 2022 Virus-like particles: fundamentals and biomedical applications *Int. J. Mol. Sci.* **23** 8579
[119] Nooraei S, Bahrulolum H, Hoseini Z S, Katalani C, Hajizade A, Easton A J and Ahmadian G 2021 Virus-like particles: preparation, immunogenicity and their roles as nanovaccines and drug nanocarriers *J. Nanobiotechnology* **19** 59
[120] Raguram A, Banskota S and Liu D R 2022 Therapeutic *in vivo* delivery of gene editing agents *Cell* **185** 2806–27
[121] Ikwuagwu B and Tullman-Ercek D 2022 Virus-like particles for drug delivery: a review of methods and applications *Curr. Opin. Biotechnol.* **78** 102785
[122] Nora L C, Westmann C A, Martins-Santana L, Alves L F, Monteiro L M O, Guazzaroni M E and Silva-Rocha R 2019 The art of vector engineering: towards the construction of next-generation genetic tools *Microb. Biotechnol.* **12** 125–47
[123] Solar G, Giraldo R, Ruiz-Echevarría M J, Espinosa M and Díaz-Orejas R 1998 Replication and control of circular bacterial plasmids *Microbiol. Mol. Biol. Rev.* **62** 434–64
[124] Al Doghaither H and Gull M 2019 Plasmids as Genetic Tools and Their Applications in Ecology and Evolution (IntechOpen)
[125] Khan S, Ullah M W, Siddique R, Nabi G, Manan S, Yousaf M and Hou H 2016 Role of recombinant DNA technology to improve life *Int. J. Genomics* **2016** 2405954
[126] Rafeeq H, Afsheen N, Rafique S, Arshad A, Intisar M, Hussain A, Bilal M and Iqbal H M N 2023 Genetically engineered microorganisms for environmental remediation *Chemosphere* **310** 136751
[127] Rodríguez-Rodríguez D R, Ramírez-Solís R, Garza-Elizondo M A, Garza-Rodríguez M L and Barrera-Saldaña H A 2019 Genome editing: a perspective on the application of CRISPR/Cas9 to study human diseases (Review) *Int. J. Mol. Med.* **43** 1559–74
[128] Rosano G L and Ceccarelli E A 2014 Recombinant protein expression in *Escherichia coli*: advances and challenges *Front. Microbiol.* **5** 172
[129] Ma Y, Lee C J and Park J S 2020 Strategies for optimizing the production of proteins and peptides with multiple disulfide bonds *Antibiotics (Basel, Switzerland)* **9** 541
[130] Wang Q, Zhong C and Xiao H 2020 Genetic engineering of filamentous fungi for efficient protein expression and secretion *Front. Bioeng. Biotechnol.* **8** 293

[131] Li Z M, Fan Z L, Wang X Y and Wang T Y 2022 Factors affecting the expression of recombinant protein and improvement strategies in chinese hamster ovary cells *Front. Bioeng. Biotechnol.* **10** 880155

[132] Rosano G L and Ceccarelli E A 2014 Recombinant protein expression in *Escherichia coli*: advances and challenges *Front. Microbiol.* **5** 172

[133] Lodish H, Berk A and Zipursky S L 2000 *Molecular Cell Biology* 4th edn (New York: Freeman)

[134] Vajo Z, Fawcett J and Duckworth W C 2001 Recombinant DNA technology in the treatment of diabetes: insulin analogs *Endocr. Rev.* **22** 706–17

[135] Gotovtsev P 2023 Microbial cells as a microrobots: from drug delivery to advanced biosensors *Biomimetics (Basel, Switzerland)* **8** 109

[136] Wells D N 2005 Animal cloning: problems and prospects *Rev. Sci. Tech.* **24** 251–64

[137] Yan X, Liu X, Zhao C and Chen G Q 2023 Applications of synthetic biology in medical and pharmaceutical fields *Signal Transduct. Target. Ther.* **8** 199

[138] Sioson V A, Kim M and Joo J 2021 Challenges in delivery systems for CRISPR-based genome editing and opportunities of nanomedicine *Biomed. Eng. Lett.* **11** 217–33

[139] Wang D, Tai P W L and Gao G 2019 Adeno-associated virus vector as a platform for gene therapy delivery *Nat. Rev. Drug Discovery* **18** 358–78

[140] Xia W, Tao Z, Zhu B, Zhang W, Liu C, Chen S and Song M 2021 Targeted delivery of drugs and genes using polymer nanocarriers for cancer therapy *Int. J. Mol. Sci.* **22** 9118

[141] Kim T K and Eberwine J H 2010 Mammalian cell transfection: the present and the future *Anal. Bioanal. Chem.* **397** 3173

[142] Carballada R, Degefa T and Esponda P 2000 Transfection of mouse eggs and embryos using DNA combined to cationic liposomes *Mol. Reprod. Dev.* **56** 360–5

[143] Liu C, Xie W, Gui C and Du Y 2013 Pronuclear microinjection and oviduct transfer procedures for transgenic mouse production methods *Mol. Biol.* **102** 710

[144] Fechheimer M, Boylan J F, Parker S, Sisken J E, Patel G L and Zimmer S G 1987 Transfection of mammalian cells with plasmid DNA by scrape loading and sonication loading *Proc. Natl Acad. Sci. USA* **84** 8463–7

[145] Maksimenko O G, Deykin A V, Khodarovich Y M and Georgiev P G 2013 Use of transgenic animals in biotechnology: prospects and problems *Acta Naturae* **5** 33–46

[146] Damak S, Su H, Jay N P and Bullock D W 1996 Improved wool production in transgenic sheep expressing insulin-like growth factor 1 *Biotechnology* **14** 185–8

[147] Imanaka T and Aiba S 1981 A perspective on the application of genetic engineering: stability of recombinant plasmid *Ann. N. Y. Acad. Sci.* **369** 1–14

[148] Kaplan J and Hukku B 1998 Cell line characterization and authentication *Methods Cell. Biol.* **57** 203–16

[149] Foote R H 1987 *In vitro* fertilization and embryo transfer in domestic animals: applications in animals and implications for humans *J. In Vitro Fertil. Embryo Transf.* **4** 73–88

[150] Wang J and Sauer M V 2006 *In vitro* fertilization (IVF): a review of 3 decades of clinical innovation and technological advancement *Ther. Clin. Risk Manag.* **2** 355–64

[151] Ashrafi M, Sadatmahalleh S J, Akhoond M R, Ghaffari F and Zolfaghari Z 2013 ICSI outcome in infertile couples with different causes of infertility: a cross-sectional study *Int. J. Fertil. Steril.* **7** 88–95

[152] Liu D Y and Baker H W 2002 Evaluation and assessment of semen for IVF/ICSI *Asian J. Androl.* **4** 281–5

[153] Canis M, Pouly J L, Tamburro S, Mage G, Wattiez A and Bruhat M A 2001 Ovarian response during IVF-embryo transfer cycles after laparoscopic ovarian cystectomy for endometriotic cysts of >3 cm in diameter *Hum. Reprod.* **16** 2583–6
[154] Ventura-Juncá P, Irarrázaval I, Rolle A J, Gutiérrez J I, Moreno R D and Santos M J 2015 *In vitro* fertilization (IVF) in mammals: epigenetic and developmental alterations. Scientific and bioethical implications for IVF in humans *Biol. Res.* **48** 68
[155] Kraemer D C 1983 Intra- and interspecific embryo transfer *J. Exp. Zool.* **228** 36371363–71
[156] Lis Q, Powers P and Smithies O 1985 Nucleotide sequence of 16-kilobase pairs of DNA 5′ to the human e-globin gene *J. Biol. Chem.* **260** 14901–10
[157] Simons J P, McClenaghan M and Clark A J 1987 Alteration of the quality of milk by expression of sheep beta-lactoglobulin in transgenic mice *Nature* **328** 530–2
[158] Wright G, Carver A, Cottom D, Reeves D, Scott A, Simons P, Wilmut I and Garner Colman A 1991 High level expression of active human alpha-1-antitrypsin in the milk of transgenic sheep *Biotechnology* **9** 830–4
[159] Pursel V G, Bolt D J, Miller K F, Pinkert C A, Hammer R E, Palmiter R D and Brinster R L 1990 Expression and performance in transgenic pigs *J. Reprod. Fertil. Suppl.* **40** 235–45
[160] Wang R, Zhang P, Gong Z and Hew C L 1995 Expression of the antifreeze protein gene in transgenic goldfish (Carassius auratus) and its implication in cold adaptation *Mol. Mar. Biol. Biotechnol.* **4** 20–6
[161] Weissmann C 1982 Structure and expressions of human alpha-interferon genes *Abstr. ICN-UCLA Symp. on Chem. Biol. Interf.:Relat. Ther.* **299** 7–28
[162] Brown J B 1969 Factors involved in the induction of fertile ovulation with human gonadotrophins *J. Obstetr. Gynaecol. Brit. Commonw* **76** 298–307
[163] Quinn P, Barros C and Whittingham D G 1982 Preservation of hamster oocytes to assay the fertilizing capacity of human spermatozoa *J. Reprod. Fertil* **66** 161–8
[164] Nancarrow C D, Marshall J T and Ward K A 1993 Production of transgenic sheep *Transgenesis Techniques. Methods in Molecular Biology vol 18* (Humana Press)
[165] Hammer R E, Pursel V G, Rexroad C E J, Wall R J, Bolt D J, Ebert K M, Palmiter R D and Ralph L 1985 Brinster production of transgenic rabbits, sheep and pigs by micro-injection *Nature* **315** 680–3
[166] McCreath K J, Howcroft J, Campbell K H, Colman A, Schnieke A E and Kind A J 2000 Production of gene-targeted sheep by nuclear transfer from cultured somatic cells *Nature* **405** 1066–9
[167] Schnieke A E, Kind A J, Ritchie W A, Mycock K, Scott A R, Ritchie M, Wilmut I, Colman A and Campbell K H 1997 Human factor IX transgenic sheep produced by transfer of nuclei from transfected fetal fibroblasts *Science* **278** 2130–3
[168] Cornetta K, Tessanne K, Long C, Yao J, Satterfield C and Westhusin M 2013 Transgenic sheep generated by lentiviral vectors: safety and integration analysis of surrogates and their offspring *Transgen. Res.* **22** 737–45
[169] Chang K 2002 Effective generation of transgenic pigs and mice by linker-based sperm-mediated gene transfer *BMC Biotechnol.* **2** 5
[170] Saeki K 2004 Functional expression of a Δ12 fatty acid desaturase gene from spinach in transgenic pigs *Proc. Natl Acad. Sci. USA* **101** 6361–6
[171] Milan D 2000 A mutation in PRKAG3 associated with excess glycogen associated with excess glycogen content in pig skeletal muscle *Science* **288** 1248–51

[172] Andersson L 1994 Genetic mapping of quantitative trait loci for growth and fatness in pigs *Science* **263** 1771–4
[173] Nezer C, Moreau L, Brouwers B, Coppieters W, Detilleux J, Hanset R, Karim L, Kvasz A, Leroy P and Georges M 1999 *Nat. Genet.* **21** 155–6
[174] Yan Q, Yang H, Yang D, Zhao B, Ouyang Z, Liu Z, Fan N, Ouyang H, Gu W and Lai L 2014 Production of transgenic pigs over-expressing the antiviral gene Mx1 *Cell Regen. (Lond.)* **3** 11
[175] Lai L 2002 Production of alpha-1,3-galactosyltransferase knockout pigs by nuclear transfer cloning *Science* **295** 1089–9
[176] Park J K 2006 Recombinant human erythropoietin produced in milk of transgenic pigs *J. Biotechnol.* **122** 362–71
[177] Swindle M M 2007 *Swine in the Laboratory: Surgery, Anesthesia, Imaging, and Experimental Techniques* 2nd edn (Boca Raton, FL: CRC Press)
[178] Bendixen E K, Danielsen M, Larsen K and Bendixen C 2010 Advances in porcine genomics and proteomics—a toolbox for developing the pig as a model organism for molecular biomedical research *Brief Funct. Genom* **9** 208–19
[179] Klymiuk N, Aigner B, Brem G and Wolf E 2010 Genetic modification of pigs as organ donors for xenotransplantation *Mol. Reprod. Dev* **77** 209–21
[180] Morrow T 2009 Transgenic goats are key to antithrombin production *Manag Care* **18** 46–7
[181] Baldassarre H, Wang B, Keefer C L, Lazaris A and Karatzas C N 2004 State of the art in the production of transgenic goats *Reprod. Fertil. Dev.* **16** 465–70
[182] Yekta A A 2013 Production of transgenic goats expressing human coagulation factor IX in the mammary glands after nuclear transfer using transfected fetal fibroblast cells *Transgen. Res.* **22** 131–42
[183] Cammuso C 2000 Hormonal induced lactation in transgenic goats *Anim. Biotechnol.* **11** 1–17
[184] Cooper C A, Klobas L C G, Maga E A and Murray J D 2013 Consuming transgenic goats' milk containing the antimicrobial protein lysozyme helps resolve diarrhea in young pigs *PLoS One* **8** e58409
[185] Yu H, Chen J, Liu S, Zhang A, Xu X, Wang X, Lu P and Cheng G 2013 Large-scale production of functional human lysozyme in transgenic cloned goats *J. Biotechnol.* **168** 676–83
[186] Carneiro I S, Menezes J N R, Maia J A, Miranda A M, Oliveira V B S, Murray J D, Maga E A, Bertolini M and Bertolini L R 2018 Milk from transgenic goat expressing human lysozyme for recovery and treatment of gastrointestinal pathogens *Eur. J. Pharm. Sci.* **112** 79–86
[187] Bao Z, Gao X I, Zhang Q, Lin J, Hu W, Yu H, Chen J, Yang Q and Yu Q 2015 The effects of GH transgenic goats on the microflora of the intestine, feces and surrounding soil *PLoS One* **10** e0139822
[188] Baruah G L, Nayak A, Winkelman E and Belfort G 2006 Purification of monoclonal antibodies derived from transgenic goat milk by ultrafiltration *Biotechnol. Bioeng.* **93** 747–54
[189] Wall R J, Powell A M, Paape M J, Kerr D E, Bannerman D D, Pursel V G, Wells K D, Talbot N and Hawk H W 2005 Genetically enhanced cows resist intramammary *Staphylococcus aureus* infection *Nat. Biotechnol.* **23** 445–51
[190] Hyvönen P, Suojala L, Orro T, Haaranen J, Simola O, Røntved C and Pyörälä S Transgenic cows that produce recombinant human lactoferrin in milk are not protected from experimental *Escherichia coli* intramammary infection *Infect. Immun* **74** 6206–12

[191] Cooper G M 2000 *The Cell: A Molecular Approach* 2nd edn (Sunderland (MA): Sinauer Associates)
[192] Gewely M R 1995 Biotechnology domain *Biotechnol. Annu. Rev.* **1** 5–68
[193] Evens R P and Witcher M 1993 Biotechnology: an introduction to recombinant DNA technology and product availability *Ther. Drug Monit.* **15** 514–20
[194] Stryjewska A, Kiepura K, Librowski T and Lochyński S 2013 Biotechnology and genetic engineering in the new drug development. Part II. Monoclonal antibodies, modern vaccines and gene therapy *Pharmacol. Rep.* **65** 1086–101
[195] Bowey-Dellinger K *et al* 2017 Introducing mammalian cell culture and cell viability techniques in the undergraduate biology laboratory *J. Microbiol. Biol. Educ.* **18** 1–7
[196] Trunfio N, Lee H, Starkey J, Agarabi C, Liu J and Yoon S 2017 Characterization of mammalian cell culture raw materials by combining spectroscopy and chemometrics *Biotechnol. Prog.;* **33** 1127–38
[197] Stacey G, Bolton B, Doyle A *et al* 1992 DNA fingerprinting—a valuable new technique for the characterisation of cell lines *Cytotechnology* **9** 211–6
[198] Kaplan J and Hukku B 1998 Cell line characterization and authentication *Methods Cell. Biol.* **57** 20316203–16
[199] Foote R H 1987 *In vitro* fertilization and embryo transfer in domestic animals: applications in animals and implications for humans *J. In Vitro Fertil. Embryo Transf* **4** 73–88
[200] Murray J and Anderson G 2000 Genetic engineering and cloning may improve milk, livestock production Calif *Agr* **54** 57–65
[201] Steptoe P C and Edwards R G 1978 Birth after the reimplantation of a human embryo *Lancet* **2** 366
[202] Foote R H 1987 *In vitro* fertilization and embryo transfer in domestic animals: applications in animals and implications for humans *J. In Vitro Fertil. Embryo. Transf* **4** 73–88
[203] McKnight K and McKenzie L J 2000 *Evaluation of Infertility, Ovulation Induction and Assisted Reproduction Endotext* ed L J De Groot (South Dartmouth, MA: MDText.com)
[204] Chandra A, Martinez G M, Mosher W D, Abma J C and Jones J 2005 Fertility, family planning, and reproductive health: data from the 2002 national survey of family growth *Vital Health Statist.* **23** 25
[205] Pursel V G, Bolt D J, Miller K F, Pinkert C A, Hammer R E, Palmiter R D and Brinster R L 1990 Expression and performance in transgenic pigs *J. Reprod. Fertil. Suppl* **40** 235–45
[206] Sotrel G 2009 Is surgical repair of the fallopian tubes ever appropriate? *Rev. Obstet. Gynecol.* **2** 176–85
[207] Medikare V, Kandukuri L R, Ananthapur V, Deenadayal M and Nallari P 2011 The genetic bases of uterine fibroids. a review *J. Reprod. Infertil* **12** 181–91
[208] Kulkarni M M, Deshmukh S D, Hol K and Neha N 2015 A rare case of Mayer–Rokitansky–Kuster– Hauser syndrome with multiple leiomyomas in hypoplastic uterus *J. Hum. Reprod. Sci.* **8** 242–4
[209] Atmaca R, Germen A T, Burak F and Kafkasli A 2005 Acute abdomen in a case with noncommunicating rudimentary horn and unicornuate uterus *JSLS* **9** 235–7
[210] Sadeghi M R 2015 Unexplained infertility, the controversial matter in management of infertile couples *J. Reprod. Infertil* **16** 121–2
[211] Isaksson R and Tiitinen A 2004 Present concept of unexplained infertility *Gynecol. Endocrinol.* **18** 278–90

[212] Slama R 2012 Estimation of the frequency of involuntary infertility on a nation-wide basis *Hum. Reprod.* **27** 1489–98

[213] Harris I D, Fronczak C, Roth L and Meacham R B 2011 Fertility and the aging male *Rev. Urol.* **13** e18490e184

[214] Anderson J E, Farr S L, Jamieson D J, Warner L and Macaluso M 2009 Infertility services reported by men in the United States: national survey data *Fertil. Steril.* **91** 2466–70

[215] Liu D Y and Baker H W 2002 Evaluation and assessment of semen fo IVF/ICSI *Asian J. Androl.* **4** 281–5

[216] Park Y S, Lee S H, Song S J, Jun J H, Koong M K and Seo J T 2003 Influence of motility on the outcome of *in vitro* fertilization/intracytoplasmic sperm injection with fresh vs frozen testicular sperm from men with obstructive azoospermia *Fertil. Steril.* **80** P526–30

[217] Erenpreiss J, Spano M, Erenpreisa J, Bungum M and Giwercman A 2006 Sperm chromatin structure and male fertility: biological and clinical aspects *Asian J. Androl.* **8** 11–29

[218] Kumaran A, Narayan P K, Pai P J, Ramachandran A, Mathews B and Kumar A S 2015 Oocyte retrieval at 140-mmHg negative aspiration pressure: a promising alternative to flushing and aspiration in assisted reproduction in women with low ovarian reserve *J. Hum. Reprod. Sci.* **8** 98–102

[219] Bénard J, Duros S, Hachem H, Sonigo C, Sifer C and Grynberg M 2016 Freezingoocytes or embryos after controlled ovarian hyperstimulation in cancer patients: the state-of-the-art *Future Oncol* **12** 1731–41

[220] Kamphuis E(for the Evidence Based IVF Group) 2014 Are we overusing IVF? *Bri. Med.* J **348** 252

[221] Menkveld R 2001 Semen parameters, including WHO and strict criteria morphology, in a fertile and subfertile population: an effort towards standardization of *in vivo* thresholds *Hum. Reprod.* **16** 1165–71

[222] Gunalp S, Onculoglu C, Gurgan T, Kruger T F and Lombard C J 2001 A study of seme parameters with emphasis on sperm morphology in a fertile population:an attempt to develop clinical thresholds *Hum. Reprod.* **16** 110–4

[223] Tomlinson M J 2010 Validation of a novel computer-assisted sperm analysis (CASA) system using multitarget-tracking algorithms *Fertil. Steril.* **93** 1911–20

[224] Jayaprakasan K 2007 Does 3D ultrasound offer any advantage in the pretreatment assessment of ovarian reserve and prediction of outcome after assisted reproduction treatment? *Hum. Reprod.* **22** 1932–41

[225] Allersma T, Farquhar C and Cantineau A E 2013 Natural cycle *in vitro* fertilisation (IVF) for subfertile couples *Cochrane Database Syst. Rev.* **2013** CD010550

[226] Bodri D 2017 *Natural Cycle IVF with Spontaneous LH Surge Development of* In Vitro *Maturation for Human Oocytes* ed R C Chian, G Nargund and J Huang (Cham: Springer)

[227] Matsuura T, Takehara Y, Kaijima H, Teramoto S and Kato O 2008 Natural IVF cycles may be desirable for women with repeated failures by stimulated IVF cycles *J. Assist. Reprod. Genet* **25** 163–7

[228] Shaulov T, Vélez M P, Buzaglo K, Phillips S J and Kadoch I J 2015 Outcomes of 1503 cycles of modified natural cycle *in vitro* fertilization: a single-institution experience *J. Assist. Reprod. Genet* **32** 1043–8

[229] Kadoch I J, Phillips S J and Bissonnette F 2011 Modified natural-cycle *in vitro* fertilization should be considered as the first approach in young poor responders *Fertil. Steril.* **96** 1066–8

[230] Pelinck M J, Hoek A, Simons A H *et al* 1995 Efficacy of natural cycle IVF: a review of the literature. 2002 *Database of Abstracts of Reviews of Effects (DARE): Quality-assessed Reviews* (York: Centre for Reviews and Dissemination (UK)) https://ncbi.nlm.nih.gov/books/NBK69177/

[231] Allersma T, Farquhar C and Cantineau A E 2013 Natural cycle *in vitro* fertilisation (IVF) for subfertile couples *Cochrane Database Syst. Rev.* **2013** CD010550

[232] Pelinck M J, Hoek A, Simons A H and Heineman M J 2002 Efficacy of natural cycle IVF: a review of the literature *Hum. Reprod. Update* **8** 129–39

[233] Jirge P R, Patil M M, Gutgutia R, Shah J, Govindarajan M, Roy V S, Kaul-Mahajan N and Sharara F I 2022 Ovarian stimulation in assisted reproductive technology cycles for varied patient profiles: an indian perspective *J. Hum. Reprod. Sci.* **15** 112–25

[234] Baerwald A R, Walker R A and Pierson R A 2009 Growth rates of ovarian follicles during natural menstrual cycles, oral contraception cycles, and ovarian stimulation cycles *Fertil. Steril.* **91** 440–9

[235] Ferraretti A P, Gianaroli L, Magli M C and Devroey P 2015 Mild ovarian stimulation with clomiphene citrate launch is a realistic option for *in vitro* fertilization *Fertil. Steril.* **104** 333–8

[236] Segawa T, Kato K, Miyauchi O, Kawachiya S, Takehara Y and Kato O 2007 Evaluation of minimal stimulation IVF with clomiphene citrate and hMG *Fertil. Steril.* **88** S286

[237] Verberg M F 2009 The clinical significance of the retrieval of a low number of oocytes following mild ovarian stimulation for IVF: a meta-analysis *Hum. Reprod. Update* **15** 5–12

[238] Frederikke B L, Gitte J A and Svend L 2013 Low ovarian stimulation using Tamoxifen/FSH compared to conventional IVF: a cohort comparative study in conventional IVF treatments *Reprod. Syst. Sex Disord* **S5** 005

[239] Gurgan T and Demirol A 2004 Why and how should multiple pregnancies be prevented in assisted reproduction treatment programmes? *Reprod. Biomed. Online* **9** 237–44

[240] Le Lannou D, Griveau J F, Laurent M C, Gueho A, Veron E and Morcel K 2006 Contribution of embryo cryopreservation to elective single embryo transfer in IVF–ICSI *Reprod. Biomed Online* **13** 368–75

[241] Ghobara T and Vanderkerchove P 2017 Cycle regimens for frozen-thawed embryo transfer The Cochrane Library (www.cochrane.org/CD003414/MENSTR_cycle-regimens-frozen-thawed-embryo-transfer) (Accessed 17 September 2017)

[242] Weissman A, Levin D, Ravhon A, Eran H and Golan A L 2009 What is the preferred method for timing natural cycle frozen–thawed embryo transfer? *Reprod. Biomed. Online* **19** 66–71

[243] Salama S, Torre A, Paillusson B, Thomin A, Ben Brahim F, Muratorio C, Bailly M and Wainer R 2011 Ovarian stimulation monitoring: past, present and perspectives *Gynecol. Obstet. Fertil.* **39** 245–54

[244] Ritchie W G 1985 Ultrasound in the evaluation of normal and induced ovulation *Fertil. Steril.* **43** 167–81

[245] Odell W V D, Ross G T and Rayford P L 1967 Radioimmunoassay for luteinizing hormone in human plasma or serum: physiological studies *J. Clin. Investig* **46** 248–55

[246] Lossl K, Andersen A N, Loft A, Freiesleben N L, Bangsboll S and Andersen C Y 2006 Androgen priming using aromatase inhibitor and hCG during early-follicular-phase GnRH antagonist down-regulation in modified antagonist protocols *Hum. Reprod.* **21** 2593–600

[247] Durnerin C I 2008 Effects of recombinant LH treatment on folliculogenesis and responsiveness to FSH stimulation *Hum. Reprod.* **23** 421–6

[248] Gembruch U, Diedrich K, Welker B, Wahode J, van der Ven H, Al-Hasani S and Krebs D 1988 Transvaginal sonographically guided oocyte retrieval for *in vitro* fertilization *Hum. Reprod.* **3** 59–63

[249] Wiseman D A, Short W B, Pattinson H A, Taylor P J, Nicholson S F, Elliott P D, Fleetham J A and Mortimer S T 1989 Oocyte retrieval in an *in vitro* fertilization- embryo transfer program: comparison of four methods *Radiology* **173** 99–102

[250] Knight D C, Tyler J P and Driscoll G L 2001 Follicular flushing at oocyte retrieval: a reappraisal *Aust. N. Z. J. Obstet. Gynaecol* **41** 210–3

[251] Hill M J and Levens E D 2010 Is there a benefit in follicular flushing in assisted reproductive technology? *Curr. Opin. Obstet. Gynecol.* **22** 208–12

[252] Nezhat F 2003 Triumphs and controversies in laparoscopy: the past, the present, and the future *JSLS* **7** 151–5

[253] Kaiser A M and Corman M L 2001 History of laparoscopy *Surg. Oncol. Clin. N. Am* **10** 483–92

[254] Dubois F, Icard P, Berthelot G and Levard H 1990 Coelioscopic cholecystectomy. Preliminary report of 36 cases *Ann. Surg.* **211** 60–2

[255] Kelley W E 2003 Surgical robotics: vascular surgery applications *Probl. Gen. Surg.* **20** 65–72

[256] Kelley W E 2008 The evolution of laparoscopy and the revolution in surgery in the decade of the 1990s *JSLS* **12** 351–7

[257] Quinn P, Barros C and Whittingham D G 1982 Preservation of hamster oocytes assay the fertilizing capacity of human spermatozoa *J. Reprod. Fertil* **66** 161–8

[258] Henke R R and Schill W B 2003 Sperm preparation for ART Reprod *Biol. Endocrinol.* **1** 108

[259] Harris L H 2006 *Challenging Conception: A Clinical and Cultural History of* in vitro *Fertilization in the United States* (University of Michigan)

[260] Bärnreuther S 2016 Innovations 'out of place': controversies over IVF beginnings in India between 1978 and 2005 *Med. Anthropol.* **35** 73–89

[261] Simon A, Safran A, Revel A, Aizenman E, Reubinoff B, Porat-Katz A, Lewin A and Laufer N 2003 Hyaluronic acid can successfully replace albumin as the sole macromolecule in a human embryo transfer medium *Fertil. Steril.* **79** 1434–8

[262] Kim S M and Kim J S 2017 A review of mechanisms of implantation *Dev. Reprod.;* **21** 351–9

[263] Choe J and Shanks A L 2023 *In Vitro Fertilization* (Treasure Island, FL: StatPearls Publishing)

[264] Leese H J 1988 The formation and function of oviduct fluid *J. Reprod. Fertil* **82** 843–56

[265] Stojkovic M 2002 Effects of high concentrations of hyaluronan in culture medium on development and survival rates of fresh and frozen-thawed bovine embryos produced *in vitro Reproduction* **124** 141–53

[266] Stojkovic M, Kölle S, Peinl S, Stojkovic P, Zakhartchenko V, Thompson J G, Wenigerkind H, Reichenbach H D, Sinowatz F and Wolf E 2002 Effects of high concentrations of hyaluronan in culture medium on development and survival rates of fresh and frozen-thawed bovine embryos produced *in vitro Reproduction* **124** 141–53

[267] Singh N, Gupta M, Kriplani A and Vanamail P 2015 Role of embryo glue as a transfer medium in the outcome of fresh non-donor in-vitro fertilization cycles *J. Hum. Reprod. Sci.* **8** 214–7

[268] Gardner D K, Lane M W and Lane M 2000 EDTA stimulates cleavage stage bovine embryo development in culture but inhibits blastocyst development and differentiation *Mol. Reprod. Dev.* **57** 256–6

[269] Mansour R T and Aboulghar M A 2002 Optimizing the embryo transfer technique *Hum. Reprod.* **17** 1149–53

[270] Moini A, Kiani K, Bahmanabadi A, Akhoond M and Akhlaghi A 2011 Improvement in pregnancy rate by removal of cervical discharge prior to embryo transfer in ICSI cycles: a randomised clinical trial *Aust. N Z J. Obstet. Gynaecol.* **51** 315–20

[271] Waterstone J, Curson R and Parsons J 1991 Embryo transfer to low uterine cavity *Lancet* **337** 1413

[272] Simon A and Laufer N 2012 Assessment and treatment of repeated implantation failure (RIF) *J. Assist. Reprod. Genet.* **29** 1227–39

[273] McCue P M 1996 Superovulation *Vet. Clin. North Am.: Equine Pract.* **12** 1–11

[274] Takeo T and Nakagata N 2015 Superovulation using the combined administration of inhibin antiserum and equine chorionic gonadotropin increases the number of ovulated oocytes in C57BL/6 female mice *PLoS One* **10** e0128330

[275] Gemzell C A, Diczfalusy E and Tillinger G 1958 Clinical effect of human pituitary follicle-stimulating hormone (FSH) *J. Clin. Endocrinol. Metab* **18** 1333–48

[276] Hirayama H, Kageyama S, Moriyasu S, Sawai K and Minamihashi A 2013 Embryo sexing and sex chromosomal chimerism analysis by loop-mediated isothermal amplification in cattle and water buffaloes *J. Reprod. Dev* **59** 321–6

[277] Illmensee K and Levanduski M 2010 Embryo splitting *Mid. East Fertil. Soc. J.* **15** 57–63

[278] Park J H, Lee J H, Choi K M, Joung S Y, Kim J Y, Chung G M and Im K S 2001 Rapid sexing of preimplantation bovine embryo using consecutive and multiplex polymerase chain reaction (PCR) with biopsied single blastomere *Theriogenology* **55** 1843–53

[279] Meraï A, Dattena M, Casu S, Rekik M and Lassoued N 2017 High-milking sheep have a lower ovulation rate and tend to yield fewer embryos in response to superovulation and intrauterine artificial insemination *Reprod. Domest. Anim.* **52** 814–8

[280] Hasler J F 2003 The current status and future of commercial embryo transfer in cattle *Anim. Reprod. Sci.* **79** 245–64

[281] Kraemer D C 1983 Intra- and interspecific embryo transfer *J. Exp. Zool* **228** 363–71

[282] Scenna F N, Hockett M E, Towns T M, Saxton A M, Rohrbach N R, Wehrman M E and Schrick F N 2005 Influence of a prostaglandin synthesis inhibitor administered at embryo transfer on pregnancy rates of recipient cows *Prostaglandins Other Lipid Mediat.* **78** 38–45

[283] Hayakawa H, Hirai T, Takimotoa A, Ideta A and Aoyagi Y 2009 Superovulation and embryo transfer in Holstein cattle using sexed sperm *Theriogenology* **71** 68–73

[284] Saragusty J and Arav A 2011 Current progress in oocyte and embryo cryopreservation by slow freezing and vitrification *Reproduction* **141** 1–19

[285] Bertipaglia E C A, Roberto Gomes da Silva Cardoso V and Fries L A 2007 Hair coat characteristics and sweating rate of braford cows in brazil *Livest. Sci.* **112** 99–108

[286] Bagath M, Krishnan G, Devaraj C, Rashamol V P, Pragna P, Lees A M and Sejian V 2019 The impact of heat stress on the immune system in dairy cattle: a review *Res. Vet. Sci.* **126** 94–102

IOP Publishing

Introduction to Pharmaceutical Biotechnology, Volume 1
(Second Edition)
Basic techniques and concepts
Ahmed Al-Harrasi, Saif Hameed, Zeeshan Fatima and Saurabh Bhatia

Chapter 4

Applications of stem cells in disease and gene therapy

Arshi Waseem and Syed Shadab Raza

Advancements in gene and stem cell therapy have greatly increased the range of therapeutic choices available to patients who were previously dealing with untreatable diseases and disorders. The growing significance of gene therapy and transplantation based on stem cells in the field of regenerative medicine is especially remarkable. Stem cells have the capacity to differentiate into a variety of cell types in the human body's three germ layers, making them highly valuable for therapeutic purposes. This chapter presents a current summary of the most recent clinical uses of stem cells obtained from several sources, such as bone marrow (BM), adipose tissue (AT), and the umbilical cord (UC), in treating a range of human illnesses. The investigated conditions include respiratory problems, skin burns, neurological disorders, pulmonary dysfunctions, metabolic/endocrine-related diseases, and reproductive abnormalities. Research on stem cells has advanced and opened up new possibilities for using cells to cure diseases that have been unresponsive to conventional therapies. Stem cells possess extraordinary potential for unlimited self-renewal and the aptitude to develop into many types of cells, making them a revolutionary presence in the field of regenerative medicine. The prospective applications of regenerative medicine rely on the innate transdifferentiating capacity of stem cells, which represents a dynamic and promising frontier in medical progress.

4.1 Introduction

Developments in biochemistry and molecular biology have helped us to understand the genetic basis of inherited diseases. The basic goal is to replace defective genes with good ones and finally cure genetic disorders. Gene therapy is the process of introducing genes into cells to treat diseases. The newly inserted genes will encode proteins and correct the deficiencies that occur in genetic diseases. Therefore, gene

doi:10.1088/978-0-7503-5382-3ch4

therapy primarily entails genetic manipulation in animals or humans to correct a disease, and keep the organism in good health. The initial experiments of gene therapy were carried out in animals and then later in humans. An outline of gene therapy approaches is shown in figure 4.1. The ability to transfect genes into a cell and to cause their expression has resulted in the practical emergence of human gene therapy, where functionally active genes are putatively introduced into the (somatic) cells of a person requiring the expression of a given protein. A novel version of gene therapy is the transfection of cells with non-resident genes in an attempt to accomplish *in situ* expression of a pharmacologically beneficial protein or create a site for further therapeutic intervention. It involves inserting functionally active genes into cells for specific protein production, or transfecting cells with non-resident genes to produce a therapeutic target or induce a helpful protein *in situ.* Alternatively, genes can act like drugs, generating a product with a particular pharmacological effect. In general terms, gene therapy entails the insertion of genetic material into a patient's cells to make them capable of producing a therapeutic protein. Currently, gene therapy has gone beyond its original definition [1]. Gene therapy has provided a chance to fight the root level cause of a disease rather than its symptoms. Almost 45 000 human diseases have been reported to be related directly to genetic disorders. So far various approaches have been adopted to treat genetic disorders such as enzyme storage disease or cystic fibrosis, or more to replace a missing protein. Additionally, gene therapy paves the way to either replace the missing or defective gene at the origin or arrest undesired gene expression (viral and oncogene expression) at the origin. Genetic medicines are usually based on gene expression systems that contain a therapeutic gene and a delivery system. A gene delivery system regulates the distribution and access of a gene expression unit to the target tissue, its recognition by cell surface receptors and its intracellular trafficking. With the development of gene manipulation it has now become possible to splice

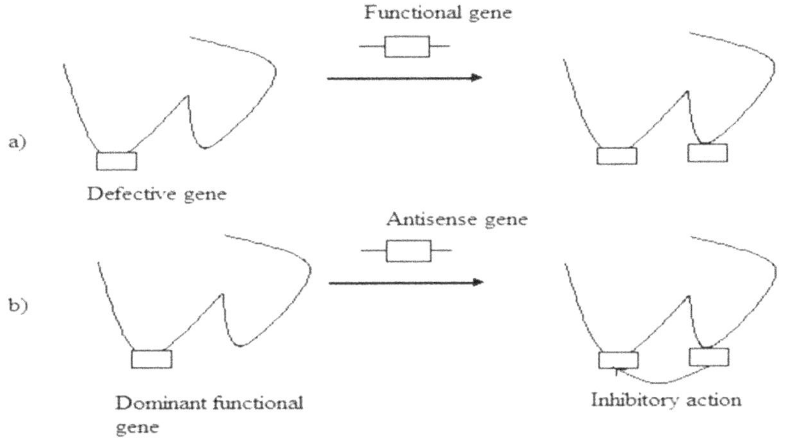

Figure 4.1. Overview of the two major gene therapy strategies, (a) gene augmentation therapy and (b) gene inhibition therapy.

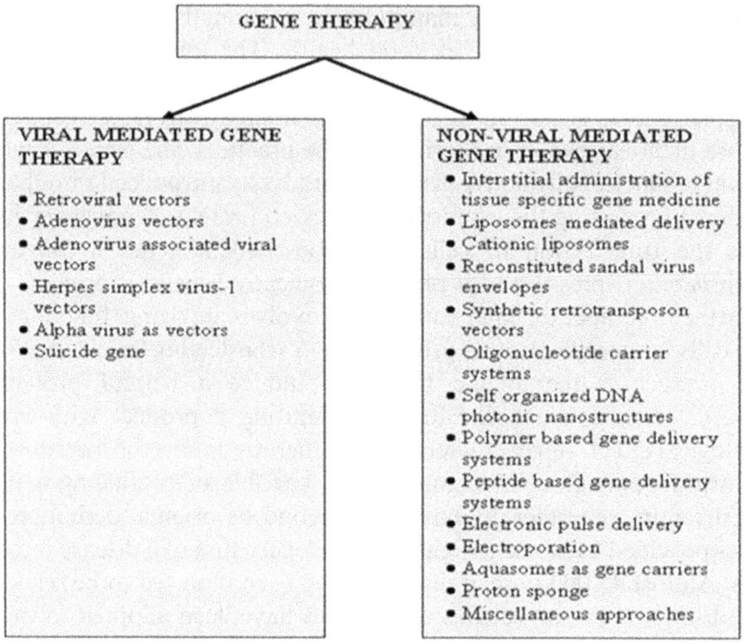

Figure 4.2. Major classification of gene therapies.

and insert human genes into viral or bacterial genomes where the latter is known as a vector. The procedure is fundamentally based on rDNA technology which facilitates the isolation of genes and their subsequent use in the production of respective proteins, as well as engineering them to be a corrective gene system. It is remarkable to note that therapeutic protein expressions have their mode of action by being in the bloodstream and exercising their effect from here. There remain some constraining factors in effective delivery, such as cell-specific gene or genome delivery. Gene therapy techniques are broadly divided into two categories, viral-mediated and non-viral-mediated, as illustrated in figure 4.2.

4.2 Types of gene therapy

Gene therapy mostly comes in two forms: one involves transferring a DNA fragment to any body cell, depending on cells that do not generate sperm or eggs; the other involves transferring a gene into cells that belong to sperm or eggs. There are numerous approaches for correcting defective genes; the most common being the insertion of a normal gene into a specific location within the genome to substitute a non-functional gene. Based on this parameter gene therapy is further classified into the following two types [2, 3]:

- Somatic gene therapy.
- Germline gene therapy.

4.2.1 Somatic gene therapy

The non-reproductive cells of an organism are known as somatic cells and include cells other than sperm or egg cells (e.g. bone marrow cells, blood cells, etc). In order to express therapeutic gene products, somatic gene therapy entails introducing novel genetic material into somatic cells. There is a lot of hope for treating inherited and acquired disorders with this new technology. Currently, all the research on gene therapy is based on the correction of genetic defects in somatic cells by introducing fully functional and expressible genes into a target somatic cell to correct a genetic disease permanently. During somatic gene therapy, the somatic cells of an individual are targeted for foreign gene transfer. In this procedure the subsequent effects caused by the foreign gene are limited to the individual patient only, and not inherited by the patient's offspring or next generations [3].

4.2.2 Germline gene therapy

Germ cells are the reproductive cells of an organism constituting the germ cell line. They encompass the introduction of DNA into germ cells which always results in the passing of traits to the next generation [2]. In this procedure, the functional genes which are to be inserted into the genomes are inserted into the germ cells, i.e. sperm or eggs. Targeting of germ cells makes the therapy heritable. Through germline gene therapy, a person's genetic variations in their reproductive cells can be corrected, and this correction will be handed down to subsequent generations. With this treatment, a genetic condition is permanently eliminated from a family line. Humans can have genetic diseases, which may be inherited from germline cells. For safety, ethical and technical reasons, germ cell gene therapy is not being attempted at present. As gene therapy involves great risk, there are different regulatory agencies whose consent must be acquired before undertaking any work related to gene therapy. Several genetic disorders and other diseases are now at various stages of gene therapy trials.

4.3 Techniques for gene therapy

When gene therapy first emerged, its primary meaning was the insertion of an exogenous complementary DNA (cDNA) copy into specific tissues or cells in order to replace or fix malfunctioning endogenous genes. Gene therapy has evolved to concentrate on changing the genetic information causing a disease or regulating the expression of a particular gene as a result of advancements in detection and technology.

4.3.1 Gene augmentation therapy (GAT)

Gene augmentation therapy (GAT) is the process by which DNA is added to the genome in order to replace a missing gene product (figure 4.3). Gene augmentation and/or gene knockdown is targeted at altering gene expression in the context of a loss-of-function mutation by incorporating the wild-type cDNA [4] or decreasing expression of or removing a toxic gain-of-function gene product [5–7]. GAT is often limited by a narrow therapeutic window due to the advanced nature of the disease,

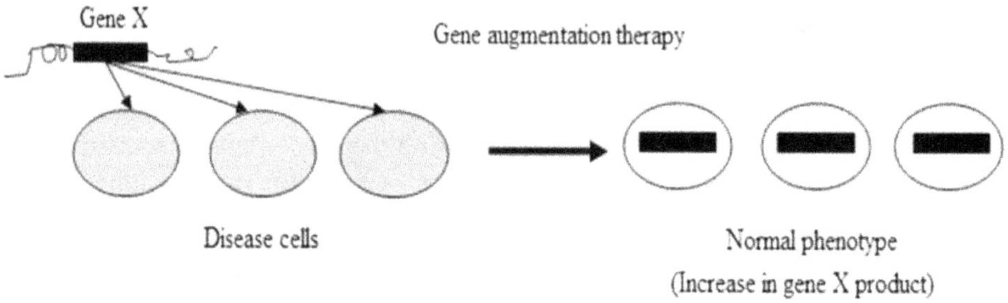

Figure 4.3. Schematic representation of a gene therapy vector that has been designed to treat the disease cells with a gene X. This vector was presented inside the disease cells by various gene transfer methods. After a successful HR the treated cells will show the presence of gene X products as well as a normal phenotype.

whereby the therapeutic target cell often degenerates and dies. When diseases are caused by loss of function of a gene, incorporating extra copies of the normal gene may possibly increase the total number of normal gene products to a level where the normal phenotype is restored (figure 4.3). Consequently GAT is targeted at clinical disorders where the pathological process is reversible. It also supports having no specific requirement for expression levels of the presented gene and a clinical response at low expression levels. GAT has been mainly applied to autosomal recessive disorders where even uncertain expression levels of an introduced gene may make a considerable difference. Autosomal dominant inheritance is much less responsive to treatment: gain-of-function mutations (dominant or semidominant) are not curable by this approach and, even if there is a loss-of-function mutation, high expression efficiency of the incorporated gene is required: individuals with 50% of normal gene product are normally affected, and so the challenge is to increase the amount of gene product towards normal levels. Basically, GAT is the addition of functional alleles to cure inherited disorders caused by genetic deficiency of a gene product, so GAT has been applied to autosomal recessive disorders. Dominantly inherited disorders are much less responsive to GAT.

4.3.2 Targeted killing of specific cells

This approach is popular in treating different types of cancers. In this process genes encoding toxic compounds (suicide genes), or prodrugs (reagents which confer sensitivity to subsequent treatment with a drug) are utilized to kill the transfected/ transformed cells [8]. Approaches that aim to remedy a deficiency by delivering a transgene that encodes a functional gene product to the cell are in contrast to targeted gene treatments. This is sometimes called 'gene replacement therapy,' despite the fact that a gene that expresses the missing gene product is used to complement the function of the damaged gene rather than actually replacing it. Genes are fixed to the target cells and then allowed to express so as to cause cell killing. Direct cell killing is only possible if the incorporated genes are expressed to produce a lethal toxin (suicide genes), or a gene encoding a prodrug is incorporated, conferring susceptibility to killing by a subsequently administered drug [8]. Otherwise, selectively lytic viruses can be used. Indirect cell killing uses immune-stimulatory genes

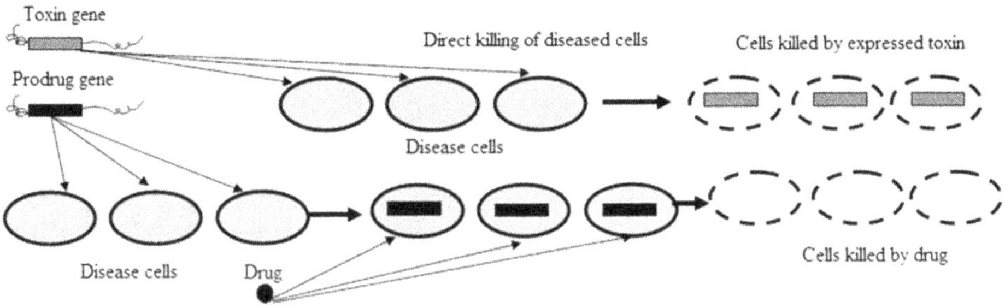

Figure 4.4. Direct killing of disease cells by two techniques. The first method is the incorporation of a toxin gene into a diseased cell so that when it expresses the toxic protein the cells die. The second method includes insertion of a certain gene (e.g. TK) into the gene therapy vector which displays a suicidal property on introducing certain drugs (e.g. GCV).

to aggravate an immune response against the target cell. This process is shown in figure 4.4.

4.3.3 Targeted inhibition of gene expression

This is done to hinder the expression of any diseased gene or a new gene from expressing a protein which is damaging for a cell [9]. It is mainly suitable for treating infectious disorders and some cancers. If disease cells show a novel gene product or inappropriate expression of a gene (as in the case of many cancers, infectious diseases, etc), a range of different systems can be used to block the expression of a single gene at the DNA, RNA or protein levels. RNA interference (RNAi) and U1 small nuclear RNA interference (snRNAi) are two methods for inhibiting gene expression. The foundation of U1i is U1 inhibitors (U1in), which are modified U1 snRNA molecules that prevent a target pre-mRNA from being polyadenylated. Allele-specific inhibition of expression may be promising in some cases, allowing treatments for some disorders ensuing from dominant-negative effects [9]. The case in figure 4.5 shows alteration of a mutation in a mutant gene by HR; but mutation correction may also be possible at the RNA level. The figure depicts the protocol involved in targeted inhibition of gene expression.

4.3.4 Targeted gene mutation correction

Targeted gene mutation correction is introduced to correct a faulty gene and restore its function, which can be done at the genetic level by HR or at the mRNA level by using therapeutic ribozymes or therapeutic RNA editing [10]. If an inherited mutation generates a dominant-negative effect, gene amplification is unlikely to help. As an alternative the resident mutation must be altered. By offering a template for homology-directed repair, targeted gene correction enables the cell's own repair mechanisms to eliminate the mutation and swap it out for the proper sequence. The illness gene is ablated by targeted gene disruption, rendering it inoperable. Due to the practical difficulties, this strategy has yet to be applied; nevertheless, in principle, it can be achieved at various levels, at the gene level (e.g. by gene targeting methods

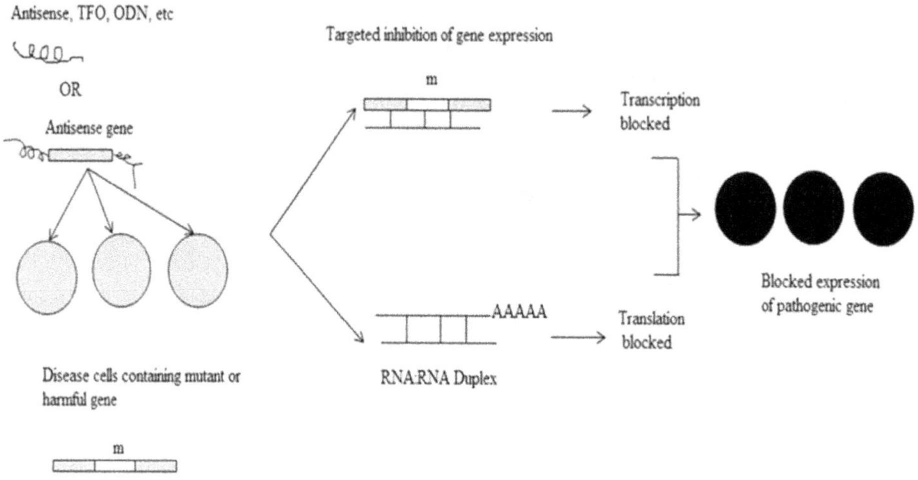

Figure 4.5. To prevent the target expression in diseased cells the antisense mRNA coding gene inserted vector triplex-forming oligonucleotides (TFOs) or antisense oligonucleotides (ODNs) can be incorporated, which will prevent the gene expression either by forming a DNA:RNA triplex inside the nucleus or forming an RNA: RNA duplex by creating a complementary mRNA strand of disease protein coding mRNA.

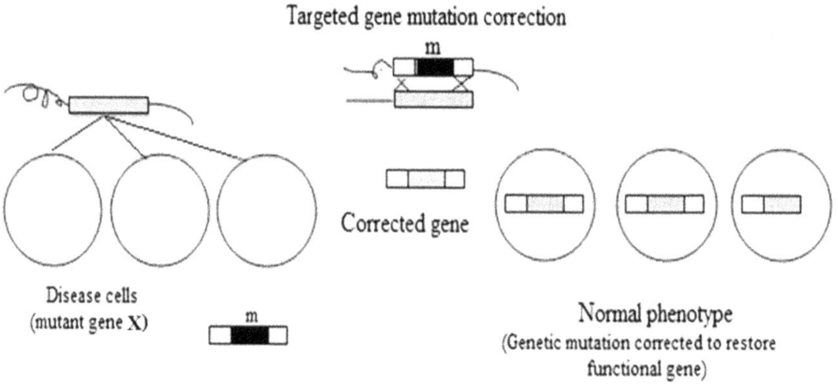

Figure 4.6. Targeted gene mutation correction (used for diseases caused by mutation). The corrected gene is swapped for the mutant gene (X). The diseased cells become normal after the correction of the mutation by gene therapy.

based on HR) or at the RNA transcript level (e.g. by using specific types of therapeutic ribozymes or therapeutic RNA editing) [10]. The protocol involved in targeted inhibition of gene expression is shown in figure 4.6.

4.4 Methods of gene therapy

There are two main approaches to the transfer of genes in gene therapy: *ex vivo* and *in vivo* gene therapy [11]. *Ex vivo* gene therapy involves the transfer of genes into cultured cells (e.g. bone marrow cells), which are then reintroduced into the patient [11].

However, *in vivo* gene therapy is done by the direct delivery of genes into the cells of a particular tissue. In short:

- Direct gene transfer to bodily cells (*in vivo* gene therapy).
- Gene transfer (*ex vivo* gene therapy) into patient cells external to the body.

4.4.1 *In vivo* gene therapy

Put simply, direct delivery of the therapeutic genes into the targeted cells of a particular tissue of a patient constitutes *in vivo* gene therapy [11]. Many tissues are potential candidates for this approach, e.g. liver, muscle, skin, spleen, lung, brain and blood cells. Gene delivery can be done by viral or non-viral vector systems. This method of gene transfer encompasses the transfer of cloned genes directly into the tissues of the patient [11]. As demonstrated by the recent approval of multiple *in vivo* gene therapy products for commercialization, for a growing number of diseases, *in vivo* genetic engineering has emerged as a potentially effective new therapeutic option. As long as the techniques are applied directly to patients, *in vivo* genetic engineering includes both the more modern genome/epigenome editing techniques and viral vector-mediated gene transfer. This is done in the case of tissues whose individual cells cannot be cultured *in vitro* in adequate numbers (e.g. brain cells) and/or where re-implantation of the cultured cells in the patient is not efficient. For this purpose, liposomes and certain viral vectors are employed because of the absence of any other mode of selection. In the case of viral vectors, cultured cells which have been infected with the recombinant retrovirus *in vitro* to regularly produce modified viral vectors are often used. These cultured cells are called vector-producing cells (VPCs). The VPCs transfer the gene to surrounding disease cells. The competence of gene transfer and expression governs the success of this approach, because of the lack of any way for selection and amplification of cells which take up and express the foreign gene. The major differences between *in vivo* and *ex vivo* gene therapy are listed in table 4.1. The various steps of gene transfer are shown in figure 4.7.

4.4.2 *Ex vivo* gene therapy

In this mode of gene therapy genes are transferred to cells grown in culture; the transformed cells are selected, multiplied and then introduced into the patient [12]. *Ex vivo* gene therapy can only be applied to selected tissues whose cells can be cultured in the laboratory. In this procedure, the patient's own cells are used for

Table 4.1. Differences between *in vivo* and *ex vivo* gene therapy.

In vivo	*Ex vivo*
Decreased control over target cells	Close control possible
Less invasive	More invasive
Safety check not possible	Safety check possible
Technically simple	Technically complex
Vectors introduced directly	No vectors introduced directly

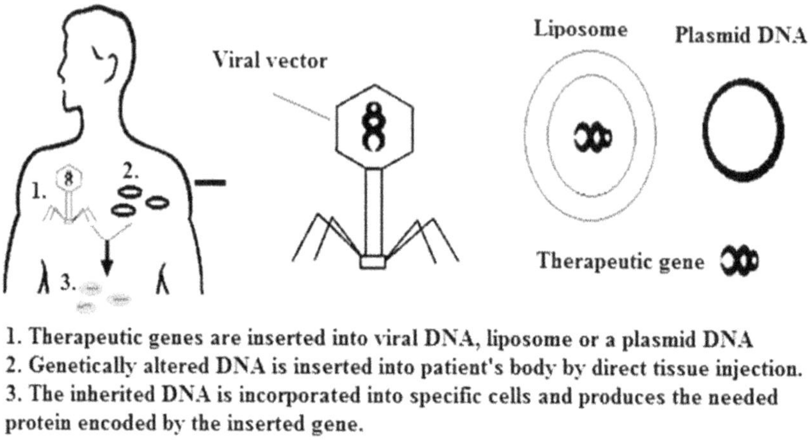

Viral vector
Liposome
Plasmid DNA
1.
2.
3.
Therapeutic gene
1. Therapeutic genes are inserted into viral DNA, liposome or a plasmid DNA
2. Genetically altered DNA is inserted into patient's body by direct tissue injection.
3. The inherited DNA is incorporated into specific cells and produces the needed protein encoded by the inserted gene.

Figure 4.7. Schematic representation of the various steps of gene transfer.

culture and genetic correction, and then returned back to the patient. Thus the technique does not produce any adverse immunological reaction after transplanting cells. The success of this procedure depends on stable and continuous expression of therapeutic genes [12]. A novel treatment approach called *ex vivo* gene therapy is particularly well-suited for treating a single organ as opposed to the entire body. This can be achieved by the use of vectors. The use of autologous cells circumvents immune system rejection of the introduced cells. The cells are sourced initially from the patient to be treated and grown in culture before being reintroduced into the same individual. This method can be applied to tissues such as hematopoietic cells and skin cells which can be easily detached from the body, genetically modified outside the body and reinserted into the patient body where they become engrafted and survive for a long period of time. Figure 4.8 shows an easily understood schematic diagram for *ex vivo* gene transfer.

4.5 Methods of gene therapy

The objective of gene therapy is to introduce new genetic material into target cells without toxicity to non-target tissues. Gene therapy has tremendous potential and can be used against various forms of cancers. For cancer treatment gene therapy can be employed to target cancer cells while sparing normal tissues. Such an approach may be useful for recurrent disease as well as in the adjuvant setting. Yet, while gene therapy holds great promise, progress in developing effective clinical protocols has been slow. The main problem lies in the development of safe and effective gene delivery systems. With the purpose of targeting cells and manufacturing the protein products via the introduced gene, the exogenous genetic material must be introduced into the cell's nucleus. This method of transfection is divided into two classes of vectors: viral and non-viral. The viral technique is related to enhance technical demands and a great risk of virus-related toxicity. Nevertheless, viral vectors have been designed for safety by making their replication useless. It is the viral ability to

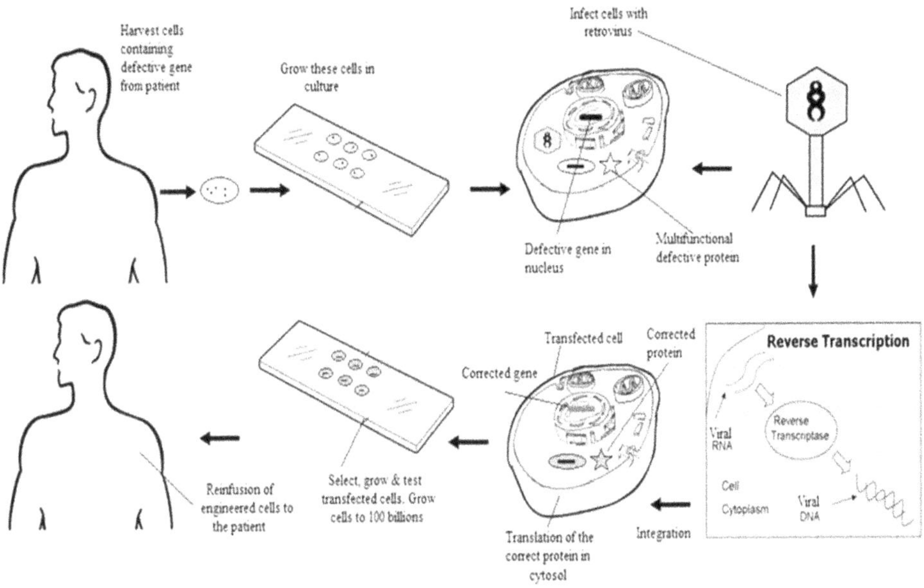

Figure 4.8. Schematic representation of *ex vivo* gene transfer which involves cellular manipulation in harvested cells.

efficiently infect cells and in this procedure to integrate DNA into the host genome without causing an immune response that makes viruses suitable as vectors. These modified viruses can be proliferated in cell lines specialized to offer the essential absent viral functions [13, 14]. Genetic material can be transferred via a vector called the vehicle, which is employed to deliver the GOI. A perfect vector would transfer a defined amount of genetic material into each target cell, thus permitting expression of the gene product without producing toxicity. A perfect vector should transfer the gene to a specific cell type, house foreign genes of adequate size, attain the level and duration of transgenic expression satisfactory to correct the defect, and be non-immunogenic and safe [15]. Gene transfer through viral vectors is known as transduction, but transfer through non-viral vectors is known as transfection [16]. Various approaches have been attempted for active transfer of genes to suitable target sites. These approaches mostly fall into four types, as shown in figure 4.9.

4.5.1 Conventional gene therapy

Conventional gene therapy, referred to as gene addition, usually encompasses introducing new genes [17]. Generally, a harmless virus is altered with the gene to be incorporated, and this 'viral vector' is mixed with cells from the patient *in vitro*. The virus enters cells and introduces the genetic material into the cells' DNA, after which the cells are transferred into the patient. Conversely, gene editing is more characterized by the fact that in a molecular cut-and-paste, scientists cut out the defective DNA sequence and then incorporate a fragment of laboratory-created

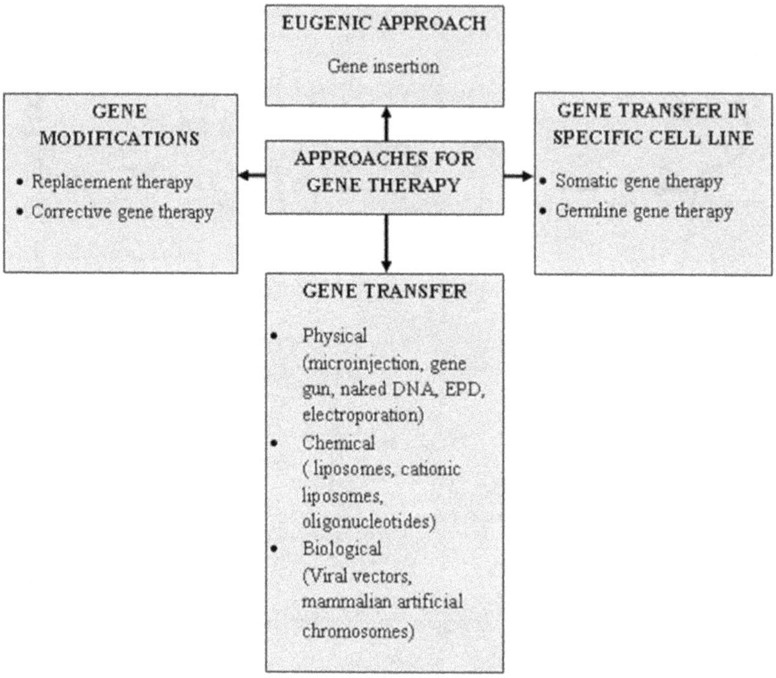

Figure 4.9. Gene therapy approaches mostly fall into four types.

DNA [17]. In both methods, the altered DNA dictates the formation of a normal, working protein. It encompasses therapeutic gene delivery and their optimum expression once inside the target cell. Because there is not a commonly recognized framework for the risk assessment procedure, biosafety specialists are essential in overseeing gene therapy research methods, estimating risk, and formulating suitable regulations. The creation of novel experimental viral vectors and developing technology serve as examples of this. The foreign genes carry out the following functions:

- Yield a toxin so that a diseased cell is killed.
- Yield a product (protein) that the patient lacks.
- Helps in destroying unhealthy cells, stimulate immune system cells.

4.5.2 Non-classical gene therapy

This encompasses the inhibition of the expression of genes linked to pathogenesis, or to correct a genetic defect and restore normal gene expression.

4.6 Vectors for gene therapy

The carrier particles or molecules used to deliver genes to somatic cells are known as vectors. Gene therapy usually encompasses the insertion of a functional gene into cells to alter a cellular dysfunction or to provide a new cellular function, such as in the case of diseases such as cystic fibrosis, combined immunodeficiency syndromes,

Table 4.2. Vectors used in gene therapy. Direct gene transfer approaches such as mechanical, electroporation or gene gun methods are also used to transfer genes into target cells.

Viral vector	Non-viral vectors
Adeno-associated virus	Peptide/protein
Adenovirus	Liposomes
Herpes simplex virus	
Lentivirus	Polymers
Retrovirus	Lipid complex
Vaccinia virus	

muscular dystrophy, hemophilia and many cancers resulting from the occurrence of defective genes [12]. In essence, vectors are vehicles created to introduce therapeutic genetic material—like a functional gene—directly into a cell. Adenoviral, lentiviral, retroviral, and adeno-associated viral are the four primary types of viral vectors; each has distinct properties, and applications. Gene therapy can be used to correct or replace the defective genes. Gene therapy has been specifically successful in the treatment of combined immunodeficiency syndromes, displaying remarkable therapeutic benefits. Vectors for gene therapy (table 4.2) can be broadly classified into two types:

- Viral vectors.
- Non-viral vectors.

4.6.1 Viral-mediated gene delivery

The vectors frequently used in gene therapy are viruses, in particular retroviruses. RNA is the genetic material in retroviruses [12]. As the retrovirus enters the host cell, it produces DNA from RNA (by reverse transcription). The so-formed viral DNA (called a provirus) is incorporated into the DNA of the host cell. The proviruses are usually harmless. However, there is a great risk that some of the retroviruses can convert normal cells into cancerous ones. Consequently it is absolutely essential to ensure that such a thing does not happen. A number of researchers employ a certain biochemical method to convert harmful retroviruses to harmless ones, before using them as vectors, e.g. by artificially removing a gene that encodes for the viral envelope, the retroviruses can be crippled and made harmless [12]. This is because, without the envelope, the retrovirus cannot penetrate the host cell. The generation of a large number of viral particles can be achieved, starting from a single envelope defective retrovirus. All viral vector genomes have had portions of their genomes deleted in order to cause deranged replication, which increases their safety. However, the system has several issues, including their high immunogenicity, which induces an inflammatory response that results in the degeneration of transduced tissue, the production of toxins, including mortality and insertional mutagenesis, and their limited capacity for transgenic growth. This is only made possible by using

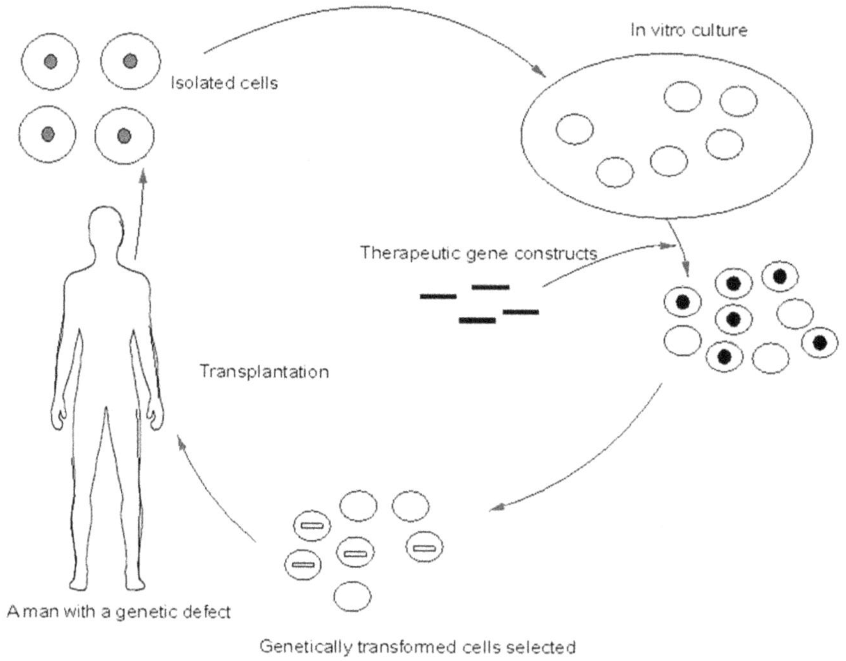

Figure 4.10. Procedure for *ex vivo* gene therapy.

helper viruses which contain the normal gene for envelope formation. Along with the helper virus, the vectors (with a defective envelope gene) can penetrate the host cell and both of them multiply. By repetitive proliferation in the host cell, billions of vector and helper viruses are produced. The vector can be isolated from the helper viruses and purified. Separation of vector viruses completely free from helper viruses is absolutely essential [12]. Infection by the helper virus is a great risk to the health of patients experiencing gene therapy.

Gene delivery has become much easier with the availability of numerous viral and non-viral delivery systems. Some of the viruses used as carriers include the Moloney murine leukemia virus, human immune deficiency virus, adenoviruses, AAV, HSV, Epstein–Barr virus, Sindbis virus, bovine and human papillomaviruses, hepatitis B virus, vaccinia virus and polyoma virus [12]. The delivery and the mechanism involved depend on the viral encoded proteins. The procedure for *ex vivo* gene therapy is demonstrated in figure 4.10. Various viral vectors used for gene therapy are listed in table 4.3.

4.6.2 Non-viral-mediated gene therapy

There are certain restrictions in using viral vectors in gene therapy. In addition to the high cost of maintaining the viruses, the viral proteins frequently induce inflammatory responses in the host [30]. Thus, there is a constant hunt by researchers to find replacements for viral vector systems. Currently, most of the approved clinical trials on gene therapy in human subjects have involved viral infection using

Table 4.3. Viral-based vectors used for gene therapy.

Vectors	Description
Retroviral vectors	Retroviruses are the usual means of delivering long-term gene therapy applications. Autologous bone marrow cells transduced *ex vivo* with gamma retrovirus vectors were utilized in the first human gene therapy trial. A retroviral vector actively inserts a genetic sequence into the host cell and multiplies in the host cell line for its own cloning. The mammalian retrovirus vectors usually used for gene transfer are categorized on the basis of their host range as they could be ecotropic, which only infects murine cells, or amphotropic, which infects both murine and non-murine cells [18, 19].
Adenovirus (AV) vectors	Adenovirus vectors are strongly immunogenic. An adenovirus vector, a non-enveloped dsDNA virus in contrast to the retrovirus, can be loaded with up to 36 kb DNA fragments and can be used *in vivo* transfection as it can also infect non-replicating cells. The AV gene remains episomal without insertion into the host genome, after gaining cell entry via endocytosis it successively releases into the cytoplasm, which eventually removes the possibility of insertional mutagenesis, the main problem with retroviral vectors [20–24]. Adenoviruses can infect an extensive variety of cell types and live AV has been used as a vaccine in US military personnel without any significant side effects [20–24].
Adenovirus associated viral (AAV) vectors	AAV is a non-pathogenic human parvovirus which has stimulated a lot of interest as a vector for gene therapy. The ability to create recombinant AAV particles—which lack viral genes but contain DNA sequences of interest for a range of therapeutic applications—has proven to be one of the safest methods of gene therapy to date. It contains a single strand of DNA infection [20–24]. It has been found that human AAV infection appears to be non-pathogenic with a majority of the population testing positive for AAV capsid protein antibodies. AAV is a dependovirus and requires a helper virus co-infection for viral replication [20–25].
HSV-1 vectors	Among the viral vectors, HSV-1 has potentially the largest DNA carrying capacity. It is capable of establishing long-term, non-cytopathic relationships with the neurons that it infects. Like AV, HSV-1 infects non-dividing cells. In addition, HSV does not generally integrate into the host geneome, providing an element of safety as there is little opportunity for insertional mutagenesis of infected cells. However, these viruses contain a genome of much greater complexity than the more retroviral gene transfer vector. This puts a considerable amount of difficulty into the development of these vectors. The ability of

	HSV-1 vectors to transfer more than 30 kbp of genetic payload to human cell nuclei is an exceptional characteristic [26].
Alpha viruses	Alpha viruses are an assembly of arthropod-borne Toga viruses that infect numerous types of host varying from mosquito to avian and mammalian species. The alpha virus genome comprises a single-stranded RNA molecule of positive polarity, i.e. a productive infection can be introduced either by infection or by transfection of a cell by the isolated RNA [27]. When alpha virus particles fuse with the plasma membrane, they are able to enter host cells and release RNA into the cytoplasm.
Epstein–Barr virus	Stable and long-term gene expressions are mandatory for certain applications that do not involve the integration of transferred DNA. For this, determined gene expression and episomal maintenance are essential [28].
Suicide gene	Suicide gene therapy is based on the insertion into tumor cells of a viral or a bacterial gene, which allows the conversion of a non-toxic compound into a lethal drug. Current research has shown that none of the DNA delivery systems existing could mediate a transfection into the cells *in vivo*. This is a major disadvantage in cases such as cancer where the treatment requires 100% selective delivery of therapeutic genes to tumor cells. By means of the suicide gene strategy's bystander effect, a small portion of the tumor cells express a suicide gene product. The system which now exists in a population of 1%–10% expresses a suicide product which transmits its toxic effect to the neighbouring tumor cells, which originally did not possess the suicide gene. Hence 100% killing of tumor cells is achieved. This approach usually involves the use of HSV-TK and cytosine deaminase [29].

viral-vector-mediated transfer [30]. In recent times, non-viral gene-based treatments have developed as potentially safe and effective gene therapy methods for a range of acquired and genetic diseases.

4.6.2.1 Direct injection/particle bombardment

DNA can be introduced parentally, which can be considered for Duchenne muscular dystrophy (DMD) [31]. It is a device that uses DNA-coated microparticles to infect target cells with foreign DNA. Direct introduction of pure DNA constructs into the targeted tissue is quite simple, but the efficiency of DNA uptake by the cells and its expression are rather low. Therefore large quantities of DNA have to be injected from time to time. The therapeutic genes synthesize the proteins in the targeted cells which enter the circulation and often become degraded. Another method uses the particle bombardment ('gene gun') technique. In this procedure DNA is coated on to metal microparticles and fired from a ballistic gun into cells/tissues. This procedure is used to transfer the foreign DNA and its transient expression in mammalian cells *in vitro* and *in vivo*. It can cross physical barriers such as skin and the muscle layer, which is why it is used for vaccination. A different tactic uses the particle bombardment (sometimes called the 'gene gun') technology, where DNA is coated on metal microparticles and fired through a ballistic cannon into tissues or cells. Particle bombardment is used to deliver drugs, fluorescent dyes, antigenic proteins, etc [31].

4.6.2.2 Microinjection

This encompasses the delivery of foreign DNA by the means of a glass micropipette into a living cell. The cell is held against a solid support or holding pipette and the microneedle containing the anticipated DNA is inserted into the cell. The tip of the pipette used is about 0.5–5 μm in diameter and looks like an injection needle [30–34]. The glass micropipette is heated until the glass becomes slightly liquefied and is rapidly stretched to resemble an injection needle. The delivery of foreign DNA is carried out under a powerful microscope (micromanipulator). Microinjection allows for the extremely exact and precise administration of even minute amounts of foreign material into the cell. The length of the DNA fragment that needs to be injected is unlimited. A schematic representation of this technique is shown in figure 4.11.

4.6.2.3 Particle bombardment method

In this method, tungsten or gold particles (microprojectiles) are coated with the foreign DNA [30–34]. High-velocity metal particles are used by using micro-projectile bombardment to transport biologically active DNA into the target cells. The macroprojectile is coated with the particles and is augmented with air pressure and shot into the target tissue. A perforated plate is used, which helps the

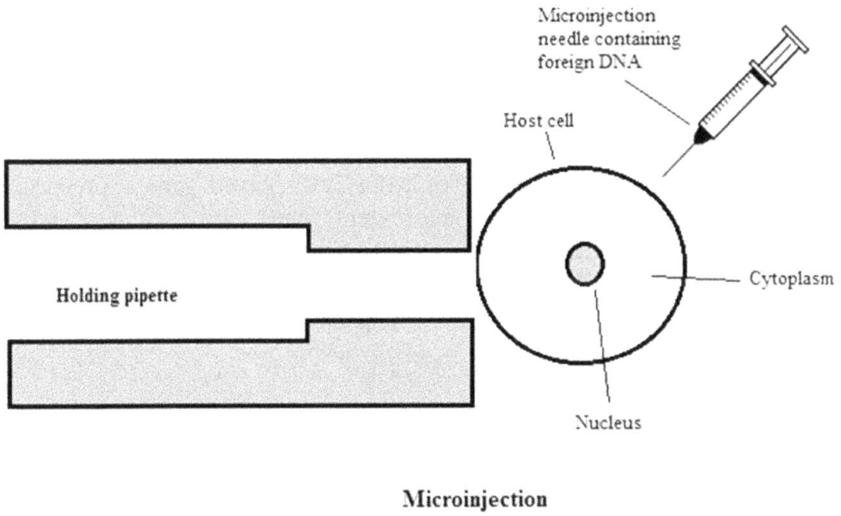

Figure 4.11. Procedure of microinjection.

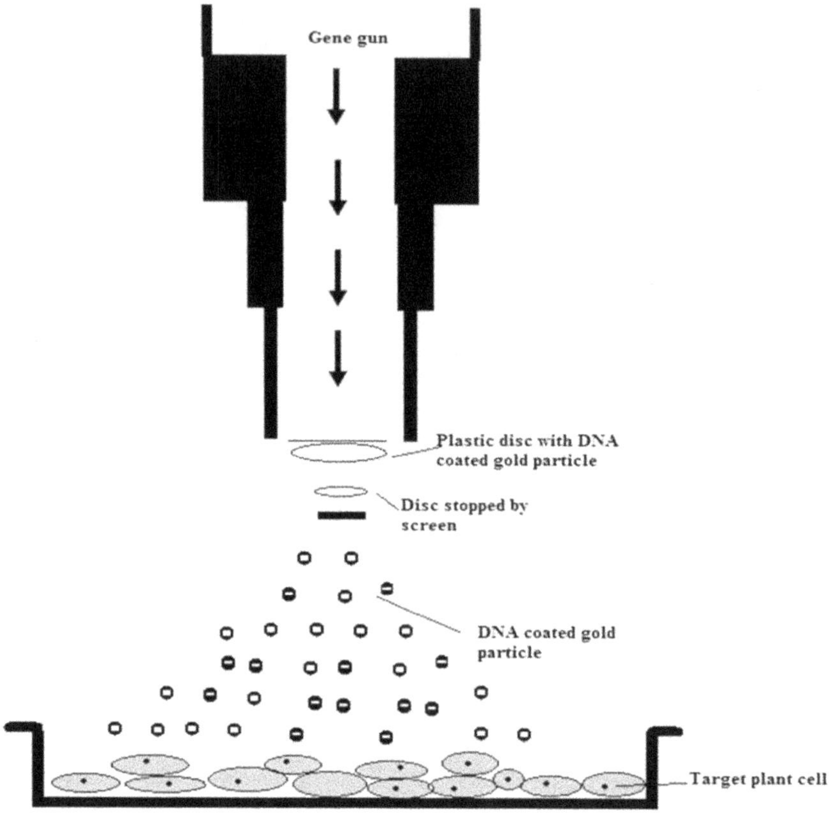

Figure 4.12. Gene-gun-mediated gene transfer.

microprojectiles cross to the cells on the other side of the plate and halts the macroprojectile. The coated particle releases the foreign gene when moving into the target cell and it incorporates into the chromosomal DNA. The fact that DNA-free genome editing is made possible by particle bombardment is one of the main benefits. It makes it possible for proteins, RNAs, and RNPs to enter the host directly. This procedure is also used to deliver genes in mammalian cells [29–33]. Mammalian cell lines, e.g. HEK 293 or MCF7, displayed gene expression when transfected with luciferase and green fluorescent genes, and their gene expression was dependent on the helium pressure, and the size and amount of gold particles and the DNA load on each particle. Cell viability depends on helium pressure [29–33]. The procedure of particle bombardment is depicted in figure 4.12.

4.6.2.4 Liposome-mediated delivery

Lipid–DNA complexes are known as lipoplexes, or more commonly liposomes. Liposomes are spherical vesicles which are fabricated with synthetic lipid bilayers that copy the structure of biological membranes [30–34]. They constitute a DNA construct surrounded by artificial lipid layers. A large number of lipoplexes have been fabricated and used. They are non-toxic and non-immunogenic. Several

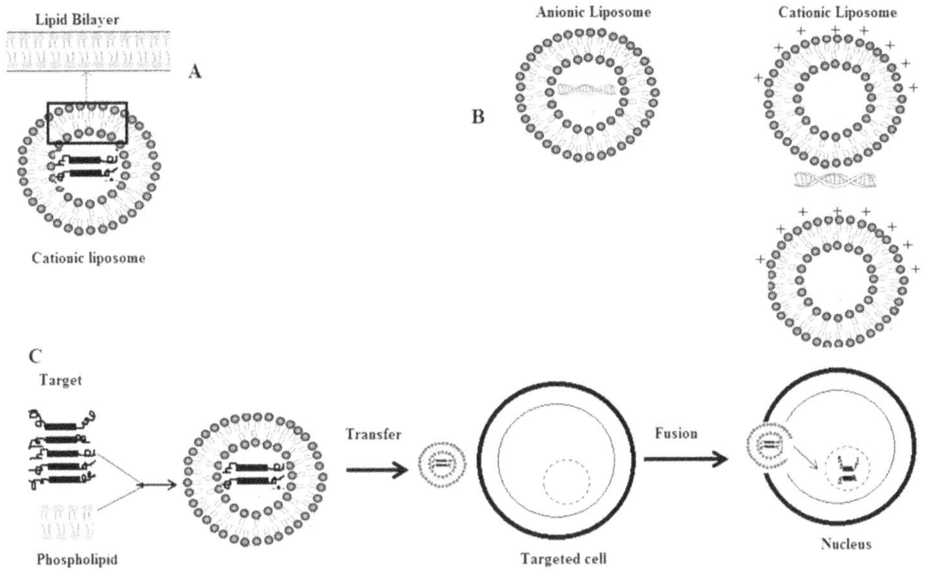

Figure 4.13. *In vivo* liposome-mediated gene transfer: (A) formation of lipid bilayer in water; (B) structure of anionic and cationic liposome; and (C) use of liposome to transfer genes into cells.

benefits of the liposomal drug delivery technology include its low toxicity, biocompatibility, resistance to chemical degradation, and site-specific targeting. The main drawback in the use of lipoplexes is that as the DNA is taken up by the cells, most of it gets degraded by the lysosomes. Consequently, the efficiency of gene delivery by liposomes is very low. A number of clinical trials using liposome CFTR gene complex showed that the gene expression was very short lived. In this method DNA to be transferred is initially packaged into the liposome *in vitro* and transferred to the targeted tissue [30–34]. Because of their adaptable physicochemical and biophysical characteristics, which make it simple to modify them to suit various delivery needs, liposomes are a desirable delivery method. The lipid coating allows the DNA to survive *in vivo* and penetrate into the cell by endocytosis. The most popular vehicles for gene transfer *in vivo* are referred to as cationic liposomes, where the positive charge on the liposomes is stabilized by binding of negatively charged DNA [30–34]. The procedure of liposome-mediated delivery is demonstrated in figure 4.13.

4.6.2.5 Electroporation

In this method, the peripheral electric field is applied to the protoplast, which alters the electrical conductivity and the permeability of the cell membrane; therefore the exogenous molecules present in the medium are taken up to either the cytoplasm (transient transfection) or into the nucleus (stable transfection) [30–34]. The effectiveness of electroporation can be enhanced by giving the cell a heat shock, prior to the application of an electric field, or by means of PEG while performing electroporation [30–34]. DNA may be efficiently delivered into cells and tissues

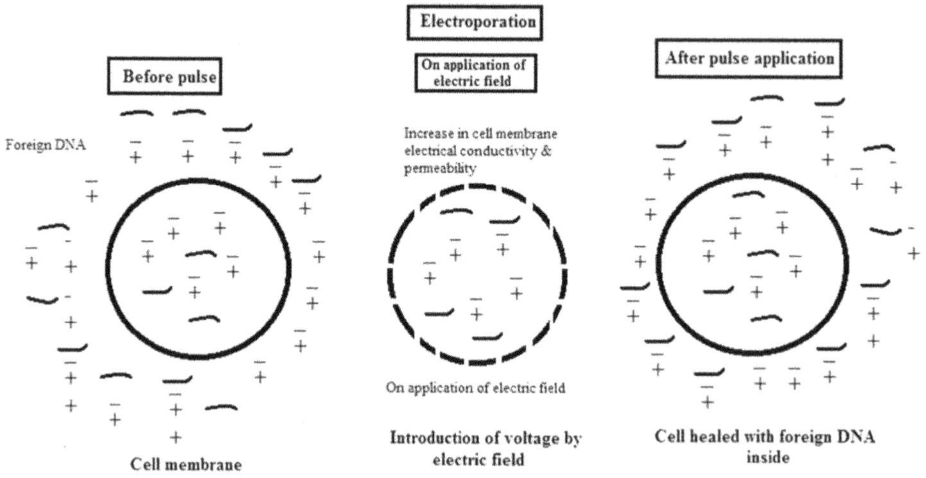

Figure 4.14. Electroporation.

using electroporation, which also improves the expression of certain proteins with immunogenic or therapeutic properties. The procedure of electroporation is depicted in figure 4.14.

4.6.2.6 Sleeping beauty transposition

Another method of gene transfer offers the benefit of stable DNA integration into the chromosomes of vertebrates [30–34]. The sleeping beauty transposition (SB transposon) system comprises a sleeping beauty transposon and a sleeping beauty transposase. The benefits of viruses and naked DNA are combined in this vector. The SB transposon system is a synthetic DNA transposon structured to integrate exactly defined DNA sequences into the chromosomes of vertebrate animals with the aim to integrate new traits and to explore new genes and their functions [30–34]. The SB transposon comprises two terminal inverted repeats present at both ends of the GOI, and the SB transposase mediates excision of the SB transposon. In addition, its integration into a chromosome site is achieved by a dinucleotide dimer TA (thymine adenine) which is based on the cut-and-paste mechanism. The SB transposon displays efficient transposition in the cells of an extensive range of vertebrates, including humans [34–36]. The procedure involved in SB transposition is illustrated in figure 4.15.

4.6.2.7 RNA–DNA chimera

Chimeric oligonucleotides, comprising RNA and DNA bases folded by complementarity into a double hairpin conformation, have been shown to change or repair single bases in plant and animal genomes [37, 38]. This procedure is based on the fusion of RNA and DNA, which is also referred to as a chimeroplast, used to correct point mutations by mismatch repair [37, 38]. These chimeric oligonucleotides contain a 68-nucleotide-long double-stranded nucleic acid molecule comprising one strand of DNA and one strand consisting of two 10-nucleotide-long 2×-O

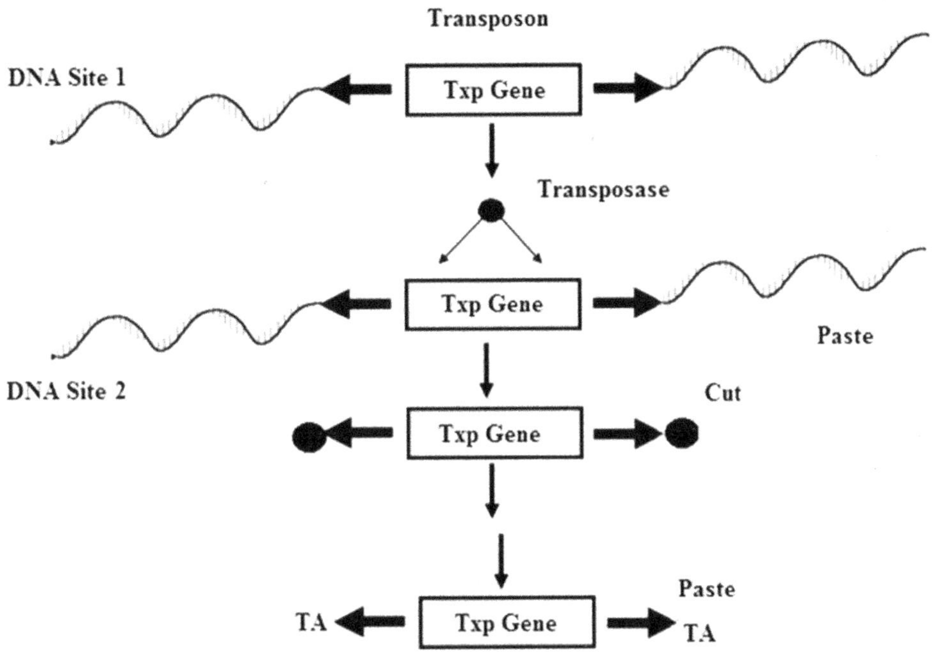

Figure 4.15. Cut-and-paste mechanism of a DNA transposon by transposase (Txp gene).

methyl RNA stretches. Each of these are separated by a five-nucleotide-long DNA stretch, as depicted in figure 4.16. The pentameric chimeric DNA transports the mismatch and the other DNA strand has its complementary bases. Moreover this RNA–DNA chimera comprises two hairpin loops and a GC clamp [37, 38]. It is evident that the method of using chimeraplasts and single-stranded oligonucleotides to correct genetic errors at pathologically significant loci has great promise and will be helpful in treating diseases for which conventional gene augmentation therapy is ineffective.

4.6.2.8 Receptor-mediated endocytosis

The so-called receptor-mediated endocytosis method can be both viral- and non-viral-mediated gene transfer [39, 40]. In this method viral vectors are attached to the surface receptors via viral surface components and are internalized. In the non-viral mode of receptor-based endocytosis DNA is initially coupled to a ligand that binds precisely to a cell surface receptor and causes transfer of the DNA into cells by endocytosis [39, 40]. Coupling is achieved by linking the receptor molecule with polylysine, pursued by reversible binding of the negatively charged DNA to the positively charged polylysine component. Transferrin receptor (a carrier protein for transferrin) which is relatively abundant in proliferating cells and hematopoietic cells is employed as a target and transferin as a ligand in this method [39, 40]. Receptor-mediated endocytosis across the blood–brain barrier is mediated by specific receptors on endothelial cells, including low-density lipoprotein (LDL),

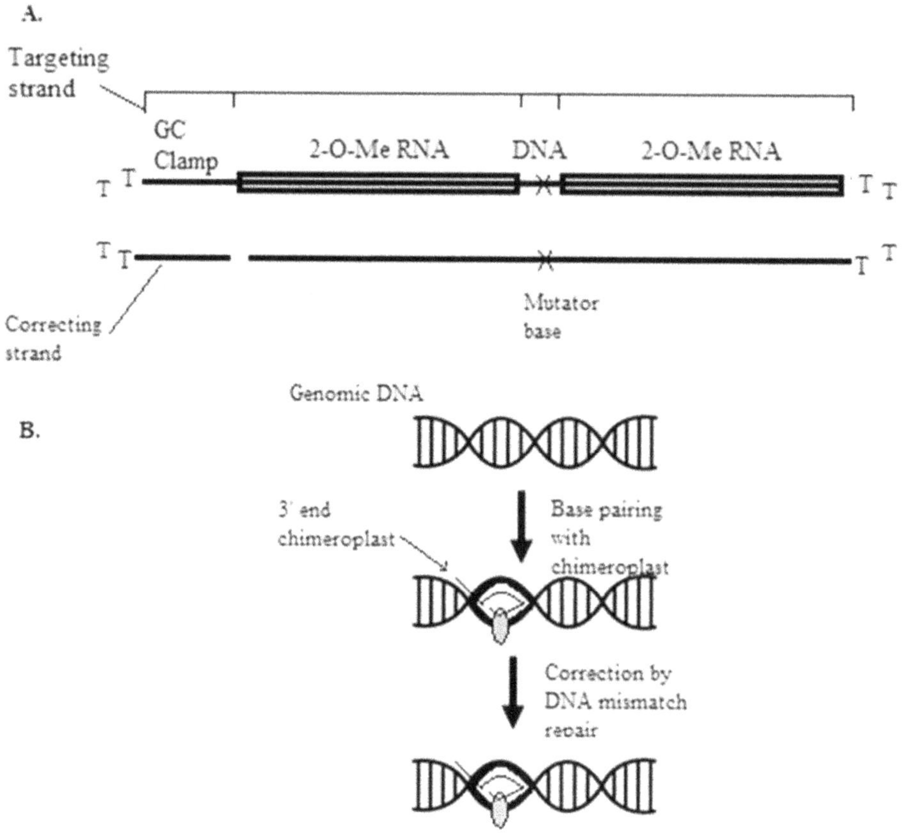

Figure 4.16. Structure and mechanism of RNA–DNA chimera.

cholesterol, integrin, iron transferrin, insulin, etc. It is essential to develop certain hybrid ligand-based carrier systems in order to deliver therapeutic cargo utilizing these particular receptors. The procedure of receptor-mediated endocytosis is shown in figure 4.17.

4.7 Target sites for gene therapy

Several ailments are caused by mutations in a single gene that prevent a somatic cell from transferring its essential functions during the course of cell transformation [41]. Targeted gene therapies have arisen as reliable approaches for the management of such diseases. These strategies depend upon rare-cutting endonucleases to cleave at specific sites in or near disease genes. Additionally, targeted gene correction offers a template for homology-directed repair, allowing the cell's own repair pathways to eliminate the mutation and substitute it with the correct sequence. Targeted gene therapy inactivates the function of the disease gene by inactivating its function. Moreover, it also encourages various areas of genome engineering, containing insertion, mutation, or gene deletion. In contrast with gene therapy, targeted gene therapies offer different potential applications [41].

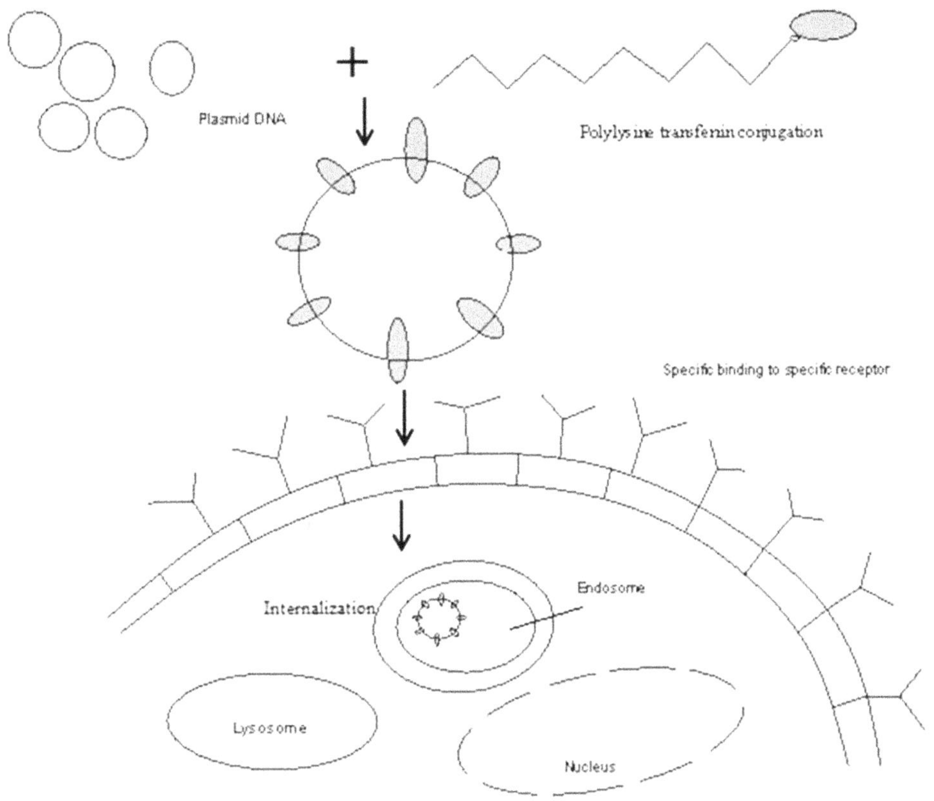

Figure 4.17. Receptor-mediated endocytosis.

4.7.1 Target cells for gene transfer

Therapeutic genes have to be delivered to specific target sites for a specific type of disease. Table 4.4 provides a list of such diseases and their target sites for gene therapy.

4.8 Gene therapy strategies for cancer

Cancer is the foremost cause of death throughout the world, despite serious treatment approaches (surgery, chemotherapy, radiation therapy). Gene therapy is a modern and new strategy for cancer treatment. With positive results from clinical trials, a variety of genes and vectors are being used in this very adaptable therapy method. A number of developments are briefly described below.

4.8.1 Tumor necrosis factor gene therapy

Tumor necrosis factor (TNF) is a protein synthesized by human macrophages [42]. TNF offers a defense against cancer cells. This is brought out by increasing the cancer-fighting ability of tumor-infiltrating lymphocytes (TILs), a special type of immune cell [42]. The TILs were altered with a TNF gene (along with a neomycin

Table 4.4. Diseases and their target sites for gene therapy.

Disease	Target cells
Cancer	Tumor cells, antigen presenting cells (APCs), blood progenitor cells, T cells, fibroblasts, muscle cells
Inherited monogenic disease	Lung epithelial cells, macrophages, T cells, blood progenitor cells, hepatocytes, muscle cells
Infectious disease	T cells, blood progenitor cells, APCs, muscle cells
Cardiovascular disease	Endothelial cells, muscle cells
Rheumatoid arthritis	Sinovial lining cells
Cubital tunnel syndrome	Nerve cells

resistant gene) and used for the management of malignant melanoma (a cancer of melanin producing cells, typically taking place in skin) [42]. TNF by itself is extremely toxic, and fortunately no toxic side effects were observed in the melanoma subjects treated with GM TILs with TNF genes. A number of improvements in the cancer patients were observed [42]. Gene therapy can be utilized to produce apoptosis-inducing ligands locally, preventing systemic toxicity. Additionally, by continuously producing the transgene, it can enhance the ligands' pharmacokinetics.

4.8.2 Suicide gene therapy

Suicide gene therapy is one of the several cancer gene therapy techniques that have garnered particular interest, it enables the targeted transformation of non-toxic substances into cytotoxic medications inside cancer cells, it has garnered significant attention. Therefore, by adding high concentrations of cytotoxic chemicals to the tumor environment with minimal effect on normal tissues, the therapeutic index can be enhanced dramatically [43]. The gene encoding the enzyme TK is frequently known as the suicide gene, and is used for the management of certain cancers [44]. TK phosphorylates nucleosides to yield nucleotides which are employed for the production of DNA during cell division. The drug GCV has a close structural similarity to certain nucleosides (thymidine). By coincidence, TK also phosphorylates GCV to yield triphosphate-GCV, a false and inappropriate nucleotide for DNA synthesis. Triphosphate-GCV DNA impedes polymerases (figure 4.18) [44]. This results in the stretching of the DNA molecule suddenly stopping at a point containing the false nucleotide 401 GCV. In addition, the triphosphate-GCV can enter and destroy the neighbouring cancer cells, known as the bystander effect. The final outcome is that the cancer cells cannot proliferate, and thus die [44]. Therefore, the drug GCV can be used to kill the cancer cells. GCV is often called a prodrug and this type of method is known as prodrug activation gene therapy. GCV has been used for the management of brain tumors (such as glioblastoma, a cancer of glial cells in brain), although with restricted success. In the suicide gene therapy, the vector used is HSV with a gene, TK, integrated into its genome. Normal brain cells

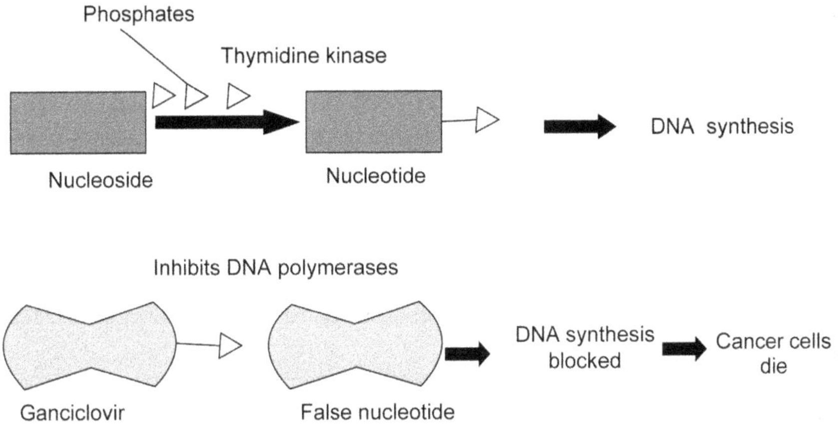

Figure 4.18. The action of GCV mediated by TK to inhibit the growth of cancer cells.

do not divide while the tumor cells go on dividing unchecked [44]. Therefore, there is a continuous DNA replication in tumor cells. By using GCV-HSV-TK suicide gene therapy, a decrease in proliferating tumor cells was reported. A number of new approaches are being introduced to enhance the delivery of the HSV-TK gene throughout a tumor.

4.8.3 Two gene cancer therapy

For management of certain cancers, two-gene systems are put together and used. For example, the TK suicide gene (i.e. GCV:HSV-TK) is conjugated with interleukin-2 gene (i.e. a gene promoting immunotherapy) [45]. Interleukin-2 stimulates an immune response. It has been observed that certain proteins are released from the tumor cells on their death. These proteins, in relationship with immune cells, influence the tumor and start immunological reactions directed against the cancer cells [45]. Two-gene treatments have been accomplished in experimental animals with colon cancer and liver cancer and the final outcomes are encouraging.

4.8.4 Gene replacement therapy

One potentially useful cancer treatment approach is gene replacement therapy, which involves swapping out a damaged gene for a functional, healthy copy of the same gene. Chemotherapy, on the other hand, often lacks selectivity and has non-specific effects [46]. A gene called p53 codes for a protein with a molecular weight of 53 kDa. p53 is treated as a tumor-suppressor gene, as the protein it encodes binds with DNA and hinders the replication process. The tumor cells of various tissues (brain, lung, skin, bladder, colon, bone) were found to have modified genes of p53 (mutated p53), producing altered proteins from the original. These modified proteins cannot prevent DNA replication. It is understood that the damaged p53 gene may be a causative reason for tumor development. Some researchers have attempted to substitute the damaged p53 gene for a normal gene by employing adenovirus vector systems. There are some promising effects in patients with liver cancer [47].

4.9 Gene therapy for AIDS

AIDS is a global disease with an alarming increase in incidence every year. It is invariably fatal, since there is no cure [48]. Attempts are being made to relieve the effects of AIDS by gene therapy. Some of the approaches are discussed below [48].

4.9.1 REV and ENV genes

A mutant strain of human immunodeficiency virus (HIV), lacking rev and env genes, has been developed [49, 50]. The regulatory and envelope proteins of HIV are separately produced by rev and env genes. Owing to lack of these genes, the virus cannot duplicate.

Scientists have used HIV deficient rev and env genes for therapeutic purposes. T-lymphocytes from HIV-infected patients are removed, and mutant viruses are incorporated into them. The modified T-lymphocytes are cultivated and injected into the patients [49, 50]. Due to the lack of essential genes, the viruses (HIV) cannot multiply, but they can stimulate the production of cluster determinant antigen 8 (CD8) cells of T-lymphocytes. CD8 cells are the killer lymphocytes. It has been demonstrated in laboratory investigations that these lymphocytes destroy the HIV-infected cells.

4.9.2 Genes of HIV proteins

Certain genes producing HIV proteins are attached to the DNA of mouse viruses. These GM viruses are administered to AIDS patients with clinical signs of the disease. It is assumed that the HIV genes trigger normal body cells to synthesize HIV proteins [51]. The latter in turn triggers the production of anti-HIV antibodies which inhibit HIV replication in AIDS patients [51].

4.9.3 Gene to inactivate gp120

gp120 is a glycoprotein (molecular weight 120 kDa) found in the envelope of HIV [52]. It is absolutely vital for the binding of the virus to the host cell and to initiate replication. Scientists have prepared a gene (called F105) to produce an antibody that can inactivate gp120 [52]. In anti-AIDS treatment, HIV-infected cells are designed to produce anti-HIV antibodies when administered into the organism. Research performed on experimental animals showed a drastic decline in the synthesis of gp120 due to anti-AIDS treatment [52]. The synthesis of HIV particles was also reduced.

4.10 Oligonucleotide therapies: antigene and antisense therapy

The developments of oligonucleotide therapies will make more progress in the next few decades, especially after the FDA-approval for antisense oligonucleotides in 2017. Complementary oligonucleotide binding to target mRNA results in the downregulation of gene expression in antisense treatment [53]. Gene silencing is a generalized term to block the expression of a gene to further prevent protein production. Gene silencing involves gene therapy which can be defined as the procedure for introducing a GOI (therapeutic value) into cells to replace a defective gene so as to correct genetic disorders. Nevertheless, several disorders such as cancer, viral and parasitic infections, and inflammatory diseases lead to the high production of certain normal proteins or defective proteins. In such cases, it is possible to block translation using a single-stranded nucleotide sequence (antigene oligonucleotide). Short single-stranded DNA sequences called antisense oligonucleotides are made to contrast with the specific 'sense' (5′ to 3′) orientation of the mRNA that codes for desired protein [53]. This single-stranded nucleotide or antigenic strand hybridizes with the specific gene, and ultimately interferes with the translation process. Sequences that are responsible for inhibition of the translation process are called antisense oligonucleotides, and this procedure is known as antisense therapy. This type of treatment involves a gene silencing technique which is quite similar to RNA interference but uses a somewhat different mechanism. Instead of repairing the gene, it aims to 'silence' the gene's function. Moreover, during this procedure it is possible to prevent the two biological processes of transcription and translation. This can be achieved by oligonucleotides, which allow the inactivation of the transcription factors that are responsible for the exact gene expression. Generally, during this procedure genes can be knocked out to define the function of that particular gene in a critical or disease pathway. So this may allow the nucleic acid based treatment (DNA/RNA/chemical analogue) to understand the role of a gene in a particular clinical condition or genetic-based diseases.

4.10.1 Antisense therapy for cancer

Targets that are increased during and causally linked to cancer growth and therapeutic resistance, and that are otherwise unresponsive to suppression with antibodies or small compounds, are the most promising for antisense therapy [54]. As discussed above, the principle of this approach is the sequence-specific binding of an antisense oligonucleotide (synthetic polymers) to target mRNA. This can result in the prevention of gene translation. One approach to treat cancer cells is to develop selective therapeutics to control/alter the expression of genes involved in the malignancies. Such genes are called oncogenes. In antisense therapy for cancer, these oncogenes can be targeted by antisense oligonucleotides. Several genes are responsible for the regulation of apoptosis, cell growth, metastasis and angiogenesis. These all are the characteristics of cancerous cells rather than normal cells, thus molecular targets can be developed for such gene functions [55]. Antisense oligonucleotides offer line of treatment to target genes involved in cancer development, particularly those that are not responsive against small-molecule or antibody inhibition. According to recent reports chemical modifications of antisense oligonucleotides increase resistance to nuclease digestion, extend tissue half-lives and improve the production procedure [54]. Antisense oligonucleotides treatment involves short, synthetic DNA which is allowed to hybridize with specific mRNA strands that resemble target genes. After binding mRNA, the antisense oligonucleotides prevent the circulation of a message by the target gene to convert into a protein. This is how the action of the gene is blocked. Currently, phosphorothioate oligonucleotides are considered as the most potential treatment in antisense therapy, as they have satisfactory physical and chemical properties and also show reasonable resistance to nucleases. New generations of these phosphorothioate oligonucleotides have been also developed. They consist of 2′-modified nucleoside building blocks to enhance RNA-binding affinity and decrease indirect toxic effects [56].

The main obstacles have been (i) insufficient affinity towards the desired target sequence, (ii) inadequate intracellular distribution to intended regions or cells, (iv) possible toxicity or off-target effects, and (v) inadequate resistance to intracellular and extracellular deterioration (primarily by action of nucleases) [57]. As most of the antisense oligonucleotides developed so far have certain limitations such as nuclease susceptibility and non-specific hybridization, thus there is an immense scope for the development of new antisense oligonucleotides that are devoid of these disadvantages. As per past nucleotide research, circular oligonucleotides, as they have no ends, are exonuclease-resistant and attach to complementary strands of RNA and DNA with greater affinity, thus are considered as superior to conventional linear oligonucleotides. By regulating gene expression for the first time in 1991, antisense technology was used for the treatment of myeloid leukemia [58].

One of the most interesting parts of antisense technology is RNA interference, which is currently considered as a potential treatment against cancer. RNA interference, often denoted as RNAi, is a member of non-coding RNA (ncRNA), which refers to the RNA that are not translated into protein; nevertheless, this does not signify that non-coding RNA supplies no performance [59]. Cancerous cells are the main targets for RNAi-based treatment. A number of *in vivo* and *in vitro* investigations showed that RNAi-based treatment can be utilized for treating single-gene disorders and those with overexpression of proteins [60]. Several small synthetic RNA can be utilized in cancer treatment such as siRNA, shRNA and bishRNA. Because of its silencing mechanism, specificity and lack of side effects this RNAi-based treatment outdoes the others [61].

In RNAi-based method, antisense RNA oligonucleotide particles are used. These antisense mRNA bind exactly to the target mRNA and prevent protein biosynthesis (translation), as shown in figure 4.19 [54]. In the first approach antisense RNA is directly introduced into the cell to prevent the translation, while in the second approach synthesized antisense cDNA can be cloned and transfected into cells to ultimately prevent the translation. Antisense mRNA is produced by transcription. In the first approach ds RNA is spliced by a dicer to produce siRNA, which will further bind with mRNA in cell to produce RISC. This hybrid formation prevents translation and ultimately protein synthesis will be inhibited. The primary goals of these chemical alterations have been to strengthen resistance to exo- and endonuclease degradation, raise affinity and, in some cases; selectivity towards target RNA/DNA sequences, and alter immunostimulation properties of the oligonucleotides.

By means of gene therapy, it is possible to treat malignant brain tumors, in fact brain tumors were the first human carcinogenicity to be targeted. This can be achieved by therapeutic transfer of nucleic acids into somatic cells (cells other than the reproductive cells) [62]. Since malignant brain tumors, especially in the adult brain, have some distinguishing features, such as high mitotic activity and the fact

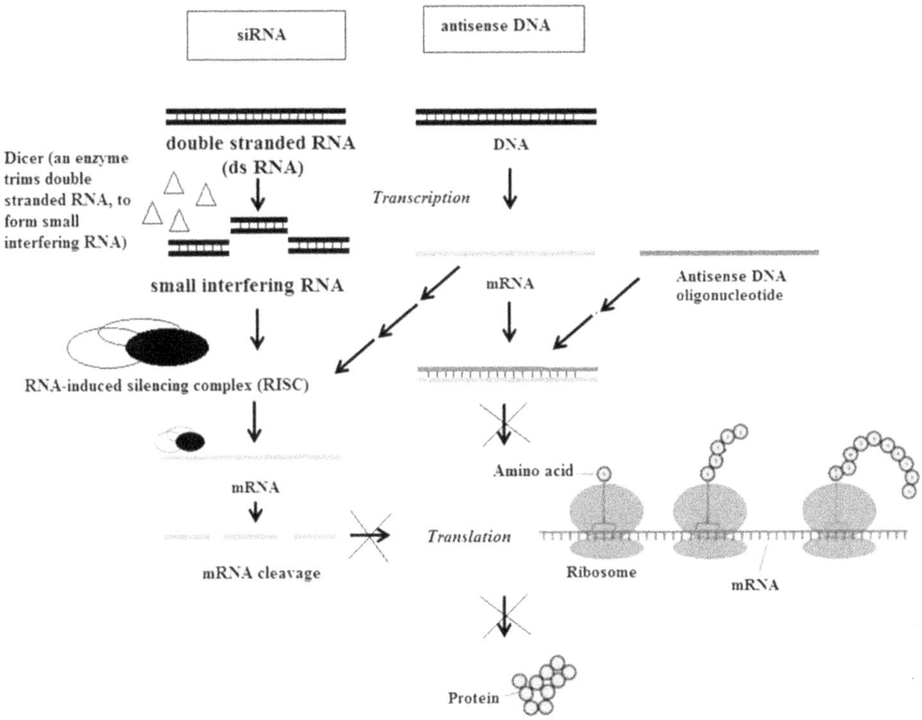

Figure 4.19. Inhibition of translation by siRNA and antisense DNA.

that the malignancy will not spread outside of the CNS (central nervous system), thus these malignant cells present in the brain offer key benefits in designing selective tumor gene therapy approaches [62]. The most advanced antisense oligodeoxynucleotide treatment of high-grade gliomas is the development of phosphorothioate-modified antisense oligodeoxynucleotides, referred to as AP 12 009 (trabedersen), which target mRNA encoding TGF-beta2 [63]. This helps in the treatment of malignant gliomas by using TGF-beta2 antisense oligonucleotides [63]. High grade malignant glioma results in the overproduction of insulin-like growth factor I, whereas prostate cancer cells also express an insulin-like growth factor receptor which may results in the high production of this protein [63, 64]. For such types of malignancies antisense cDNAs can be used to produce an antisense mRNA molecule which can further prevent translation, as shown in figure 4.19.

4.10.2 Antisense therapy for AIDS

Antisense medications can be created with particular antisense activity to block reverse transcriptase and suppress virus gene expression during the HIV cycle. Antisense therapy is being studied as an alternative approach for several infectious diseases that cannot be successfully treated using other existing treatments [65]. It involves several factors, such as nucleic acid based treatment which involves antisense DNA or RNA, RNA decoys and catalytic RNA moieties (ribozymes);

protein-based treatments such as transdominant negative proteins and single-chain antibodies; and finally immunotherapeutic-based treatments that involve genetic vaccines or pathogen-specific lymphocytes [65]. It has been already reported that HIV virus entry is facilitated by specific interaction between the viral envelope glycoprotein and the cell surface molecule CD4. These cell surface molecules are the primary receptor and act as chemokine (C–C or C–X–C motif) receptor CCR5 or CXCR4 which serves as a co-receptor [66]. It has been already reported that CCR5 is necessary for HIV-1 infection through all routes of transmission. It was also evidenced that CCR5 synthesis as well as function can be blocked by using small interfering RNAs, antisense RNAs or ribozymes [66].

Gene-based treatments suppress the expression of host or viral mRNA targets necessary for HIV-1 infection and/or replication by using RNA interference (RNAi). RNA interference (RNAi) greatly increases the number of therapeutic targets beyond the reach of combined antiretroviral therapy (cART) by enabling sequence-specific design to compensate for viral mutations and natural variants [67]. Thus RNAi-based approaches can be utilized to silence the expression of viral or host mRNA targets that are essential for HIV-1 infection and/or replication [67]. Current developments in clinical investigations have established the potential of RNAi therapeutics, supporting the idea that RNAi-based agents might offer a safe, effective and more durable strategy for the management of HIV/AIDS [67]. During antisense therapy, HIV-infected cells are targeted to insert a gene that synthesizes antisense RNA. The complementary strand of the HIV genome is produced in the form of antisense RNA by a set of particular genes. This antisense RNA is allowed to interact with HIV, in particular viral RNA, to develop double-stranded RNA–RNA hybrid particles, which cannot be utilized by the enzyme reverse transcriptase. Thus there is no scope for the development of DNA copy and integration of the HIV genome into host genome, as shown in figure 4.20.

4.11 Antisense oligonucleotides as therapeutic agents

Antisense oligonucleotides can be used to suppress the expression of specific target genes that are linked to the beginning of human disorders. It has been reported that antisense oligonucleotides can potentially prevent the expression of specific target genes involved in the development of human diseases [68]. This can be achieved by hybridization of oligodeoxynucleotides with targeted mRNA to prevent translation, which may further block specific protein synthesis. As per the above discussion, antisense oligodeoxynucleotides can potentially be utilized in cardiovascular diseases, various cancers and infectious diseases like AIDS [68]. These small fragments of antisense oligodeoxynucleotides are capable of hybridizing with various types of RNA transcripts, such as mRNAs, intron-exons and double-stranded RNAs [68, 69]. As per previous reports, unmodified phosphodiester oligodeoxynucleotides are more susceptible against nucleolytic degradation then modified phosphodiester oligodeoxynucleotides. This fact has limited their utilization as potential therapeutics. Several studies are available that demonstrate the lack of stability of unmodified oligodeoxynucleotides in biological fluids, such as their short half-lives in serum

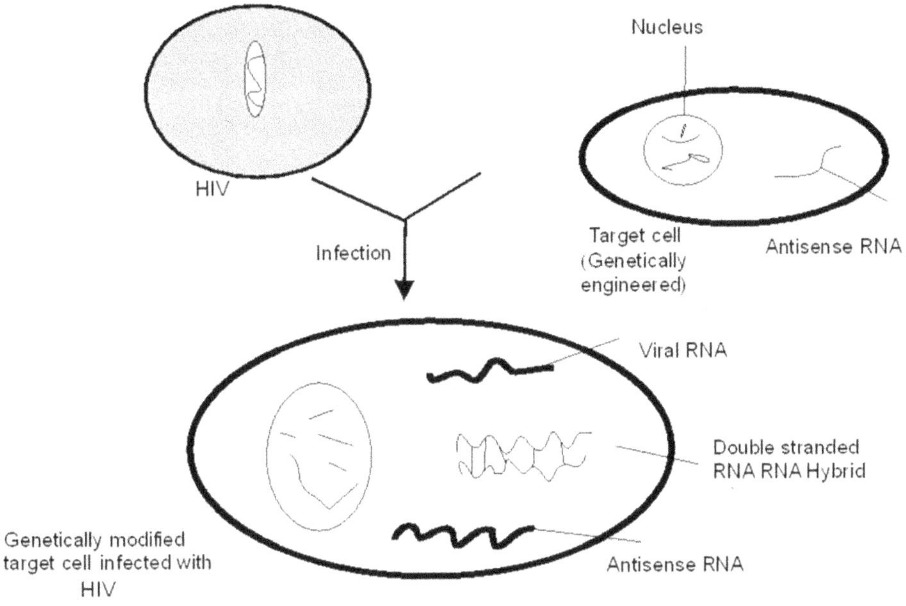

Figure 4.20. Antisense therapy to prevent AIDS.

(5 min) and in living cells (30 min) [70, 71]. Antisense oligonucleotides are made to bind to target transcripts with a high degree of affinity, but since they lack RNase H competence, they cannot cause target transcript destruction. Therefore, these oligonucleotides are either made up of nucleotides that, when combined with RNA, do not produce RNase H substrates, or they are made up of a combination of nucleotide chemistries, or 'mixmers,' which prevent runs of consecutive bases that resemble DNA [72]. In serum oligodeoxynucleotide degradation is observed due to the 3′-exonuclease activity, while in the cell both endonuclease and exonuclease activity is responsible for the degradation of these molecules [71, 73, 74]. Chemical treatment of the oligonucleotides, in particular their natural phosphodiester backbone, is considered as an excellent approach to prevent nucleolytic degradation in both the cell and serum. Such types of modifications enhance the stability of oligonucleotides in biological systems [75]. One of the most common synthetic approaches that reduce oligonucleotide sensitivity toward nucleases is the phosphorothioate analog. This can be synthesized by substituting one of the non-bridging oxygen atoms of the internucleotide linkage with sulfur. Another approach that has been reported is alternate phosphorothioate modifications with phosphodiester linkages to further enhance the stability of oligonucleotides against nucleases under *in vitro* conditions [73]. Despite having good features, phosphorothioate oligonucleotides still have potential limitations as follows: High concentrations of phosphorothioates can inhibit the activity of nucleases and polymerases [75–77].

- They bind with heparin-binding growth factors and interfere with their activity [77].
- They encourage immune-stimulatory effects in rats.

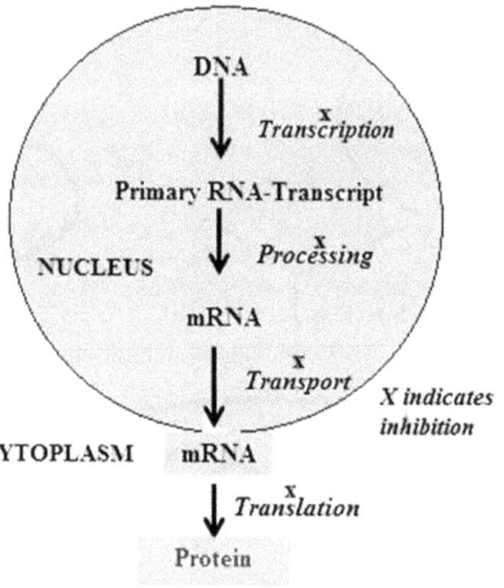

Figure 4.21. Structural modifications of antisense oligonucleotides increases their stability in intranuclear and intracellular environments.

- They are responsible for complement activation and hypotension in monkeys.
- They cause clotting problems in monkeys, which proves the direct effects on thrombin [78].

Thus necessary modifications in the oligonucleotides prevent its nucleolytic-based degradation [68, 69], such as phosphodiester bond modification (bases or sugars, phosphates) which involves the modification of sulfur group by free oxygen. This allows the modification of the phosphodiester bond, which imparts water solubility and decreased sensitivity against nuclease degradation. Such modifications of antisense oligonucleotides increase their stability in intranuclear and intracellular environments, as shown in figure 4.21. These modified antisense oligonucleotides are considered as therapeutic agents for the management of certain diseases such as cancers, bowel disease, AIDS, malaria and viral infections.

4.12 Chimeric oligonucleotides in gene correction

Gene therapy utilizing chimeric RNA/DNA oligonucleotides has the potential to become a significant therapeutic approach for hereditary diseases. In the right cells or tissues, it can provide repaired genes with normal control and persistent expression [79]. In addition to the antisense oligonucleotides, chimeric RNA/DNA oligonucleotides have emerged as a potential approach for gene therapy. These chimeras are composed of RNA and DNA bases folded by complementarity into a double hairpin conformation. This confirmation contains hairpin caps and methylated ribose sugars (at the second carbon) and is reported to alter or repair single bases in plant and animal genomes. These chimeric oligonucleotides are used to treat various genetic diseases that are due to single base pair mutations [37, 80]. One of the advantages of these hairpin caps is to shield the entire molecule from

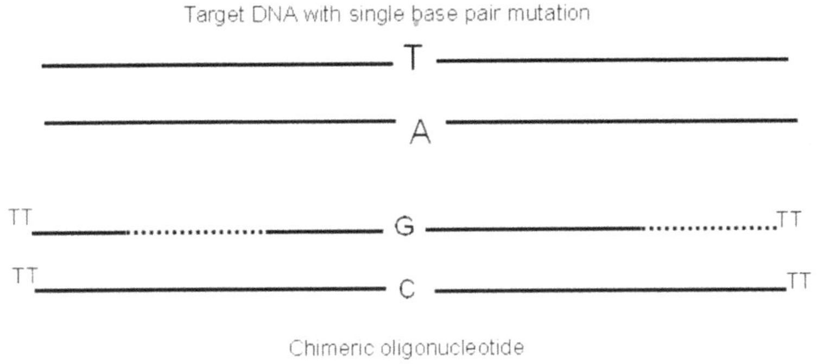

Figure 4.22. Chimeric oligonucleotides in gene correction. The dotted lines represent ribonucleotides while the continuous lines correspond to deoxyribonucleotides; the coloured base pair is the correct one to replace the mutated base.

exonucleases degradation. As reported, modification of the ribose sugar such as methylation can prevent its digestion by RNase [37]. The alteration of a single base pair mutation by using a chimeric oligonucleotide is shown in figure 4.22.

4.13 Aptamers as therapeutic agents

Aptamers can act as carriers for therapeutic medicines in addition to binding and suppressing the immunoregulatory elements of carcinogenesis. Aptamers are oligonucleotides obtained from an *in vitro* process known as SELEX (systematic evolution of ligands by exponential enrichment). The distinguishing features of aptamers allow them to bind with several molecules with high specificity and affinity for their target. In addition, properties such as their small size and their ease of production make them attractive and promising therapeutic molecules for targeting diseases. Aptamers have been developed to bind proteins which are related to some disease states [81]. Thus aptamers are oligonucleotides that can exactly bind to target proteins and not to nucleic acids. Using this approach, several powerful antagonists of such proteins can be developed. In order for these antagonists to work in animal models of disease and in humans, it is essential to alter the aptamers [81]. Aptamers can be used for diagnosis of cancer by detecting specific biomarkers, circulating cancer cells or imaging diseased tissue [82]. Alternatively, aptamers can also be utilized as therapeutic molecules because of likely antagonist activity and act as targeting agents. Consequently, they can be developed to transport anti-tumor molecules, e.g. chemotherapeutic drugs, siRNA or photodynamic therapy sensitizers to diseased tissues [82]. RNA/DNA oligonucleotide molecules known as aptamers attach themselves selectively to a particular complementary molecule. Aptamers, such as monoclonal antibodies, are potential recognition components with intriguing therapeutic and diagnostic applications that could offer a variety of alternatives for treating and diagnosing blood diseases [83]. Efforts have also been made to develop aptamer-targeted nanoplatforms to transport cargo for both imaging and therapeutic functions producing so-called nanotheragnostics agents [82].

4.14 Ribozymes as therapeutic agents

Catalytic RNA molecules known as ribozymes have a highly sequence-specific ability to recognize their target RNA. Because of this, they can be employed to fix mutant cellular RNAs or even prevent the production of harmful genes (by cleaving the target mRNA) targets include viral genomes and transcripts, as well as the mRNAs of oncogenes (caused by base mutations or chromosome translocations, such as ras or bcr-abl). Nucleic acid, in particular RNA molecules, can act as enzymes in the form of biocatalysts, also known as ribozymes. This breakthrough of RNA as a biological catalyst and genetic molecule proved that there will be a time when almost all biological reactions in the laboratory will be catalyzed by these biocatalysts rather than catalyzed by protein-based enzymes [84]. Ribozymes (ribonucleic acid enzymes) offer a platform to synthesize those catalytic RNA molecules that are capable of catalyzing specific biochemical reactions, which should be more similar to the action of protein-based enzymes. By using this approach diseases that are caused by viruses or diseases due to genetic lesions can be targeted therapeutically, however, the genetic information involved in the disease should be known [84]. To achieve this, naturally occurring ribozymes should be altered in such that they can precisely hybridize with mRNA sequences and stop translation [84].

4.15 The future of gene therapy

Ideally, gene therapy would be permanent solution for genetic diseases. But it is not as simple as it appears, since gene therapy has several inbuilt complexities. Gene therapy broadly involves isolation of a specific gene and making copies by inserting them into target tissue cells to make the desired protein. The story does not end here. It is absolutely essential to ensure that the gene is harmless to the patient and it is appropriately expressed (too much or too little will be no good). Another concern in gene therapy is the body's immune system will react to the foreign proteins produced by the new genes. The public, in general, have exaggerated expectations of gene therapy. Researchers, at least for the present, are unable to satisfy them [85]. It is encouraging to see new gene therapy therapies approved in the near future for uncommon hereditary brain and spinal cord illnesses, given the growing number of development projects and advancements. In perfect harmony with these anticipations, the FDA declared that starting in 2025, they plan to approve 10–20 gene and cell therapies annually. As per the literature, by 1999 about 1000 Americans had undergone clinical trials involving various gene therapies. Unfortunately, gene therapists are unable to categorically claim that gene therapy has permanently cured any one of these patients. A number of people in the media (including leading newspapers and magazines) have openly questioned whether it is worth continuing research into genes. It may be true that as of now, due to several limitations gene therapy has not advanced the way it was hoped, despite intensive research. But a revolution may come any time, and of course this is only likely with persistent research. A time may come (which might take some decades) when almost every disease will have a gene therapy as one of the treatment modalities and gene therapy will transform the practice of medicine. In the near future, gene therapy is

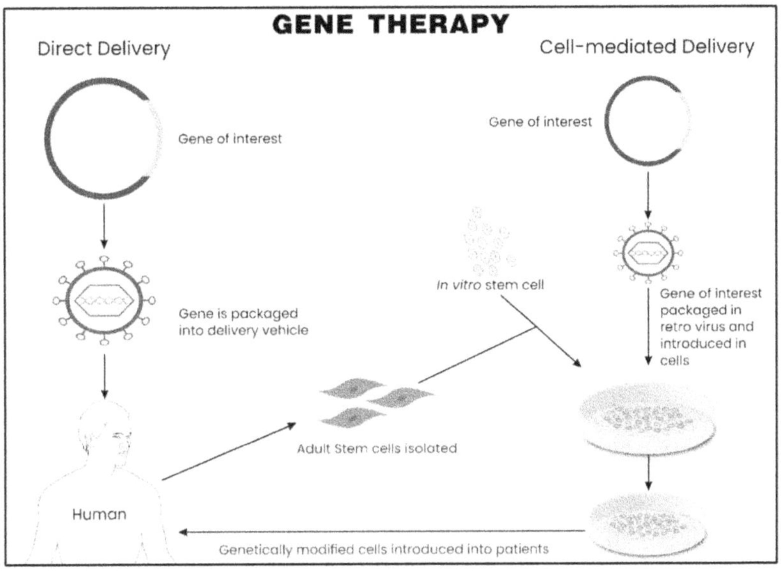

Figure 4.23. Gene therapy by direct delivery method or by stem cell mediated method. Gene therapy is mediated by direct gene delivery by encapsulating it in a delivery vehicle such as a retrovirus. In cell mediated delivery, the gene is encapsulated in a retrovirus and introduced into the cell and then administered in the patient.

anticipated to have more significance in treating uncommon brain and spinal cord disorders. Given that the great majority of medical interventions for the diseases under review only address the underlying pathological aetiology, approving additional gene therapies by regulatory bodies may significantly improve the lives of patients with rare diseases [85] (figure 4.23)

4.16 Stem cell research

Stem cells are undifferentiated cells that can develop into specialized cells. These specialized cells can further divide (through mitosis) to produce more stem cells. Based on their origin stem cells are often classified into different types of categories [86]. Stem cells are found both in the embryo and in the adult [86]. Depending on their origination, they have dissimilar properties. Stem cells can be obtained from early embryos after the formation of the blastocyst or from fetal, postnatal or adult sources. However, the complexity of stem cell-based therapies often forces researchers to search for a dependable, safe, and easily accessible source of multilineage-developing stem cells. As such, it is imperative that the type of stem cells that are suitable for therapeutic usage be carefully selected [87].

Based on the classification scheme, the three kinds of stem cells are:

- ES cells.
- Embryonic germ cells.
- Adult stem cells.

ES cells are obtained from the inner cellular mass, which is part of the early (4–5 day old) embryo called the blastocyst. After separation, the inner cellular mass can be cultured into ES cells [88]. Embryonic germ cells have features similar to ES cells. Embryonic germ cells, however, are harvested from the fetus later in the developmental process from a region called the gonadal ridge (which would ultimately develop into the sex organs). However, these cells can further develop into the three germ layers that make all the specific organs of the body. The cell types that derive from embryonic germ cells are somewhat more limited in growth pattern than those that derive from ES cells. This is simply because embryonic germ cells are further along in the developmental process [88]. Adult stem cells are derived from mature adults. These can also be further called multipotent stem cells, as the number of cell types which they can develop into is limited. Adult stem cells serve as a fresh source of cells in living organisms. They substitute cells that are required to be replaced consistently in a living organism, e.g. blood (which has a 120 day lifespan) and other connective tissues. Regarding MSCs, these cells are generally regarded as safe; nevertheless, future research should concentrate on long-term follow-up and ongoing monitoring to prevent the chance of tumor growth following therapies [89]. It is usually assumed that adult stem-cell-based treatments will balance but not replace ES cell therapies. One benefit of adult stem cells is that they offer the chance to employ small samples of adult tissues of a patient's own cells for expansion and successive implantation. This circumvents the ethical issues of ES cells, as well as the concerns that go along with allogeneic donations. No one type of stem cell is necessarily better than the other; rather, the different stem cells have different advantages [88].

4.16.1 Stem cell classification

As mentioned above, stem cells are self-renewing and undifferentiated cells that can differentiate into functional cells and can be categorized into two main types based on their source of origin: embryonic and adult stem cells. Stem cells are maybe best understood in terms of how committed they are to becoming any particular type of cell, thus cells can also be further divided according to their plasticity, or developmental versatility. The growth, development, upkeep, and restoration of our brains, bones, muscles, nerves, blood, skin, and other organs depend on them. Through laboratory research on these cells, scientists can learn the essential traits of stem cells and what sets them apart from other specialized cell types. Our knowledge of how an organism develops from a single cell and how healthy cells replace damaged ones in mature animals is still being advanced by the research of stem cells [90]. The categories into which they fall include totipotent stem cells, pluripotent stem cells, multipotent stem cells, adult stem cells (a certain type of multipotent stem cell) and unipotent stem cells [91]. Multipotent stem cells have the potential to further differentiate into all cell types within one particular lineage [92]. There are several advantages to multipotent stem cells, as they are key in the processes of development, tissue repair and protection. These cells have been used in the treatment of various disorders, e.g. rheumatoid arthritis, hematopoietic defects, spinal cord injury, bone fracture, autoimmune diseases and fertility preservation [92].

4.16.1.1 Totipotent stem cells

These are the most versatile of the stem cell types. When a sperm and egg are fertilized, they form a one-celled fertilized egg. This cell is totipotent, i.e. it has the capability to differentiate into any and all human cells, e.g. brain, liver, blood or heart cells. It can even develop into an entire functional organism. The first few cell divisions in embryonic development produce more totipotent cells. After four days of embryonic cell division, the cells begin to specialize into pluripotent stem cells [93]. These cells may eventually develop into a placenta or into any one of the three germ layers. After around four days, the blastocyst's inner cell mass becomes pluripotent. This structure is the source of pluripotent cells.

4.16.1.2 Pluripotent stem cells

Human pluripotent stem cells signify an available cell source for new cell-based clinical research and therapies [94]. With the understanding of induced pluripotent stem cells, it is now possible to produce nearly any desired cell type from any patient's cells. Current developments in gene modification approaches have unlocked the prospect of creating genetically corrected human-induced pluripotent stem cells for certain genetic diseases that could be used later in autologous transplantation [94]. Human pluripotent stem cells, which comprise human ES cells and human-induced pluripotent stem cells, can self-renew indefinitely in culture while maintaining the potential to become almost any cell type in the human body. These cells are like totipotent stem cells in that they can give rise to all tissue types. Unlike totipotent stem cells, however, they cannot give rise to an entire organism [94]. On the fourth day of development, the embryo forms into two layers, an outer layer which will become the placenta, and an inner mass which will form the tissues of the developing human body. These inner cells, although they can form nearly any human tissue, cannot do so without the outer layer; so they are not totipotent, but pluripotent. As these pluripotent stem cells continue to divide, they begin to specialize further [94]. From fully pluripotent cells like embryonic stem cells (ESCs) and induced pluripotent stem cell (iPSC) to representatives with different potencies like multi-, oligo-, or unipotent cells, they display a continuum of pluripotency. Their spectrum and activity can be assessed, for example, using the teratoma development assay. iPSCs are made intentionally from somatic cells and function similarly to PSCs. Their cultivation and application in regenerative medicine have enormous potential.

4.16.1.3 Multipotent stem cells

While pluripotent stem cells may develop into all types of cells in an organism, multipotent and unipotent stem cells remain limited to particular tissues or lineages. The strength of these stem cells can be explained by using a number of functional assays along with the assessment of various molecular markers [95]. Multipotent stem cells are cells that do not differentiate into cell types of diverse tissue origin under the usual physiological circumstances. The developing potential of unipotent stem cells is further limited and they remain able to give rise to only a single cell type, e.g. the blast forming unit-erythroid may only develop into erythrocytes [95]. Multipotent stem cells are less plastic and more differentiated stem cells. They give rise to a limited range of cells within a tissue type [95]. The offspring of the pluripotent cells become the progenitors of such cell lines as blood cells, skin cells and nerve cells. At this stage, they are multipotent. They can become one of several types of cells within a given organ e.g. multipotent blood stem cells can develop into red blood cells, white blood cells or platelets [95]. Numerous ailments, such as autoimmune disease, rheumatoid arthritis, spinal cord injuries, bone fractures, haematological abnormalities, and fertility preservation, have been treated with them [92].

4.16.1.4 Adult stem cells

An adult stem cell is a multipotent stem cell in adult humans that is used to replace cells that have died or lost function [95]. It is an undifferentiated cell present in differentiated tissue. It renews itself and can specialize to yield all cell types present in the tissue from which it originated. So far, adult stem cells have been identified for many different tissue types such as hematopoietic (blood), neural, endothelial, muscle, mesenchymal, gastrointestinal and epidermal cells [95]. Because of their proliferative nature and ability to regenerate tissue, adult stem cells hold promise for the treatment of ageing and several degenerative diseases. In addition, as stem cells are commonly thought to be the origins of malignant tumors, understanding the processes that keep their proliferative powers in control can pave the way for new cancer therapies [96].

4.16.2 Historical background of stem cell research

The historical background of stem cell research is described in table 4.5.

4.16.3 Ethical issues associated with cell lines

Stem cell studies show great promise for interpreting the basic mechanisms of human development and differentiation, as well as scope for different treatments for diseases, for example diabetes, spinal cord injury, Parkinson's disease and myocardial infarction [107]. Pluripotent stem cells maintain themselves in culture and can develop into all types of specialized cells. Researchers plan to develop pluripotent cells into specialized cells that could be used for transplantation. However, human stem cell research also raises acute ethical and political controversies. The origin of pluripotent stem cell lines from oocytes and embryos is criticized with arguments regarding the onset of human personhood and human reproduction. Several other methods of developing stem cells raise fewer ethical concerns. The reprogramming of somatic cells to create induced pluripotent stem cells (iPS cells) circumvents the ethical issues specific to ES cells. With any human stem cell (hSC) research, however, there are challenging issues, including consent to donate materials for hSC research,

Table 4.5. Historical background of stem cell research.

Year	Historical background	References
1878	First evidence of fertilizing mammalian eggs outside the body.	[97]
1959	First evidence of animals (rabbits) produced via IVF in the USA.	[97]
1960s	Investigations of teratocarcinomas in the testes of a number of inbred strains of mice show they derived from embryonic germ cells.	[98]
1968	Edwards and Bavister fertilize the first human egg *in vitro* (for the development of human *in vitro* fertilization).	[97]
1970s	ES cells introduced into mouse blastocysts produce chimeric mice.	[99]
1978	Louise Joy Brown, the first IVF baby, is born in England.	[97]
1980	Australia's first IVF baby, Candace Reed, is born in Melbourne.	[97]
1981	Martin Evans and Matthew Kaufman develop mouse ES cells from the inner cell mass of blastocysts. The first IVF baby in the USA, Elizabeth Carr, is born.	[97]
1984–88	Peter W Andrews develops pluripotent, genetically identical (clonal) cells known as embryonal carcinoma cells from Tera-2.	[100]
1989	Pera *et al* develop a clonal line of human embryonal carcinoma cells, which produces tissues from all three primary germ layers.	[101]
1994	Human blastocysts developed for reproductive purposes using IVF and donated by patients for investigation are produced from the 2-pronuclear stage.	[102]
1995–96	Non-human primate ES cells are developed and maintained *in vitro*, initially from the inner cell mass of rhesus monkeys, and later from marmosets.	[103]
1998	Human embryonic germ cells from the gonadal ridge and mesenchyma tissue (5–9 week fetal tissue) resulting from elective abortions are developed. These cells are cultured *in vitro* for approximately 20 passages, and the cells maintain normal karyotypes.	[104]
2000	Reubinoff *et al* derive pluripotent embryonic stem cells from human blastocysts.	[105]
2001	Kaufman *et al* [75] derived hematopoietic colony-forming cells from human embryonic stem cells.	[106]

early clinical trials of hSC therapies and oversight of hSC research. Table 4.6 reviews the ethical concerns that arise at different phases of stem cell research.

4.16.4 Applications of stem cell research

4.16.4.1 Stem cells can be used to study development

Stem cells may support us in understanding exactly how a complex organism develops from a fertilized egg. In the laboratory, scientists can work on stem cells as they have the capability to divide and become specialized, creating skin, bone, brain and other cell types. Recognizing the signals and mechanisms that govern whether a stem cell chooses to carry on replicating itself or differentiate into a specialized cell type, and into which cell type, will help us to know what controls normal

Table 4.6. Ethical issues at different phases of stem cell research.

Phase of research	Ethical issue
Research with human ES cells.	Destruction of embryos. Creation of embryos specifically for research purposes: • Payment to oocyte donors. • Medical risks of oocyte retrieval. • Protecting reproductive interests of women in infertility treatment.
Use of stem cell lines obtained at another institution.	Contradictory legal and ethical standards.
Stem cell clinical trials.	Possibilities and benefits of experimental intervention. Informed consent.

development. Due to their distinct capacity for regeneration, human stem cells find extensive application in biomedical research and the creation of therapies. Stem cells can be used by researchers to develop new treatments and to understand more about human biology [108]. A number of the most serious medical conditions, e.g. cancer and birth defects, are due to abnormal cell division and differentiation. A better knowledge of the genetic and molecular controls of these processes may yield information about how such diseases arise and suggest new strategies for therapy. This is a significant goal of stem cell research.

4.16.4.2 Stem cells have the ability to replace damaged cells and treat disease

This feature of stem cells is already explored in the management of extensive burns, and to restore the blood system in patients suffering from leukemia and other blood disorders. Stem cells also have the potential to replace cells lost in many other devastating diseases for which there are currently no reliable treatments. Donated tissues and organs are frequently utilized to replace damaged tissue, but the requirement for transplantable tissues and organs far outweighs the available supply. In stem cell transplants, the donor's immune system fights blood-related diseases such multiple myeloma, leukaemia, lymphoma, and neuroblastoma, or the stem cells heal either diseased or chemotherapy-damaged cells. These transplants employ either umbilical cord blood or adult stem cells [109].

4.16.4.3 Stem cells could be used to study disease

In numerous cases it is challenging to obtain cells that have been damaged by a disease, and to examine them in detail. Stem cells, either carrying the disease gene or engineered to contain disease genes, offer a viable alternative. Researchers could use stem cells to model disease processes in the laboratory, and better understand what goes wrong. Diverse types of stem cells have diverse potential uses in cell treatment and disease modelling because of differences in their cell origins, proliferation, and differentiation capacities [110].

4.16.4.4 Stem cells could offer a resource for testing new medical treatments
New medications could be tested for safety on specialized cells generated in large numbers from stem cell lines—reducing the need for animal testing. Other kinds of cell lines are already used in this way. Cancer cell lines, for example, are used to screen potential anti-tumor drugs.

4.16.5 Human ES cells

'Stem cells' are cells with the capacity to divide and develop into more identical stem cells or to specialize and form specific cells of somatic tissues. From donated embryos, hundreds of hESC lines have been produced [111]. Usually, there are two types of stem cells: ES cells which can only be developed from pre-implantation embryos and have a reported potential to yield cells of all tissues of the adult organism (called 'pluripotent'), and 'adult' stem cells, which are present in a range of tissues in the fetus and after birth and are, under normal conditions, more specialized ('multipotent') with a significant function in tissue replacement and repair. hES cells are obtained from the so-called 'inner cell mass' of blastocyst stage embryos that develop in culture within five days of fertilization of the oocyte [105, 112]. Although hES cells can form all somatic tissues, they cannot form all of the other 'extraembryonic' tissues essential for complete growth, e.g. the placenta and membranes, so that they cannot develop into complete new organisms. They are thus dissimilar from the 'totipotent' fertilized oocyte and blastomere cells developing from the first cleavage divisions. hES cells are also remarkable, expressing great levels of a gene known as telomerase, the protein product of which guarantees that the telomere ends of the chromosomes are reserved at each cell division and the cells do not experience senescence. Human hESCs' capacity to develop specialized cells to replace damaged tissue in patients with a variety of degenerative diseases has the most therapeutic promise. The only other cells with established pluripotency comparable to that of ES cells are embryonic germ cells, which as their name implies, have been obtained from 'primordial germ cells' that would finally form the gametes if the fetus had not been aborted. In humans, human embryonic germ (hEG) cells were first identified in culture in 1998, just after the first hES cells, from tissue derived from an aborted fetus [104]. Naturally, hEG cells have many features in common with hES cells [113]. In the adult organism, a diversity of tissues have also been found to harbor stem cell populations, e.g. umbilical cord blood, brain, skeletal muscle and bone marrow, while the heart, in contrast, contains no stem cells after birth [114]. These adult stem cells have usually been observed as having the ability to form only the cell types of the organ in which they are found, but in recent times they have been revealed to display a surprising versatility [115]. The evidence is strongest in animal experiments, but is increasing in humans, that adult stem cells originating in one germ layer can form a variety of other derivatives of the same germ layer (e.g. bone marrow-to-muscle within the mesodermal lineage), as well as transdifferentiate to derivatives of other germ layers (e.g. bone marrow-to-brain between the mesodermal and ectodermal lineages). Even though the discussion here concerns hES cells and the use of embryos, the logical state-of-the-art on other types of stem cell is significant with regard to the 'subsidiarity principle'.

4.17 Applications of stem cells in diseases

At the vanguard of contemporary medical progress, regenerative medicine employs functional recovery of organs or tissues to address severe injuries or chronic diseases. Developments in the study of stem cells have created prospects in the creation of treatments based on cells that target conditions that are unmanageable with conventional methods. Stem cells, due to their infinite ability to regenerate themselves and their capability of differentiating in various cell types, represent the prospective frontier of regenerative medicine. The versatility of regenerative medicine applications is also contingent upon the transdifferentiating capacity of the stem cells utilized as a source. Stem cells not only serve as the fundamental support for all tissue and organ systems in the body, but they also perform a variety of functions in the development, progression, and recovery of diseases within the host. Based on their capacity for transdifferentiation, stem cells are classified as (1) unipotent, (2) multipotent, (3) pluripotent, or (4) totipotent [91]. Additionally, given their potential for use in regenerative applications, stem cells can be categorized as follows: ESCs, bone marrow stem cells (BM-SCs), umbilical cord stem cells (UC-SCs), mesenchymal stem cells (MSCs), tissue-specific progenitor stem cells (TSPSCs), and iPSCs.

When it comes to regenerative medicine, recent advancements emphasize the importance of stem cell-based therapies, like multipotent MSCs and human pluripotent stem cells (hPSCs). In the case of terminally ill patients, for whom conventional treatments primarily aim at disease management rather than curative measures, stem cell therapy emerges as an encouraging prospect. A fundamental component of regenerative medicine, the main goal of stem cell therapy is to increase the body's capacity for self-healing through stimulation, regulation, and alteration in number of endogenous stem cells, and replenishment of cell numbers in a manner that promotes tissue homeostasis and regeneration [116]. Since inception of the stem cell concept, which is based on the recognition of its potential therapeutic capabilities of self-renewal and differentiation, extensive basic and clinical research has been conducted on these cells. Regenerative medicine is a field that aims to accomplish cellular replacement and tissue regeneration through the utilization of diverse stem cell types—progenitor cells, multipotent stem cells, and hPSCs—among others. Stem cell therapy is a cutting-edge treatment strategy that makes use of stem cells' special characteristics, such as their capacity for differentiation and self-renewal to repair or substitute impaired human body cells and tissues with fresh, healthy ones [88]. This is achieved by introducing exogenous cells into the patient. Stem cells function as the foundational components of all bodily organs and tissue systems, assuming a multitude of functions in the development, advancement, and restoration of pathological conditions within the host. Stem cell therapy has demonstrated its efficacy in regenerating many physiological systems and conditions, such as autoimmune diseases, cardiovascular disease, digestive system

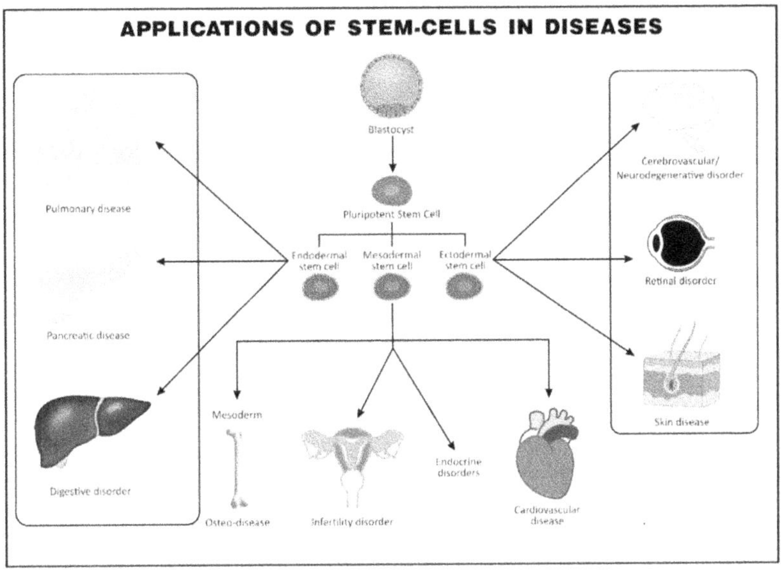

Figure 4.24. Applications of stem cells in various diseases.

disorder, liver disease, arthritis, cancer treatment, pulmonary fibrosis, endocrine disorder, acute respiratory distress syndrome, skin burn, and wound healing, neurodegenerative disorder, chronic obstructive pulmonary disease, asthma, and idiopathic pulmonary fibrosis (figure 4.24).

Stem cells derived from blastocyst divide into PSCs that differentiate into endodermal, ectodermal and mesodermal stem cells. These are employed in the management of various diseases.

4.17.1 Applications of stem cells in cardiovascular diseases

More than seventeen million deaths annually are ascribed to cardiovascular disease on a global scale, positioning it as the leading cause of mortality. The American Heart Association estimates that the global mortality toll from cardiovascular causes will surpass 23 million by 2030 [117]. While contemporary therapies for ischemic heart disease strive to decrease premature mortality rates, avert additional harm to the heart muscle, and lower the likelihood of subsequent myocardial infarctions, it is expected that the majority of patients will encounter a decline in quality of life characterized by increased frequency of hospitalization. To ultimately ameliorate clinical conditions, therefore, a therapeutic approach that either replaces the damaged heart cells or improves cardiac function is required. The potential therapeutic utility of stem cell-based cardiac tissue regeneration has been recognized [118].

Recent developments indicate that direct conversion is achievable of somatic cells into cardiomyocytes, albeit with an extremely weak effect. Isomi *et al* (2021) demonstrated that induced cardiomyocytes (iCMs), which mature into contracting cardiomyocytes, can be generated from fibroblasts via transgenic expression of three transcription factors specific to the heart (Gata4, Mef2c, and Tbx5) [119].

iPSC-derived progenitor cells have undergone differentiation into cardiomyocytes, which are responsible for the formation of contracting regions in the cardiac tissue of rodents. Notwithstanding the lack of mature donor cardiomyocytes that were precisely aligned, advantageous remodelling and improved ventricular function were detected [120]. In another investigation, particular growth factors, such as GSK3 and BMP, were used to promote the development of cardiac progenitor cells [121]. The embryoid body technique was employed in electrophysiological experiments to validate the cardiac differentiation of these cells into cells of the nodal, atrial, and ventricular types [122]. Successful differentiation of iPSCs in smooth muscle cells, vascular endothelium, and cardiomyocytes was observed in the heart of a rat following injection [123]. This differentiation was accompanied by a reduction in fibrosis and an increase in the ejection fraction. Cardiomyocytes, smooth muscle cells, and endothelial cells produced from human-induced pluripotent stem cells (hiPSCs) were introduced into the host myocardium in a pig model via means of transplanting microspheres into the heart. This procedure resulted in enhancements to left ventricular function, infarct size, and myocardial metabolism [124]. The ejection fraction was maintained in a larger animal model where sheep hearts that had been infarcted and implanted with cardiac-committed ESCs indicated a successful engraftment [125]. Additionally, MSCs are present in umbilical cord blood, adipose tissue, placenta, and bone marrow. Myeloid-derived suppressor cells are a valuable source of donor cells on a global scale due to their immunomodulatory properties and ability to elude immune cell recognition via the unique distribution of surface signals. In addition to MHC class I, they lack MHC class II molecules and have diminished quantities of costimulatory CD40, CD80, and CD86 [126]. Even in the absence of sufficient differentiation into cardiomyocytes and minimal cellular retention, transplanted MSCs have been shown to enhance heart function, according to studies [127]. This suggests that transplanted MSCs may operate via a paracrine mechanism. Among the cardioprotective factors secreted by MSCs are angiogenic, homing, apoptotic, mitogenic, and apoptotic factors [128]. The significance of hepatocyte growth factor (HGF) in cardiomyocyte proliferation and angiogenesis was emphasized in one study. In addition, through a paracrine pathway, MSC implantation stimulated endogenous cardiac progenitor cells, resulting in their proliferation, migration, and prevention of cell mortality; increased expression of genes associated with cardiomyocytes was also observed [129].

After injury, stem cells from various locations go to the organ damage site, where they undergo differentiation and contribute to the process of organ restoration. In their investigation, Orlic *et al* examined the feasibility of scar regeneration through the remote injection of stem cells into the heart. The results indicated that the myocardium of infarcted rodents could undergo repair with local administration of autologous BM-SCs [130]. MSCs' capacity to develop into cardiomyocytes *in vitro* was confirmed through their co-cultivation with ventricular myocytes in neonates [131]. In animal models, MSCs derived from bone marrow exhibited successful engraftment and differentiation into vascular and cardiomyogenic phenotypes after being injected into hearts of mice and rats subsequent to myocardial infarction [132]. Myocytes were thought to be incapable of regenerating. Despite this, myocytes are capable of mitotic division following myocardial ischemia, according to research [133]. Early hallmarks of cardiogenesis (platelet-derived growth factor receptor-α) and mesenchymal stem cell (MSC) markers (CD90, CD105) were detected on these cells, along with embryonic stem cell markers (Rex1, Nanog, Sox2) [134]. Consistently, research on animals has shown that it is possible for cardiac stem cells to differentiate into cardiac lineage cells, thereby more efficiently taking on the anatomical features of arteries and myocytes [135]. Enhanced left ventricular function (LVEF) was observed in animal experiments where human-derived cells were injected into the infarcted myocardium [136]. The procurement of cardiac stem cells presents a significant obstacle, as the majority of studies have relied on autologous cardiac stem cells that have been culture-grown subsequent to their extraction from the ventricles, atrial appendages, or epicardial biopsies [137]. The 'Stem Cell Infusion in Patients with Ischemic Cardiomyopathy' (SCIPIO) phase I clinical trial provides coronary artery bypass grafting (CABG) patients with heart failure autologous cardiac stem cells. At four and twelve months after infusion, preliminary results indicate an increase in LVEF and a reduction in infarct size [138].

4.17.2 Applications of stem cells in digestive system diseases

The gastrointestinal tract is protected by a single layer of epithelial cells, which serves as a barrier against dangerous substances found in the gut. The cells demonstrate a significant ability to regenerate in response to damage and regular cell replacement [139]. Under normal circumstances, these epithelial cells have fast regeneration, occurring about every two to seven days, and more quickly after inflammation and tissue damage. The ability to proliferate quickly is attributed to a certain group of stem cells that are closely confined within intestinal crypts [140]. The susceptibility of the gastrointestinal system to harm, inflammation of tissues, and diseases becomes more noticeable when the protective layer of mucosal lining is weakened, resulting in obvious clinical symptoms [141]. An investigation carried out by Rashed and colleagues in 2016 assessed the combined effect of MSCs generated from bone marrow and a nitric oxide (NO) inducer on damaged gastric mucosa in a rat model [142]. After intravenously infusing MSCs and a nitric oxide inducer, histopathological examinations were performed. The group that received both stem cells and NO had changes in the process of mucosal regeneration and achieved full recovery of gastric ulcers. BM-SCs can accelerate healing process and improve efficacy in ulcer treatment by releasing vascular endothelial growth factor (VEGF) [143].

Inflammatory bowel disease (IBD) primarily presents as Crohn's disease (CD) and ulcerative colitis, impacting the gastrointestinal system. CD is a persistent and unmanageable inflammatory condition that affects inner lining of the intestines. It is defined by the presence of granulomas and inflammation that extends across the entire thickness of the intestinal wall in certain segments [144]. Ulcerative colitis is a chronic inflammatory bowel illness that mostly affects colon and rectum. It is characterized by ongoing inflammation of the rectum that spreads to the colon [145]. According to recent studies, hematopoietic stem cell (HSC) recruitment is not enhanced by high dosages of cyclophosphamide, but they do increase likelihood of bladder and heart damage. Autologous hematopoietic stem cell transplants (HSCTs) have shown long-lasting clinical remission in certain individuals with CD, although not in all cases [146, 147]. This sparked interest in utilizing HSCTs for the treatment of CD, leading to the largest group of CD patients with treatment-resistant symptoms getting HSCT as part of the Autologous Stem Cell Transplantation International Crohn Disease trial (ASTIC) in 2015 [148]. Despite the presence of high toxicity, a further reassessment of the outcomes of the ASTIC study revealed that the approach had endoscopic and clinical benefits, despite a considerable number of adverse events [149]. A recent systematic analysis, conducted by Wang *et al* (2021), examined 18 human trials including 360 persons with Crohn's disease (CD) [150]. The HSCT groups showed an improvement over the control group in the Crohn's disease activity score that was statistically significant. Concerns regarding the application of HSCT for refractory CD patients have emerged due to significant toxicity linked with the procedure. One of the main areas of research for CD treatment has been the safety of stem cell-based therapy, with special attention given to the increased susceptibility to infection in CD patients compared to those receiving treatment for cancer or other conditions. It is widely accepted that people with genetic predispositions and dysregulated immune responses are the source of inflammatory and immunologically mediated bowel diseases. The rising occurrence and frequency of chronic illnesses in Western populations have a substantial effect on public health.

4.17.3 Applications of stem cells in intestinal fibrosis

Stem cell transplantation appears to be a viable treatment option for intestinal fibrosis, according to some research. According to Luo *et al*, BM-MSC transplantation can cause them to migrate to injured liver regions, boosting the M2/M1 macrophage ratio [151]. This action therefore has an effect on the mortality of HSCs [151]. Ly6Chi/lo macrophages and other macrophage subtypes are seen in the liver. In contrast to the highly inflammatory and fibrotic Ly6Chi, Ly6Clo has the potential to attenuate liver inflammation and fibrosis through its ability to produce particular cytokines. According to Li *et al*, BM-MSCs limit the recruitment of Ly6Chi and regulate the conversion of Ly6Chi to Ly6Clo, lowering liver fibrosis [152]. MSCs have been shown in animal experiments to have antiapoptotic [153] antioxidant [154] antifibrotic [155] angiogenic [156] and immunosuppressive effects in macrophages, dendritic cells, and T cells. Patients with liver cirrhosis were given injections of bone marrow-derived MSCs (BM-MSCs) in studies conducted by Kantarcioglu *et al* [157] and Mohamadnejad *et al* [158] but no therapeutic results were detected. Kharaziha *et al*, on the other hand, described phase I–II clinical trials against liver cirrhosis of different aetiologies, exhibiting improvement in liver function, employing autologous BM-MSCs [159]. Suk *et al* reported a phase II trial and a pilot study using autologous BM-MSCs delivered into the hepatic artery to treat alcoholic liver cirrhosis [160]. There was an improvement in liver function and histology liver fibrosis trials using autologous BM-MSCs to treat hepatitis B virus-associated cirrhosis, confirming improved liver function, decreased Th17 cells, and increased regulatory T cells [161]. Trials including umbilical cord-derived MSCs in people with chronic hepatitis B who had primary biliary cirrhosis or decompensated liver cirrhosis [162, 163]. In a trial of hepatitis B-related acute or chronic liver failure, MSCs markedly increased survival rates [164]

4.17.4 Applications of stem cells in liver diseases

Around the world, hundreds of millions of patients suffer from liver problems, with liver failure resulting from severe hepatic injury that prevents the liver from carrying out its metabolic processes—typical, physiological, and synthetic. Liver failure has conventionally been classified as either acute (ALF) or chronic (CLF). ALF is distinguished by the abrupt onset of coagulopathy, hepatic encephalopathy, and hyperbilirubinemia in the absence of any pre-existing liver disease. Polson *et al* [165] describe this syndrome as dramatic, unpredictable, and connected to a high rate of morbidity and death. Acute-on-chronic liver failure (AoCLF) is a condition characterized by episodes of acute decompensation, which are initiated by factors such as upper gastrointestinal hemorrhage or infection. These episodes serve to worsen the pre-existing chronic liver disease [166]. In order to investigate the potential therapeutic applications of BM-SCs, Autologous $CD133^{+}$ cells were intraportally transplanted into liver cancer patients by Terai *et al* [167] before they had extensive liver resection (LR) due to portal embolization. Autologous BM-SC transplantation prior to LR has recently demonstrated enhanced hepatocellular carcinoma and cirrhosis patients' liver function [168].

HGF, fibroblast growth factor 2 (FGF2), fibroblast growth factor 4 (FGF4), and bone morphogenetic protein 4 (BMP4) regulate hepatic specification in MSC. At the mature stage, dexamethasone, ITS premix, and oncostatin M (OSM) are frequently required [169]. To monitor hepatic development, numerous genes, including early and ultimate hepatic maturation markers such as alpha-fetoprotein (AFP), alpha-1-antitrypsin (A1AT), and ALB, can be selectively upregulated or downregulated. After undergoing hepatic differentiation, HLCs derived from MSCs exhibited increased levels of AFP, MRP2, CYP1A2, CYP3A4, and UTG1A6, in addition to decreased levels of CD73 [170]. Liver function was enhanced in both the group treated with MSCs and the group treated with HLC, although MSCs demonstrated superior performance across multiple metrics [171]. As described by Kollet *et al* [172], proteolytic enzymes, chemokines, and cytokines aided HSC migration into the wounded liver. Diffusion of HSCs was found to be essential for liver repair. HSCs stimulated with G-CSF exhibited hepatocyte proliferation, migration to the site of injury in the liver, and tissue regeneration potential [173]. At the 12-month follow-up, the repeated HSC infusion group demonstrated more pronounced enhancements in liver functions and a sustained continuance of clinical efficacy in comparison to the single HSC infusion group. According to a study by Lu *et al* [174], MSCs have the ability to proliferation, prevent hepatocyte apoptosis, and decrease mortality. It was discovered that MSCs increase hepatocyte proliferation in models of liver failure; PGE2 emitted by MSCs stimulates hepatocyte proliferation via YAP and mTOR signalling [174].

4.17.5 Applications of stem cells in osteoarthritis

Osteoarthritis (OA) is a dynamic condition resulting from an imbalance between joint deterioration and repair, rather than just a passive degenerative illness [175]. The main cause of the rising incidence of OA in recent years is changes in the environment. Obesity, metabolic syndrome, dietary changes, and physical inactivity are the four main environmental variables that contribute to the genesis of osteoarthritis. Due to the increased weight loading pressure on weight-bearing joints, obesity is regarded as a key risk factor, especially for knee OA [176]. Three main goals of OA treatment are to reduce pain, postpone joint degradation, and maintain or improve mobility function.

The most popular therapeutic MSC source is BM-MSCs, they are appreciated for their ease of application, rapid cell division, capacity for prolonged differentiation, and reduced immunological exclusion [177]. Superior scores on arthroscopy and histological grading after 42 weeks were found in a 20-year clinical trial using BM-MSC transplantation for knee osteoarthritis, indicating possible efficacy [178]. Autologous BM-MSC transplantation showed improved scores in a 2-year follow-up trial following high tibial osteotomy and microfracture, suggesting that it is an effective treatment for osteoarthritis [179]. Increased meniscal volume and pain reduction without side effects were seen in another trial using allogeneic BM-MSCs following partial medial meniscectomy [180]. Therapeutic MSCs can benefit from the use of adipose tissue-derived MSCs (AD-MSCs), since their potential is higher for differentiation and proliferation than BM-MSCs [181]. Low-dose AD-MSCs dramatically decreased pain and enhanced function in osteoarthritis patients in a phase I dosage-escalation experiment [182]. Better tissue healing and pain alleviation were observed in a 24-month experiment that compared AD-MSCs with microfracture therapy [183]. After six months of treatment with AD-MSCs, patients with knee OA showed increased function, a lower WOMAC score, safety, and less discomfort [184]. MSCs produced from umbilical cord (UC-MSCs), an additional intriguing source for stem cell treatment, which have been shown to have higher proliferation capability, active differentiation ability, and improved immunomodulatory potential [185]. Clinical trials show that UC-MSCs may be useful in the treatment of osteoarthritis; a 6-month experiment that included 36 patients found that the cell therapy group had improved Lysholm, WOMAC, and SF-36 ratings without experiencing a recurrence of knee pain at follow-up [186].

4.17.6 Applications of stem cells in cancer

When discussing cancer treatment, the term ‘stem cell therapy’ needs to be carefully considered and used with caution. It is imperative that medical professionals and researchers shield healthy people and cancer patients from potentially expensive, dangerous, or useless stem cell treatments. In an effort to treat cancer, unreliable stem cell facilities frequently use three main cell-based therapies: stromal vascular fraction (SVF), autologous HSCs, and multipotent stem cells like MSCs. HSCs derived from allogeneic donors are recognized for their ‘graft-versus-tumor effects,’ which include the capacity to generate donor lymphocytes that support the targeting of solid tumors and the regression and suppression of haematological malignancies [187]. In their efforts to manage cancer, clinics using stem cells in experimentation have employed the main cell-based therapies: autologous HSCs, multipotent stem cells, and stem cell fraction. Targeting solid tumors and suppressing and regressing hematological malignancies are both made possible by allogeneic HSCs' special capacity to produce 'graft-versus-tumor effects' [187]. In addition to the specific C–X–C chemokine receptor type 4 (CXCR4), MSCs express other chemokine receptors, such as CCR1, CCR2, CCR4, and CCR7, which are necessary for reacting to environmental cues [188]. Moreover, MSCs can adhere, rotate, migrate, and pierce blood channel lumens to infiltrate injured tissues because of adherent proteins expressed on their surface, such as CD49d, CD44, CD54, CD102, and CD106 [189].

4.17.7 Applications of stem cells in endocrine disorders

To maintain function and homeostatic balance, the human body produces and releases a variety of hormones through an intricate network of endocrine glands. The development of diabetes, thyroid issues, irregular growth patterns, reproductive dysfunction, and other metabolic illnesses are mostly caused by dysregulation of the endocrine system. Adult stem cells as a template for the regeneration of tissues and organs are a central idea in regenerative medicine. These stem cells' activities are controlled by endocrine signals from hormones, growth factors, and cytokines as well as microenvironmental cues from nervous system (rapid response). This organized and choreographed system directly regulates tissue homeostasis and post-injury repair through a symphony of signals. In recent years, type 1 diabetes mellitus (T1DM) and type 2 diabetes (T2DM) have emerged as two main endocrinology research topics. Using MSCs is now a practical therapeutic approach to be investigated. Insulin resistance plus dysfunction of the insulin-producing pancreatic cells identify T2DM, whereas autoimmune death of pancreatic β-cells characterizes T1DM. The main goal of regenerative medicine is to restore damaged or lost β-cells to patients' bodies in order to normalize their blood glucose levels. According to http://www.clinicaltrials.gov, 28 clinical studies were conducted using MSCs to treat type 1 diabetes as of October 2021. Out of these, three trials with allogeneic AT-MSCs (NCT03920397) [190], autologous BM-MSCs (NCT01068951) [191], and allogeneic BM-MSCs (NCT00690066) [192] were finished. Fascinatingly, UC-MSCs were the most favoured MSCs in the clinical trials. The studies have demonstrated that MSC therapy for type 1 diabetes is safe and does not cause any adverse effects. According to Carlsson *et al* [193], using autologous BM-MSCs, the first trial revealed that patients randomized to the group administering the MSC responded to a mixed-meal tolerance test with higher C-peptide levels than did the control group. Regretfully, there was no discernible drop in insulin level needs, HbA1C, or C-peptide. Better HbA1C results were seen six months following therapy, and using autologous AT-MSCs in conjunction with vitamin D was found to be safe. The main use of MSCs as a treatment for T1DM with recent onset was observed three and six months after injection, when Wharton's Jelly (WJ)-MSCs significantly improved both HbA1C and C-peptide levels in contrast to the control group [194]. Autologous BM-derived mononuclear cells enhanced insulin production and decreased insulin needs in T1DM patients when paired with allogeneic WJ-MSCs [195]. 23 studies related to type 2 diabetes were identified when clinicaltrials.gov was searched in October 2021; six of these studies were completed (three of those used BM-MSCs and three used allogeneic UC-MSCs). The results of studies that used MSCs to treat T2DM indicated the safety of MSCs because no significant side effects were observed [196]. It was shown that MSC therapy increased C-peptide levels and may have lowered HbA1C and fasting blood glucose levels. However, the effects of MSCs were only transient, requiring many dosages to maintain. It is interesting to note that both diminished stemness and functional characteristics were observed in BM-MSCs and AT-MSCs isolated from patients with diabetes. This complicates the autologous MSC strategy to treat patients with diabetes generally [197]. Therefore, the allogeneic strategy—which employs MSCs from healthy donors—offers a different approach to using stem cell therapy to treat diabetic patients.

4.17.8 Applications of stem cells in infertility and reproductive function recovery

The inability to conceive following more than a year of unprotected sexual activity is known as infertility, and it is a problem that is becoming more and more prevalent in modern society [198]. This problem has grown to be a major global health and social burden. *In vitro* fertilization and assisted reproduction procedures are the most successful methods for treating infertility. Their restricted application, however, presents difficulties for individuals who are sperm-deficient or who experience problems with implantation during pregnancy. Furthermore, these methods are linked to intricacies, substantial expenses, temporal limitations, and ethical dilemmas in some situations [199].

Premature ovarian failure (POF) is a serious concern. It affects 1%–2% of fertile women and is characterized by diminished ovarian function before the age of 40 [200]. Huhtaniemi *et al* [201] have identified several factors that contribute to POF, such as autoimmune disorders, genetic factors, environmental impacts, and iatrogenic and idiopathic conditions. Preclinical research using animal models of POF produced by chemotherapy has demonstrated encouraging outcomes in improving ovarian function with the use of MSCs derived from adipose tissue, bone marrow, and umbilical cord. Notably, in an early trial, BM-MSCs showed better follicular regeneration, which resulted in elevated levels of anti-Müllerian hormone (AMH), a successful pregnancy, and a healthy baby born [202]. Two women with POF showed improved ovarian volume and baseline estrogen levels after receiving autologous BM-MSC treatment, which also relieved menopausal symptoms [203]. Subsequent trials using a similar methodology also showed favourable effects, even though these early trials entailed invasive procedures like laparoscopy and BM aspiration [204]. Using bone marrow-derived stem cells, the autologous stem cell ovarian transplantation (ASCOT) experiment demonstrated positive signals of increased ovarian performance in 81.3% of patients, building on good results from animal models. The antral follicle count (AFC), elevated AMH levels, six pregnancies, and the safe delivery of three children were among these. In 20 people with POF under 39 years old, a random study sought to investigate the results of the ASCOT trial in more detail [205]. Nonetheless, there are not many studies evaluating MSCs produced from adipose tissue and umbilical cords for the therapy of POF, perhaps because the illness is uncommon. Although it is rare—affecting only 1% of women under 40—new developments in assisted reproductive technologies, such as stem cell transplantation, provide patients hoping to regain reproductive function a variety of options [206].

4.17.9 Applications of stem cells in skin burns and wound healing

Burns rank fourth among the world's most prevalent injuries with roughly 11 million occurrences and 180 000 patient fatalities each year,and are divided into four severity levels. The amount of burned surface area, burn depth, location, and patient age all affect the severity of a burn [207]. The severity of burns, as well as the quality of therapy, have a direct impact on postburn recovery, which can range from quick recovery over a few weeks to a slow process lasting many months, sometimes resulting in scarring and functional impairment. Burn injuries are distinguished from other types of injury by the presence of both mechanical and biological damage, such as oxidative stress, spontaneous apoptosis, prolonged inflammation, and decreased tissue perfusion [208]. While complete reversal of severe burn damage remains a challenge in modern medicine, stem cell therapy offers an alternate treatment option. The first case study, which involved a patient, 45 years old, who had 40% burns and was treated with BM-MSCs, showed reduced scarring and better vascularization at the wound site [209]. Following research, autologous or allogeneic BM-MSCs were used to treat deep second- and third-degree burns. MSCs were either sprayed onto burn sites or mixed into a layer of dermal matrix covering the injury. The outcomes showed that MSC-based therapy may be helpful in reducing pain, increasing blood flow, and accelerating healing without reinfection [210]. A 2017 study revealed using autologous BM-MSCs or UC-MSCs in patients with 10%–25% burns depicted a quicker recovery and shorter hospital stays for both MSC types [211]. Despite the disadvantages of invasive BM-MSC harvesting procedures that cause pain and problems, allogeneic MSCs obtained from healthy donors, for example AT-MSCs and UC-MSCs, emerge as preferable burn treatment choices. While the most effective MSCs for burn tissue regeneration are unknown, research suggests that AT-MSCs have advantageous biological qualities, such as boosting keratinocyte proliferation and secretion patterns that considerably accelerate the skin regeneration process [212].

4.17.10 Stem cell applications in neurodegenerative diseases

Neurodegenerative diseases are typified by a progressive decrease in the quantity of neurons, anatomical alterations, and a loss of function in brain or spinal cord. These diseases include Parkinson's disease (PD), Alzheimer's disease (AD), Huntington's disease (HD), amyotrophic lateral sclerosis (ALS), and frontotemporal dementia (FTD). Regretfully, there aren't many treatment choices available right now to stop these neurodegenerative processes [213]. Our comprehension of the harmful processes and the creation of efficient remedies are significantly hampered by the intricacy of the pathways linked with neuronal loss and various physiological explanations of these illnesses.

Regenerative therapy, often known as stem cell therapy, uses stem cells or their derivatives to improve the ability of injured and dysfunctional tissues to regenerate. Restoring lost cells or enhancing the environment are the main objectives of stem cell treatments. Stem cell therapy has transformed medicine over time and presents significant opportunities for the management of several ailments, including neurological disorders [214]. When PD patients had fetal mesencephalic tissue transplantation in the 1980s, the possibility of stem cell therapy for neurological disorders was initially shown [215]. Neuronal populations are lost in neurodegenerative illnesses such PD, AD, HD, ALS, and FTD that typified by disruptions in protein homeostasis. These inclusion bodies are formed of unfolded and insoluble proteins. Slow paralysis and the progressive loss of motor neurons, senses, and cognitive function result from this degenerative trend. There are currently no detectable markers or viable treatments to halt the progression of neurodegenerative illnesses, despite significant investments in clinical trials and developments in our knowledge of the underlying processes [216]. The purpose of stem cell therapy for neurodegenerative diseases is to produce specific neural subtypes and recreate a brain network similar to the one that has been lost as a result of the illness. Building new neural networks surrounding injured areas or improving the environment to produce neurotrophic and scavenging chemicals that help host neurons are two other strategies [217]. *De novo* production and administration of growth factors that are neuroprotective, such as VEGF, brain-derived neurotrophic factor (BDNF), insulin-like growth factor-1 (IGF-1), and glial-derived neurotrophic factor (GDNF), at the site of disease to enhance the environment, are two popular stem cell-based strategies.

4.17.10.1 Applications of stem cells in Parkinson's disease

The symptoms of PD include movement-related symptoms that are caused by a reduction in dopamine levels in the striatum as a result of the selective death of dopaminergic neurons in the substantia nigra pars compacta [218]. Additional non-motor symptoms are caused by neurodegeneration in other areas, like the cerebral cortex [219]. PD first presents as bradykinesia, stiffness, rest tremor, and later on, postural instability and convulsions. Dopamine (DA), a crucial neurotransmitter that promotes signal transmission between neurons, is largely responsible for motor control. PD is caused by impairments in DA in the striatum due to the substantia nigra's dopamine-producing neurons dying off [220]. Deep brain stimulation and drugs that raise dopamine levels by utilizing DA precursors, such as levodopa, are the current therapy for PD. In the past 20 years, scientists have looked into ways to raise DA levels using dopaminergic neuron substitutes made from stem cells. To create adult dopaminergic neurons, researchers use iPSCs, NSCs, and ESCs [221]. Human fetal brain cells are being transplanted into patients in clinical studies as a means of optimizing benefits and reducing side effects from stem cell treatment, which has demonstrated promise in treating PD in animal models [222].

Research involving dopaminergic neurons produced from monkey ESCs transplanted into the brains of PD patients showed functional recovery [223]. In a PD rat model, undifferentiated ESCs were essential for functional recovery [224]. Parthenogenetic stem cells' safety and tolerability for treating PD were evaluated in phase I clinical studies [225]. Positive results have been shown for both ESCs and NSCs; NSCs reduce PD symptoms by releasing DA [226]. MSCs have shown promise in PD animal model in repairing damaged striatal dopaminergic nerve terminals [227]. Bladder dysfunction was alleviated *in vivo* by stem cell therapy employing MSCs and human amniotic fluid stem cells [228]. Better dyskinesias and functional recovery without side effects were shown in an early clinical trial utilizing MSC transplants [229]. PD patients' motor function was enhanced by modified MSCs infused into the substantia nigra artery [224].

For patients with PD, iPSCs have shown promise in producing DA replacement. iPSC-derived dopaminergic neurons have demonstrated long-lasting integration into the host with advantageous functional outcomes [230]. Reprogrammed iPSC transplantation into dopaminergic neurons enhanced *in vivo* cell integration and functional deficits [231]. In preclinical studies, iPSC-derived DA progenitors showed efficacy and safety for long-term survival and functionality [232]. Altogether, stem cell therapy for PD may be highly beneficial when paired with environmental enrichment and cellular replacement therapy. This makes PD a prime target for stem cell therapy. However, as long-term transplantation studies have shown, care must be taken when assessing the hazards related to graft-induced dyskinesias [233].

4.17.10.2 Applications of stem cells in Alzheimer's disease

AD is a neurodegenerative disorder defined by neuronal loss in the neocortex and hippocampal regions, along with synaptic degradation. The disease usually manifests itself with symptoms like memory loss, impaired judgment, communication problems, and difficulty solving problems, dementia, and eventually death [234, 235]. AD includes early-onset familial types resulting from genetic defects that affect people under the age of 65, as well as sporadic forms that affect people over 65. Gene polymorphisms, age, type 2 diabetes, Down's syndrome, stroke, and traumatic brain injury are linked to late-onset AD [224]. With an emphasis on neurogenesis, neuron replacement, and improving the environment, stem cell therapy has the potential to slow the course of AD.

It has been demonstrated that NSCs upregulate the expression of cognition-related proteins *in vivo*, which may enhance synaptic plasticity, lessen illness symptoms, and alleviate memory issues in AD mouse models [236]. Nonetheless, no discernible reduction in tau or Aβ pathology was seen, suggesting that NSCs might modulate degenerative processes without treating the underlying illness [237]. In the hippocampal region of an animal model of AD, transplanted NSCs enhanced memory deficits, produced BDNF, and suppressed pro-inflammatory cytokines, and stimulated neuroplasticity and endogenous neural precursors. They underwent differentiation into distinct brain cells, such as neurons, oligodendrocytes, glutamatergic, and astrocytes, indicating possible advantages in promoting neurogenesis and cognitive function [238]. According to recent research, the implantation of iPSC-produced progenitors of cholinergic neurons in the hippocampal area can restore spatial memory impairment in transgenic AD mice. Despite the fact that these precursors matured into cholinergic neurons, there remains a non-negligible risk of tumor development due to the extremely proliferating nature of iPSCs [239]. According to several studies, MSCs improve synaptogenesis and/or microglial activation in AD models, decrease accumulation, encourage cognitive recovery, stimulate neurogenesis, and induce neuronal differentiation. For example, Ma *et al* demonstrated that MSCs altered microglial activation, upregulating VEGF and IL-10, and improving memory impairments and Aβ levels in animal AD models [240]. Furthermore, Kan *et al* showed that endogenous NSCs were induced to proliferate, differentiate, and mature towards a neuronal phenotype by MSCs implanted into an AD model [241]. According to Martinez-Morales *et al*, MSCs can generate neurotrophic factors, which promote angiogenesis, endogenous neurogenesis, and brain defence systems [242].

4.17.10.3 Applications of stem cells in Huntington's disease

HD is a neurological disorder inherited in an autosomal dominant manner. It is characterized by the degeneration of certain brain regions, including the brain stem, cortex, hippocampus, and GABAergic inhibitory spiny neurons in striatum of the forebrain [243]. The underlying etiology of HD is the improper differentiation of cytosine-adenine-guanine (CAG) encoded repeats at the N-terminal of the huntingtin protein (Htt). The spread of this condition specifically causes the striatal medium spiny neurons' specific degeneration, leading to impairments in cognitive and emotional functioning, involuntary motor movements, and the development of dementia [217]. Therapeutic strategies based on stem cells have garnered a lot of interest as potential remedies for HD, with replacing depleted or impaired neurons and altering extended CAG repeats in mutant genes. Ebert *et al* [243] employed HD-infected mice to discover that NSCs from the mice could produce GDNF, which prevented the death of neurons and the ensuing damage of motor function. MSCs are excellent cells for treating HD because they can prevent immune cells from malfunctioning, reduce apoptosis, increase compensatory neurogenesis, assist cells survive, and improve mitochondrial function [243]. Genetically engineered MSCs that overexpressed nerve growth factor (NGF) or BDNF were discovered to lessen neuronal loss in the striatum and enhance neurological function with behavioural problems in the YAC 128 mouse model of HD in 2010 [244]. Introducing BDNF-rich MSCs into the striatum may make it a more pleasant place to dwell, thereby slowing neuronal degeneration [214]. Snyder *et al* [245] found injecting MSCs derived from human into HD-infected rats boosted the development and differentiation of endogenous NSCs in the hippocampus's dentate gyrus. Lin *et al* [246] demonstrated that human-derived MSCs protected and restored neurons through neurotrophic support, neuronal differentiation, and antiapoptotic actions, resulting in a notable improvement in the motor dysfunction of an HD mouse model. Dental pulp stem cells (DPSCs) have also been considered as a potential treatment for HD due to a decreased rate of immunological rejection following transplantation [247]. Giving HD animals NPCs via the striatum produced similar functional results [217]. As part of a study that looked into mHTT clustering at 33 weeks, mice brains were implanted with iPSC-derived NSCs in the lateral ventricle. Autologous transplantation of cells from HD patients with the Htt mutation appeared to contribute to the HD phenotype and persistent cell death. An *et al* used an iPSC gene from a person with HD to generate human neural stem cells, which were subsequently transplanted into a mouse model of HD. The transplanted cells not only survived but also matured into motor neurons [248].

4.17.10.4 Applications of stem cells in amyotrophic lateral sclerosis (ALS)
ALS, commonly referred to as Lou Gehrig's disease, is a progressive and incurable neurodegenerative illness characterized by the death of motor neurons in the spinal cord's ventral horn and motor cortex. As the condition worsens, symptoms include stiffness, twitching, loss of voluntary control, and motor weakness appears [234]. For the previous 20 years, the only genetic anomaly associated with familial ALS was a mutation in Cu–Zn superoxide dismutase 1 (SOD1), recent research has identified additional anomalies connected to the start of sporadic ALS and non-SOD1 familial ALS, such as the degenerative effects of non-neuronal cells, protein instability, toxicity to motor neurons, breakdown and aggregation of proteins that bind DNA and RNA, and impaired neuronal cytoskeletal function [249, 250].

The basic ideas behind using stem cells to treat ALS are theoretically similar to those used to treat other neurodegenerative diseases: (1) repair motor neurons that are injured or dead; (2) regulate inflammation; and (3) stimulate the synthesis of neurotrophic agents. The main objective of treatment is to stop the degradation of existing motor neurons by providing an integrated neuronal component and required environmental enrichment [205]. Neural progenitor cells (NPCs) from fetal spinal cord were used in the first FDA-approved clinical study at Emory University in 2010 to treat patients with ALS. The purpose of the trial was to determine if it would be safe to implant NSCs into the spinal cords of eighteen patients [251]. Additionally, safety evaluations of the 67 ALS patients' frontal motor cortex stem cell transplantation were conducted [242]. In a nine-year study following dorsal spinal cord implantation, clinical trials examining intraspinal, intrathecal, and intracerebral MSC transplantation for ALS evaluated safety and viability and found no issues, either short- or long-term [252, 253]. According to Minguell *et al* [254] these investigations shed important light on the feasibility and security of MSC-based autologous treatments in patients with ALS. It was also required to assess the effectiveness of the treatment. A study on 11 ALS patients in Spain revealed that MSC implantation enhanced the number of motor neurons and reduced ubiquitin accumulation [254]. Exogenous NSC transplantation is the subject of ongoing clinical trials, which are based on credible findings that the course of ALS is delayed in patients by infusing foetal NSCs into their spinal cords [255]. The potential of stem cells to release growth factors and enrich the environment, as well as the neuroprotective effects of growth factors on motor neurons that survive, are also being investigated in current research. For instance, to explore the potential advantages of MSCs' neurotrophic, pro-angiogenic, anti-inflammatory, and immunomodulatory components, Brainstorm Therapeutics is developing an intrathecal delivery method for MSCs into the fluid surrounding ALS patients' brains and spinal cords [256].

4.17.10.5 Applications of stem cells in frontotemporal dementia

The most frequent cause of neurodegenerative dementia, FTD, primarily affects people under 65 [257]. FTD, which is characterized by increasing problems in language, behaviour, cognition, and personality, is caused by neurodegeneration in the frontotemporal cortex and selective neurodegeneration in the cerebral cortex [258]. FTD shares clinical features with motor neuron disease (FTD-MND or FTD-ALS), parkinsonian disorders (FTD-PD), corticobasal syndrome (CBS), and progressive supranuclear palsy (PSP) [259]. FTD exists in both familial and sporadic variants, making it a genetically and pathologically complicated illness [260]. Approximately 20%–30% of FTD cases are familial variations, with MAPT gene, which encodes microtubule-associated protein tau, altered in 15%–25% of these cases [261, 262]. The growing frequency of FTD, combined with its societal impact and the lack of effective treatments, emphasizes the importance of unravelling its pathogenic mechanisms in order to identify biomarkers, improve diagnostic criteria, and investigate new therapy targets.

Uncertainty surrounds the genetic cause of a sizeable portion of familial and sporadic FTD cases, making it difficult to construct reliable disease models that adequately replicate the complicated pathologies associated with FTD. Cell lines and animal models are examples of existing models that are unable to reproduce the intricate alterations in patterns observed in the adult human central nervous system (CNS). Furthermore, studies using tau overexpression models frequently produce symptoms that are too extreme to truly represent endogenous tau expression in FTD [259]. With the introduction of iPSCs, an encouraging method for simulating FTD pathogenic mechanisms has emerged, overcoming earlier hurdles. Reprogramming somatic cells into iPSCs provides an appealing paradigm for studying the molecular mechanisms behind FTD since it allows for the replication of clinical symptoms seen in FTD patients [257, 263] The creation and characterization of iPSCs derived from patients with familial FTD have been documented in recent studies. For example, Lee *et al* [264] collected FTD patient PBMCs that were utilized in integration-free factors that contribute to CytoTune-iPSC Sendai reprogramming including Oct Sendai virus particles, Sox2, Klf4, and c-Myc (Yamanaka factors), to generate iPSCs. This innovation in iPSC technology holds great potential for understanding the pathogenic mechanisms of FTD and speeding medication discovery.

4.17.10.6 Applications of stem cells in spinal cord injury

Spinal cord injury (SCI) stands as one of the most perilous neurological conditions globally, contributing significantly to societal financial burdens due to the high prevalence of associated disabilities [265]. The pathogenic mechanism of spinal cord damage encompasses primary injury and secondary injury. 'Primary injury' refers to nerve damage in the spinal cord caused by contusion, tearing, and compression from external forces, or vascular injury-induced infarction [266]. Subsequent to the initial damage, there is a substantial loss of nerve cells, accompanied by the breach of the spinal cord–blood barrier. A cascade reaction including vasospasm, bleeding, the generation of reactive oxygen species (ROS), inflammation, lipid peroxidation, and apoptosis causes this damage to worsen [267]. Presently, the main approaches for SCI treatment include physical therapy, hyperbaric oxygen therapy, medication treatment, and surgery; however, the outcomes for SCI patients remain insufficient [268]. Stem cell transplantation emerges as a potential solution for repairing injured nerve cells and tissues, aiming to restore the functionality and integrity of the nerve conduction system. Stem cells, including neurons and glial cells, transplanted into the injured site can induce the formation of new synapses, promote axon sprouting, and release neurotrophic factors, thereby modifying the microenvironment and accelerating axon growth [269]. Stem cell transplantation after SCI has been shown to upregulate genes with neuroprotective properties and downregulate genes associated with apoptosis and inflammation, thus shielding spinal neurons from further harm [270]. Additionally, stem cells have the ability to develop into glial cells, which helps people with SCI recover functionally by myelinating areas of their brains [271].

The potential application of ESCs to treat SCI by promoting their differentiation into neurons and glial cells has been explored in recent studies [272]. When Manley *et al* implanted human embryonic cell-derived oligodendrocyte progenitor cells into rats with spinal cord injuries, the animals showed no negative effects and showed improvements in motor function, axon survival, and parenchymal cavity size [273]. Hwang *et al* transplanted ESCs intrathecally into SCI rats, promoting spinal GABAergic neuron differentiation and greatly reduced chronic neuropathic pain [274]. Numerous studies have shown that BM-MSCs transplantation for SCI can reduce neurological abnormalities and promote neurological functioning restoration [275]. Gu *et al* [276] showed that BM-MSCs can reduce apoptosis, strengthen motor skills, and diminish CHOP expression in rats with SCI. Other research has shown that BM-MSCs can stimulate the formation of nerve fibres in the spinal cord, improving motor function [277], as well as reduce inflammatory responses and improve neurological performance [278]. Furthermore, Yousefifard *et al* [279] determined the possible advantages of HUC-MSCs transplantation for treating neuropathic pain symptoms and increasing rehabilitation of motor function following SCI. In an SCI model in rats, transplanting human UC-MSCs reduced inflammation and improved axon survival [280]. In clinical settings, Zhao *et al* implanted a nerve regeneration scaffold containing human UC-MSCs into patients with chronic SCI, resulting in improved sensory and motor function and neuron regeneration [281].

Other stem cell types have showed promise in preclinical and clinical research for SCI treatment, including NSCs, iPSCs, dental pulp stem cells (DPSCs), and olfactory ensheathing cells (OECs). NSCs transplantation improved neurological function after SCI by promoting proliferation and differentiation [282–284]. In rats after SCI, iPSCs from older donors displayed axon extension and survival [285]. DPSCs developed into Schwann-like glial cells, secreting neurotrophic factors and increasing neurite proliferation and survival [286, 287]. By suppressing neuro-inflammation and encouraging neurological recovery, OEC transplantation provided significant neuroprotection against SCI [288–290]. In summary, numerous stem cell types have demonstrated encouraging results in preclinical and clinical research for SCI treatment, opening up new paths for improving outcomes and fostering recovery in affected patients.

4.17.10.7 Applications of stem cells in stroke

Stroke, the second leading global cause of death, claims over 5.5 million lives annually and impacts 13.7 million individuals. Ischemic strokes, constituting 87% of cases, saw a rise from 1990 to 2016 due to lack of improved treatments. Primary hemorrhages occur in most cases, with subsequent hemorrhages in 10%–15%. While modern therapies like thrombectomy and thrombolysis transform treatment, challenges persist. Ischemic strokes often result from blood artery obstruction, causing downstream deprivation. Collateral vessels, attempting compensation, often fall short, leaving areas near the blockage vulnerable. The irreversibly damaged ischemic core and the salvageable penumbra define the brain injury. Transplanted cells exhibit neuro- and vascular-protective effects, aiding neural network reconfiguration, reducing glial scarring, and promoting regeneration. These effects stem from cell differentiation and paracrine factor secretion. Survival is possible in the penumbra if blood flow is swiftly restored, but the ischemic core faces irreparable damage. Stroke fatalities (85%) result from ischemic occlusions, with stem cell therapy showing promise for improved outcomes. Stem cells aim to restore damaged tissue in the chronic stage and preserve brain tissue acutely. Various stem cells enhance neurological outcomes in animal stroke models, with pluripotent and multipotent cells playing key roles.

Studies exist on the potential for treating ischemic stroke with BM-MSCs [291]. By promoting endogenous cerebral repair mechanisms, BM-MSCs release neurotrophic factors like HGF, NGF, BDNF, VEGF, bFGF, and IGF-1, which contribute to functional improvements [292, 293]. Moreover, BM-MSCs have anti-inflammatory properties, lower apoptosis rates, and promote endogenous neurogenesis and angiogenesis [291, 294]. Operating outside of the framework of cell replacement theory, BM-MSC exosomes, which include neurotrophic factors, regenerative microRNAs, and anti-inflammatory cytokines, have demonstrated therapeutic promise [295]. In stroke pathophysiology, EPCs have shown therapeutic promise [296]. Regional cortical blood flow, cerebral microvascular density, and functional recovery are all improved by EPC transplantation. During the acute phase, EPCs release neuroprotective growth factors that may aid in the rebuilding of the brain's architecture and have anti-inflammatory effects [297]. Through a variety of neuroprotective, neurogenic, and anti-inflammatory pathways, DPSCs, AD-MSCs, and iPSCs have also showed promise in the treatment of stroke [298, 299]. In summary, stem cell therapy offers a comprehensive strategy to tackle the intricacies of ischemic stroke, with potential advantages in both acute and chronic phases through advancement of neuroprotection, neurogenesis, angiogenesis, and anti-inflammatory reactions. The complex mechanisms underpinning the various stem cell types' therapeutic potential are still being uncovered by ongoing research, which gives patients with ischemic stroke hope for better results.

4.17.11 Applications of stem cells in pulmonary fibrosis

A form of interstitial lung illness known as pulmonary fibrosis (PF) is characterized by the extracellular matrix's (ECM) proliferative and myofibroblastic fibroblasts, which cause damage to the alveolar architecture and replace the normal structure of the lungs. Lung tissue damage and the development of PF are influenced by a range of risk factors and fibrogenic triggers. These include smoking, viral infections, radiation, immunological reactions, aging, genetics, and exposure to environmental substances including silica and asbestos. The lungs, an intricate organ responsible for the exchange of oxygen and carbon dioxide, are often subjected to detrimental compounds that might damage the alveolar epithelial cells [300]. Through the synchronization of several biological processes, the lungs are capable of repairing damaged alveolar cells [301]. PF arises from the combination of various risk factors, with the interplay between epithelial cells, mesenchymal cells, and ECM affecting the intricacy of the disease [302].

Stem cells, possessing the ability to undergo differentiation into diverse cell lineages, play a crucial part in the management of illnesses including lung injury. At present, the treatment of idiopathic pulmonary fibrosis (IPF) is dependent on pharmacological drugs, supplemental oxygen, and organ transplants. There are only two pharmaceuticals, pirfenidone and nintedanib, that have been approved by the FDA for this purpose [300]. Different categories of stem cells, including endocrine stem/progenitor cells, iPSCs, MSCs, and ESCs, show potential in the treatment of disorders such as PD. Lung stem/progenitor cells are essential for lung development and alveolar balance maintenance. Lung regeneration is aided by distal airway stem cells (DASCs), which express the transcription factors KRT5 and p63 that are confined to basal cells [303]. Human iPSCs possess the capacity of undergoing differentiation into lung and airway progenitor cells, providing a restorative strategy for fibrotic lung disorders. Nevertheless, there are some obstacles in the practical application of this technique, such as apprehensions over safety, the laborious process of generating cell lines, and the potential for immunological reactions and tumorigenicity [304]. Preclinical studies have demonstrated the potential of reprogramming iPSCs to produce alveolar epithelial cells and basal cells for the treatment of lung injury. Transplantation of iPSC-derived cells, such as human iPSC-derived alveolar type II (hiPSC-ATII) cells, has been shown to be safe and successful in treating PF. This treatment preserves normal lung function and does not lead to the formation of tumors [305]. Furthermore, research conducted by Wang *et al* (2010) has demonstrated that MSCs generated from human umbilical cords have exhibited therapeutic properties in both the prevention and reversal of lung injury induced by bleomycin [306]. Systemic administration of MSCs effectively remedied fibrotic scarring in the lung tissue of mice. Ultimately, stem cell therapy, encompassing iPSCs and MSCs, exhibits substantial promise in the treatment of pulmonary fibrosis through the facilitation of lung regeneration and the prevention of fibrotic scarring. Nevertheless, it is imperative to tackle the obstacles concerning safety and feasibility in order to achieve a successful clinical application.

4.17.12 Applications of stem cell therapy in acute respiratory distress syndrome (ARDS)

Acute respiratory distress syndrome (ARDS) is a serious medical condition that causes respiratory failure. It occurs when there is inflammation and fluid build-up in the lungs due to damage to the alveolar–epithelial barrier. As the condition progresses, it enters a fibrotic stage characterized by an increase in fibroblasts, matrix deposition, myofibroblasts, and type II pneumocytes after the initial 'exudative phase'. Although other pharmacologic therapies, including ibuprofen, ketoconazole, simvastatin, and inhaled synthetic surfactants, have been investigated, none have effectively decreased the elevated mortality rate associated with ARDS, which ranges from 34 to 44% [307].

Recent preclinical studies indicate that the secretomes of MSCs may prove to be significant and useful ARDS therapeutic tools. Severe sepsis frequently results in ARDS, especially when gram-negative bacteria are involved [308]. MSC therapy effectively prevented the progression of ARDS in animal models of sepsis induced by lipopolysaccharide (LPS) derived from *Escherichia coli*, as demonstrated by Curley *et al* in 2017. The introduction of MSCs through the bloodstream in a mouse model with LPS-induced ARDS resulted in a notable decrease in inflammation and damage to the air sacs (alveoli) [309]. The presence of MSCs resulted in a decrease in the generation of inflammatory cytokine TNF-α by immune cells that had invaded the lungs. Additionally, MSCs blocked the entry of neutrophils into the lungs by a mechanism that is dependent on the signalling molecule IL-10, which acts locally (paracrine) [305]. MSCs exerted a protective effect on endothelial cells by preventing their programmed cell death. They also assisted the restoration of the barrier between the epithelium and alveoli, and promoted the regeneration of ATII cells in lung injury associated with ARDS. These beneficial effects were achieved by production of growth factors such as KGF, VEGF, and HGF [310, 311] The mice treated with MSCs showed decreased swelling, enhanced oxygen levels, and prolonged lifespan [312]. In addition, MSCs increased the efficiency of macrophages to produce anti-inflammatory IL-10 through a process that relies on PGE2. This mechanism further aids in the prevention of ARDS that is linked to sepsis, as demonstrated by Curley *et al* in 2017. The pathological changes in the lung environment caused by ARDS have an adverse effect on MSC proliferation and ATII cell differentiation [313]. Wilson *et al* (2015) conducted clinical research to investigate the utilization of MSCs in patients with ARDS [314]. They found positive outcomes in nine patients who received intravenous administration of MSCs obtained from bone marrow. A study conducted by Zheng and colleagues discovered that administering intravenous allogeneic MSCs to patients with ARDS was a safe but ultimately useless treatment approach [315]. Further, MSCs have demonstrated the capacity to improve the phagocytic capability of alveolar macrophages and alleviate symptoms of pneumonia caused by Gram-negative *Escherichia coli* by generating microvesicles [316]. In addition, MSCs have the ability to directly inhibit the growth of bacteria in infected lungs and generate antimicrobial proteins. The administration of MSCs directly into the trachea resulted in a notable decrease in lung injury and inflammation, as well as an increase in the lifespan of mice suffering from bacterial pneumonia. This effect was achieved by enhancing the elimination of germs, which was reliant on the presence of lipocalin-2 [317]. Activation of TLR-4 by LPS in MSCs enhances the synthesis of lipocalin-2, which binds to bacterial ferric siderophores, reduces iron uptake, and hampers bacterial growth [318]. An investigation conducted by Gupta *et al* (2018) discovered that the therapeutic effectiveness of MSCs was significantly diminished in an experimental model of bacterial pneumonia when a TLR-4 mutation was present [319].

4.17.13 Applications of stem cell therapy in asthma

Globally, bronchial asthma impacts more than 300 million individuals, as indicated by epidemiological data [320]. The chronic inflammation of the airways can trigger recurrent episodes of airflow constriction and bronchial hyperresponsiveness in susceptible individuals, potentially leading to long-term structural changes. A thorough understanding of the pathophysiology of asthma, a chronic inflammatory lung disease, is necessary for the purpose of looking into the possible therapeutic uses of MSCs.

MSCs have the capacity to suppress the production of IgE in plasma cells, prevent the activation of mast cells in laboratory conditions that rely on IgE, and impede the proliferation and activity of $CD4^{+}$Th2 cells. Multiple research teams showed evidence that MSCs can mitigate inflammation in the airways, modify the structure of the airways, and improve lung function in animals with asthma [321, 322]. The anti-inflammatory actions of MSCs are primarily mediated via soluble substances they generate. According to Cruz *et al*, in a model of airway allergic inflammation, MSC exosomes—tiny extracellular vesicles that carry proteins, lipids, microRNA, and DNA fragments—have the power to alter the properties of antigen-specific $CD4^{+}$T cells. These exosomes target various types of cells such as endothelial cells, immune cells, pericytes, and other cells found in tissues [321]. In addition, a study discovered that exosomes obtained from MSCs had a beneficial effect on asthma and inflammation. They enhanced the growth of Treg cells and their ability to suppress the immune response. Moreover, these exosomes increased the production of anti-inflammatory cytokines by asthmatic patients' peripheral blood mononuclear cells (IL-10 and TGF-β) [323]. Within an environment characterized by a prevalence of Th2 cells and allergies, the transplanted MSCs were stimulated by IL-4/IL-13, which activated the STAT6 pathway. This activation resulted in an augmentation of TGF-β production. In addition to the expansion of Tregs by heme oxygenase-1 produced from MSCs, this process effectively prevents the ongoing lung inflammation induced by Th2 cells [324]. Administration of MSCs via intravenous injection caused the blood levels of IgG1 and IgE to drop, as well as a reduction in eosinophil infiltration and mucus formation in the lungs. A study by Nemeth *et al* (2010) found that bronchial lavage resulted in a reduction in Th2 cytokines, specifically IL-4, IL-5, and IL-13 [325]. Braza *et al* emphasized the ability of MSCs to decrease bronchial asthma by interacting with alveolar macrophages in diseased lungs [326]. After MSC transplantation, alveolar macrophages undergo a process called phagocytosis, which leads to their alternative activation and acquisition of an M2 phenotype that is anti-inflammatory and immunosuppressive [326]. Li and colleagues discovered that placenta-derived human MSCs (PL-MSCs) decreased the presence of Th17 cells, eosinophils, macrophages, and neutrophils in the lungs of asthmatic rats. Additionally, PL-MSCs increased the overall population of Tregs that produce IL-10 [327]. The apparent inconsistency in these findings might be ascribed to the divergence in molecular pathways employed by human and murine MSCs in the generation and proliferation of Treg cells [328] as well as the varying impact of different sources of MSCs on immune cells [329].

4.17.14 Applications of stem cell therapy in chronic obstructive pulmonary disease (COPD)

Chronic respiratory symptoms and impaired breathing brought on by the deterioration of lung parenchyma and terminal bronchioles (emphysema) are the hallmarks of chronic obstructive pulmonary disease (COPD), primarily caused by prolonged exposure to noxious particles or gases [330]. Contributing factors to the advancement of this severe condition encompass smoking, respiratory infections throughout childhood, a familial predisposition to asthma, and heightened sensitivity of the airways [331]. The main pathological alterations in people with COPD are a progressive and uninterrupted constriction of airflow, coupled with a persistent inflammatory reaction in the lungs and airways. The alterations in oxidative stress functions, influx of immune cells into the lungs, and unbalanced activity of proteases and their inhibitors are responsible for these modifications [332]. MSCs are regarded as promising therapeutic agents for cell-based treatment of COPD because they may effectively reduce detrimental immunological reactions, preserve oxidative equilibrium, and control the function of matrix-degrading enzymes. Multiple clinical and experimental investigations have provided evidence of the advantageous impact of MSCs in the treatment of COPD [333]. Administration of BM-MSCs and AT-MSCs has been shown to be a safe treatment method with positive effects on the structure and function of the respiratory system in animal models of COPD induced by cigarette smoke exposure or elastase instillation. The cells are typically administered intrabronchially, intratracheally, or intravenously, with a minimum of 5×10^4 cells per animal [333]. The administration of BM-MSCs through the trachea produced superior outcomes compared to MSCs obtained from lung tissue. Remarkably, animals experienced instantaneous death after receiving LT-MSCs through intravenous injection, which did not occur when BM-MSCs or AT-MSCs were delivered intravenously [334]. Within a day, MSCs administered intravenously and intratracheally moved and successfully engrafted into the lungs of COPD-stricken experimental mice [335, 336]. The transplantation of MSCs effectively decreased the damage and loss of alveoli, which are characteristic of emphysematous alterations, in mice used in the experiment [337]. The study conducted by

Liu *et al* (2013) found transplanted MSCs have the ability to transform into functional, ATII-like cells that express SPC [338]. This transformation occurs through the canonical Wnt/β-catenin pathway, and it was observed both in laboratory conditions (*in vitro*) and in lung tissue affected by emphysema. Corroborating these results, Zhen *et al* documented that transplanted MSCs successfully integrated into the lungs, transformed into cells resembling ATII, and exhibited preventative effects against pulmonary emphysema [339].

4.17.15 Applications of stem cell therapy in idiopathic pulmonary fibrosis (IPF)

IPF is typified by an excessive accumulation of extracellular matrix components such as collagen components in the alveolar septa, which thickens the septal interstitium. The outcome of this procedure can vary in terms of lung structure damage and the presence of fibrotic masses, depending on its severity. IPF is the predominant kind of interstitial lung fibrosis, characterized by unknown origins and usually impacting adults aged 50 and above. The histopathologic/radiologic pattern of typical interstitial pneumonia (UIP) is demonstrated [340]. Transplanting MSCs at various doses (ranging from 0.1×10^6 to 4×10^6 cells) has shown to provide protection against lung damage and fibrosis caused by bleomycin. This protection is evident through notable improvements in histopathology, reduced lung inflammation, decreased collagen build-up, reduced pulmonary edema, suppressed activation of MMP-2, MMP-9, and MMP-13 enzymes, and a significant decrease in mortality rates among animals treated with MSCs [341]. Ortiz and his colleagues have discovered a distinct subgroup of MSCs that exhibit the expression of interleukin-1 receptor antagonist (IL-1Ra). In a study conducted by Lee *et al* in 2010, it was found that MSCs were able to effectively reduce inflammation and lung fibrosis in mice that had been wounded by bleomycin [342]. This effect was reliant on the presence of IL-1Ra. The binding of IL-1Ra derived from MSCs to IL-1R prevents several inflammatory processes caused by the binding of IL-1 to IL-1R. These processes involve the synthesis and release of inflammatory cytokines and chemokines, also increase in neutrophil, macrophage, and lymphocyte movement. Ultimately, this leads to a decrease in inflammation and fibrosis [343]. Multiple clinical trials have evaluated the effectiveness and safety of therapy using MSCs for persons with IPF [344]. A phase 1b trial, done in Australia (NCT01385644) [345], investigated the therapeutic efficacy of intravenously delivered PL-MSCs in patients with IPF. While both dosages of PL-MSCs were well-tolerated and resulted in only minor and transitory alterations in gas exchange and peri-infusion hemodynamics, the therapy with PL-MSCs did not provide relief for IPF. The intravenous administration of PL-MSCs did not produce any significant changes in the monitored parameters over the course of the six-month follow-up period. These parameters included computed tomography (CT), diffusing lung capacity for carbon monoxide (DLCO), forced vital capacity (FVC), fibrosis score, and the six-minute walk test (6MWT) [344]. On the other hand, a different phase 1b clinical trial produced more positive outcomes. It demonstrated a notable enhancement in quality-of-life indicators for 14 patients with IPF after receiving AT-MSCs through endobronchial administration [346]. Significantly, a recent study showed that the transplantation of AT-MSCs into the bronchial tubes was a safe treatment method. No significant adverse effects were observed, even after two years of initial MSCs administration, even in patients whose IPF condition worsened after receiving MSCs treatment [347].

4.17.16 Applications of stem cell therapy in osteoporosis

Osteoporosis, a prevalent condition affecting predominantly the elderly, is observed in both developed and developing nations. The escalating impact of osteoporosis on human and financial resources underscores the urgency for innovative approaches. The pathophysiology of osteoporosis is significantly influenced by stem cells, specifically in relation to their development into osteoblasts. The decrease in osteoblast quantity and function associated with osteoporosis suggests that stem cell activation and transplantation may restore bone demineralization. As a chronic bone condition more prevalent in older adults, osteoporosis leads to fractures by diminishing bone mass and mineral density, particularly in individuals over 65 (men) and 55 (women) [348–350]. Osteoporosis is a degenerative skeletal illness that is characterized by poor bone density and microarchitectural deterioration. It is believed to be caused by imbalances in bone cell function [351]. While pharmacological treatments like bisphosphonates, hormone replacement therapy, selective estrogen receptor denosumab, modulators, and teriparatide exist, non-pharmacological options such as nutritional therapy, physical exercise, vertebroplasty, and kyphoplasty also have therapeutic benefits but may present drawbacks [352].

Regenerative medicine and stem cell treatment have emerged as major methods for addressing the clinical demand for new therapeutic approaches in controlling chronic diseases [353]. Stem cell therapy for osteoporosis utilizes many types of stem cells, such as embryonic and iPSCs, together with their secreted factors [354]. The reduced involvement of naturally occurring MSCs in osteoporosis highlights their importance in therapy. Human skeletal stem cells (SSCs) are a type of cells that have the ability to differentiate into many types of cells such as stroma, cartilage, and bone precursors. These cells are also capable of self-renewal, meaning they may produce more of themselves [355]. The ability of MSCs to develop into bone cells and to multiply is significantly impacted by osteoporosis, which leads to a decline in bone production, especially in elderly adults [356–358]. The pathophysiology of osteoporosis is modulated by chemicals such as glucocorticoids and estrogen, which have an impact on the formation of MSCs. The presence of estrogen receptors in osteoblasts and the ability of estrogen to stimulate the proliferation of MSCs and promote their differentiation into bone cells highlight their importance in maintaining bone homeostasis [359, 360]. Estradiol promotes the synthesis of bone morphogenetic protein 2, which increases the growth and formation of osteoblasts from MSCs [361]. Various studies have shown that stem cell therapies using ADSCs and UCB-derived cells have the ability to improve bone regeneration and prevent bone loss in animal models [354, 362, 363]. The placenta and amniotic fluid, which are part of the fetal adnexa, provide new sources of nonembryonic stem cells that have the ability to proliferate into several cell types [364, 365]. Transplanting MSCs from a different donor has been proven to have therapeutic advantages. Research investigations have demonstrated that this approach leads to improvements in patients with osteogenesis imperfecta and hypophosphatasia [366–368]. Transplantation of allogeneic MSCs has been shown to be safe and effective, and there is promise for prenatal allogeneic MSCs transplantation [369]. According to Taketani *et al* (2015), the introduction of *ex vivo* grown allogeneic MSCs has a positive impact on the health status of individuals suffering from severe hypophosphatasia [368].

4.17.17 Applications of stem cell therapy in autoimmune disease

As a result of an aberrant immune response to self-antigens, autoimmune disorders arise when the immune system unintentionally targets its own tissues. Individuals with autoimmune illnesses frequently have abnormal antibodies targeting biological tissues, which contributes to autoimmune diseases being the third most significant disease burden, following cancer and heart disease. These conditions impact around 6% of the population [369]. By utilizing the target antigen's location and clinical characteristics, these illnesses can be classified as either systemic or organ-specific. Diabetes mellitus (DM) is a condition marked by high levels of glucose in the blood due to either the body's resistance to insulin or inadequate production of insulin. The four categories of diabetes include T1DM, T2DM, gestational diabetes mellitus (GDM), and monogenic diabetes mellitus [370, 371]. The autoimmune disease known as T1DM is typified by the degeneration of islet β-cells, which is brought on by autoreactive T-lymphocytes targeting pancreatic β-cells. As a result, there is a need for exogenous insulin and impaired glucose metabolism [372]. The replacement of β-cells through islet or pancreatic transplantation has been investigated as an effective therapy for T1DM. This approach has the potential to restore insulin production in a regulated manner, hence reducing the risk of hypoglycemia and long-term consequences [373].

MSCs show potential as viable cell choices for the treatment of T1DM. MSCs have the ability to shield β-cells, improve insulin production, and reduce glycemia in individuals with T1DM via regulating the immune system. Research conducted on animal models has shown that MSCs are beneficial in treating autoimmune illnesses by suppressing the growth of T cells and regulating immune cells [374, 375]. MSC therapy has demonstrated favourable results in diminishing the invasion of inflammatory cells and enhancing the condition of autoimmune diabetes in animal models [376]. The immune-modulating characteristics of MSCs, such as their ability to absorb and break down antigens, heightened expression of HLA-DR, and improved immunosuppressive effects, provide additional evidence for their potential in the treatment of T1DM [377, 378]. An *in vitro* study conducted by Montanucci *et al* indicates that immunoisolatory microcapsules (CpS-hUCMS) have the ability to act as an artificial biohybrid system in regulating immunological responses in patients with T1DM. This result recommends that further research can be conducted to explore the therapeutic advantages of these microcapsules [379]. Human clinical trials have shown that MSC transplantation has positive effects on T1DM, including enhanced protection of β-cells and increased stability of the immune system [380]. Recent studies have shown that autologous hematopoietic stem cell transplantation can effectively restore normal blood sugar levels in individuals who have just been diagnosed with T1DM. In addition, laboratory experiments have demonstrated that this procedure can enhance the immune system's capabilities [381, 382]. Implanting ESCs or iPSCs into people with T1DM can transform into islet organoids, insulin-producing cells, interspecific pancreatic chimeras, and pancreatic progenitors. It has potential to regenerate islet β-cells and increase β-cell mass [383–385]. The progress highlights the diverse strategies employed in stem cell therapy for autoimmune conditions such as T1DM.

4.17.18 Applications of stem cell therapy in renal diseases

Prevalence of renal disease on a global scale is seeing a rapid escalation, presenting a substantial issue in terms of public health. These diseases affect more than 10% of the worldwide population [386]. The conventional multidrug therapy commonly used for kidney illnesses frequently proves ineffective in preventing the advancement to end-stage renal disease (ESRD), thus requiring the implementation of renal replacement therapies such as transplantation or maintenance dialysis [387]. The scarcity of organ donors and the potential for organ rejection impose limitations on the utilization of kidney transplantation. Hence, it is imperative to investigate innovative and enhanced therapeutic options in order to effectively manage, treat, or even avert renal disorders and improve patient longevity. Stem cell therapy presents favourable treatment possibilities in order to treat renal disease owing to its advantageous characteristics, including adaptability, simplicity of genetic manipulation, and limitless multiplication. Stem cells exhibit therapeutic potential in the restoration of renal damage, preservation of renal structure and function, and prolongation of animal survival in models of chronic kidney disease (CKD) and acute kidney injury (AKI). An effective method to activate regeneration mechanisms involves the incorporation of stem cells that have ability to replace impaired tissues by undergoing differentiation, engraftment, migration, and paracrine actions. MSCs and EPCs have demonstrated potential in preclinical studies for CKD, as seen by reduced proteinuria and urea levels, indicating a decrease in glomerulosclerosis and interstitial fibrosis [388]. Although MSCs and EPCs have advantages, they may encounter diminished pro-angiogenic activity and circulating cell count, indicating possible difficulties in their sustained performance. MSCs release cytokines, growth factors, and extracellular vesicles that affect neighbouring parenchymal cells and stimulate tissue regeneration [389, 390]. Research shows that MSCs have the ability to safeguard kidney function and alleviate kidney damage in several situations, including diabetic nephropathy, chronic allograft nephropathy, and partial nephrectomy [391, 392]. Administering MSCs directly into the kidney, particularly when paired with renal revascularization, enhances the functioning and blood flow of the kidney while decreasing cell death, scarring, loss of small blood vessels, oxygen deprivation, inflammation, and oxidative damage [393, 394]. The low immunogenicity and immunoregulatory characteristics of MSCs make them beneficial for kidney transplantation. They efficiently manage the immune system and assist in the recovery of the kidneys [395]. Clinical trials, including those evaluating the safety and efficacy of MSCs infusion following kidney transplantation in the absence of severe clinical rejection, emphasize the continuous investigation of MSCs in transplantation scenarios [396]. Studies testing the safety and effectiveness of using autologous BM-MSCs after kidney transplantation have demonstrated positive outcomes in terms of graft performance, despite temporary decreases in renal function [397]. Furthermore, research comparing typical immunosuppressive treatments with procedures that reduce responsiveness by employing donor-specific AD-MSCs show promising advantages in the survival of transplanted organs [398]. To summarize, stem cell therapy, namely with MSCs, has potential for treating renal disorders by activating regeneration pathways and facilitating tissue restoration. Current investigations and clinical trials persist in examining the safety, effectiveness, and enduring advantages of stem cell treatments in relation to renal ailments and organ transplantation.

4.17.19 Applications of stem cell therapy in retinal disease

Retinal diseases are becoming more common as causes of vision impairment, and the present treatments for retinal degeneration are not effective enough in restoring the injured retina. The genesis of retinal degenerative diseases involves a combination of hereditary and non-genetic causes, resulting in the deterioration of photoreceptor cells and retinal pigment epithelium (RPE) cells. Conventional therapies focus on boosting the regeneration and repair of damaged retinal tissue in order to produce a long-term benefit. Aside from traditional therapy, researchers have investigated the use of stem cell therapies to revitalize and restore the impaired retina, due to its inherent limited ability to regenerate [399]. Extensive preclinical and clinical research has thoroughly examined the potential of stem cell treatment to regenerate and repair damaged retinal cells. These researches have evaluated several types of stem cells to determine their effectiveness in reversing retinal degeneration.

ESCs, known for their remarkable ability to multiply and transform into multiple cell types, have been utilized as a cellular resource for the treatment of retinal degeneration. Injecting RPE cells produced from hESC into an animal model of age-related macular degeneration (AMD) showed no tumor formation. The transplanted cells were still present and identifiable seven months after the injection. The cells successfully formed a single layer of RPE on the existing layer, demonstrating encouraging outcomes [400]. The transplantation of RPE cells derived from hESC resulted in enhanced visual acuity for individuals with AMD and Stargardt macular dystrophy (SMD), without any abnormal proliferation [401]. Researchers have investigated iPSCs as a potential solution. The transplantation of retina produced from iPSC into rats with retinitis pigmentosa and monkeys with laser-induced retinal injury led to enhanced visual capacities and successful integration of the transplanted cells into the recipient retina, as reported by [402]. In a study conducted by Zhu *et al* in 2020, it was shown that transplanting RPE spheroids produced from iPSC into an animal model of retinitis pigmentosa resulted in a delay in the thinning of the retinal outer nuclear layer (ONL) [403]. Furthermore, there was a decrease in apoptosis and infiltration of microglial cells. The combined transplantation of retinal progenitor cells (RPCs) and RPE cells produced from iPSCs in a rat model of retinal degeneration demonstrated improved visual response and maintained ONL integrity, as compared to the transplantation of each cell type individually [404]. MSCs have been thoroughly examined for their capacity to address different retinal disorders. The effectiveness of MSCs has been proven in recent research employing preclinical models of retinal degeneration. Rat BM-MSCs maintained the thickness of the ONL by enhancing the process of autophagy. On the other hand, human dental pulp-derived mesenchymal stem cells DP-MSCs enhanced retinal function in a rat model of retinal degeneration [405]. Manuguerra-Gagne *et al* (2013) found that in a mouse model of glaucoma, the introduction of BM-MSCs or the release of paracrine substances from BM-MSCs into the front part of the eye resulted in enhanced regeneration of the eye, stimulating the growth of the ciliary body's precursor cells [406]. In addition, the introduction of UC-MSCs and exosomes from UC-MSCs directly into the eye of mice with retinal injury resulted in a decrease in inflammation and an enhancement of visual capacities [407]. Administration of MSC through intravenous injection resulted in a reduction in microvascular permeability associated with diabetes in a rat model [408]. The introduction of AD-MSCs into the vitreous cavity of diabetic rats with retinopathy resulted in the preservation of retinal ganglion cells (RGCs) and an elevation in the levels of neurotrophic factors [409]. Multiple preclinical and clinical investigations have examined the utilization of MSCs and their products for the management of ocular conditions. Studies examining the use of PD-MSCs transplanted into the subtenon space for traumatized optic neuropathy, and intravitreal autologous BM-MSCs for retinopathy (RP), have demonstrated encouraging outcomes in enhancing visual acuity and safeguarding retinal ganglion cells [410, 411]. A study conducted by Kahraman *et al* found that implanting UC-MSCs into the suprachoroidal area of patients with retinitis pigmentosa during Phase III clinical trials resulted in better vision in a large number of eyes [412]. Importantly, no negative side effects were reported. Furthermore, the administration of UC-MSCs through intravenous injection in individuals with retinitis pigmentosa led to improved visual acuity, without any negative consequences [413]. To summarize, the investigation of stem cell treatments, such as ESCs, iPSCs, and MSCs, presents hopeful opportunities for the regeneration and restoration of impaired retinal tissue. Continuous research, encompassing both preclinical and clinical studies, persists in enhancing our comprehension of the potential advantages and difficulties linked to these stem cell-derived methods for addressing retinal degenerative disorders.

4.17.20 Applications of stem cell therapy in hearing loss

Depending on where the impairment occurs, hearing loss can be categorized as sensorineural hearing loss (SNHL) or conductive hearing loss (HL). While conductive hearing loss mostly affects the outer and middle ears, SNHL typically affects the inner ear and auditory nerve [414]. Currently, the primary methods of treating

SNHL involve administering injections or oral drugs. Therapeutic options for SNHL include cochlear implants, hearing aids, hyperbaric oxygen chamber rehabilitation, local hormone injections, and other interventions [415].

Recently developed stem cells treatment in order to treat hearing loss is promising. Clarke *et al* (2000) discovered that neural stem cells develop into functioning auditory neurons [416]. Neural precursor cells, dorsal root ganglion cells, inner ear-isolated precursor or stem cells, immortalized auditory neuroblasts, embryonic stem cells, and their derived neural stem cells. Also, bone marrow stromal cells treated with retinoic acid and Shh, have all been reported as sources of neural stem cells implanted in the inner ear [417]. Michael *et al* constructed an *in vitro* organoid culture system using the *in vivo* embryonic development paradigm [418]. By blocking TGF-β and turning on BMP, they produced non-neuroectoderm using mouse mESCs without generating mesoderm. By inhibiting activated FGF2 and BMP, pre-placodal ectode (PPE) and otic placode development were created. Serum-free 2D Matrigel was used to form and differentiate spiral ganglia. 15 days of BDNF and NT-3 therapy produced normal spiral ganglia shape and activity in the tissues [418]. To create mouse embryonic neural stem cells, Koehler and colleagues used the quickly aggregated serum-free embryonic body technique (SFEBq). They controlled the expression of BMP, FGF, and TGF-β at different points in the cell population to create non-neuroectoderm, PPE, and otic placode epithelial cells. Wnt, Notch, Hippo, Shh, and MAPK signalling pathways were activated, resulting in the formation of many hair cells with a distinct function and shape capable of sensing mechanical pressure [419, 420]. Furthermore, NGF was found to be important in the survival and development of neural stem cells, increasing their ability to differentiate in an NGF-containing media [421].

4.17.21 Applications of stem cell therapy in HIV-AIDS

When the HIV epidemic broke out in 1981, it signalled the discovery of a new disease state characterized by immune system deficiencies [422]. AIDS was characterized by hypergammaglobulinemia, enhanced B-cell proliferation, and a dramatic decrease in $CD4^+$ cell numbers [422]. AIDS's causative culprit, later identified as HIV, is a retrovirus with two identical single-stranded RNA molecules in its genome [423]. Innovative therapeutic techniques are being pursued to address a wide range of safety and efficacy concerns, with the goal of establishing infection remission for life. Stem cell transplants employing natural or synthetic resistant cell resources, genetic manipulation methodologies, and cytotoxic anti-HIV effector cells have expedited HIV cell management advancements [424].

Red blood cells with receptor integration are to be altered in a potential treatment approach based on BM-MSCs, which would remove and contain HIV infections that are already in circulation. This entails modifying red blood cell membrane C–C chemokine receptor type 5, C–X–C chemokine receptor type 4, and CD4 receptor co-receptors to preferentially bind circulating HIV particles [425, 426]. Recent research reveals tremendous progress in the clinical usage of stem cell-based HIV treatment methods, particularly in the conduct of large phase II HSC-based gene therapy trials. Adult autologous HSCs are transduced with a retroviral vector encoding a tat-vpr-specific anti-HIV ribozyme to develop cells that are less susceptible to infection. Despite having a minor impact on virus loads, the technique is considered a more established and successful therapy [427, 428]. In clinical trials, other RNA-based techniques, such as a TAR segment decoy, shRNA targeting tat/rev transcripts, and ribozyme targeting CCR5, have been used [429]. Using B-cells derived from HSCs to generate HIV-neutralizing antibodies is a well-known tactic. Even while a single customized antibody might not offer total protection, research on animals and some HIV-positive individuals has shown promise [430]. Allogeneic hematopoietic stem cell transplantation (HSCT) using donor cells containing the CCR5 gene has been shown to be effective in HIV-cured patients, indicating the need for myeloablative procedures to diminish the viral reservoir [431–433]. hUC-MSCs were used to treat HIV/AIDS immunological non-responders in a randomized clinical study, exhibiting success in boosting $CD4^+$ T cells in both high and low-dose groups [434]. Researchers at UC Davis have discovered that MSCs are a type of stem cell that can increase the immune system's antiviral activity, offering a potential route for HIV treatment that calls for specific delivery methods and stringent cell quality control.

4.17.22 Applications of stem cells in dental diseases

One of the main reasons for anomalies in the hard tissue of the teeth is dental caries originating from oral bacteria demineralizing tooth enamel and affecting its structure [435]. Non-carious lesions like abfraction, abrasion, erosion, and chemical degradation can cause tooth tissue wear due to a variety of reasons such as normal, abnormal, or pathological wear [436]. Effective repair or regeneration of damaged areas can provide patients with physiological and psychological benefits [437]. Current tissue rehabilitation therapies include flap transplants in conjunction with dental implants or obturators. However, research into better functionality and aesthetics in these systems is underway [437, 438].

Alveolar bone, teeth, and periodontal tissues are all important components in dental regeneration. Dental tissue-derived iPSCs have piqued the interest of researchers because of its potential for dental tissue regeneration. To construct tooth-like structures, mouse iPSCs were combined with mesenchymal and embryonic dental epithelial cells to resemble both dental pulp and bone areas [439]. The connection between neural-crest-derived mesenchymal cells and ectoderm-derived epithelial cells is required for tooth germ development, indicating that iPSCs have the capacity to differentiate into odontogenic lineages [440]. d'Aquino *et al* (2007) extracted DPSCs from adult dental pulp tissue and demonstrated their odontogenic capacity in the same way that bone marrow cells do [441]. However, stem cell-based regenerative therapy for orofacial bone repair is still in its infancy, with little knowledge of the full process, including transplantation events [442]. While dental stem cells show potential for immunological and regenerative therapy [443], research on transplanted cells' immunological effects and clinical results is scarce. DESCs and DMSCs were coupled to generate tooth germs, which were implanted into recipient alveolar bone and demonstrated proliferation, budding, and transformation into functional teeth [444]. Recent research in mice models have revealed that functioning teeth with entire roots are possible, as is the ability of *de novo* regenerated teeth to fully integrate into the alveolar bone [445, 446]

4.18 Limitations of stem cell therapy

There are various limits to stem cell therapies that affect their effectiveness and practical use. The following are the major challenges:

(a) **Limited stem cell supply:** The availability of stem cells is limited, making extensive therapeutic application difficult. This constraint is especially noticeable in the case of MSCs in bone marrow, which decline dramatically with age and require culture expansion [447]. *Ex vivo* cultivation, on the other hand, may cause senescence and loss of stem cell characteristics, limiting their therapeutic potential [448].

(b) **Ideal window of opportunity:** For maximum efficacy, stem cell treatments must be administered on time. The optimal cell dosage and delivery technique for various illnesses, including cardiovascular problems, is still being debated [449]. In the case of stroke, key components such as microRNAs, trophic factors, and chemokines are more concentrated in the infarcted brain at this time [450].

(c) **Adult stem cell genetic limitations:** Adult stem cells, particularly MSCs, show genetic variety and variability in terms of proliferation, trophic support, and differentiation potentials. Because of lower quantities of NSCs and bone marrow MSCs, the aged population may have a diminished capacity for neurorestorative therapy [447]. Furthermore, genetic constraints may have an impact on the efficacy of stem cell therapy.

(d) **Teratoma development:** There is a possibility of teratoma creation when undifferentiated stem cells are transplanted. The connection between cancer and stem cells raises concerns about uncontrolled proliferation, which may be more dangerous than the original sickness. The transplanted stem cells have the potential to grow into malignancies, offering a serious risk to patients [451].

(e) **Immunological rejection:** Stem cell transplantation may cause immune system responses, resulting in donor cell rejection. While ESCs were always thought to be immune privileged, current research has revealed rejection after transplantation in immunocompetent hosts. The rejection of stem cell-based therapies can restrict their therapeutic impact [452].

(f) **Engraftment, long-term viability, and toxicity:** It is vital to ensure the engraftment, long-term viability, and safety of transplanted stem cells. Donor stem cells, with their unlimited ability to proliferate, may avoid immunological rejection but represent a risk of malignant transformation. To solve this issue, the construction of a 'kill-switch' to limit stem cell multiplication is proposed [453].

(g) **Concerns about safety:** Safety concerns, such as the danger of teratoma formation, arrhythmogenic effects, and immunological rejection, must be prioritized alongside effectiveness and clinical accessibility. Carcinogenesis after stem cell transplantation, particularly with ESCs and iPSCs, remains a substantial hurdle that necessitates mitigation techniques [454].

To summarize, overcoming these restrictions is critical for furthering the field of stem cell therapies and optimizing their therapeutic potential in a variety of medical problems. Continuous research and technology breakthroughs are critical to overcome these obstacles and enhance the safety and efficacy of stem cell-based therapies.

4.19 Conclusion

Finally, stem cell technology's unique dual position as a therapeutic and diagnostic tool emphasizes its remarkable promise. The development of strong *in vitro* models for disease research using iPS cells and their derivatives is a significant accomplishment. Patient-specific iPS cell models have considerable promise for furthering toxicology and drug development research. With their ability to restore damaged tissue and assist the regeneration of functioning structures, stem cells have enormous therapeutic potential. Furthermore, stem cell-based treatments have the potential to improve the body's natural self-healing mechanisms. Despite these outstanding characteristics, the actual use of stem cell therapies faces significant hurdles that must be carefully considered. The identification of stem cell populations capable of continuous cultivation in sufficient proportions to satisfy the considerable amounts necessary for therapeutic efficacy is a top priority. Furthermore, the possible hazards of immunologic rejection and malignant transformation demand thorough exploration, especially as these elements have received little attention to date. The urgency with which these issues must be addressed emphasizes the significance of meticulous testing; *in vitro* and *in vivo*, using appropriate animal models before widespread implementation of stem cell therapy. While stem cell technology is still in its early stages, fundamental research insights into stem cell culture, derivation, and differentiation methods, combined with advances in engraftment, transplantation, and survival strategies, will undoubtedly contribute to the future evolution of safer and more effective stem cell-based therapies.

References

[1] Roemer K and Friedmann T 1992 Concepts and strategies for human gene therapy *Eur. J. Biochem.* **208** 211–25

[2] Matthews Q L and Curiel D T 2007 Gene therapy: human germline genetic modifications—assessing the scientific, socioethical, and religious issues *South Med. J.* **100** 98–100

[3] Bank A 1996 Human somatic cell gene therapy *Bioessays* **18** 999–1007

[4] Den Hollander A I, Black A, Bennett J and Cremers F P 2010 Lighting a candle in the dark: advances in genetics and gene therapy of recessive retinal dystrophies *J. Clin. Invest.* **120** 3042–53

[5] Farrar G J, Millington-Ward S, Chadderton N, Humphries P and Kenna P F 2012 Gene-based therapies for dominantly inherited retinopathies *Gene Ther.* **19** 137–44
[6] Millington-Ward S *et al* 2011 Suppression and replacement gene therapy for autosomal dominant disease in a murine model of dominant retinitis pigmentosa *Mol. Ther.* **19** 642–9
[7] Jiang L, Zhang H, Dizhoor A M, Boye S E, Hauswirth W W, Frederick J M and Baehr W 2011 Long-term RNA interference gene therapy in a dominant retinitis pigmentosa mouse model *Proc. Natl Acad. Sci. USA* **108** 18476–81
[8] Westphal E M 2002 Melchner Hv Hv. Gene therapy approaches for the selective killing of cancer cells *Curr. Pharm. Des.* **8** 1683–94
[9] Rubinstein N, Alvarez M, Zwirner N W, Toscano M A, Ilarregui J M, Bravo A, Mordoh J, Fainboim L, Podhajcer O L and Rabinovich G A 2004 Targeted inhibition of galectin-1 gene expression in tumor cells results in heightened T cell-mediated rejection; a potential mechanism of tumor-immune privilege *Cancer Cell.* **5** 241–51
[10] Parekh-Olmedo H, Ferrara L, Brachman E and Kmiec E B 2005 Gene therapy progress and prospects: targeted gene repair *Gene Ther.* **12** 639–46
[11] Mali S 2013 Delivery systems for gene therapy *Indian J. Hum. Genet.* **19** 3–8
[12] Scheller E L and Krebsbach P H 2009 Gene therapy: design and prospects for craniofacial regeneration *J. Dent. Res.* **88** 585–96
[13] Shillitoe E J 2009 Gene therapy: the end of the rainbow? *Head Neck Oncol.* **1** 7
[14] Gardlík R, Pálffy R, Hodosy J, Lukács J, Turna J and Celec P 2005 Vectors and delivery systems in gene therapy *Med. Sci. Monit* **11** RA110–21
[15] Kay M A, Liu D and Hoogerbrugge P M 1997 Gene therapy *Proc. Natl Acad. Sci. USA* **94** 12744–6
[16] Biçeroğlu S and Memiş A 2005 Gene therapy: applications in interventional radiology *Diagn. Interv. Radiol.* **11** 113–8
[17] Gammon K 2014 Gene therapy: editorial control *Nature* **515** S11–3
[18] Kurian K M, Watson C J and Wyllie A H 2000 Retroviral vectors *Mol. Pathol.* **53** 173–6
[19] Buchschacher G L 2001 Introduction to retroviruses and retroviral vectors *Somat. Cell Mol. Genet.* **26** 1–11
[20] ROWE W P, HUEBNER R J and BELL J A 1957 Definition and outline of contemporary information on the adenovirus group *Ann. N. Y. Acad. Sci.* **67** 255–61
[21] Zhang X and Godbey W T 2006 Viral vectors for gene delivery in tissue engineering *Adv. Drug Deliv. Rev.* **58** 515–34
[22] Ginsberg H S 1999 The life and times of adenoviruses *Adv. Virus Res.* **54** 1–13
[23] Barnett B G, Crews C J and Douglas J T 2002 Targeted adenoviral vectors *Biochim. Biophys. Acta.* **1575** 1–14
[24] Russell W C 2000 Update on adenovirus and its vectors *J. Gen. Virol.* **81** 2573–604
[25] Carter B J 2005 Adeno-associated virus vectors in clinical trials *Hum. Gene Ther.* **16** 541–50
[26] Epstein A L 2022 HSV-1's contribution as a vector for gene therapy *Nat. Biotechnol.* **40** 1316
[27] Lundstrom K 2009 Alphaviruses in gene therapy *Viruses* **1** 13–25
[28] Delecluse H J and Hammerschmidt W 2000 The genetic approach to the epstein-barr virus: from basic virology to gene therapy *Mol. Pathol* **53** 270–9
[29] Duarte S, Carle G, Faneca H, De Lima M C and Pierrefite-Carle V 2012 Suicide gene therapy in cancer: where do we stand now? *Cancer Lett.* **324** 160–70

[30] Ramamoorth M and Narvekar A 2015 Non viral vectors in gene therapy- an overview *J. Clin. Diagn. Res.* **9** GE01–6

[31] Nayerossadat N, Maedeh T and Ali P A 2012 Viral and nonviral delivery systems for gene delivery *Adv. Biomed. Res.* **1** 27

[32] Al-Dosari M S and Gao X 2009 Nonviral gene delivery: principle, limitations, and recent progress *AAPS J.* **11** 671–81

[33] Manjila S B, Baby J N, Bijin E N, Constantine I, Pramod K and Valsalakumari J 2013 Novel gene delivery systems *Int. J. Pharm. Investig.* **3** 1–7

[34] Kamimura K, Suda T, Zhang G and Liu D 2011 Advances in gene delivery systems *Pharmaceut. Med.* **25** 293–306

[35] Izsvák Z and Ivics Z 2004 Sleeping beauty transposition: biology and applications for molecular therapy *Mol. Ther.* **9** 147–56

[36] Hackett P B, Ekker S C, Largaespada D A and McIvor R S 2005 Sleeping beauty transposon-mediated gene therapy for prolonged expression *Adv. Genet.* **54** 189–232

[37] Lai L W and Lien Y H 2002 Chimeric RNA/DNA oligonucleotide-based gene therapy *Kidney Int.* **61** S47–51

[38] Wu X S, Liu D P and Liang C C 2001 Prospects of chimeric RNA-DNA oligonucleotides in gene therapy *J. Biomed. Sci.* **8** 439–45

[39] Ziello J E, Huang Y and Jovin I S 2010 Cellular endocytosis and gene delivery *Mol. Med.* **16** 222–9

[40] Guy J, Drabek D and Antoniou M 1995 Delivery of DNA into mammalian cells by receptor-mediated endocytosis and gene therapy *Mol. Biotechnol.* **3** 237–48

[41] Humbert O, Davis L and Maizels N 2012 Targeted gene therapies: tools, applications, optimization *Crit. Rev. Biochem. Mol. Biol.* **47** 264–81

[42] Mauceri H J, Hanna N N, Wayne J D, Hallahan D E, Hellman S and Weichselbaum R R 1996 Tumor necrosis factor alpha (TNF-alpha) gene therapy targeted by ionizing radiation selectively damages tumor vasculature *Cancer Res.* **56** 4311–4

[43] Karjoo Z, Chen X and Hatefi A 2016 Progress and problems with the use of suicide genes for targeted cancer therapy *Adv. Drug Deliv. Rev.* **99** 113–28

[44] Beck C, Cayeux S, Lupton S D, Dörken B and Blankenstein T 1995 The thymidine kinase/ganciclovir-mediated 'suicide' effect is variable in different tumor cells *Hum. Gene Ther.* **6** 1525–30

[45] O'Malley B W, Sewell D A, Li D, Kosai K, Chen S H, Woo S L and Duan L 1997 The role of interleukin-2 in combination adenovirus gene therapy for head and neck cancer *Mol. Endocrinol.* **11** 667–73

[46] Das S K, Menezes M E, Bhatia S, Wang X Y, Emdad L, Sarkar D and Fisher P B 2015 Gene therapies for cancer: strategies, challenges and successes *J. Cell. Physiol.* **230** 259–71

[47] Roth J A, Swisher S G and Meyn R E 1999 p53 tumor suppressor gene therapy for cancer *Oncology (Williston Park)* **13** 148–54

[48] Strayer D S, Akkina R, Bunnell B A, Dropulic B, Planelles V, Pomerantz R J, Rossi J J and Zaia J A 2005 Current status of gene therapy strategies to treat HIV/AIDS *Mol. Ther.* **11** 823–42

[49] Hammarskjöld M L, Heimer J, Hammarskjöld B, Sangwan I, Albert L and Rekosh D 1989 Regulation of human immunodeficiency virus env expression by the rev gene product *J. Virol.* **63** 1959–66

[50] Rossi J J, June C H and Kohn D B 2007 Genetic therapies against HIV *Nat. Biotechnol.* **25** 1444–54
[51] Karn J and Stoltzfus C M 2012 Transcriptional and posttranscriptional regulation of HIV-1 gene expression *Cold Spring Harb. Perspect. Med.* **2** a006916
[52] Chertova E *et al* 2002 Envelope glycoprotein incorporation, not shedding of surface envelope glycoprotein (gp120/SU), Is the primary determinant of SU content of purified human immunodeficiency virus type 1 and simian immunodeficiency virus *J. Virol.* **76** 5315–25
[53] Dhuri K, Bechtold C, Quijano E, Pham H, Gupta A, Vikram A and Bahal R 2020 Antisense Oligonucleotides: an emerging area in drug discovery and development *J. Clin. Med.* **9** 2004
[54] Gleave M E and Monia B P 2005 Antisense therapy for cancer *Nat. Rev. Cancer* **5** 468–79
[55] Stahel R A and Zangemeister-Wittke U 2003 Antisense oligonucleotides for cancer therapy-an overview *Lung. Cancer* **41 Suppl 1** S81–8
[56] Jansen B and Zangemeister-Wittke U 2002 Antisense therapy for cancer—the time of truth *Lancet. Oncol.* **3** 672–83
[57] Moreno P M and Pêgo A P 2014 Therapeutic antisense oligonucleotides against cancer: hurdling to the clinic *Front. Chem.* **2** 87
[58] Rowley P T, Kosciolek B A and Kool E T 1999 Circular antisense oligonucleotides inhibit growth of chronic myeloid leukemia cells *Mol. Med.* **5** 693–700
[59] Gesteland R F, Cech T R and Atkins J F 2006 *The RNA World* 3rd edn (New York: Cold Spring Harbor Laboratory)
[60] Dykxhoorn D M and Lieberman J 2006 Knocking down disease with siRNAs *Cell* **126** 231–5
[61] Rao D D, Vorhies J S, Senzer N and Nemunaitis J 2009 siRNA vs. shRNA: similarities and differences *Adv. Drug Deliv. Rev.* **61** 746–59
[62] Rainov N G and Ren H 2003 Gene therapy for human malignant brain tumors *Cancer J.* **9** 180–8
[63] Hau P, Jachimczak P and Bogdahn U 2009 Treatment of malignant gliomas with TGF-beta2 antisense oligonucleotides *Expert Rev. Anticancer Ther.* **9** 1663–74
[64] Burfeind P, Chernicky C L, Rininsland F, Ilan J and Ilan J 1996 Antisense RNA to the type I insulin-like growth factor receptor suppresses tumor growth and prevents invasion by rat prostate cancer cells *in vivo Proc. Natl Acad. Sci. USA* **93** 7263–8
[65] Bunnell B A and Morgan R A 1998 Gene therapy for infectious diseases *Clin. Microbiol. Rev.* **11** 42–56
[66] Nazari R and Joshi S 2008 CCR5 as target for HIV-1 gene therapy *Curr. Gene Ther.* **8** 264–72
[67] Bobbin M L, Burnett J C and Rossi J J 2015 RNA interference approaches for treatment of HIV-1 infection *Genome Med.* **7** 50
[68] Galderisi U, Cascino A and Giordano A 1999 Antisense oligonucleotides as therapeutic agents *J. Cell. Physiol.* **181** 251–7
[69] Stein C A and Cheng Y C 1993 Antisense oligonucleotides as therapeutic agents—is the bullet really magical? *Science* **261** 1004–12
[70] Cazenave C, Chevrier M, Nguyen T T and Hélène C 1987 Rate of degradation of [alpha]- and [beta]-oligodeoxynucleotides in Xenopus oocytes. Implications for anti-messenger strategies *Nucleic Acids Res.* **15** 10507–21

[71] Shaw J P, Kent K, Bird J, Fishback J and Froehler B 1991 Modified deoxyoligonucleotides stable to exonuclease degradation in serum *Nucleic Acids Res.* **19** 747–50

[72] Roberts T C, Langer R and Wood M J A 2020 Advances in oligonucleotide drug delivery *Nat. Rev. Drug Discov* **19** 673–94

[73] Hoke G D, Draper K, Freier S M, Gonzalez C, Driver V B, Zounes M C and Ecker D J 1991 Effects of phosphorothioate capping on antisense oligonucleotide stability, hybridization and antiviral efficacy versus herpes simplex virus infection *Nucleic Acids Res.* **19** 5743–8

[74] Crooke S T *et al* 1996 Pharmacokinetic properties of several novel oligonucleotide analogs in mice *J. Pharmacol. Exp. Ther.* **277** 923–37

[75] Cook P D 1991 Medicinal chemistry of antisense oligonucleotides—future opportunities *Anticancer Drug Des.* **6** 585–607

[76] Gao W Y, Han F S, Storm C, Egan W and Cheng Y C 1992 Phosphorothioate oligonucleotides are inhibitors of human DNA polymerases and RNase H: implications for antisense technology *Mol. Pharmacol.* **41** 223–9

[77] Crooke S T, Lemonidis K M, Neilson L, Griffey R, Lesnik E A and Monia B P 1995 Kinetic characteristics of *Escherichia coli* RNase H1: cleavage of various antisense oligonucleotide-RNA duplexes *Biochem. J.* **312** 599–608

[78] Galbraith W M, Hobson W C, Giclas P C, Schechter P J and Agrawal S 1994 Complement activation and hemodynamic changes following intravenous administration of phosphorothioate oligonucleotides in the monkey *Antisense Res. Dev.* **4** 201–6

[79] Ghosh A, Myacheva K, Riester M, Schmidt C and Diederichs S 2022 Chimeric oligonucleotides combining guide RNA and single-stranded DNA repair template effectively induce precision gene editing *RNA Biol.* **19** 588–93

[80] Gamper H B, Parekh H, Rice M C, Bruner M, Youkey H and Kmiec E B 2000 The DNA strand of chimeric RNA/DNA oligonucleotides can direct gene repair/conversion activity in mammalian and plant cell-free extracts *Nucleic Acids Res.* **28** 4332–9

[81] Brody E N and Gold L 2000 Aptamers as therapeutic and diagnostic agents *J. Biotechnol.* **74** 5–13

[82] Lassalle H P, Marchal S, Guillemin F, Reinhard A and Bezdetnaya L 2012 Aptamers as remarkable diagnostic and therapeutic agents in cancer treatment *Curr. Drug Metab.* **13** 1130–44

[83] Aljohani M M, Cialla-May D, Popp J, Chinnappan R, Al-Kattan K and Zourob M 2022 Aptamers: potential diagnostic and therapeutic agents for blood diseases *Molecules* **27** 383

[84] Phylactou L A, Kilpatrick M W and Wood M J 1998 Ribozymes as therapeutic tools for genetic disease *Hum. Mol. Genet.* **7** 1649–53

[85] Rubanyi G M 2001 The future of human gene therapy *Mol. Aspects Med.* **22** 113–42

[86] Weiner L P 2008 Definitions and criteria for stem cells *Methods Mol. Biol.* **438** 3–8

[87] De Luca M, Aiuti A, Cossu G, Parmar M, Pellegrini G and Robey P G 2019 Advances in stem cell research and therapeutic development *Nat. Cell Biol.* **21** 801–11

[88] Biehl J K and Russell B 2009 Introduction to stem cell therapy *J. Cardiovasc. Nurs.* **24** 98–103

[89] Volarevic V, Markovic B S, Gazdic M, Volarevic A, Jovicic N, Arsenijevic N, Armstrong L, Djonov V, Lako M and Stojkovic M 2018 Ethical and safety issues of stem cell-based therapy *Int. J. Med. Sci.* **15** 36–45

[90] Zakrzewski W, Dobrzyński M, Szymonowicz M and Rybak Z 2019 Stem cells: past, present, and future *Stem Cell Res. Ther.* **10** 68
[91] Fortier L A 2005 Stem cells: classifications, controversies, and clinical applications *Vet. Surg.* **34** 415–23
[92] Sobhani A, Khanlarkhani N, Baazm M, Mohammadzadeh F, Najafi A, Mehdinejadiani S and Sargolzaei Aval F 2017 Multipotent stem cell and current application *Acta. Med. Iran* **55** 6–23
[93] Mitalipov S and Wolf D 2009 Totipotency, pluripotency and nuclear reprogramming *Adv. Biochem. Eng. Biotechnol.* **114** 185–99
[94] Simara P, Motl J A and Kaufman D S 2013 Pluripotent stem cells and gene therapy *Transl. Res.* **161** 284–92
[95] Singh V K, Saini A, Kalsan M, Kumar N and Chandra R 2016 Describing the stem cell potency: the various methods of functional assessment and *in silico* diagnostics *Front. Cell Dev. Biol.* **4** 134
[96] Cable J *et al* 2020 Adult stem cells and regenerative medicine-a symposium report *Ann. N. Y. Acad. Sci.* **1462** 27–36
[97] Trounson A O 2000 *Handbook of In Vitro Fertilization* (Boca Raton, FL: CRC Press)
[98] Friedrich T D, Regenass U and Stevens L C 1983 Mouse genital ridges in organ culture: the effects of temperature on maturation and experimental induction of teratocarcinogenesis *Differentiation* **24** 60–4
[99] Martin G R 1980 Teratocarcinomas and mammalian embryogenesis *Science* **209** 768–76
[100] Andrews P W 1988 Human teratocarcinomas *Biochim. Biophys. Acta* **948** 17–36
[101] Pera M F, Cooper S, Mills J and Parrington J M 1989 Isolation and characterization of a multipotent clone of human embryonal carcinoma cells *Differentiation* **42** 10–23
[102] Bongso T A, Fong C Y, Ng C Y and Ratnam S S 1994 Blastocyst transfer in human *in vitro* fertilization: the use of embryo co-culture *Cell Biol. Int.* **18** 1181–9
[103] Thomson J A, Kalishman J, Golos T G, Durning M, Harris C P, Becker R A and Hearn J P 1995 Isolation of a primate embryonic stem cell line *Proc. Natl Acad. Sci. USA* **92** 7844–8
[104] Shamblott M J, Axelman J, Wang S, Bugg E M, Littlefield J W, Donovan P J, Blumenthal P D, Huggins G R and Gearhart J D 1998 Derivation of pluripotent stem cells from cultured human primordial germ cells *Proc. Natl Acad. Sci. USA* **95** 13726–31
[105] Reubinoff B E, Pera M F, Fong C Y, Trounson A and Bongso A 2000 Embryonic stem cell lines from human blastocysts: somatic differentiation *in vitro Nat. Biotechnol.* **18** 399–404
[106] Kaufman D S, Hanson E T, Lewis R L, Auerbach R and Thomson J A 2001 Hematopoietic colony-forming cells derived from human embryonic stem cells *Proc. Natl Acad. Sci. USA* **98** 10716–21
[107] Lo B and Parham L 2009 Ethical issues in stem cell research *Endocr. Rev.* **30** 204–13
[108] Mahla R S 2016 Stem cells applications in regenerative medicine and disease therapeutics *Int. J. Cell Biol.* **2016** 6940283
[109] Lennard A L and Jackson G H 2001 Stem cell transplantation *West J. Med.* **175** 42–6
[110] Bai X 2020 Stem cell-based disease modeling and cell therapy *Cells* **9** 2193
[111] Cowan C A *et al* 2004 Derivation of embryonic stem-cell lines from human blastocysts *N. Engl. J. Med.* **350** 1353–6
[112] Thomson J A, Itskovitz-Eldor J, Shapiro S S, Waknitz M A, Swiergiel J J, Marshall V S and Jones J M 1998 Embryonic stem cell lines derived from human blastocysts *Science* **282** 1145–7

[113] Shamblott M J, Axelman J, Littlefield J W, Blumenthal P D, Huggins G R, Cui Y, Cheng L and Gearhart J D 2001 Human embryonic germ cell derivatives express a broad range of developmentally distinct markers and proliferate extensively *in vitro Proc. Natl Acad. Sci. USA* **98** 113–8

[114] Spradling A, Drummond-Barbosa D and Kai T 2001 Stem cells find their niche *Nature* **414** 98–104

[115] Sanchez-Ramos J *et al* 2000 Adult bone marrow stromal cells differentiate into neural cells *in vitro Exp. Neurol.* **164** 247–56

[116] O'Brien T and Barry F P 2009 Stem cell therapy and regenerative medicine *Mayo Clin. Proc.* **84** 859–61

[117] Benjamin E J, Blaha M J, Chiuve S E *et al* American Heart Association Statistics Committee and Stroke Statistics Subcommittee 2017 Heart disease and stroke statistics-2017 update: a report from the American Heart Association *Circulation* **135** e146–603

[118] Fernández-Avilés F, Sanz-Ruiz R, Climent A M *et al* TACTICS Writing Group 2018 Global overview of the transnational alliance for regenerative therapies in cardiovascular syndromes (TACTICS) recommendations: a comprehensive series of challenges and priorities of cardiovascular regenerative medicine *Circ. Res.* **122** 199–201

[119] Isomi M, Sadahiro T, Yamakawa H *et al* 2021 Overexpression of Gata4, Mef2c, and Tbx5 generates induced cardiomyocytes via direct reprogramming and rare fusion in the heart *Circulation* **143** 2123–5

[120] Mauritz C, Martens A, Rojas S V *et al* 2011 Induced pluripotent stem cell (iPSC)-derived Flk-1 progenitor cells engraft, differentiate, and improve heart function in a mouse model of acute myocardial infarction *Eur. Heart J.* **32** 2634–41

[121] Tian S, Liu Q, Gnatovskiy L *et al* 2015 Heart regeneration with embryonic cardiac progenitor cells and cardiac tissue engineering *J. Stem Cell Transplant. Biol.* **1** 104

[122] Zhang J, Wilson G F, Soerens A G *et al* 2009 Functional cardiomyocytes derived from human induced pluripotent stem cells *Circ. Res.* **104** e30–41

[123] Citro L, Naidu S, Hassan F *et al* 2014 Comparison of human induced pluripotent stem-cell derived cardiomyocytes with human mesenchymal stem cells following acute myocardial infarction *PLoS One* **9** e116281

[124] Ye L, Chang Y H, Xiong Q *et al* 2014 Cardiac repair in a porcine model of acute myocardial infarction with human induced pluripotent stem cell-derived cardiovascular cells *Cell Stem Cell* **15** 750–61

[125] Ménard C, Hagège A A, Agbulut O *et al* 2005 Transplantation of cardiac-committed mouse embryonic stem cells to infarcted sheep myocardium: a preclinical study *Lancet* **366** 1005–12

[126] Le Blanc K, Tammik C, Rosendahl K, Zetterberg E and Ringdén O 2003 HLA expression and immunologic properties of differentiated and undifferentiated mesenchymal stem cells *Exp. Hematol.* **31** 890–6

[127] Zhang Y, Zhang Z, Gao F *et al* 2015 Paracrine regulation in mesenchymal stem cells: the role of Rap1 *Cell Death Dis.* **6** e1932

[128] Zhang M, Mal N, Kiedrowski M *et al* 2007 SDF-1 expression by mesenchymal stem cells results in trophic support of cardiac myocytes after myocardial infarction *FASEB J.* **21** 3197–207

[129] Nakanishi C, Yamagishi M, Yamahara K, Hagino I, Mori H, Sawa Y, Yagihara T, Kitamura S and Nagaya N 2008 Activation of cardiac progenitor cells through paracrine effects of mesenchymal stem cells *Biochem. Biophys. Res. Commun.* **374** 11–6

[130] Orlic D *et al* 2001 Bone marrow cells regenerate infarcted myocardium *Nature* **410** 701–5

[131] Li X, Yu X, Lin Q *et al* 2007 Bone marrow mesenchymal stem cells differentiate into functional cardiac phenotypes by cardiac microenvironment *J. Mol. Cell. Cardiol.* **42** 295–303

[132] Rota M, Kajstura J, Hosoda T *et al* 2007 Bone marrow cells adopt the cardiomyogenic fate *in vivo Proc. Natl Acad. Sci. USA* **104** 17783–8

[133] Beltrami A P, Barlucchi L, Torella D *et al* 2003 Adult cardiac stem cells are multipotent and support myocardial regeneration *Cell* **114** 763–76

[134] Tateishi K, Ashihara E, Honsho S *et al* 2007 Human cardiac stem cells exhibit mesenchymal features and are maintained through Akt/GSK-3beta signaling *Biochem. Biophys. Res. Commun.* **352** 635–41

[135] Li T S, Cheng K, Malliaras K *et al* 2012 Direct comparison of different stem cell types and subpopulations reveals superior paracrine potency and myocardial repair efficacy with cardiosphere-derived cells *J. Am. Coll. Cardiol.* **59** 942–53

[136] Smith R R, Barile L, Cho H C *et al* 2007 Regenerative potential of cardiosphere-derived cells expanded from percutaneous endomyocardial biopsy specimens *Circulation* **115** 896–908

[137] Dixit P and Katare R 2015 Challenges in identifying the best source of stem cells for cardiac regeneration therapy *Stem Cell Res. Ther.* **6** 26

[138] Chugh A R, Beache G M, Loughran J H *et al* 2012 Administration of cardiac stem cells in patients with ischemic cardiomyopathy: the SCIPIO trial: surgical aspects and interim analysis of myocardial function and viability by magnetic resonance *Circulation* **126** S54–64

[139] Okamoto R, Matsumoto T and Watanabe M 2006 Regeneration of the intestinal epithelia: regulation of bone marrow-derived epithelial cell differentiation towards secretory lineage cells *Hum. Cell.* **19** 71–5

[140] Gehart H and Clevers H 2019 Tales from the crypt: new insights into intestinal stem cells *Nat. Rev. Gastroenterol. Hepatol.* **16** 19–34

[141] Santos A J M, Lo Y H, Mah A T and Kuo C J 2018 The intestinal stem cell niche: homeostasis and adaptations *Trends Cell Biol.* **28** 1062–78

[142] Rashed L, Gharib D M, Hussein R E *et al* 2016 Combined effect of bone marrow derived mesenchymal stem cells and nitric oxide inducer on injured gastric mucosa in a rat model *Tissue Cell* **48** 644–52

[143] Wang G, Li C, Fan X *et al* 2015 [Effect of bone marrow mesenchymal stem cells on gastric ulcer repairing] *Zhongguo Xiu Fu Chong Jian Wai Ke Za Zhi* **29** 889–92 (in Chinese)

[144] Hendrickson B A, Gokhale R and Cho J H 2002 Clinical aspects and pathophysiology of inflammatory bowel disease *Clin. Microbiol. Rev.* **15** 79–94

[145] Kobayashi T, Siegmund B, Le Berre C *et al* 2020 Ulcerative colitis *Nat. Rev. Dis. Primers* **6** 74

[146] Hurley J M, Lee S G, Andrews R E *et al* 1985 Separation of the cytolytic and mosquitocidal proteins of *Bacillus thuringiensis* subsp. israelensis *Biochem. Biophys. Res. Commun.* **126** 961–5

[147] Hasselblatt P, Drognitz K, Potthoff K *et al* 2012 Remission of refractory Crohn's disease by high-dose cyclophosphamide and autologous peripheral blood stem cell transplantation *Aliment. Pharmacol. Ther.* **36** 725–35

[148] Hawkey C J, Allez M, Clark M M *et al* 2015 Autologous hematopoetic stem cell transplantation for refractory crohn disease: a randomized clinical trial *JAMA* **314** 2524–34

[149] Lindsay J O, Allez M, Clark M *et al* ASTIC Trial Group; European Society for Blood and Marrow Transplantation Autoimmune Disease Working Party; European Crohn's and Colitis Organisation 2017 Autologous stem-cell transplantation in treatment-refractory Crohn's disease: an analysis of pooled data from the ASTIC trial *Lancet Gastroenterol. Hepatol.* **2** 399–406

[150] Wang R, Yao Q, Chen W *et al* 2021 Stem cell therapy for Crohn's disease: systematic review and meta-analysis of preclinical and clinical studies *Stem Cell Res. Ther.* **12** 463

[151] Luo X Y, Meng X J, Cao D C *et al* 2019 Transplantation of bone marrow mesenchymal stromal cells attenuates liver fibrosis in mice by regulating macrophage subtypes *Stem Cell Res. Ther.* **10** 16

[152] Li Y H, Shen S, Shao T *et al* 2021 Mesenchymal stem cells attenuate liver fibrosis by targeting $Ly6C^{hi/lo}$ macrophages through activating the cytokine-paracrine and apoptotic pathways *Cell Death Discov.* **7** 239

[153] Jin S, Li H, Han M *et al* 2016 Mesenchymal stem cells with enhanced Bcl-2 expression promote liver recovery in a rat model of hepatic cirrhosis *Cell. Physiol. Biochem.* **40** 1117–28

[154] Quintanilha L F, Takami T, Hirose Y *et al* 2014 Canine mesenchymal stem cells show antioxidant properties against thioacetamide-induced liver injury *in vitro* and *in vivo Hepatol. Res.* **44** E206–17

[155] Volarevic V, Nurkovic J, Arsenijevic N and Stojkovic M 2014 Concise review: therapeutic potential of mesenchymal stem cells for the treatment of acute liver failure and cirrhosis *Stem Cells* **32** 2818–23

[156] Xia X, Tao Q, Ma Q *et al* 2016 Growth hormone-releasing hormone and its analogues: significance for MSCs-mediated angiogenesis *Stem Cells Int.* **2016** 8737589

[157] Kantarcıoğlu M, Demirci H, Avcu F *et al* 2015 Efficacy of autologous mesenchymal stem cell transplantation in patients with liver cirrhosis *Turk. J. Gastroenterol.* **26** 244–50

[158] Mohamadnejad M, Alimoghaddam K, Bagheri M *et al* 2013 Randomized placebo-controlled trial of mesenchymal stem cell transplantation in decompensated cirrhosis *Liver Int.* **33** 1490–6

[159] Kharaziha P, Hellstrom P M, Noorinayer B *et al* 2009 Improvement of liver function in liver cirrhosis patients after autologous mesenchymal stem cell injection: a phase I-II clinical trial *Eur. J. Gastroenterol. Hepatol.* **21** 1199–205

[160] Suk K T, Yoon J H, Kim M Y *et al* 2016 Transplantation with autologous bone marrow-derived mesenchymal stem cells for alcoholic cirrhosis: phase 2 trial *Hepatology* **64** 2185–97

[161] Xu L, Gong Y, Wang B *et al* 2014 Randomized trial of autologous bone marrow mesenchymal stem cells transplantation for hepatitis B virus cirrhosis: regulation of Treg/Th17 cells *J. Gastroenterol. Hepatol.* **29** 1620–8

[162] Zhang Z, Lin H, Shi M *et al* 2012 Human umbilical cord mesenchymal stem cells improve liver function and ascites in decompensated liver cirrhosis patients *J. Gastroenterol. Hepatol.* **27** 112–20

[163] Wang L, Li J, Liu H *et al* 2013 Pilot study of umbilical cord-derived mesenchymal stem cell transfusion in patients with primary biliary cirrhosis *J. Gastroenterol. Hepatol* **28** 85–92

[164] Shi M, Zhang Z, Xu R *et al* 2012 Human mesenchymal stem cell transfusion is safe and improves liver function in acute-on-chronic liver failure patients *Stem Cells Transl. Med.* **1** 725–31

[165] Polson J and Lee W MAmerican Association for the Study of Liver Disease 2005 AASLD position paper: the management of acute liver failure *Hepatology* **41** 1179–97

[166] Jalan R and Williams R 2002 Acute-on-chronic liver failure: pathophysiological basis of therapeutic options *Blood Purif.* **20** 252–61
[167] Terai S, Ishikawa T, Omori K *et al* 2006 Improved liver function in patients with liver cirrhosis after autologous bone marrow cell infusion therapy *Stem Cells* **24** 2292–8
[168] Ismail B E and Cabrera R 2013 Management of liver cirrhosis in patients with hepatocellular carcinoma *Chin. Clin. Oncol.* **2** 34
[169] Snykers S, De Kock J, Tamara V and Rogiers V 2011 Hepatic differentiation of mesenchymal stem cells: *in vitro* strategies *Methods Mol. Biol.* **698** 305–14
[170] Choi J, Kang S, Kim B *et al* 2021 Efficient hepatic differentiation and regeneration potential under xeno-free conditions using mass-producible amnion-derived mesenchymal stem cells *Stem Cell Res. Ther.* **12** 569
[171] Ewida S F, Abdou A G, El-Rasol Elhosary A A and El-Ghane Metawe S A 2017 Hepatocyte-like versus mesenchymal stem cells in CCl4-induced liver fibrosis *Appl. Immunohistochem. Mol. Morphol.* **25** 736–45
[172] Kollet O, Shivtiel S, Chen Y Q *et al* 2003 HGF, SDF-1, and MMP-9 are involved in stress-induced human CD34+ stem cell recruitment to the liver *J. Clin. Invest.* **112** 160–9
[173] Yannaki E, Athanasiou E, Xagorari A *et al* 2005 G-CSF-primed hematopoietic stem cells or G-CSF per se accelerate recovery and improve survival after liver injury, predominantly by promoting endogenous repair programs *Exp. Hematol.* **33** 108–19
[174] Lu W, Qu J, Yan L *et al* 2023 Efficacy and safety of mesenchymal stem cell therapy in liver cirrhosis: a systematic review and meta-analysis *Stem Cell Res. Ther.* **14** 301
[175] Fu K, Robbins S R and McDougall J J 2018 Osteoarthritis: the genesis of pain *Rheumatology (Oxford)* **57** iv43–50
[176] Berenbaum F, Wallace I J, Lieberman D E and Felson D T 2018 Modern-day environmental factors in the pathogenesis of osteoarthritis *Nat. Rev. Rheumatol.* **14** 674–81
[177] Volarevic V, Gazdic M, Simovic Markovic B *et al* 2017 Mesenchymal stem cell-derived factors: immuno-modulatory effects and therapeutic potential *Biofactors* **43** 633–44
[178] Wakitani S, Imoto K, Yamamoto T *et al* 2002 Human autologous culture expanded bone marrow mesenchymal cell transplantation for repair of cartilage defects in osteoarthritic knees *Osteoarthr. Cartil.* **10** 199–206
[179] Wong K L, Lee K B, Tai B C *et al* 2013 Injectable cultured bone marrow-derived mesenchymal stem cells in varus knees with cartilage defects undergoing high tibial osteotomy: a prospective, randomized controlled clinical trial with 2 years' follow-up *Arthroscopy* **29** 2020–8
[180] Vangsness C T Jr., Farr J 2nd, Boyd J *et al* 2014 Adult human mesenchymal stem cells delivered via intra-articular injection to the knee following partial medial meniscectomy: a randomized, double-blind, controlled study *J. Bone Joint Surg. Am.* **96** 90–8
[181] Chen H T, Lee M J, Chen C H *et al* 2012 Proliferation and differentiation potential of human adipose-derived mesenchymal stem cells isolated from elderly patients with osteoporotic fractures *J. Cell. Mol. Med.* **16** 582–93
[182] Pers Y M, Rackwitz L, Ferreira R *et al* ADIPOA Consortium 2016 Adipose mesenchymal stromal cell-based therapy for severe osteoarthritis of the knee: a phase I dose-escalation trial *Stem Cells Transl. Med.* **5** 847–56
[183] Koh Y G, Kwon O R, Kim Y S *et al* 2016 Adipose-derived mesenchymal stem cells with microfracture versus microfracture alone: 2-year follow-up of a prospective randomized trial *Arthroscopy* **32** 97–109

[184] Lee W S, Kim H J, Kim K I *et al* 2019 Intra-articular injection of autologous adipose tissue-derived mesenchymal stem cells for the treatment of knee osteoarthritis: a phase IIb, randomized, placebo-controlled clinical trial *Stem Cells Transl. Med.* **8** 504–11

[185] Saghahazrati S, Ayatollahi S A M, Kobarfard F and Minaii Zang B 2020 The synergistic effect of glucagon-like peptide-1 and chamomile oil on differentiation of mesenchymal stem cells into insulin-producing cells *Cell J.* **21** 371–8

[186] Wang Y, Jin W, Liu H *et al* 2016 [Curative effect of human umbilical cord mesenchymal stem cells by intra-articular injection for degenerative knee osteoarthritis] *Zhongguo Xiu Fu Chong Jian Wai Ke Za Zhi* **30** 1472–7 (in Chinese)

[187] Barisic S and Childs R W 2022 Graft-versus-solid-tumor effect: from hematopoietic stem cell transplantation to adoptive cell therapies *Stem Cells* **40** 556–63

[188] Fu X, Liu G, Halim A *et al* 2019 Mesenchymal stem cell migration and tissue repair *Cells* **8** 784

[189] Zachar L, Bačenková D and Rosocha J 2016 Activation, homing, and role of the mesenchymal stem cells in the inflammatory environment *J. Inflamm. Res.* **9** 231–40

[190] https://classic.clinicaltrials.gov/ct2/show/NCT03920397

[191] https://classic.clinicaltrials.gov/ct2/show/NCT01068951

[192] https://classic.clinicaltrials.gov/ct2/show/NCT00690066

[193] Carlsson P O, Schwarcz E, Korsgren O and Le Blanc K 2015 Preserved β-cell function in type 1 diabetes by mesenchymal stromal cells *Diabetes* **64** 587–92

[194] Hu J, Yu X, Wang Z *et al* 2013 Long term effects of the implantation of Wharton's jelly-derived mesenchymal stem cells from the umbilical cord for newly-onset type 1 diabetes mellitus *Endocr. J.* **60** 347–57

[195] Cai J, Wu Z, Xu X *et al* 2016 Umbilical cord mesenchymal stromal cell with autologous bone marrow cell transplantation in established type 1 diabetes: a pilot randomized controlled open-label clinical study to assess safety and impact on insulin secretion *Diabetes Care* **39** 149–57

[196] Huang Q, Huang Y and Liu J 2021 Mesenchymal stem cells: an excellent candidate for the treatment of diabetes mellitus *Int. J. Endocrinol.* **2021** 9938658

[197] Nguyen L T, Hoang D M, Nguyen K T *et al* 2021 Type 2 diabetes mellitus duration and obesity alter the efficacy of autologously transplanted bone marrow-derived mesenchymal stem/stromal cells *Stem Cells Transl. Med.* **10** 1266–78

[198] Agarwal A, Baskaran S, Parekh N *et al* 2021 Male infertility *Lancet* **397** 319–33

[199] Farquhar C and Marjoribanks J 2018 Assisted reproductive technology: an overview of Cochrane reviews *Cochrane Database Syst. Rev.* **8** CD010537

[200] Fenton A J 2015 Premature ovarian insufficiency: pathogenesis and management *J. Midlife Health* **6** 147–53

[201] Huhtaniemi I, Hovatta O, La Marca A *et al* 2018 Advances in the molecular pathophysiology, genetics, and treatment of primary ovarian insufficiency *Trends Endocrinol. Metab.* **29** 400–19

[202] Gupta S, Lodha P, Karthick M S and Tandulwadkar S 2018 Role of autologous bone marrow-derived stem cell therapy for follicular recruitment in premature ovarian insufficiency: review of literature and a case report of world's first baby with ovarian autologous stem cell therapy in a perimenopausal woman of age 45 year *J. Hum. Reprod. Sci.* **11** 125–30

[203] Igboeli P, El Andaloussi A, Sheikh U *et al* 2020 Intraovarian injection of autologous human mesenchymal stem cells increases estrogen production and reduces menopausal symptoms

in women with premature ovarian failure: two case reports and a review of the literature *J. Med. Case Rep.* **14** 108
[204] Ulin M, Cetin E, Hobeika E *et al* 2021 Human mesenchymal stem cell therapy and other novel treatment approaches for premature ovarian insufficiency *Reprod. Sci.* **28** 1688–96
[205] Herraiz S, Romeu M, Buigues A *et al* 2018 Autologous stem cell ovarian transplantation to increase reproductive potential in patients who are poor responders *Fertil. Steril.* **110** 496–505.e1
[206] Wang M Y, Wang Y X, Li-Ling J and Xie H Q 2022 Adult stem cell therapy for premature ovarian failure: from bench to bedside *Tissue Eng. Part B. Rev.* **28** 63–78
[207] Kaddoura I, Abu-Sittah G, Ibrahim A *et al* 2017 Burn injury: review of pathophysiology and therapeutic modalities in major burns *Ann. Burns Fire Disast.* **30** 95–102
[208] Jeschke M G, van Baar M E, Choudhry M A *et al* 2020 Burn injury *Nat. Rev. Dis. Primers* **6** 11
[209] Rasulov M F, Vasilchenkov A V, Onishchenko N A *et al* 2005 First experience of the use bone marrow mesenchymal stem cells for the treatment of a patient with deep skin burns *Bull. Exp. Biol. Med.* **139** 141–4
[210] Mansilla E, Marín G H, Berges M *et al* 2015 Cadaveric bone marrow mesenchymal stem cells: first experience treating a patient with large severe burns *Burns Trauma* **3** 17
[211] Abo-Elkheir W, Hamza F, Elmofty A M *et al* 2017 Role of cord blood and bone marrow mesenchymal stem cells in recent deep burn: a case-control prospective study *Am. J. Stem Cells* **6** 23–35
[212] Zhou Y, Zhao B, Zhang X L *et al* 2021 Combined topical and systemic administration with human adipose-derived mesenchymal stem cells (hADSC) and hADSC-derived exosomes markedly promoted cutaneous wound healing and regeneration *Stem Cell Res. Ther.* **12** 257
[213] Katsuno M, Sahashi K, Iguchi Y and Hashizume A 2018 Preclinical progression of neurodegenerative diseases *Nagoya J. Med. Sci.* **80** 289–98
[214] Sakthiswary R and Raymond A A 2012 Stem cell therapy in neurodegenerative diseases: from principles to practice *Neural Regen. Res.* **7** 1822–31
[215] Shariati A, Nemati R, Sadeghipour Y *et al* 2020 Mesenchymal stromal cells (MSCs) for neurodegenerative disease: a promising frontier *Eur. J. Cell Biol.* **99** 151097
[216] Karussis D, Petrou P and Kassis I 2013 Clinical experience with stem cells and other cell therapies in neurological diseases *J. Neurol. Sci.* **324** 1–9
[217] Lunn J S, Sakowski S A, Hur J and Feldman E L 2011 Stem cell technology for neurodegenerative diseases *Ann. Neurol.* **70** 353–61
[218] Dickson D W 2012 Parkinson's disease and Parkinsonism: neuropathology *Cold Spring Harb. Perspect. Med.* **2** a009258
[219] Selikhova M, Williams D R, Kempster P A *et al* 2009 A clinico-pathological study of subtypes in Parkinson's disease *Brain* **132** 2947–57
[220] Ford E, Pearlman J, Ruan T, Manion J, Waller M, Neely G G and Caron L 2020 Human pluripotent stem cells-based therapies for neurodegenerative diseases: current status and challenges *Cells* **9** 2517
[221] Kim H J 2011 Stem cell potential in Parkinson's disease and molecular factors for the generation of dopamine neurons *Biochim. Biophys. Acta* **1812** 1–11
[222] Schwarz J and Storch A 2010 Transplantation in Parkinson's disease: will mesenchymal stem cells help to reenter the clinical arena? *Transl. Res.* **155** 55–6

[223] Takagi Y, Takahashi J, Saiki H *et al* 2005 Dopaminergic neurons generated from monkey embryonic stem cells function in a Parkinson primate model *J. Clin. Invest.* **115** 102–9
[224] Reddy A P, Ravichandran J and Carkaci-Salli N 2020 Neural regeneration therapies for Alzheimer's and Parkinson's disease-related disorders *Biochim. Biophys. Acta, Mol. Basis Dis.* **1866** 165506
[225] Garitaonandia I, Gonzalez R, Christiansen-Weber T *et al* 2016 Neural stem cell tumorigenicity and biodistribution assessment for phase I clinical trial in Parkinson's disease *Sci. Rep.* **6** 34478
[226] Deleidi M, Cooper O, Hargus G *et al* 2011 Oct4-induced reprogramming is required for adult brain neural stem cell differentiation into midbrain dopaminergic neurons *PLoS One* **6** e19926
[227] Wang Y, Ji X, Leak R K *et al* 2017 Stem cell therapies in age-related neurodegenerative diseases and stroke *Ageing Res. Rev.* **34** 39–50
[228] Soler R, Füllhase C, Hanson A *et al* 2012 Stem cell therapy ameliorates bladder dysfunction in an animal model of Parkinson disease *J. Urol.* **187** 1491–7
[229] Venkataramana N K, Kumar S K, Balaraju S *et al* 2010 Open-labeled study of unilateral autologous bone-marrow-derived mesenchymal stem cell transplantation in Parkinson's disease *Transl. Res.* **155** 62–70
[230] Cave J W, Wang M and Baker H 2014 Adult subventricular zone neural stem cells as a potential source of dopaminergic replacement neurons *Front. Neurosci.* **8** 16
[231] Barker R A, Drouin-Ouellet J and Parmar M 2015 Cell-based therapies for Parkinson disease—past insights and future potential *Nat. Rev. Neurol.* **11** 492–503
[232] Doi D, Magotani H, Kikuchi T *et al* 2020 Pre-clinical study of induced pluripotent stem cell-derived dopaminergic progenitor cells for Parkinson's disease *Nat. Commun.* **11** 3369
[233] Politis M, Oertel W H, Wu K *et al* 2011 Graft-induced dyskinesias in Parkinson's disease: high striatal serotonin/dopamine transporter ratio *Mov. Disord.* **26** 1997–2003
[234] Gan L and Johnson J A 2014 Oxidative damage and the Nrf2-ARE pathway in neurodegenerative diseases *Biochim. Biophys. Acta* **1842** 1208–18
[235] Bangde P, Atale S, Dey A *et al* 2017 Potential gene therapy towards treating neurodegenerative disea ses employing polymeric nanosystems *Curr. Gene Ther.* **17** 170–83
[236] Duncan T and Valenzuela M 2017 Alzheimer's disease, dementia, and stem cell therapy *Stem Cell Res. Ther.* **8** 111
[237] Ager R R, Davis J L, Agazaryan A *et al* 2015 Human neural stem cells improve cognition and promote synaptic growth in two complementary transgenic models of Alzheimer's disease and neuronal loss *Hippocampus* **25** 813–26
[238] Kern D S, Maclean K N, Jiang H *et al* 2011 Neural stem cells reduce hippocampal tau and reelin accumulation in aged Ts65Dn Down syndrome mice *Cell Transplant.* **20** 371–9
[239] Guo Z, Zhang L, Wu Z *et al* 2014 In vivo direct reprogramming of reactive glial cells into functional neurons after brain injury and in an Alzheimer's disease model *Cell Stem Cell* **14** 188–202
[240] Ma T, Gong K, Ao Q *et al* 2013 Intracerebral transplantation of adipose-derived mesenchymal stem cells alternatively activates microglia and ameliorates neuropathological deficits in Alzheimer's disease mice *Cell Transplant.* **22** S113–26
[241] Kan I, Barhum Y, Melamed E and Offen D 2011 Mesenchymal stem cells stimulate endogenous neurogenesis in the subventricular zone of adult mice *Stem Cell Rev. Rep.* **7** 404–12

[242] Martínez-Morales P L, Revilla A, Ocaña I *et al* 2013 Progress in stem cell therapy for major human neurological disorders *Stem Cell Rev. Rep.* **9** 685–99
[243] Ebert A D, Barber A E, Heins B M and Svendsen C N 2010 Ex vivo delivery of GDNF maintains motor function and prevents neuronal loss in a transgenic mouse model of Huntington's disease *Exp. Neurol.* **224** 155–62
[244] Dey N D, Bombard M C, Roland B P *et al* 2010 Genetically engineered mesenchymal stem cells reduce behavioral deficits in the YAC 128 mouse model of Huntington's disease *Behav. Brain Res.* **214** 193–200
[245] Snyder B R, Chiu A M, Prockop D J and Chan A W 2010 Human multipotent stromal cells (MSCs) increase neurogenesis and decrease atrophy of the striatum in a transgenic mouse model for Huntington's disease *PLoS One* **5** e9347
[246] Lin Y T, Chern Y, Shen C K *et al* 2011 Human mesenchymal stem cells prolong survival and ameliorate motor deficit through trophic support in Huntington's disease mouse models *PLoS One* **6** e22924
[247] Snyder B R, Cheng P H, Yang J *et al* 2011 Characterization of dental pulp stem/stromal cells of Huntington monkey tooth germs *BMC Cell Biol.* **12** 39
[248] An M C, Zhang N, Scott G *et al* 2012 Genetic correction of Huntington's disease phenotypes in induced pluripotent stem cells *Cell Stem Cell* **11** 253–63
[249] Sivandzade F, Prasad S, Bhalerao A and Cucullo L 2019 NRF2 and NF-κB interplay in cerebrovascular and neurodegenerative disorders: molecular mechanisms and possible therapeutic approaches *Redox Biol.* **21** 101059
[250] Lin C Y, Wu C L, Lee K Z, C *et al* 2019 Extracellular Pgk1 enhances neurite outgrowth of motoneurons through Nogo66/NgR-independent targeting of NogoA *Elife* **8** e49175
[251] Raore B, Federici T, Taub J *et al* 2011 Cervical multilevel intraspinal stem cell therapy: assessment of surgical risks in Gottingen minipigs *Spine (Phila Pa 1976)* **36** E164–71
[252] Chiò A, Mora G, L, Bella V *et al* STEMALS Study Group 2011 Repeated courses of granulocyte colony-stimulating factor in amyotrophic lateral sclerosis: clinical and biological results from a prospective multicenter study *Muscle Nerve* **43** 189–95
[253] Mazzini L, Mareschi K, Ferrero I, Miglioretti M *et al* 2012 Mesenchymal stromal cell transplantation in amyotrophic lateral sclerosis: a long-term safety study *Cytotherapy* **14** 56–60
[254] Minguell J J, Allers C and Lasala G P 2013 Mesenchymal stem cells and the treatment of conditions and diseases: the less glittering side of a conspicuous stem cell for basic research *Stem Cells Dev.* **22** 193–203
[255] Mazzini L, Gelati M, Profico D C *et al* 2015 Human neural stem cell transplantation in ALS: initial results from a phase I trial *J. Transl. Med.* **13** 17
[256] Petrou P, Gothelf Y, Argov Z *et al* 2016 Safety and clinical effects of mesenchymal stem cells secreting neurotrophic factor transplantation in patients with amyotrophic lateral sclerosis: results of phase 1/2 and 2a clinical trials *JAMA Neurol.* **73** 337–44
[257] Guo W, Fumagalli L, Prior R *et al* 2017 Current advances and limitations in modeling ALS/FTD in a dish using induced pluripotent stem cells *Front. Neurosci.* **11** 671
[258] Greaves C V and Rohrer J D 2019 An update on genetic frontotemporal dementia *J. Neurol.* **266** 2075–86
[259] Lines G, Casey J M, Preza E *et al* 2020 Modelling frontotemporal dementia using patient-derived induced pluripotent stem cells *Mol. Cell Neurosci.* **109** 103553

[260] Capozzo R, Sassi C, Hammer M B *et al* 2017 Clinical and genetic analyses of familial and sporadic frontotemporal dementia patients in Southern Italy *Alzheimers Dement.* **13** 858–69
[261] Ferrari R, Manzoni C and Hardy J 2019 Genetics and molecular mechanisms of frontotemporal lobar degeneration: an update and future avenues *Neurobiol. Aging* **78** 98–110
[262] Kim E J, Kim Y E, Jang J H *et al* 2018 Analysis of frontotemporal dementia, amyotrophic lateral sclerosis, and other dementia-related genes in 107 Korean patients with frontotemporal dementia *Neurobiol. Aging* **72** 186.e1–7
[263] Karch C M, Kao A W, Karydas A *et al* 2019 A comprehensive resource for induced pluripotent stem cells from patients with primary tauopathies *Stem Cell Rep.* **13** 939–55
[264] Lee H K, Morin P, Wells J *et al* 2015 Induced pluripotent stem cells (iPSCs) derived from frontotemporal dementia patient's peripheral blood mononuclear cells *Stem Cell Res.* **15** 325–7
[265] van den Berg M E, Castellote J M, Mahillo-Fernandez I and de Pedro-Cuesta J 2010 Incidence of spinal cord injury worldwide: a systematic review *Neuroepidemiology* **34** 184–92 discussion 192
[266] Silva N A, Sousa N, Reis R L and Salgado A J 2014 From basics to clinical: a comprehensive review on spinal cord injury *Prog. Neurobiol.* **114** 25–57
[267] Stenudd M, Sabelström H and Frisén J 2015 Role of endogenous neural stem cells in spinal cord injury and repair *JAMA Neurol.* **72** 235–7
[268] Fehlings M G, Tetreault L A, Wilson J R *et al* 2017 A clinical practice guideline for the management of acute spinal cord injury: introduction, rationale, and scope *Global Spine J.* **7** 84S–94S
[269] De Feo D, Merlini A, Laterza C and Martino G 2012 Neural stem cell transplantation in central nervous system disorders: from cell replacement to neuroprotection *Curr. Opin. Neurol.* **25** 322–33
[270] Oliveri R S, Bello S and Biering-Sørensen F 2014 Mesenchymal stem cells improve locomotor recovery in traumatic spinal cord injury: systematic review with meta-analyses of rat models *Neurobiol. Dis.* **62** 338–53
[271] Cusimano M, Biziato D, Brambilla E *et al* 2012 Transplanted neural stem/precursor cells instruct phagocytes and reduce secondary tissue damage in the injured spinal cord *Brain* **135** 447–60
[272] Shroff G and Gupta R 2015 Human embryonic stem cells in the treatment of patients with spinal cord injury *Ann. Neurosci.* **22** 208–16
[273] Manley N C, Priest C A, Denham J, Wirth E D and Lebkowski J S 2017 Human embryonic stem cell-derived oligodendrocyte progenitor cells: preclinical efficacy and safety in cervical spinal cord injury *Stem Cells Transl. Med.* **6** 1917–29
[274] Hwang I, Hahm S C, Choi K A *et al* 2016 Intrathecal transplantation of embryonic stem cell-derived spinal GABAergic neural precursor cells attenuates neuropathic pain in a spinal cord injury rat model *Cell Transplant.* **25** 593–607
[275] Wang Y, Kong Q J, Sun J C *et al* 2018 Protective effect of epigenetic silencing of CyclinD1 against spinal cord injury using bone marrow-derived mesenchymal stem cells in rats *J. Cell. Physiol.* **233** 5361–9
[276] Gu C, Li H, Wang C *et al* 2017 Bone marrow mesenchymal stem cells decrease CHOP expression and neuronal apoptosis after spinal cord injury *Neurosci. Lett.* **636** 282–9

[277] Zhou Y J, Liu J M, Wei S M *et al* 2015 Propofol promotes spinal cord injury repair by bone marrow mesenchymal stem cell transplantation *Neural Regen. Res.* **10** 1305–11
[278] Han D, Wu C, Xiong Q *et al* 2015 Anti-inflammatory mechanism of bone marrow mesenchymal stem cell transplantation in rat model of spinal cord injury *Cell Biochem. Biophys.* **71** 1341–7
[279] Yousefifard M, Nasirinezhad F, Shardi Manaheji H *et al* 2016 Human bone marrow-derived and umbilical cord-derived mesenchymal stem cells for alleviating neuropathic pain in a spinal cord injury model *Stem Cell Res. Ther.* **7** 36
[280] Zhilai Z, Biling M, Sujun Q *et al* 2016 Preconditioning in lowered oxygen enhances the therapeutic potential of human umbilical mesenchymal stem cells in a rat model of spinal cord injury *Brain Res.* **1642** 426–35
[281] Zhao Y, Tang F, Xiao Z *et al* 2017 Clinical study of neuroregen scaffold combined with human mesenchymal stem cells for the repair of chronic complete spinal cord injury *Cell Transplant.* **26** 891–900
[282] Liu Y, Tan B, Wang L *et al* 2015 Endogenous neural stem cells in central canal of adult rats acquired limited ability to differentiate into neurons following mild spinal cord injury *Int. J. Clin. Exp. Pathol.* **8** 3835–42
[283] Cheng Z, Zhu W, Cao K *et al* 2016 Anti-inflammatory mechanism of neural stem cell transplantation in spinal cord injury *Int. J. Mol. Sci.* **17** 1380
[284] You Y, Che L, Lee H Y *et al* 2015 Antiapoptotic effect of highly secreted GMCSF from neuronal cell-specific GMCSF overexpressing neural stem cells in spinal cord injury model *Spine (Phila Pa 1976)* **40** E1284–91
[285] Lu P, Woodruff G, Wang Y *et al* 2014 Long-distance axonal growth from human induced pluripotent stem cells after spinal cord injury *Neuron* **83** 789–96
[286] Choo A M, Liu J, Dvorak M, Tetzlaff W and Oxland T R 2008 Secondary pathology following contusion, dislocation, and distraction spinal cord injuries *Exp. Neurol.* **212** 490–506
[287] Martens W, Sanen K, Georgiou M *et al* 2014 Human dental pulp stem cells can differentiate into Schwann cells and promote and guide neurite outgrowth in an aligned tissue-engineered collagen construct *in vitro FASEB J.* **28** 1634–43
[288] Zhang L, Zhuang X, Chen Y and Xia H 2019 Intravenous transplantation of olfactory bulb ensheathing cells for a spinal cord hemisection injury rat model *Cell Transplant.* **28** 1585–602
[289] Wright A A, Todorovic M, Tello-Velasquez J *et al* 2018 Enhancing the therapeutic potential of olfactory ensheathing cells in spinal cord repair using neurotrophins *Cell Transplant.* **27** 867–78
[290] Czyz M, Tabakow P, Hernandez-Sanchez I *et al* 2015 Obtaining the olfactory bulb as a source of olfactory ensheathing cells with the use of minimally invasive neuroendoscopy-assisted supraorbital keyhole approach—cadaveric feasibility study *Br. J. Neurosurg.* **29** 362–70
[291] Lee J Y, Kim E, Choi S M *et al* 2016 Microvesicles from brain-extract-treated mesenchymal stem cells improve neurological functions in a rat model of ischemic stroke *Sci. Rep.* **96** 33038
[292] Chen Q H, Liu A R, Qiu H B *et al* 2015 Interaction between mesenchymal stem cells and endothelial cells restores endothelial permeability via paracrine hepatocyte growth factor *in vitro Stem Cell Res. Ther.* 24 **6** 44

[293] Shichinohe H, Ishihara T, Takahashi K *et al* 2015 Bone marrow stromal cells rescue ischemic brain by trophic effects and phenotypic change toward neural cells *Neurorehabil. Neural Repair* **29** 80–9

[294] Li G, Yu F, Lei T *et al* 2016 Bone marrow mesenchymal stem cell therapy in ischemic stroke: mechanisms of action and treatment optimization strategies *Neural Regen. Res.* **11** 1015–24

[295] Kong D, Zhu J, Liu Q *et al* 2017 Mesenchymal stem cells protect neurons against hypoxic-ischemic injury via inhibiting parthanatos, necroptosis, and apoptosis, but not autophagy *Cell Mol. Neurobiol.* **37** 303–13

[296] Gao L, Li P, Zhang J *et al* 2014 Novel role of kallistatin in vascular repair by promoting mobility, viability, and function of endothelial progenitor cells *J. Am. Heart Assoc.* **3** e001194

[297] Garbuzova-Davis S, Haller E, Williams S N *et al* 2014 Compromised blood–brain barrier competence in remote brain areas in ischemic stroke rats at the chronic stage *J. Comp. Neurol.* **522** 3120–37

[298] Eckert M A, Vu Q, Xie K *et al* 2013 Evidence for high translational potential of mesenchymal stromal cell therapy to improve recovery from ischemic stroke *J. Cereb. Blood Flow Metab.* **33** 1322–34

[299] Leong W K, Henshall T L, Arthur A *et al* 2012 Human adult dental pulp stem cells enhance poststroke functional recovery through non-neural replacement mechanisms *Stem Cells Transl. Med.* **1** 177–87

[300] Lederer D J and Martinez F J 2018 Idiopathic pulmonary fibrosis *N. Engl. J. Med.* **378** 1811–23

[301] Parekh K R, Nawroth J, Pai A *et al* 2020 Stem cells and lung regeneration *Am. J. Physiol. Cell Physiol.* **319** C675–93

[302] Martinez F J, Collard H R, Pardo A *et al* 2017 Idiopathic pulmonary fibrosis *Nat. Rev. Dis. Primers* **3** 17074

[303] Zuo W, Zhang T, Wu D Z *et al* 2015 p63(+)Krt5(+) distal airway stem cells are essential for lung regeneration *Nature* **517** 616–20

[304] Cao J, Li X, Lu X *et al* 2014 Cells derived from iPSC can be immunogenic—yes or no? *Protein Cell* **5** 1 3

[305] Yan Q, Quan Y, Sun H *et al* 2014 A site-specific genetic modification for induction of pluripotency and subsequent isolation of derived lung alveolar epithelial type II cells *Stem Cells* **32** 402–13

[306] Wang D, Morales J E, Calame D G *et al* 2010 Transplantation of human embryonic stem cell-derived alveolar epithelial type II cells abrogates acute lung injury in mice *Mol. Ther.* **18** 625–34

[307] Phua J, Badia J R, Adhikari N K *et al* 2009 Has mortality from acute respiratory distress syndrome decreased over time?: A systematic review *Am. J. Respir Crit. Care Med.* **179** 220–7

[308] Devaney J, Horie S, Masterson C *et al* 2015 Human mesenchymal stromal cells decrease the severity of acute lung injury induced by *E. coli* in the rat *Thorax* **70** 625–35

[309] Gupta N, Su X, Popov B *et al* 2007 Intrapulmonary delivery of bone marrow-derived mesenchymal stem cells improves survival and attenuates endotoxin-induced acute lung injury in mice *J. Immunol.* **179** 1855–63

[310] Yang Y, Hu S, Xu X *et al* 2016 The vascular endothelial growth factors-expressing character of mesenchymal stem cells plays a positive role in treatment of acute lung injury *in vivo Mediators Inflamm.* **2016** 2347938

[311] Hu S, Li J, Xu X *et al* 2016 The hepatocyte growth factor-expressing character is required for mesenchymal stem cells to protect the lung injured by lipopolysaccharide *in vivo Stem Cell Res. Ther.* **7** 66

[312] Curley G F, Jerkic M, Dixon S *et al* 2017 Cryopreserved, xeno-free human umbilical cord mesenchymal stromal cells reduce lung injury severity and bacterial burden in rodent *Escherichia coli*-induced acute respiratory distress syndrome *Crit. Care Med.* **45** e202–12

[313] Antebi B, Walker K P, Mohammadipoor A *et al* 2018 The effect of acute respiratory distress syndrome on bone marrow-derived mesenchymal stem cells *Stem Cell Res. Ther.* **9** 251

[314] Wilson J G, Liu K D, Zhuo H *et al* 2015 Mesenchymal stem (stromal) cells for treatment of ARDS: a phase 1 clinical trial *Lancet Respir. Med.* **3** 24–32

[315] Zheng G, Huang L, Tong H *et al* 2014 Treatment of acute respiratory distress syndrome with allogeneic adipose-derived mesenchymal stem cells: a randomized, placebo-controlled pilot study *Respir. Res.* **15** 39

[316] Park J, Kim S, Lim H *et al* 2019 Therapeutic effects of human mesenchymal stem cell microvesicles in an *ex vivo* perfused human lung injured with severe *E. coli* pneumonia *Thorax* **74** 43–50

[317] Monsel A, Zhu Y G, Gennai S *et al* 2015 Therapeutic effects of human mesenchymal stem cell-derived microvesicles in severe pneumonia in mice *Am. J. Respir. Crit. Care Med.* **192** 324–36

[318] Gupta N, Krasnodembskaya A, Kapetanaki M *et al* 2012 Mesenchymal stem cells enhance survival and bacterial clearance in murine *Escherichia coli* pneumonia *Thorax* **67** 533–9

[319] Gupta N, Sinha R, Krasnodembskaya A *et al* 2018 The TLR4-PAR1 axis regulates bone marrow mesenchymal stromal cell survival and therapeutic capacity in experimental bacterial pneumonia *Stem Cells* **36** 796–806

[320] Masoli M, Fabian D, Holt S and Beasley RGlobal Initiative for Asthma (GINA) Program 2004 The global burden of asthma: executive summary of the GINA Dissemination Committee report *Allergy* **59** 469–78

[321] Cruz F F, Borg Z D, Goodwin M *et al* 2015 Systemic administration of human bone marrow-derived mesenchymal stromal cell extracellular vesicles ameliorates aspergillus hyphal extract-induced allergic airway inflammation in immunocompetent mice *Stem Cells Transl. Med.* **4** 1302–16

[322] Zhang L B and He M 2019 Effect of mesenchymal stromal (stem) cell (MSC) transplantation in asthmatic animal models: a systematic review and meta-analysis *Pulm. Pharmacol. Ther.* **54** 39–52

[323] Du Y M, Zhuansun Y X, Chen R *et al* 2018 Mesenchymal stem cell exosomes promote immunosuppression of regulatory T cells in asthma *Exp. Cell. Res.* **363** 114–20

[324] Li J G, Zhuan-sun Y X, Wen B *et al* 2013 Human mesenchymal stem cells elevate CD4 +CD25+CD127low/- regulatory T cells of asthmatic patients via heme oxygenase-1 *Iran. J. Allergy Asthma Immunol.* **12** 228–35

[325] Nemeth K, Keane-Myers A, Brown J M *et al* 2010 Bone marrow stromal cells use TGF-beta to suppress allergic responses in a mouse model of ragweed-induced asthma *Proc. Natl Acad. Sci. USA* **107** 5652–7

[326] Braza F, Dirou S, Forest V *et al* 2016 Mesenchymal stem cells induce suppressive macrophages through phagocytosis in a mouse model of asthma *Stem Cells* **34** 1836–45

[327] Li Y, Li H, Cao Y *et al* 2017 Placenta-derived mesenchymal stem cells improve airway hyperresponsiveness and inflammation in asthmatic rats by modulating the Th17/Treg balance *Mol. Med. Rep.* **16** 8137–45

[328] Gazdic M, Volarevic V, Arsenijevic N and Stojkovic M 2015 Mesenchymal stem cells: a friend or foe in immune-mediated diseases *Stem Cell Rev. Rep.* **11** 280–7

[329] Abreu S C, Antunes M A, Xisto D G *et al* 2017 Bone marrow, adipose, and lung tissue-derived murine mesenchymal stromal cells release different mediators and differentially affect airway and lung parenchyma in experimental asthma *Stem Cells Transl. Med.* **6** 1557–67

[330] Janczewski A M, Wojtkiewicz J, Malinowska E and Doboszyńska A 2017 Can youthful mesenchymal stem cells from wharton's jelly bring a breath of fresh air for COPD? *Int. J. Mol. Sci.* **18** 2449

[331] Antunes M A, Lapa E Silva J R and Rocco P R 2017 Mesenchymal stromal cell therapy in COPD: from bench to bedside *Int. J. Chron. Obstruct. Pulmon. Dis.* **12** 3017–27

[332] Berg K and Wright J L 2016 The pathology of chronic obstructive pulmonary disease: progress in the 20th and 21st centuries *Arch. Pathol. Lab. Med.* **140** 1423–8

[333] Liu X, Fang Q and Kim H 2016 Preclinical studies of mesenchymal stem cell (MSC) administration in chronic obstructive pulmonary disease (COPD): a systematic review and meta-analysis *PLoS One* **11** e0157099

[334] Antunes M A, Abreu S C, Cruz F F *et al* 2014 Effects of different mesenchymal stromal cell sources and delivery routes in experimental emphysema *Respir. Res.* **15** 118

[335] Gu W, Song L, Li X M *et al* 2015 Mesenchymal stem cells alleviate airway inflammation and emphysema in COPD through down-regulation of cyclooxygenase-2 via p38 and ERK MAPK pathways *Sci. Rep.* **5** 8733

[336] Katsha A M, Ohkouchi S, Xin H *et al* 2011 Paracrine factors of multipotent stromal cells ameliorate lung injury in an elastase-induced emphysema model *Mol. Ther.* **19** 196–203

[337] Kennelly H, Mahon B P and English K 2016 Human mesenchymal stromal cells exert HGF dependent cytoprotective effects in a human relevant pre-clinical model of COPD *Sci. Rep.* 6 38207

[338] Liu A R, Liu L, Chen S *et al* 2013 Activation of canonical Wnt pathway promotes differentiation of mouse bone marrow-derived MSCs into type II alveolar epithelial cells, confers resistance to oxidative stress, and promotes their migration to injured lung tissue *in vitro J. Cell. Physiol.* **228** 1270–83

[339] Zhen G, Liu H, Gu N *et al* 2008 Mesenchymal stem cells transplantation protects against rat pulmonary emphysema *Front. Biosci.* 3415–22

[340] Miravitlles M, Cosío B G, Arnedillo A *et al* 2017 A proposal for the withdrawal of inhaled corticosteroids in the clinical practice of chronic obstructive pulmonary disease *Respir. Res.* **18** 198

[341] Tzouvelekis A, Toonkel R, Karampitsakos T *et al* 2018 Mesenchymal stem cells for the treatment of idiopathic pulmonary fibrosis *Front. Med. (Lausanne)* **5** 142

[342] Lee S H, Jang A S, Kim Y E *et al* 2010 Modulation of cytokine and nitric oxide by mesenchymal stem cell transfer in lung injury/fibrosis *Respir. Res.* **11** 16

[343] Ortiz L A, Dutreil M, Fattman C *et al* 2007 Interleukin 1 receptor antagonist mediates the antiinflammatory and antifibrotic effect of mesenchymal stem cells during lung injury *Proc. Natl Acad. Sci. USA* **104** 11002–7

[344] Chambers D C, Enever D, Ilic N *et al* 2014 A phase 1b study of placenta-derived mesenchymal stromal cells in patients with idiopathic pulmonary fibrosis *Respirology* **19** 1013–8

[345] https://clinicaltrials.gov/study/NCT01385644

[346] Tzouvelekis A, Paspaliaris V, Koliakos G *et al* 2013 A prospective, non-randomized, no placebo-controlled, phase Ib clinical trial to study the safety of the adipose derived stromal cells-stromal vascular fraction in idiopathic pulmonary fibrosis *J. Transl. Med.* **11** 171

[347] Ntolios P, Manoloudi E, Tzouvelekis A *et al* 2018 Longitudinal outcomes of patients enrolled in a phase Ib clinical trial of the adipose-derived stromal cells-stromal vascular fraction in idiopathic pulmonary fibrosis *Clin. Respir. J.* **12** 2084–9

[348] Sözen T, Özışık L and Başaran N Ç 2017 An overview and management of osteoporosis *Eur. J. Rheumatol.* **4** 46–56

[349] Compston J E, McClung M R and Leslie W D 2019 Osteoporosis *Lancet* **393** 364–76

[350] Cummings S R and Melton L J 2002 Epidemiology and outcomes of osteoporotic fractures *Lancet* **359** 1761–7

[351] Bawa S 2010 The significance of soy protein and soy bioactive compounds in the prophylaxis and treatment of osteoporosis *J. Osteoporos.* **2010** 891058

[352] Cramer J A, Gold D T, Silverman S L and Lewiecki E M 2007 A systematic review of persistence and compliance with bisphosphonates for osteoporosis *Osteoporos. Int.* **18** 1023–31

[353] Goodarzi P, Aghayan H R, Soleimani M *et al* 2014 Stem cell therapy for treatment of epilepsy *Acta Med. Iran* **52** 651–5

[354] Li F, Zhou C, Xu L *et al* 2016 Effect of stem cell therapy on bone mineral density: a meta-analysis of preclinical studies in animal models of osteoporosis *PLoS One* **11** e0149400

[355] Chan C K F, Gulati G S, Sinha R *et al* 2018 Identification of the human skeletal stem cell *Cell* **175** 43–56.e21

[356] Wang Q, Zhao B, Li C *et al* 2014 Decreased proliferation ability and differentiation potential of mesenchymal stem cells of osteoporosis rat *Asian Pac. J. Trop. Med.* **7** 358–63

[357] Katsara O, Mahaira L G, Iliopoulou E G *et al* 2011 Effects of donor age, gender, and *in vitro* cellular aging on the phenotypic, functional, and molecular characteristics of mouse bone marrow-derived mesenchymal stem cells *Stem Cells Dev.* **20** 1549–61

[358] Kiernan J, Davies J E and Stanford W L 2017 Concise review: musculoskeletal stem cells to treat age-related osteoporosis *Stem Cells Transl. Med.* **6** 1930–9

[359] Yuan F L, Xu R S, Jiang D L *et al* 2015 Leonurine hydrochloride inhibits osteoclastogenesis and prevents osteoporosis associated with estrogen deficiency by inhibiting the NF-κB and PI3K/Akt signaling pathways *Bone* **75** 128–37

[360] Martin A, Xiong J, Koromila T *et al* 2015 Estrogens antagonize RUNX2-mediated osteoblast-driven osteoclastogenesis through regulating RANKL membrane association *Bone* **75** 96–104

[361] Kim R Y, Yang H J, Song Y M *et al* 2015 Estrogen modulates bone morphogenetic protein-induced sclerostin expression through the Wnt signaling pathway *Tissue Eng. Part A* **21** 2076–88

[362] Ye X, Zhang P, Xue S *et al* 2014 Adipose-derived stem cells alleviate osteoporosis by enhancing osteogenesis and inhibiting adipogenesis in a rabbit model *Cytotherapy* **16** 1643–55
[363] Aggarwal R, Lu J, Kanji S *et al* 2012 Human umbilical cord blood-derived CD34+ cells reverse osteoporosis in NOD/SCID mice by altering osteoblastic and osteoclastic activities *PLoS One* **7** e39365
[364] Gucciardo L, Lories R, Ochsenbein-Kölble N *et al* 2009 Fetal mesenchymal stem cells: isolation, properties and potential use in perinatology and regenerative medicine *BJOG* **116** 166–72
[365] Heo J S, Choi Y, Kim H S and Kim H O 2016 Comparison of molecular profiles of human mesenchymal stem cells derived from bone marrow, umbilical cord blood, placenta and adipose tissue *Int. J. Mol. Med.* **37** 115–25
[366] Horwitz E M, Gordon P L, Koo W K *et al* 2002 Isolated allogeneic bone marrow-derived mesenchymal cells engraft and stimulate growth in children with osteogenesis imperfecta: implications for cell therapy of bone *Proc. Natl Acad. Sci. USA* **99** 8932–7
[367] Götherström C, Westgren M, Shaw S W *et al* 2014 Pre- and postnatal transplantation of fetal mesenchymal stem cells in osteogenesis imperfecta: a two-center experience *Stem Cells Transl. Med.* **3** 255–64
[368] Taketani T, Oyama C, Mihara A *et al* 2015 *Ex vivo* expanded allogeneic mesenchymal stem cells with bone marrow transplantation improved osteogenesis in infants with severe hypophosphatasia *Cell Transplant.* **24** 1931–43
[369] Siatskas C, Chan J, Field J *et al* 2006 Gene therapy strategies towards immune tolerance to treat the autoimmune diseases *Curr. Gene Ther.* **6** 45–58
[370] Quansah D Y, Gross J, Gilbert L *et al* 2022 Cardiometabolic and mental health in women with early gestational diabetes mellitus: a prospective cohort study *J. Clin. Endocrinol. Metab.* **107** e996–e1008
[371] Wang J, Lv B, Chen X *et al* 2021 An early model to predict the risk of gestational diabetes mellitus in the absence of blood examination indexes: application in primary health care centres *BMC Pregnancy Childbirth* **21** 814
[372] Chiang J L, Kirkman M S, Laffel L M and Peters A L 2014 Type 1 Diabetes Sourcebook Authors. Type 1 diabetes through the life span: a position statement of the American Diabetes Association *Diabetes Care* **37** 2034–54
[373] Ryan A J, O'Neill H S, Duffy G P and O'Brien F J 2017 Advances in polymeric islet cell encapsulation technologies to limit the foreign body response and provide immunoisolation *Curr. Opin. Pharmacol.* **36** 66–71
[374] Domouky A M, Hegab A S, Al-Shahat A and Raafat N 2017 Mesenchymal stem cells and differentiated insulin producing cells are new horizons for pancreatic regeneration in type I diabetes mellitus *Int. J. Biochem. Cell Biol.* **87** 77–85
[375] Shigemoto-Kuroda T, Oh J Y, Kim D K *et al* 2017 MSC-derived extracellular vesicles attenuate immune responses in two autoimmune murine models: type 1 diabetes and uveoretinitis *Stem Cell Rep.* **8** 1214–25
[376] Bassi Ê J, Moraes-Vieira P M, Moreira-Sá C S *et al* 2012 Immune regulatory properties of allogeneic adipose-derived mesenchymal stem cells in the treatment of experimental autoimmune diabetes *Diabetes* **61** 2534–45
[377] Gerace D, Martiniello-Wilks R, Habib R *et al* 2019 *Ex vivo* expansion of murine MSC impairs transcription factor-induced differentiation into pancreatic β-cells *Stem Cells Int.* **2019** 1395301

[378] van Megen K M, van 't Wout E T, Lages Motta J *et al* 2019 Activated mesenchymal stromal cells process and present antigens regulating adaptive immunity *Front. Immunol.* **10** 694
[379] Montanucci P, Alunno A, Basta G *et al* 2016 Restoration of t cell substes of patients with type 1 diabetes mellitus by microencapsulated human umbilical cord Wharton jelly-derived mesenchymal stem cells: an *in vitro* study *Clin. Immunol.* **163** 34–41
[380] Lu J, Shen S M, Ling Q *et al* 2021 One repeated transplantation of allogeneic umbilical cord mesenchymal stromal cells in type 1 diabetes: an open parallel controlled clinical study *Stem Cell Res. Ther.* **12** 340
[381] Ben Nasr M, D'Addio F, Malvandi A M *et al* 2018 Prostaglandin E2 stimulates the expansion of regulatory hematopoietic stem and progenitor cells in type 1 diabetes *Front Immunol.* **9** 1387
[382] Gu B, Miao H, Zhang J *et al* 2018 Clinical benefits of autologous haematopoietic stem cell transplantation in type 1 diabetes patients *Diabetes Metab.* **44** 341–5
[383] Rezania A, Bruin J E, Arora P *et al* 2014 Reversal of diabetes with insulin-producing cells derived *in vitro* from human pluripotent stem cells *Nat. Biotechnol.* **32** 1121–33
[384] Maehr R, Chen S, Snitow M *et al* 2009 Generation of pluripotent stem cells from patients with type 1 diabetes *Proc. Natl Acad. Sci. USA* **106** 15768–73
[385] Korytnikov R and Nostro M C 2016 Generation of polyhormonal and multipotent pancreatic progenitor lineages from human pluripotent stem cells *Methods* **101** 56–64
[386] Saran R, Li Y, Robinson B *et al* 2016 US renal data system 2015 annual data report: epidemiology of kidney disease in the United States *Am. J. Kidney Dis.* **67** Svii S1–305
[387] Schoonover K L, Hickson L J, Norby S M *et al* 2013 Risk factors for hospitalization among older, incident haemodialysis patients *Nephrology (Carlton)* **18** 712–7
[388] Papazova D A, Oosterhuis N R, Gremmels H *et al* 2015 Cell-based therapies for experimental chronic kidney disease: a systematic review and meta-analysis *Dis. Model. Mech.* **8** 281–93
[389] Eirin A, Riester S M, Zhu X Y *et al* 2014 MicroRNA and mRNA cargo of extracellular vesicles from porcine adipose tissue-derived mesenchymal stem cells *Gene* **551** 55–64
[390] Collino F, Bruno S, Incarnato D *et al* 2015 AKI recovery induced by mesenchymal stromal cell-derived extracellular vesicles carrying microRNAs *J. Am. Soc. Nephrol.* **26** 2349–60
[391] Eirin A and Lerman L O 2014 Mesenchymal stem cell treatment for chronic renal failure *Stem Cell Res. Ther.* **5** 83
[392] Choi S, Park M, Kim J *et al* 2009 The role of mesenchymal stem cells in the functional improvement of chronic renal failure *Stem Cells Dev.* **18** 521–9
[393] Ebrahimi B, Eirin A, Li Z *et al* 2013 Mesenchymal stem cells improve medullary inflammation and fibrosis after revascularization of swine atherosclerotic renal artery stenosis *PLoS One* **8** e67474
[394] Peichev M, Naiyer A J, Pereira D *et al* 2000 Expression of VEGFR-2 and AC133 by circulating human CD34(+) cells identifies a population of functional endothelial precursors *Blood* **95** 952–8
[395] Squillaro T, Peluso G and Galderisi U 2016 Clinical trials with mesenchymal stem cells: an update *Cell Transplant.* **25** 829–48
[396] Pileggi A, Xu X, Tan J and Ricordi C 2013 Mesenchymal stromal (stem) cells to improve solid organ transplant outcome: lessons from the initial clinical trials *Curr. Opin. Organ. Transplant.* **18** 672–81

[397] Perico N, Casiraghi F, Introna M *et al* 2011 Autologous mesenchymal stromal cells and kidney transplantation: a pilot study of safety and clinical feasibility *Clin. J. Am. Soc. Nephrol.* **6** 412–22
[398] Vanikar A V, Trivedi H L, Feroze A *et al* 2011 Effect of co-transplantation of mesenchymal stem cells and hematopoietic stem cells as compared to hematopoietic stem cell transplantation alone in renal transplantation to achieve donor hypo-responsiveness *Int. Urol. Nephrol.* **43** 225–32
[399] Shen Y 2020 Stem cell therapies for retinal diseases: from bench to bedside *J. Mol. Med. (Berl)* **98** 1347–68
[400] Mazzilli J L, Snook J D, Simmons K *et al* 2020 A preclinical safety study of human embryonic stem cell-derived retinal pigment epithelial cells for macular degeneration *J. Ocul. Pharmacol. Ther.* **36** 65–9
[401] Song W K, Park K M, Kim H J *et al* 2015 Treatment of macular degeneration using embryonic stem cell-derived retinal pigment epithelium: preliminary results in Asian patients *Stem Cell Rep.* **4** 860–72
[402] Tu H Y, Watanabe T, Shirai H *et al* 2019 Medium- to long-term survival and functional examination of human iPSC-derived retinas in rat and primate models of retinal degeneration *EBioMedicine* **39** 562–74
[403] Zhu D, Xie M, Gademann F *et al* 2020 Protective effects of human iPS-derived retinal pigmented epithelial cells on retinal degenerative disease *Stem Cell Res. Ther.* **11** 98
[404] Salas A, Duarri A, Fontrodona L *et al* 2021 Cell therapy with hiPSC-derived RPE cells and RPCs prevents visual function loss in a rat model of retinal degeneration *Mol. Ther. Methods Clin. Dev.* **20** 688–702
[405] Alsaeedi H A, Koh A E, Lam C *et al* 2019 Dental pulp stem cells therapy overcome photoreceptor cell death and protects the retina in a rat model of sodium iodate-induced retinal degeneration *J. Photochem. Photobiol.,* B **198** 111561
[406] Manuguerra-Gagné R, Boulos P R, Ammar A *et al* 2013 Transplantation of mesenchymal stem cells promotes tissue regeneration in a glaucoma model through laser-induced paracrine factor secretion and progenitor cell recruitment *Stem Cells* **31** 1136–48
[407] Yu B, Shao H, Su C *et al* 2016 Exosomes derived from MSCs ameliorate retinal laser injury partially by inhibition of MCP-1 *Sci. Rep.* **6** 34562
[408] Yu C, Yang K, Meng X *et al* 2020 Downregulation of long noncoding RNA MIAT in the retina of diabetic rats with tail-vein injection of human umbilical-cord mesenchymal stem cells *Int. J. Med. Sci.* **17** 591–8
[409] Ezquer M, Urzua C A, Montecino S *et al* 2016 Intravitreal administration of multipotent mesenchymal stromal cells triggers a cytoprotective microenvironment in the retina of diabetic mice *Stem Cell Res. Ther.* **7** 42
[410] Sung Y, Lee S M, Park M *et al* 2020 Treatment of traumatic optic neuropathy using human placenta-derived mesenchymal stem cells in Asian patients *Regen. Med.* **15** 2163–79
[411] Tuekprakhon A, Sangkitporn S, Trinavarat A *et al* 2021 Intravitreal autologous mesenchymal stem cell transplantation: a non-randomized phase I clinical trial in patients with retinitis pigmentosa *Stem Cell Res. Ther.* **12** 52
[412] Kahraman N S and Oner A 2020 Umbilical cord derived mesenchymal stem cell implantation in retinitis pigmentosa: a 6-month follow-up results of a phase 3 trial *Int. J. Ophthalmol.* **13** 1423–9

[413] Zhao T, Liang Q, Meng X *et al* 2020 Intravenous infusion of umbilical cord mesenchymal stem cells maintains and partially improves visual function in patients with advanced retinitis pigmentosa *Stem Cells Dev.* **29** 1029–37
[414] Weissman J L 1996 Hearing loss *Radiology* **199** 593–611
[415] Chandrasekhar S S, Tsai Do B S, Schwartz S R *et al* 2019 Clinical practice guideline: sudden hearing loss (update) *Otolaryngol. Head Neck Surg.* **161** S1–S45
[416] Clarke D L, Johansson C B, Wilbertz J *et al* 2000 Generalized potential of adult neural stem cells *Science* **288** 1660–3
[417] Lang H, Schulte B A, Goddard J C *et al* 2008 Transplantation of mouse embryonic stem cells into the cochlea of an auditory-neuropathy animal model: effects of timing after injury *J. Assoc. Res. Otolaryngol.* **9** 225–40
[418] Perny M, Ting C C, Kleinlogel S *et al* 2017 Generation of otic sensory neurons from mouse embryonic stem cells in 3D culture *Front Cell Neurosci.* **11** 409
[419] Susanto E, Marin Navarro A, Zhou L *et al* 2020 Modeling SHH-driven medulloblastoma with patient iPS cell-derived neural stem cells *Proc. Natl. Acad. Sci. USA* **117** 20127–38
[420] Koehler K R, Mikosz A M, Molosh A I *et al* 2013 Generation of inner ear sensory epithelia from pluripotent stem cells in 3D culture *Nature* **500** 217–21
[421] Han Z, Wang C P, Cong N *et al* 2017 Therapeutic value of nerve growth factor in promoting neural stem cell survival and differentiation and protecting against neuronal hearing loss *Mol. Cell. Biochem.* **428** 149–59
[422] Levy J A 2009 HIV pathogenesis: 25 years of progress and persistent challenges *AIDS* **23** 147–60
[423] Fanales-Belasio E, Raimondo M, Suligoi B and Buttò S 2010 HIV virology and pathogenetic mechanisms of infection: a brief overview *Ann. Ist. Super. Sanita* **46** 5–14
[424] Hütter G 2016 Stem cell transplantation in strategies for curing HIV/AIDS *AIDS Res Ther.* **13** 31
[425] Fackler O T, Murooka T T, Imle A and Mempel T R 2014 Adding new dimensions: towards an integrative understanding of HIV-1 spread *Nat. Rev. Microbiol.* **12** 563–74
[426] Archin N M, Sung J M, Garrido C *et al* 2014 Eradicating HIV-1 infection: seeking to clear a persistent pathogen *Nat. Rev. Microbiol.* **12** 750–64
[427] Mitsuyasu R T, Zack J A, Macpherson J L and Symonds G P 2011 Phase I/II clinical trials using gene-modified adult hematopoietic stem cells for HIV: lessons learnt *Stem Cells Int.* **2011** 393698
[428] Kitchen S G and Zack J A 2011 Stem cell-based approaches to treating HIV infection *Curr. Opin. HIV AIDS* **6** 68–73
[429] DiGiusto D L, Krishnan A, Li L *et al* 2010 RNA-based gene therapy for HIV with lentiviral vector-modified CD34(+) cells in patients undergoing transplantation for AIDS-related lymphoma *Sci. Transl. Med.* **2** 36–43
[430] Luo X M, Maarschalk E, O'Connell R M *et al* 2009 Engineering human hematopoietic stem/progenitor cells to produce a broadly neutralizing anti-HIV antibody after *in vitro* maturation to human B lymphocytes *Blood* **113** 1422–31
[431] Saglio F, Hanley P J and Bollard C M 2014 The time is now: moving toward virus-specific T cells after allogeneic hematopoietic stem cell transplantation as the standard of care *Cytotherapy* **16** 149–59

[432] Gupta R K, Peppa D, Hill A L *et al* 2020 Evidence for HIV-1 cure after CCR5Δ32/Δ32 allogeneic haemopoietic stem-cell transplantation 30 months post analytical treatment interruption: a case report *Lancet HIV* 7 e340–7
[433] Henrich T J, Hanhauser E, Marty F M *et al* 2014 Antiretroviral-free HIV-1 remission and viral rebound after allogeneic stem cell transplantation: report of 2 cases *Ann. Intern. Med.* **161** 319–27
[434] Wang L, Zhang Z, Xu R *et al* 2021 Human umbilical cord mesenchymal stem cell transfusion in immune non-responders with AIDS: a multicenter randomized controlled trial *Signal Transduct. Target. Ther.* **6** 217
[435] Soares T R, Fidalgo T K, Quirino A S *et al* 2017 Is caries a risk factor for dental trauma? a systematic review and meta-analysis *Dent. Traumatol.* **33** 4–12
[436] Mjör I A 2001 Pulp-dentin biology in restorative dentistry. Part 5: clinical management and tissue changes associated with wear and trauma *Quintessence Int.* **32** 771–88
[437] Mertens C, Freudlsperger C, Bodem J *et al* 2016 Reconstruction of the maxilla following hemimaxillectomy defects with scapular tip grafts and dental implants *J. Craniomaxillofac. Surg.* **44** 1806–11
[438] Wijbenga J G, Schepers R H, Werker P M *et al* 2016 A systematic review of functional outcome and quality of life following reconstruction of maxillofacial defects using vascularized free fibula flaps and dental rehabilitation reveals poor data quality *J. Plast. Reconstr. Aesthet. Surg.* **69** 1024–36
[439] Wen Y, Wang F, Zhang W *et al* 2012 Application of induced pluripotent stem cells in generation of a tissue-engineered tooth-like structure *Tissue Eng. Part* A **18** 1677–85
[440] Ning F, Guo Y, Tang J *et al* 2010 Differentiation of mouse embryonic stem cells into dental epithelial-like cells induced by ameloblasts serum-free conditioned medium *Biochem. Biophys. Res. Commun.* **394** 342–7
[441] d'Aquino R, Graziano A, Sampaolesi M *et al* 2007 Human postnatal dental pulp cells co-differentiate into osteoblasts and endotheliocytes: a pivotal synergy leading to adult bone tissue formation *Cell Death Differ.* **14** 1162–71
[442] Meijer G J, de Bruijn J D, Koole R and van Blitterswijk C A 2007 Cell-based bone tissue engineering *PLoS Med.* **4** e9
[443] Yamaza T, Kentaro A, Chen C *et al* 2010 Immunomodulatory properties of stem cells from human exfoliated deciduous teeth *Stem Cell Res. Ther.* **1** 5
[444] Ikeda E and Tsuji T 2008 Growing bioengineered teeth from single cells: potential for dental regenerative medicine *Expert Opin. Biol. Ther.* **8** 735–44
[445] Oshima M and Tsuji T 2014 Functional tooth regenerative therapy: tooth tissue regeneration and whole-tooth replacement *Odontology* **102** 123–36
[446] Otsu K, Kumakami-Sakano M, Fujiwara N *et al* 2014 Stem cell sources for tooth regeneration: current status and future prospects *Front. Physiol.* **5** 36
[447] Caplan A I 2009 Why are MSCs therapeutic? New data: new insight *J. Pathol.* **217** 318–24
[448] Bonab M M, Alimoghaddam K, Talebian F *et al* 2006 Aging of mesenchymal stem cell *in vitro BMC Cell Biol.* **7** 14
[449] Golpanian S, Schulman I H, Ebert R F *et al* Cardiovascular Cell Therapy Research Network 2016 Concise review: review and perspective of cell dosage and routes of administration from preclinical and clinical studies of stem cell therapy for heart disease *Stem Cells Transl. Med.* **5** 186–91

[450] Hill W D, Hess D C, Martin-Studdard A *et al* 2004 SDF-1 (CXCL12) is upregulated in the ischemic penumbra following stroke: association with bone marrow cell homing to injury *J. Neuropathol. Exp. Neurol.* **63** 84–96
[451] Vierbuchen T, Ostermeier A, Pang Z P *et al* 2010 Direct conversion of fibroblasts to functional neurons by defined factors *Nature* **463** 1035–41
[452] Swijnenburg R J, Schrepfer S, Govaert J A *et al* 2008 Immunosuppressive therapy mitigates immunological rejection of human embryonic stem cell xenografts *Proc. Natl Acad. Sci. USA* **105** 12991–6
[453] Li S C and Zhong J F 2009 Twisting immune responses for allogeneic stem cell therapy *World J. Stem Cells* **1** 30–5
[454] Kooreman N G and Wu J C 2010 Tumorigenicity of pluripotent stem cells: biological insights from molecular imaging *J. R. Soc. Interface* **7 Suppl 6** S753–63

IOP Publishing

Introduction to Pharmaceutical Biotechnology, Volume 1
(Second Edition)
Basic techniques and concepts
Ahmed Al-Harrasi, Saif Hameed, Zeeshan Fatima and Saurabh Bhatia

Chapter 5

Transgenic animals in biotechnology

Muskan Kumari, Abdullah Faizaan, Sneh Shalini and Anil Kumar

5.1 Introduction

Humans rely heavily on animals such as cows, sheep, poultry, pigs, and fish for various purposes (milk, meat, eggs, wool, etc). Genetic improvement of traits in livestock and other farm animals has traditionally been achieved through selective breeding methods. One of the first reports on transgenic animals, published in December 1982, involved the introduction of the GH gene fused to the promoter of the mouse metallothionein 1 (MT) gene [1]. Since then, many transgenic animals have been created and will continue to be used for a variety of purposes. The genome of a transgenic animal contains one or more genes introduced by one or another transfection technique. Genes introduced by transfection are called transgenes. Transfection can also be defined as the insertion of a DNA segment (naked or incorporated into a vector) into an animal cell. Previously, this term was criticized for being similar to the phenomenon of metamorphosis in all other living organisms. Nevertheless, transformation has long been used in animals to express changes from normal cells, i.e. non-tumor cells, to tumor-like cells in culture. Therefore, it was important to use the word 'transfection' to avoid confusion. There are two types of transfection: transient or permanent (stable). When the inserted gene is progressively lost from the daughter cells of transfected cells, the phenomenon is known as transient transfection, whereas in stable transfection, the introduced gene(s) are held and expressed in almost all cells resulting from the transfected cells. We will look at how vectors are introduced to transgenic animals. This includes a wide range of precision gene manipulation approaches, including microinjections, mass gene transfers with gametes, as well as specialized techniques like somatic cell nuclear transfers. These techniques have allowed scientists to genetically modify animals, providing insight into the function of particular genes and paving the way for transgenic animal development for research purposes. However, many ethical issues

doi:10.1088/978-0-7503-5382-3ch5

arise when transgenesis is used, such as using surrogate mothers (mice) for embryonic stem microinjection. However, once these issues are resolved, transgenesis has the potential to revolutionize medicine and medical treatments, potentially leading to novel treatments for diseases.

As the majority of the animal vectors are unstable (i.e. are gradually lost) in their extrachromosomal state, stable transfections are ordinarily owing to the incorporation of the introduced gene into the cell genome.

Transgenic animals have become a powerful tool not only to improve genetic characteristics but also to study gene expression and growth processes in higher organisms. As per current research, transgenic animals offer excellent models for understanding human disease. In addition, various proteins produced by transgenic animals are essential for medical and pharmaceutical applications. Therefore, transgenic farm animals are a component of the profitable global biotechnology industry, with huge benefits to mankind. Transgenesis is significant for developing the quality and quantity of egg, meat, milk, and wool production, in addition to creating disease-resistant animals.

5.2 Major objectives of gene transfer

Different goals for which transgenic cells/animals are generated can be abridged into the following six categories:

- Gene transfer also aims at improving or even reducing the symptoms and resulting miseries of genetic diseases. In this case, normal and functional copies of the defective gene that produced the genetic disease are transferred into the patient. This process is known as gene therapy.
- Genes have been inserted into animals to achieve large-scale production of the proteins encoded by these genes in the milk, urine, or blood of such animals; such animals are often known as bioreactors, this kind of approach is called molecular farming or sometimes gene farming. The accurate expression of definite genes, for instance, p-globin and a-fetoprotein, is negatively affected by the existence of bacterial vector sequences. However, the expression of various other genes is not so sensitive to these sequences. Most researchers regularly remove prokaryotic sequences to circumvent probable adverse effects.
- Genes have been transfected and allowed to express into cultured cell lines to obtain the proteins encoded by them.
- Genetic alteration of animals can also be intended for improving the production of milk, meat, wool, etc.
- Most genetic insertion aims at investigation of promoter functions, reporter gene expression, regulation of gene expression, functions of transferred genes/ DNA sequences, etc.
- Ultimately, definite transgenic animal strains or lines are produced to accomplish specialized experimental and/or biomedical needs. An excellent case of such animals is 'knockout' mice strains in which precise genes have been replaced or knocked out by their disordered counterparts via the process

of HR. In general, the approach is as follows. The knocked out gene, e.g. the TK gene, is cloned first and is disrupted by the introduction of another DNA sequence (e.g. the neo gene of *E. coli*, within its coding region). This disrupted gene is utilized to transfect embryonic stem cells where it could replace the normal TK gene present in the genome of ES cells through HR. The ES cells including such recombination can be chosen by an appropriate experimental design.

5.3 Cloning vectors

Generally cloning vectors are plasmids that are mainly used to amplify or propagate DNA. For cloning purposes or to create multiple copies of foreign DNA fragments of a GOI or therapeutic gene, the large genome that contains the therapeutic gene should initially be treated with a restriction enzyme to convert it into small pieces of DNA. Since the whole genome cannot be inserted into the cloning vector as it contains certain undesirable sequences and is too large. Thus, by means of the restriction enzyme the large sequences of genetic material are converted into small pieces by splicing at particular restriction sites (which are present in the genetic material). After splicing these restriction enzymes produce sticky ends in the DNA fragments (the therapeutic genes). These small fragments of therapeutic gene can be inserted into a cloning vector such as virus, plasmid, or any cell of a higher organism, where they can be stably maintained in an organism. Again, for the successful introduction of therapeutic genes, prior treatment with a restriction enzyme is required to produce sticky ends at both sides in the cloning vector. It is well known that a cloning vector acts as a backbone for the DNA insert (therapeutic gene) to be reproduced and multiplied inside the bacteria; nevertheless, these cloning vectors are only beneficial for storing a genetic sequence. Independently they are not capable of performing the transcription and translation of the gene into a functional protein product. Some of the main characteristics required of cloning vectors are that it carries a selectable marker gene (antibiotic resistant and lacZ gene), an origin of replication which allows vector propagation and a multiple cloning site (MCS) or polylinker that contains several restriction sites to clone foreign DNA. These MCSs with restriction sites are used for introducing a DNA fragment.

All these important features are covered by expression vectors. Expression vectors are prepared to perform transcription of the cloned gene and ultimately translation into protein. Both cloning and expression vectors have some common features as they both contain an MCS and a selectable marker. But the cloning vectors are only used for propagating DNA, whereas expression vectors tend to have fewer copies within cells and they rarely have a screenable marker. As per the definition of expression vectors, they are prepared to perform transcription of the cloned gene and ultimately translation into a protein, whereas the primary purpose of a cloning vector is to multiply a desirable gene. In addition, expression vectors contain certain important additional features which allow them to express genes and make proteins, such as MCS, a fusion tag often present to help in purification steps, a promoter gene (that initiates transcription of a particular gene), a ribosome-binding site, an ATG start codon (the first codon of a messenger mRNA transcript translated by a ribosome), a translation initiation sequence, a transcription termination sequence and termination codons (or stop codons that terminates translation). The assembly of whole genome libraries is now possible with the development of cloning vectors. Therapeutic genes can be identified and isolated from these libraries by means of hybridization or other detection methods. Currently, different types of cloning vectors are available, such as genetically engineered plasmids and bacteriophages (such as phage λ). In addition, various cloning vectors are derived from animal viruses, such as SV40 vectors, bovine papillomavirus vectors, etc, for which a complete nucleotide sequence and a detailed understanding of transcription are available. An SV40 vector is considered as the first eukaryotic DNA virus, capable of infecting a number of mammalian species. The important characteristics of some of these vectors are listed in table 5.1.

Table 5.1. Various types of vectors used for gene transfers in animals.

Vector	Derived from	Features
SV40 vectors		
Early-region replacement vectors	Replacement of large-T gene of SV40	1. Produce virions, which infect host cells. 2. Transient gene expression. 3. Mammalian cells are hosts of SV40.
Late-region replacement vectors	Replacement of VP1, VP2 and VP3 genes of SV40, e.g. SVGT-5	
Plasmid vectors	Origin of replication and large-T gene of SV40	
Shuttle plasmid vectors	Plasmid vector lus pBR322 origin and amp× gene, e.g. pSV2, pSV3, etc	Strong expression of the marker gene.
	Rous sarcoma virus promoter in place of SV40 early promoter, e.g. pRSV SV40 transcription regulatory and polyadenylation sequences, plus pBR322 origin and amp × gene	Shuttle vectors; used for gene integration in mammalian cells.
Bovine papillomavirus (BPV) vectors	Bovine papillomavirus 'transforming region' + pBR322	Shuttle vector; often pBR322 sequence deleted prior to transfection; plasmid-like vector.

Retrovirus vectors	pBR322 + retrovirus sequences	Shuttle vector; integrates as provirus into mammalian genome; produces virions; used in gene therapy.
Polyomavirus vectors	Polyomavirus origin and early region + pBR322 sequences	Similar to SV40 vectors; mouse cells used as host.
Vaccinia virus	DNA insert placed within the TK gene of virus by a process of recombination	Promising as live vaccines; DNA insert is a pathogen gene encoding an antigen.
P element vectors	*Drosophila* transposable element P; minimum of 31 by inverted repeat borders and the neighboring regions, plus an *E. coli* vector, e.g. pUC8; DNA inserts of up to 40 kb placed within the two borders	Gene transfer in *Drosophila*; a helper P element is needed to provide the transposase necessary for transposition or insertion of the recombinant P vector into the *Drosophila* genome.
Baculovirus vectors(versatile vectors for protein expression in insect and mammalian cells)	Nuclear polyhedroma virus (NPV) polyhedrin gene replaced by DNA insert; e.g. *Autographa californica* NPV (AcNPV) and *Bombyx mori* NPV (BmNPV) vectors	Produce virions; expression vector for production of transgenic proteins in silkworm larvae (BmNPV vectors) and in *Spodoptera frugiperda* larvae or cultured cells (AcNPV vectors).

It perhaps indicated that a number of the mammalian vectors, for example simian vacuolating virus 40 (SV40 vectors) as either early or late region helper vectors generate virions. These virions (virus particles that contain a core and capsid, in which the core imparts infectivity, and the capsid offers specificity) which are further utilized to infect the host cells. Some other vectors, such as bacterial plasmids, have unique features, and thus are often used as cloning vectors in genetic engineering. *E. coli* is considered as the first cloning vector source, and the most common cloning vectors in *E. coli* include plasmids, cosmids (a hybrid plasmid that contains a lambda phage cos sequence), bacteriophages (viruses that infect and replicate within a bacterium such as phage λ) and bacterial artificial chromosomes (a DNA construct, based on a functional fertility plasmid). Some additional plasmids, such as polyomavirus-based shuttle vectors, SV40 vectors, and bovine papillomavirus vectors, can be utilized to transfect mammalian cells, using a suitable transfection technique, to propagate the desirable gene.

5.3.1 Fish vectors in molecular genetics and biotechnology

A typical fish vector, e.g. pRSV (figure 5.1), is a plasmid, usually including a selectable marker, (e.g. ampicillin resistance), the origin of replication (ori) from *E.*

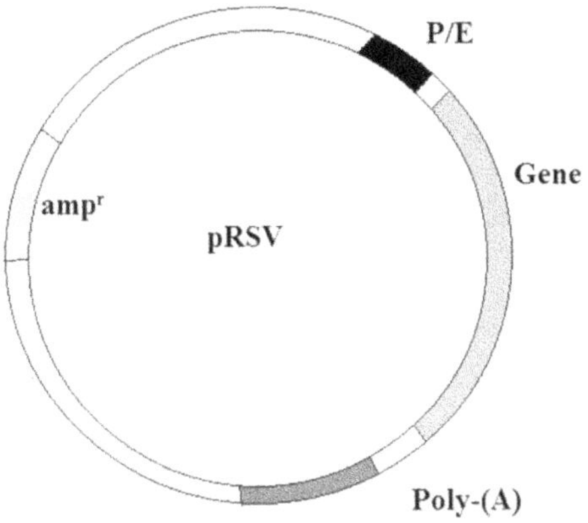

Figure 5.1. A systematic illustration of a plasmid vector with a selectable marker (reporter) (ampr) gene. This is a prototype for fish (amp, ampicillin resistance; P/E, promoter/enhancer; Poly(A), polyadenylation site; ori, origin of DNA replication).

coli plasmid pBR322 and an enhancer/promoter sequence (SV40 or Roux sarcoma virus promoter). It also includes a multiple cloning site for insertion of the DNA insert and a termination site including the polyadenylation site. Moreover, it has the SV40 origin of replication as well.

5.3.2 P element vectors/transposon

Transposons, small fragments of DNA smaller than 10 kb, are often present in all kinds of organisms, whereas P transposable elements are eukaryotic mobile DNA elements that are only present in metazoans (animals of the metazoa division). These were initially discovered as a cause for hybrid dysgenesis, which takes place between the germline of flies by crosses between females lacking P elements and males carrying P elements. This syndrome results in a unique pattern of maternal inheritance. P transposable elements can be utilized as vectors for gene transfer. Moreover, eukaryotic cut-and-paste-transposition (the target site is cleaved and ligated after the integration of the transposon) can also be investigated by the P element transposition reaction. This major breakthrough was based on a study conducted on flies (e.g. *Drosophila*) belonging to the metazoa division. It has been observed that plasmids are not present in *Drosophila*, so there was immense scope for the development of suitable vectors for *Drosophila*.

It was observed that just like mammalian cells these organisms are more vulnerable against viral infection, thus this factor cannot be considered for generating cloning vectors for *Drosophila*. However cloning in *Drosophila* is possible using the P element. One of the most important features of the transposon is that it can easily move from one site to another in the chromosomes of a cell. So, a transposon tagging technique can be utilized to introduce the P element to further clone sequences from the su(s) region of *Drosophila*. There are many types of small P elements (2.9 kb) present in *Drosophila* that encode for 87-kD transposase protein and carry three different genes preceded by short inverted report sequences (31 bp) at

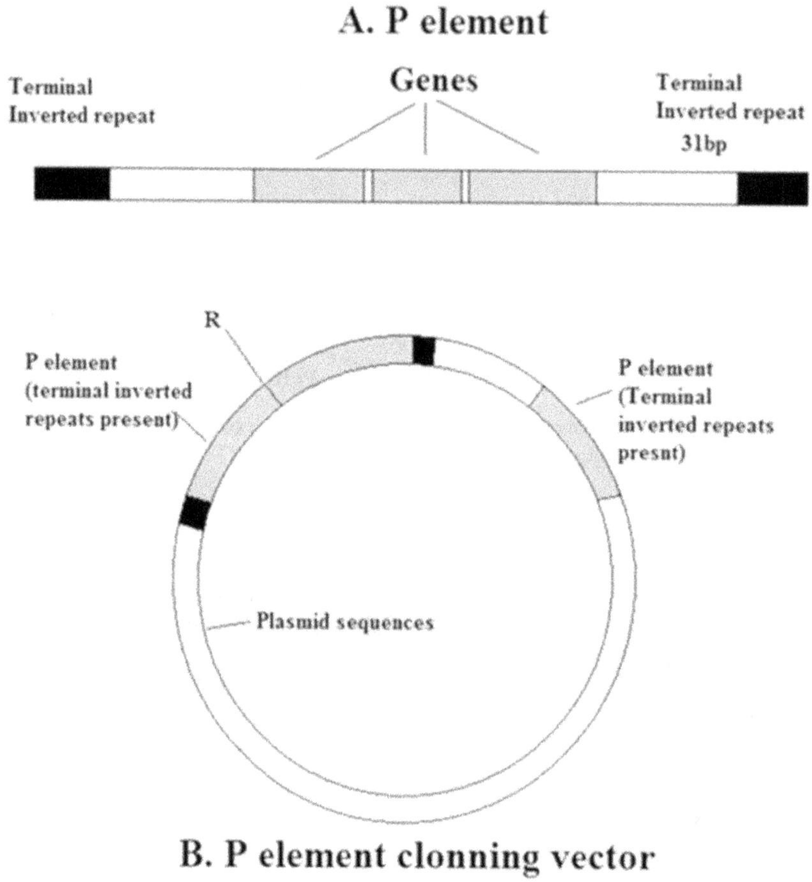

Figure 5.2. A cloning vector for *Drosophila.* (A) association of a P element; (B) a cloning vector based on P element; and R, the exclusive restriction site within a gene encoding transposase into which the DNA insert is incorporated.

either end of the element, as shown in figure 5.2(A). The P transposable element in *D. melanogaster* has been considered as a useful tool as strains whose genomes are free of this element exist [2]. Moreover, movement of these elements in the chromosome can be controlled by restricting the availability of its transposase (the enzyme that catalyzes the movement of the transposon) [3]. Additionally, modified elements can be prepared under *in vitro* conditions and reinserted into the genome [4]. The expression of transposase (transposase synthesis) is usually limited to germline cells because splicing of the P element third intron (IVS3) only takes place in the germline or, in other words, this polypeptide is limited to the germline as the last of the element's three introns is eliminated from P RNA only in that particular tissue [5]. Inside germline cells three introns are united in the P transcript resulting in the production of transposase. The gene responsible for the synthesis of transposase recognizes the terminal repeats and effects transposition of the P elements.

The P element cloning vector is primarily a bacterial plasmid vector that contains two P elements. P element transposition, like bacterial transposons, necessitates the action of a transposase. This action is in the form of action on inverted repeat sequences at the ends of the element. Since one of these P elements carries terminal repeats, it is removed so it cannot be recognized by the transposase, whereas the other P element has its terminal repeats intact, it can easily be identified by transposase to transpose. The desired DNA is incorporated in the transposase gene of this element (figure 5.2(B)). A shuttle vector (usually a plasmid) is prepared to propagate in two different host species.

P element vectors are shuttle vectors; like YACs, they are propagated in *E. coli*, and are used for gene cloning in *Drosophila*. After the DNA insert is integrated in the P element with intact terminal repeats, the plasmid DNA is microinjected into fruit fly embryos. Transposase is produced by the other P element that lacks the terminal repeats; this transposase directs the transposition of the DNA insert containing the P element into the *Drosophila* genome. If such a transposition occurs within a germline nucleus of an embryo, the resulting adult fly will carry copies of the cloned gene in all its germinal cells. P elements were first used for cloning in the 1980s; their use has made several important contributions to *Drosophila* genetics. DNA inserts of up to 40 kb have been cloned using some P element vectors.

5.3.3 Baculovirus as versatile vectors for protein expression in insects

As is well-known, gene expression in insect cells is more time-consuming than in bacteria. Baculovirus vectors are one of the most widely used systems for expressing proteins in insect and mammalian cells [6]. The baculovirus expression system was developed for virus production and expression of recombinant proteins from baculovirus-infected insect cells. The type of expression system allows the utilization of recombinant baculoviruses (insect viruses) and their capability to generate a high amount of protein in cultured insect cells or insect larvae.

Such expression vector system vectors have been developed for the transfection of insects. Two expression systems belonging to nuclear polyhedrosis viruses (NPVs) (viruses that are not capable of infecting humans in the way they can infect insects, as human cells are acidic and NPV requires an alkaline cell to replicate), Autographa californica NPV and Bombyx mori NPV, have been frequently exploited for this purpose. The genome of the nuclear polyhedrosis virus of B. mori contains the gene encoding for a viral occlusion body protein called polyhedrin. The polyhedrin gene has a powerful promoter, so the polyhedrin protein is synthesized in large amounts. As this protein is not required for virus infection of cultured insect cells, the polyhedrin promoter gene can be utilized to synthesize recombinant proteins. To achieve this, the polyhedrin coding sequence is deleted and substituted by cDNA that encodes for protein expression. Thus, in this approach, the polyhedrin promoter encourages the expression of the transgene [6]. Numerous baculoviruses are currently used. One of the most common is the multiple nuclear polyhedrosis virus, which can potentially infect several insects and also replicate well in various cultured insect cell lines. The fall armyworm (Spodoptera frugiperda) derived cell line is considered to have the most potential to propagate baculovirus as it yields a high amount of polyhedron. Thus the polyhedrin promoter gene is responsible for the particularly high production of recombinant proteins in this cell line.

As per table 5.1, several animal vectors are developed to replicate expression in mammalian cells; only the passive transducing SV40 vectors are incompetent in replication. The introduction of retrovirus and transposon vectors into the genomes of host cells is quite similar to natural retroviruses and transposons. Both circular (vectors are by nature circular and because of the helical nature of DNA can resemble a knot) and linearized vectors can assimilate into the host genome, nevertheless, the latter (linearized vectors) are far more quickly integrated than the former. It has also been reported that the occurrence of additional vector DNA along with the integrated gene construct obstructs the expression of inserted genes or transgenes. Therefore, it is important to incorporate the transgene with a minimum of vector DNA associated with it.

5.3.3.1 Conclusion

Baculovirus vectors are one of the most commonly used systems to express proteins in insect and mammalian cells. The baculovirus expression system was developed for virus production and recombinant protein expression from baculovirus-infected insect cells. The nature of the expression system allows the use of recombinant baculoviruses (insect viruses) and the ability to produce large amounts of protein in cultured insect cells or insect larvae. Nuclear polyhedral virus (NPV) (a virus that cannot infect humans in the same way it infects insects because human cells are acidic and NPV requires alkaline cells for replication), *Autographa californica* NPV and *Bombyx mori* Two expression systems belonging to capital values were often utilized for this purpose. B nuclear polyhedral virus genome mori contains a gene that encodes a viral occluder protein called polyhedrin. The polyhedrin gene has a strong promoter, which allows polyhedrin protein to be synthesized in large amounts. Because this protein is not required for viral infection of cultured insect cells, the polyhedrin promoter gene can be used to synthesize recombinant proteins. Therefore, in this approach, the polyhedrin promoter drives transgene expression [6]. One of the most prevalent is poly nucleopolyhedrosis virus, which can infect multiple insects and also replicate well in a variety of cultured insect cell lines. Therefore, the polyhedrin promoter gene is responsible for particularly high recombinant protein production in this cell line.

5.4 Efficient and versatile mammalian virus vectors

The polyomavirus simian virus 40 (SV40) is a DNA tumor virus, and is considered as an emergent human pathogen. SV40 vectors were the first viral vectors to be used for transfection and can be replicated in different mammalian species. The SV40 papovavirus was considered as the first animal vector, and was developed from monkeys and utilized for cloning in 1979. Since then, vectors have been produced from many other viruses, e.g. papillomavirus, the Epstein–Barr herpes virus, adenoviruses, vaccinia viruses (all for mammals) and baculoviruses (for insects). Mammalian artificial chromosomes (MACs) and artificial chromosomes (HACs) were also developed later.

5.4.1 SV40 vectors

SV40 vectors are spherical viruses with a circular, double-stranded 5243 bp chromosome. This chromosome is encoded for five proteins: small-T, large-T (both early proteins), VP1, VP2 and VP3 (VP is the virion protein). It has an origin of replication (about 80 bp) and is complexed with histones to form chromatin. These plasmids can be packaged only if their DNA is within the range of 3900–5300 bp. Large-T is necessary for viral replication, whereas VP1, VP2 and VP3 form the viral capsid. In the laboratory, it is multiplied in cultured kidney cells from the African green monkey. Infected cells lyse after four days releasing up to 10^5 virions/cell. SV40 has been established to offer a sole vector for gene therapy which has several merits over any of the currently existing viral vectors [7]. The SV40 genome (figure 5.3(A)) has been utilized to develop chiefly the following three kinds of vectors:

- Plasmid vectors.
- Transducing vectors.
- Transforming vectors.

5.4.1.1 Using SV40 transducing vectors to transduce foreign genes

SV40 vectors can be packaged only if their DNA is within the range of 3900–5300 bp. As these small genomes do not have much expendable DNA, it is just about impracticable to construct a functional vector with any added genes. Luckily, functions offered by helper DNA molecules might help to surmount these problems. SV40 has been investigated as a viral vector with a focus on the ease of generating

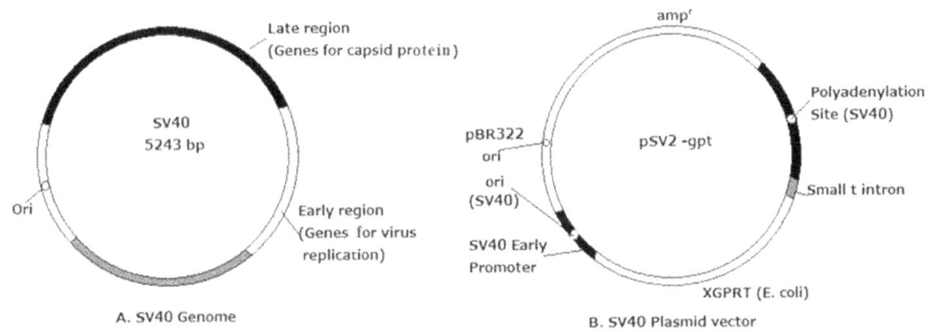

Figure 5.3. SV40-based plasmid vector. (A) SV40 genome. (B) shuttle vector with origin and amp^r gene from pBR322 (for function in *E. coli*), and the following SV40 segments: the origin and the neighboring transcriptional control sequences including the early promoter, and the polyadenylation site. This vector works as a plasmid vector in host cells with the large-T gene, e.g. the COS cell line, but as a non-replicative vector in other host cells.

high-titer stocks and its potential to transduce genes. After infecting monkey cells, these vectors manufacture viral particles. As information about SV40s genome association, sequence, and expression grew and the rDNA technology for breaking down and reassembling DNA molecules advanced, it was expected that SV40 DNA would be suitable as a possible vector for delivering foreign DNA segments into mammalian cells.

All SV40 transducing vectors have the following three features:

- Genes encoding large-T, VP1, VP2 and VP3. This leaves very little room for DNA inserts. However, the genes encoding the necessary proteins, i.e. large-T, VP1, VP2, and VP3, can be nearby in another virus or within the host genome. This suppleness is an advantage for solving the size and selection issues.
- The SV40 origin comprises the surrounding region including the transcriptional regulatory signals (i.e. regions at which splicing and polyadenylation take place).
- Total size (including that of the DNA insert) between 3900 bp and 5300 bp for packaging into virions.

5.4.1.2 SV40 vector with early gene replacement

SV40 late replacement vectors offer an excellent means for expressing large amounts of proteins from cDNAs of less than 2400 bp. The region encoding VP1, VP2, and VP3 may be substituted in the vector by a DNA insert; such a vector is known as a late-region replacement vector, e.g. SVGT-5. A vector of this kind comprises the following:

- The entire early region of the SV40 genome.
- The origin of replication.
- The regions at which splicing and polyadenylation occur.

This vector is utilized for infection of host cells in combination with another virus, known as a helper virus, which has the VP1, VP2 and VP3 genes intact but has a defective large-T gene (a gene in the early region). The large-T function is intact and offered by the late replacement vector. Thus, in this procedure, only those host cells that are infected by both the vector and the helper virus will lyse and produce virions while cells infected by either the vector or the helper virus alone will not support packaging or replication (respectively) of the virus. This characteristic is very useful as all the plaques formed on monkey cell monolayers contain the vector. Late-region replacement vectors have been utilized to investigate post-transcriptional RNA processing and stability. The presence of an intron in the late-region primary transcript was essential in a number of cases (but not in others), for the production of cytoplasmic mRNA, the reasons for this being unknown.

5.4.1.3 SV40 early replacement vectors for effective gene transfer

Early replacement vectors, like their late counterparts, must be structured with proper regard for the position of viral transcription. Important genes missing from the vector may exist within the genome of host cells. For instance, the COS (CV-I, the origin of SV40; CV-I is a monkey cell line) cell line of African green monkey kidney cell cultures holds in its genome the gene for large-T of SV40. Thus, a vector containing the origin of replication and genes for VP1, VP2, and VP3 will replicate and create virions in COS cell line cells. In such a case, no helper virus is necessary. As in such a vector the early genes (large-T gene) are substituted by the DNA insert, it is known as an early-region replacement vector.

The main benefits of both late- and early-region replacement SV40 vectors are as below:

- The rDNA generates virions, which allows the transfer of the DNA into host cells by infecting them like SV40 virions.
- The rDNA replicates to a high copy number, which is a distinct benefit.

However, these vectors have the following disadvantages:

- The expression of transgene is transient in the infected cells.
- The maximum size of DNA insert is -2.5 kb.

5.4.1.4 SV40 plasmid vector based gene transfer

As per reports SV40 is a polyomavirus which is present in both monkeys and humans. Polyomavirus simian virus, abbreviated as SV40, is named for the effect it produced on an infected green monkey kidney cell line (Vero), which developed an abnormal number of vacuoles. Similarly to other polyomaviruses, SV40 is an oncogenic DNA virus that can cause tumors in animals, however, it is often responsible for long-term persistent infection. After the breakthrough of SV40, from 1955 to 1963 about 90% of children and many adults in the USA were administered with SV40-contaminated polio vaccines. SV40 contains the origin of replication and the large-T encoding gene (the large-T gene is not necessary for multiplication in COS cells). SV40 contains a single origin of replication which is opposite to mammalian cells as they contain many origins of replication. SV40 contains circular DNA which replaces from the origin of replication and forms replication forks which ultimately form a bubble. Since the replication is bidirectional, it can lead to the formation of two replication forks in opposite directions, that ultimately form a bubble, the size of which keeps on increasing. SV40 cannot replicate separately if the replication origin (ori) is defective. SV40 replicates extensively in primary African green monkey kidney cells and assimilates into the genetic material of the green monkey cells, and then replicates along with the chromosomal DNA. With regard to the cellular chromosomes the SV40 DNA is integrated at random positions and for viral DNA the exact integration site also seems to be random. Nevertheless, SV40 integration in all transformed cell lines is such that the SV40 early promoter and T antigen coding sequences are intact. This may thus assure uninterrupted T antigen expression. These vectors replicate inside the monkey cells but do not get packaged into virions. SV40 can replicate in monkey cell lines and can replicate to a high copy number, and this is a significant discovery since there is no size limitation on the foreign DNA and the SV40 replicons are not packed into viral capsids. Since there is no size limit on such vectors, these vectors synthesize a high copy number per COS cell. Thus, permanent COS cell lines encompassing rDNA are not obtained, but transient expression of cloned genes can be investigated.

The shuttle vectors are utilized to multiply the rDNA in *E. coli*, which are then incorporated into monkey cells to investigate the expression of DNA inserts. By using the features (origin of replication and the early region of polyomavirus) of SV40, plasmid vectors can be constructed by using, in the place of SV40, e.g. pSV (plasmid simian virus). pSV vectors are made by incorporating the SV40 sequences into pBR322. For this type of construction, the bacterial XGPRT gene (or mouse DHFR gene or bacterial neomycin phosphotransferase gene) integrated after the SV40 early promoter sequence. This particular gene is called a selectable marker, and further helps in the selection of the transformed cells. One of the series derived from pSV vectors is pRSV vectors. They are also called derivatives of pSV vectors. A major difference between these two vectors is that in pRSV SV40 an early promoter sequence is replaced by a 524 bp long fragment from the long terminal repeat (LTR) sequence. This sequence is derived from another virus known as retrovirus Rous sarcoma virus (RSV). This sequence contains the retroviral promoter sequence, which is more powerful than the SV40 promoter in various cell types. According to various reports, in monkey cells plasmid vectors are unstable and are generally used for transient transfection only. In the case that the large-T function is provided by COS cells, these vectors can be stably maintained and the vector has a selectable marker, e.g. the *E. coli* neo gene, and the host cells are maintained under the selection environment, in this case on G-418. The plasmid derived from such vectors integrates into the host cell genome with a frequency of $10–10^{-3}$. This results in stable transfection. Plasmid vectors derived from such an origin can be utilized to investigate sequences involved in transcriptional and post-transcriptional regulation. This investigation helps in understanding elements of SV40, such as SV40 enhancer sequences and its characteristics. Stable transfection of COS cell lines can be developed by utilizing several approaches such as:

- The gene encoding the large T protein, present in the COS cell line, should be a temperature-sensitive mutant.
- The wild-type allele (which refers to the phenotype of the typical form of a species) of the large-T gene is positioned under the control of a metallothionein gene promoter.

In both of these cases the SV40-based plasmid is stably maintained as an episome (a non-essential genetic element) at a low copy number. Nevertheless they do allow the activity of the large-T protein to be increased. This leads to an increase in plasmid production and in the level of expression of the transgene contained in the plasmid.

5.4.1.5 Conclusion

To conclude, this polyomavirus simian virus, abbreviated as SV40, is called for the impact it produced on an infected green monkey kidney molecular line (Vero), which advanced a peculiar variety of vacuoles. SV40 carries the beginning of replication and the large-T encoding gene (the large-T gene is not vital for multiplication in COS cells). SV40 carries round DNA which replaces the origin of replication and forms replication forks which in the long run shape a bubble. Nevertheless, SV40 integration in all transformed molecular strains is such that the SV40 early promoter and T antigen coding sequences are intact. These vectors mirror the monkey cells, however, now no longer get packaged into virions. SV40 can mirror in monkey molecular strains and might mirror to an excessive replica variety, and that is a sizable discovery due to the fact there is no length dilemma at the foreign DNA and the SV40 replicons are not packed into viral capsids. Since there is no length restriction on such vectors, those vectors synthesize an excessive replica variety in line with COS molecular. Thus, everlasting COS molecular strains encompassing rDNA are not obtained, however, temporary expression of cloned genes may be investigated. *E.coli* can be then integrated into monkey cells to research the expression of DNA inserts. By the usage of the features (beginning of replication and the early vicinity of polyomavirus) of SV40, plasmid vectors may be built with the usage of Simian Virus large T antigen (SVLT), inside the area of SV40, e.g. pSV (plasmid simian virus). pSV vectors are made with the aid of incorporating the SV40 sequences into pBR322. For this sort of construction, the bacterial XGPRT gene (or mouse DHFR gene or bacterial neomycin phosphotransferase gene) is included after the SV40 early promoter sequence. They also are known as derivatives of PSV vectors. According to numerous reports, in monkey cells, plasmid vectors are volatile and are typically used for temporary transfection only. In the case that the large-T feature is furnished with the aid of using COS cells, those vectors may be stably maintained and the vector has a selectable marker, *E.coli* neo gene, and the host cells are maintained beneath the choice environment, in this example on G-418. The plasmid derived from such vectors integrates into the host molecular genome with a frequency of 10–10-3. Plasmid vectors derived from such a beginning may be applied to research sequences worried in transcriptional and post-transcriptional regulation.

5.4.1.6 Non-replicating viral vectors

These vectors do not replicate. An array of non-replicating virus vectors have been explored for vaccine and gene therapy applications [8]. Various important features of replicating and non-replicating vaccine vectors are listed in table 5.2.

SV40 vectors serve as vehicles for transfecting DNAs, which might be incorporated into the host DNA; such vectors are known as passive transfecting vectors. Generally these vectors are shuttle vectors. They are initially cloned in *E. coli* to separate rDNA and then are utilized to transfect a variety of mammalian cells, as they need not be limited to monkey cells in view of their lack of replication. The SV40 segments used in these vectors are generally the transcription regulatory

Table 5.2. Key features of replicating and non-replicating vaccine vectors.

Viral vector	Type	Insert	Advantages	Disadvantages
Adenovirus	Non-replicating; dsDNA	7–8 kb	Common features: Targets mucosal inductive sites. Infects dividing, non-dividing and dendritic cells. No integration. Physically and genetically stable. Specific for non-replicating vectors. Safe. Long history of gene therapy use. Multiple serotypes and chimeric forms.	Prior immunity to Ad5. High doses needed to elicit immunity.
Adeno-associated virus	Non-replicating; ssDNA	<5 kb	Resistant to acid; physically stable. Alternate serotypes available. Tropic for dendritic cells. Non-pathogenic.	Difficult production uses helper virus. Possible integration. Prior immunity to prevalent AAV2.
Alphavirus	Non-replicating; +ssRNA	<8 kb	No integration. Does not elicit anti-vector immunity. Targets dendritic cells. Highly immunogenic.	Safety concerns regarding VEE. Difficult to produce.
Pox viruses: NYVAC; MVA	Non-replicating; ds DNA	>10 kb	Excellent immunogenicity; more immunogenic than avian pox viruses.	Prior immunity.
Pox viruses: ALVAC; FPV	Non-replicating; ds DNA	>10 kb	No prior immunity.	Less immunogenic than mammalian pox viruses.

sequences and the polyadenylation sites. Permanent transfectants are chosen on the basis of selectable markers in the vector.

The selectable markers need not be covalently linked to the DNA insert or the transfecting DNA. Still, when two separate DNA fragments comprising separate genes are selected and used for transfection, more than 50% of the permanently transfected cells contain both genes, generally integrated side by side. The two DNA segments are likely to become joined after entering the animal cells. This is the cause for their co-transformation, i.e. assimilation of the two genes together in the genome.

5.4.2 BPV (bovine papillomavirus) DNA vectors

BPV is a class of DNA viruses of the family *Papillomaviridae* that are widespread in cattle. Infection causes warts (papillomas and fibropapillomas) of the alimentary tract and skin, and on the odd occasion cancers of the urinary bladder and alimentary tract [9]. Papillomavirus is affiliated to the papovavirus class and has a circular 7.9 kb genome organized in nucleosomes. BPV replicates as a stable plasmid in rodents and many bovine cells. The cells are not killed; the virus acts like a multicopy plasmid (up to 100 copies per cell) and is transferred to daughter cells on cell division. The viral genome transforms cells which act like tumor cells and form piled up colonies of cells instead of the typical monolayer. The transformed condition is owing to the genes in the 'transforming region' (about 5500 bp) of the virus genome. The virus genome is usually used to generate shuttle vectors by means of the transforming region of the genome. Eukaryotic DNA fragments are initially cloned in *E. coli* to choose rDNA. After that the *E. coli* plasmid, e.g. pBR322, is deleted from the rDNA. Then the remaining linear rDNA is incorporated into animal cells. After this genetic introduction the vector becomes circular and replicates as a plasmid. The *E. coli* neo gene may be incorporated within the vector. This incorporation allows easy selection of transfected cells by culturing them on a medium containing the aminoglycoside G-418. The BPV-derived vector offers permanent cell lines that hold the rDNA either episomally or integrated into the cell genome at high copy numbers. Moreover, these vectors can carry large DNA inserts [9].

5.4.3 Retrovirus vectors and their use

Viral vectors are common tools utilized by molecular biologists to transport genetic material into cells. This whole process can be conducted within a living organism (*in vivo*) or in cell culture (*in vitro*). Viruses have developed particular molecular mechanisms to proficiently deliver their genomes within the cells they infect. All retroviruses have single-stranded RNA genomic structures. Each individual virus has two copies of the genome, which appear like eukaryotic mRNAs. The genome of a virus is reverse transcribed by reverse transcriptase into a DNA double-stranded copy within the host cells. The DNA copy assimilates into the host genome to become a provirus. This causes stable transfection of the cells. The provirus genome is transcribed and expressed, resulting in the formation of virions and finally extradition into the medium. The subsequent characteristics of retroviruses are significant in their use as vectors:

- Broad host range (birds, mammals and animals).
- Infected cells are not destroyed and they persist to synthesize virus particles over a longer time.
- The presence of strong promoters.
- Promoter action regulation in the case of a number of viruses, e.g. murine mammary tumor virus. Retroviral vectors are made from cloned DNA genomes of retroviruses.

Viral vectors have three important properties:

- The vector has viral sequences for replication, gene expression and packaging (xv sequences).
- DNA inserts may either replace or be located in the non-essential coding region of the viral genome, e.g. it may replace the gag gene.
- The vector and the rDNA are packaged into virions and used as transducing viruses.
- The viral proteins are usually provided by a helper virus or a provirus.
- DNA copies of the retrovirus genomes are utilized as vectors, generally as shuttle vectors (figure 5.4).

A typical vector has the following sequences:

- At least one distinctive restriction site for the insertion of DNA fragments (figure 5.4) without interrupting any of the main sequences.
- It also has R, U5, U3, P and Pu encoding sequences (reverse transcription).
- It contains pBR322 on and a selectable marker for cloning in *E. coli.*

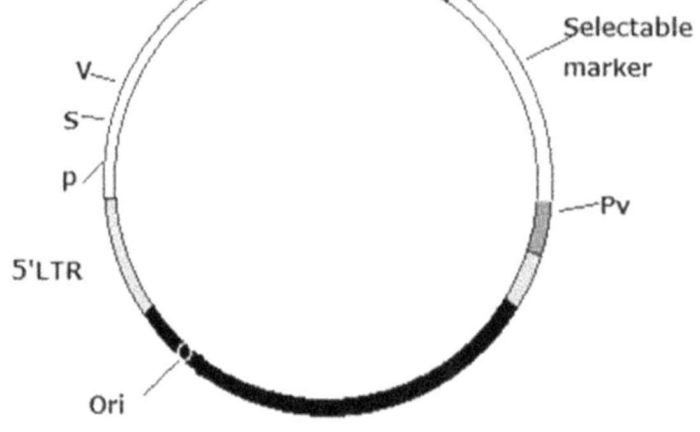

Figure 5.4. A retroviral shuttle vector. Note that the pBR322 segment is placed outside 5′LTR and 3′LTR (RE, unique endonuclease site).

- Retroviral 5′LTR and 3′LTR (long terminal direct repeats) are needed for efficient delivery of proviral DNA and for generating the 3′-end of transcripts. LTRs are also necessary for incorporation of the proviral DNA into the host sequences involved in retroviral replication which are located between 5′LTR and the gag gene, the env gene and the 3′LTR.
- The LTR sequence (necessary for packaging into virions).

The rDNA is structured and initially cloned in *E. coli*; after that it is isolated and transferred into animal cells using, say, trapped calcium-phosphate-mediated transfection. Within the animal cells the complete vector, apart from the *E. coli* plasmid sequence, is transcribed. This transcript holds an RNA copy of the DNA insert, and is packaged into virions, which is usually not that effective in animal cells. As the vector does not predetermine the viral capsid proteins, they must be supplied by a helper virus or provirus. If the provirus or helper virus lacks the w sequence, its genome will not be packaged into virions. The cell line containing the helper provirus is called the helper cell line. For instance, psi-2 is a 3T3 mouse cell line with a transfected provirus obtained from Moloney murine leukemia virus. This provirus has a defective psi sequence. As a result, all the virions are collected from the medium containing the RNA copy of rDNA. This RNA copy of the rDNA can be utilized in further experiments. The rDNA can incorporate as a provirus into the host genome; the transfected cells can be simply selected either as piled up colonies of cells (if the rDNA retains an oncogene) or due to the expression of an *E. coli* gene, for example, gene neo presenting resistance to the drug G-418. These transfected cell lines include the recombinant provirus. The provirus sequences, including the DNA insert, are transcribed and the transgenes are expressed. However, these RNA transcripts are not packaged into virions since the rDNA lacks sequences encoding the capsid proteins. The host collection of the recombinant retrovirus will depend on that of the helper retrovirus or the provirus present in the helper cell line. Therefore, the helper virus is said to be a pseudotype of the recombinant. Thus, helper cell lines have been constructed utilizing such strains of retroviruses that can replicate in an extensive variety of cells. This has been done with Moloney-Mu LV; these helper cell lines permit the delivery of retroviral rDNAs to human cells. It is also likely to produce a non-defective recombinant virus that has a complete set of all essential genes. This has been accomplished with the derivatives of avian virus, RSV, which possibly indicates that the retrovirus life-cycle, as a rule, removes introns present in the original DNA insert. Consequently, the DNA insert present in a recombinant retrovirus recovered by transfection of host cells lacks introns.

5.4.4 Vaccinia virus vectors: new approach for producing recombinant vaccines

Vaccinia virus is a complex, large, enveloped virus belonging to the poxvirus family, with a linear, dsDNA genome which encodes approximately 250 genes. The vaccinia virus genome has been utilized to construct vectors for the cloning of genes of pathogen origin that allow the use of recombinant vaccinia viruses as live vaccines.

5.4.5 Adenovirus vectors (for gene therapy, vaccination and cancer gene therapy)

Adenovirus vectors are the most frequently utilized vectors for cancer gene therapy. They are also utilized for other gene therapies and as vaccines to express foreign antigens. Adenovirus vectors can be replication defective. Certain important viral genes are removed and substituted by a cassette that expresses a foreign therapeutic gene. Such vectors are utilized for gene therapy, as vaccines and for cancer therapy [9].

Adenoviruses are medium-sized DNA viruses; non-enveloped, icosahedral viruses composed of a nucleocapsid and a linear dsDNA genome, and their genome is dsDNA of 36 kb.

In recombinant viruses, a DNA insert substitutes genes EIA/E1B. These genes control transcription and are necessary for virus replication. Thus, recombinant viruses are multiplied in a transfected cell line that collaboratively expresses EIA/E1B genes. In adenoviruses gene E3 is usually deleted in addition to EIA/E1B. Gene E3 down controls the immune response of the host animal, but is not required for virus replication in cultured cells. The largest insert size for such vectors is 6–8 kb. The recombinant virus continues in susceptible cells as an episome for comparatively extensive periods, e.g. from days up to months in post-mitotic brain cells *in vivo*. Adenoviruses infect the respiratory tract. Recombinant adenoviruses have been used to transfect respiratory tract cells for somatic gene therapy of cystic fibrosis, and for gene transfer into skeletal muscle.

5.5 Mammalian artificial chromosome (MAC) vectors for somatic gene therapy

Each and every vector system at present available for gene therapy has some limitations and advantages. The utilization of viral vectors such as lentiviral and retroviral vectors allows for an enhanced period of therapeutic gene expression by their superficial integration into the host genome, but are plagued by safety issues, e.g. malignant transformation. In contrast, non-viral vectors are identified to be non-pathogenic, but less efficient at introducing and maintaining the transgene expression [10]. Mammalian artificial chromosome (MAC) and human artificial chromosome (HAC) vectors are linear vectors that include centromeres, telomeres, origin (of replication) recognition sequences and transcriptionally active chromosomal domains. These vectors are very similar to microchromosomes and mitotically and cytogenetically stable in the absence of any selection. MACs and HACs can be developed in cultured cells by artificially modifying the structure of natural chromosomes. On the other hand, cloned chromosomal elements may be delivered into cultured cells resulting in *de novo* formation of MACs and HACs. The different approaches utilized for *de novo* MAC/HAC construction are as follows:

- Long synthetic ranges of alpha satellite DNA are combined with telomeric DNA and genomic DNA. This approach was utilized to offer the first generation of HACs in human HT1080 cells. In this scheme, there is *de novo* formation of centromere activity; the HACs so derived are maintained steadily during mitosis, i.e. act as native chromosomes.

- Telomere repeats and selectable markers are incorporated into a YAC that has human centromeric DNA, including centromere protein B (CENP-B) boxes.
- The PAC vector is utilized to obtain high concentrations of centromeres, telomeres, origins of replication and structural gene sequences. These sequences are joined together *in vitro* within agarose plugs using site-specific recombination, and transformed into mammalian cells, where *de novo* MAC/HAC formation takes place.

The chromosomal sequences essential for *de novo* construction of MACs and HACs are such that their cloning in a single molecule is very complex. Instability during cloning of telomeric and centromeric DNA further complicates MAC/HAC construction. Moreover, such DNA molecules are not stable in solution. Thus, their isolation, manipulation and delivery are difficult.

5.6 DNA constructs

A gene construct is a synthetically designed fragment of nucleic acid that is going to be 'transplanted' into a target tissue or cell. Genetic incorporation into animal cells is achieved either for offering transgenic cells/animals or for molecular biology studies. The goals of studies in molecular biology may simply be limited to gaining an understanding of the functions of different genes in animal development and regulation of their action. However, this may be expanded to a diversity of individual investigations, on topics such as promoter functions during transcription and translation, expression of reporter genes, products of any identified or unknown DNA sequences of interest, actions of oncogenes, regulation of gene expression, biological functions of hormones in relation to development, the identification of transcription and translation factors, analysis of the consequences of site-directed mutagenesis in DNA, and replacement or 'knockout' of functional genes and marking genes for identification and developmental lineages. Most of these molecular investigations are easily conducted using *Xenopus laevis* oocytes. The approach to complete genetic studies using an organism or cell that is different from the one whose genes are being studied is known as surrogate genetics. The use of *Xenopus* oocytes for molecular biology investigations is an excellent example of replacement genetics.

A transgene must be incorporated into the host genome for obtaining transgenic cells/animals, whereas for molecular biology investigations the transgenes are normally there in an extrachromosomal state. But in both cases, the transgene must be there in an appropriate direction in relation to and in organization with the various sequences essential for its competent transcription and translation in the host cells. The different sequences necessary for gene expression may be listed as follows:

- An efficient promoter/enhancer.
- The translation initiation codon (AUG in mRNA, and ATG in DNA).
- The chain termination codon(s).
- Transcription termination sequence.
- Polyadenylation cleavage/addition site (figure 5.5).

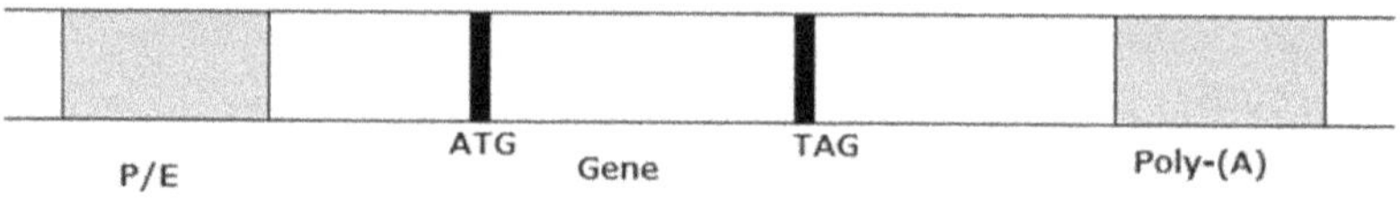

Figure 5.5. A simple representation of a gene construct for expression in animal/plant cells. P/E, promoter/enhancer sequence; ATG (=AUG), the initiation codon; gene, the gene (may contain introns) that is to be expressed; TAG, chain termination signal (during translation); Poly(A), transcription termination including poly(A) addition/deletion site. Suitable signal sequences must be included for protein translocation, if required.

A proper expression vector usually includes a promoter, transcription termination sequence and, typically, a polyadenylation site, for example pRSV vectors (figure 5.2). In addition, some marker genes have to be utilized for recognition and selection of the transfected cells; such genes are called reporter genes. Moreover, the gene must contain suitable signaling sequences for the transport etc of the protein encoded by it.

5.6.1 Promoter sequences

Promoter sequences are those DNA sequences that characterize where transcription of a gene by RNA polymerase commences [11]. Promoter sequences are usually to be found directly upstream or at the 5′ end of the transcription initiation site. These are the sequences at which RNA polymerase first binds during the initiation of transcription. The RNA polymerase affinity to the promoter sequences is several orders of scale higher than that for other DNA sequences. Fundamentally, the occurrence of a promoter sequence is extremely important for the transcription of a DNA segment. In this process the promoter must be located at the end of the gene which has the initiation codon AUG, i.e. upstream of the coding region of the gene [11]. In contrast, an enhancer sequence is itself not the site of RNA polymerase binding, but it enhances the activity of the promoter located in its area, often up to several kilobases away. The promoter sequence evaluates not only the level of transcription of a gene but also the tissue or cell type where the gene will be expressed; it also determines the developmental stage at which the gene will be expressed and, if applicable, to which stimuli the expression will respond. For instance, SV40 early promoter is a constitutive promoter which means it is expressed in a broad number of mammalian cells. Similarly, the RSV promoter is also constitutive; however, it is much more dominant than the SV40 promoter. The activity of the promoter, e.g. RSV and other retroviruses, is positioned in their LTR sequences. The RSV promoter utilized in pRSV vectors is a 524 base pairs (bp) sequence isolated from one LTR of RSV; it substitutes the SV40 early promoter of the pSV series plasmids. In contrast, 13-lactoglobulin promoter/enhancer is a mammary-gland tissue-specific promoter, such that the genes fused with and, as a result, driven by this promoter are expressed only in the mammary glands and the proteins encoded by them are secreted in milk [11].

5.6.2 Selectable reporter or marker genes

A gene utilized in molecular biology to decide if a nucleic acid sequence has been effectively inserted into an organism's DNA is called a marker gene. A selectable marker (antibiotics) and a marker for screening (green fluorescent protein, or GFP) are two types of marker genes. A gene that attaches to a regulatory sequence of another GOI in cell culture, animals or plants is called a reporter gene (often simply a reporter). Certain genes are selected as reporters as the characteristics they present on organisms expressing them are easily identified and determined (GFP), or because they are selectable markers (antibiotics). It can be a selectable marker that exerts some selection pressure such as an antibiotics, or a screenable marker, such as GFP, GUS or blue/white screening A reporter gene is utilized to examine the strength and/or regulation of a regulatory sequence that they are fused to, e.g. after incorporating the fragment of DNA (e.g. plasmid) into the organism (with the help of antibiotic marker gene), the cells are exposed to various conditions or treatments, and their green fluorescence is measured, if the plasmid has on it the GFP used for some promoters of interest. A marker or reporter gene offers a phenotype, which is either easily or specifically determined or that allows a differential multiplication of the cells. The former is known as a scorable marker, whereas the latter is called a selectable marker. The different marker genes utilized in animals are summarized in table 5.3. Scorable markers are utilized for investigating promoter/enhancer movement, whereas selectable markers utilized to select for transfected cells, e.g. of scorable markers, include the chloramphenicol acetyltransferase (CAT) gene from *E. coli* transposon Tn9, 13-galactosidase gene from *E. coli* and bacterial luciferase gene.

The enzyme CAT catalyzes transfer of acetyl groups from acetyl-CoA to chloramphenicol to initially yield a mixture of monoacetylated forms, which are ultimately converted into 1,3-acetyl-chloramphenicol. The CAT activity is assayed by incubating cell/tissue homogenate with 14C-labeled chloramphenicol. Thin layer chromatography separates the substrate and the products, which are examined by autoradiography. This assay is rapid, simple and highly sensitive. Firefly (*Photinus pyralis*) luciferase serves as a scorable marker both in animals and plants. This luciferase has a single polypeptide of 550 amino acids. It catalyzes oxidation of luciferin; this reaction entails adenosine triphosphate (ATP) and produces a yellow-green light. When surplus substrate is supplemented under controlled conditions, there is a flash of light that is proportional to the quantity of luciferase. The light emission decays rapidly to give an extended period of low emission. ATP can be replaced by coenzyme-A in the reaction. When coenzyme A is utilized, the emission of light does not decay so rapidly as it does when ATP is used. The light emission can be detected with luminometers, by utilizing a scintillation counter as a luminometer or even by using photographic film. This recognition is highly sensitive so that lactiferase assays are much more sensitive than CAT assays. Luciferases from other insects may offer more versatile tools. For instance, tropical click beetle luciferases elicit bioluminescence of various colors; these genes have already been cloned. GFP, encoded by a gene from Pacific jellyfish (*Aequoria victoria*), gives out green fluorescence when exposed to UV light. Consequently, it can be utilized to score

Table 5.3. A record of promoter/enhancer sequences utilized for driving transgenes in various transgenic animal species. A promoter/enhancer sequence is usually designated by the gene with which it is naturally associated.

Promoter/enhancer	Source	Animal species used in	Gene expression sequence in the tissue
Metallothionein promoter	1. Fish 2. Mouse 3. Sheep 4. Human	Fish Fish, mouse, pig Sheep Rabbit, pig	Stimulus-specific
β-actin	1. Fish 2. Chicken	Fish Fish	
cd-crystallin SV	SV40	Fish	All tissues
SV40 early promoter	SV40	Mammalian cells, Fish	All tissues
Moloney murine leukemia virus (MLV)	MLV	Pig	All tissues
RSV promoter	RSV	Mammalian cells, fish	All tissues
TK promoter	HSV	Mammalian cells	All tissues
SV40 enhancer	72 bp sequence with tandem repeats near SV40 origin	Enhances transcription of all genes transcribed by RNA polymerase II	All tissues
Antifreeze protein promoter	Fish	Fish	Mammary tissue
β-casein promoter	Mouse	Goat	Mammary tissue
β-lactoglobulin promoter	Sheep	Sheep	Mammary tissue
Prolactin promoter	Cow	Pig	
Immunoglobulin heavy chain promoter	Rabbit	Rabbit	

living cells/tissues, and also for cell sorting by fluorescence-activated cell sorting (FACS). Storable reporter genes are utilized for analyzing transient gene expression. These analyses can serve different purposes, e.g. recognition of sequences that regulate transcription, monitoring of promoter activity, etc

5.6.2.1 TK as a marker/reporter gene

TK has a main role in the production of DNA [12]. So far two isoenzymes have been described. TK1 and TK2; TK1 is cell cycle-dependent and present in the cytoplasm whereas TK2—located in mitochondria—is cell cycle-independent [12]. The DNA nucleotides dATP, dGTP and dTTP are offered by two separate pathways:

- Salvage pathway.
- Endogenous pathway.

In the endogenous pathway, amino acids, e.g. glycine (for dATP and dGTP) and aspartate (for dTTP), and dihydrofolate are used to produce new nucleotides. But the salvage pathway, as suggested by its name, recycles the purine and pyrimidine nucleosides produced from degradation of nucleic acids. The enzyme TK belongs to the salvage pathway; it phosphorylates thymidine to yield thymidine monophosphate (tdTMP), which is subsequently converted into thymidine triphosphate (dTTP). Thymidine kinase deficient (TK-) cells are killed on hypoxanthine-aminopterin-thymidine (HAT) medium, which contains the DNA nucleosides hypoxanthine and thymidine plus the drug aminopterin. Aminopterin blocks the endogenous pathway of nucleotide production by inhibiting the enzyme dihydrofolate reductase (DHFR), which catalyzes the first reaction in the utilization of dihydrofolate in nucleotide biosynthesis. Additionally, the TK cells are incapable of utilizing the thymidine present in the medium for nucleotide production. Consequently, TK cells die of nucleotide starvation on the HAT medium; thus, the HAT medium acts as a tremendously efficient selection agent for TK cells. The thymidine kinase gene can be utilized as a selectable marker only when TK host cells are utilized for transfection. The transfected cells are cultured on the HAT medium on which only TK+ cells can survive and multiply. The requirement for TK host cells is a serious limitation as it restricts the application of this marker. Consequently, selectable markers with more general applicability to non-mutant animal cell lines have been produced; such markers are known as dominant selectable markers.

5.6.2.2 Dihydrofolate reductase gene amplification

Gene amplification is one of the most frequent signs of genomic instability in human tumors. Additionally they play a significant role in tumor progression and acquisition of drug resistance [13]. Dihydrofolate reductase (DHFR) is an enzyme that decreases dihydrofolic acid to tetrahydrofolic acid production, using nicotinamide adenine dinucleotide phosphate (NADPH) as an electron donor, which can be transformed to the variety of tetrahydrofolate cofactors used in 1-carbon transfer chemistry. The DHFR enzyme (in humans) is encoded by the DHFR gene.

It has been observed that the cultured cells (normal non-mutant) are very responsive to methotrexate (Mtx) at even about 0.1 $\mu g\ ml^{-1}$ [14]. Mtx is a strong non-specific inhibitor of DHFR. This dihydrofolate reductase is also involved in endogenous production of nucleotides dATP, dTTP and dGTP. The Mtx-resistant cell lines developed via selection show one of the following three characteristics:

- Changed DHFR with decreased affinity with Mtx.
- Overproduction of DHFR.
- Reduced Mtx uptake.

In cell lines overproducing DHFR, the related gene is highly amplified, which means it is present in several copies per genome compared to the normal one. This copy number may be up to 1000 per cell which may either be integrated into the genome or be present as extrachromosomal elements known as double minute chromosomes.

5.6.2.3 CAD genes in N-(phosphonacetyl)-L-aspartate

The protein CAD activates the transcription of various target genes. CAD protein (encoded by the gene Cad) is a multifunctional enzyme that is present in various eukaryotes and contains domains for three enzymes of pyrimidine biosynthesis [15]. It catalyzes the first three reactions of endogenous pyrimidine synthesis, out of which one is inhibited by N-phosphonacetyl-L-aspartate (PALA). Most mammalian cells are sensitive to PALA. PALA-resistant cell lines developed through selection overproduce CAD protein due to high amplification of the relevant Cad gene [15, 16]. Cad genes isolated from Syrian hamsters serve as a dominant marker making normal mammalian cells resistant to high concentrations of PALA. This gene, like the DHFR gene, becomes highly amplified in the stably transfected cell lines [15, 16].

5.6.2.4 Xanthine guanine-phosphoribosyltransferase marker gene/mycophenolic acid

The enzyme XGPRT (bacterial) is similar to the mammalian enzyme hypoxanthine guanine-phosphoribosyltransferase (HGPRT) [17]. These salvage pathway enzymes (XGPRT and HGPRT) convert hypoxanthine and inosine monophosphate (IMP) and finally into guanosine monophosphate (GMP). In addition they also convert guanine into GMP, but XGPRT also changes xanthine into xanthine monophosphate and finally into GMP [17]. Normal mammalian cells are very sensitive to mycophenolic acid, which inhibits HGPRT catalyzed conversion of IMP to xanthosine monophosphate (XMP). This sensitivity is drastically increased by the presence of aminopterin, which obstructs endogenous purine biosynthesis. The XGPRT (bacterial) gene, which has been isolated and cloned, acts as a dominant selectable marker on a culture medium containing mycophenolic acid, aminopterin, adenine and xanthine. Ordinary mammalian cells cannot survive as HGPRT is not capable of exploiting xanthine for producing cGMP. Nevertheless, mammalian cells producing bacterial XGPRT can exploit xanthine in the medium to synthesize GMP, and thus are able to stay alive and propagate [17].

5.6.2.5 Neomycin phosphotransferase (selection of transformed organisms)

Neomycin is an aminoglycoside antibiotic present in many topical medications. Neomycin resistance is presented by either one of two aminoglycoside phosphotransferase genes. A neo gene is commonly incorporated into DNA plasmids which are ultimately used by molecular biologists to produce stable mammalian cell lines expressing cloned proteins in culture; many commercially available protein expression plasmids contain neo as a selectable marker. Non-transfected cells will ultimately not survive when the culture is treated with neomycin or similar antibiotics. Neomycin can be used for prokaryotes, however geneticin (G-418) is usually required for eukaryotes. Ordinary mammalian cells are responsive to the aminoglycoside antibiotic G-418 (an analog of neomycin), which obstructs protein synthesis. Neomycin phosphotransferase (encoded by the aph gene of bacterial transposons Tn5 and Tn601) presents resistance to G-418. A variety of constructs (plasmid, cosmid) of the neomycin phosphotransferase gene have been synthesized and utilized for transfection of an array of mammalian cell lines. Transfected cells are efficiently selected for use on a medium containing the antibiotic G-418, which is a dominant selection agent. This marker gene is also functional in yeast and plants.

5.7 Transfection methods using transgenesis techniques: an approach towards mammalian cell transfection

Transgenesis is the introduction of a transgene into another organism through different kinds of genetically engineered techniques, changing the phenotype of an organism. There are three steps in the transgenesis process: identifying, isolating, and transforming.

(1) **Identification**—in this first step, we identify the gene with the specific trait.
(2) **Isolation**—in the second step, The target DNA sequence has been extracted from the ruptured cells, replicated, and injected into the bacterial genome to generate the vectors.
(3) **Transformation**—The last step involves inserting the transgene-carrying vector within the desired animal.

The first step is to identify the gene that carries the particular trait. The second step is to extract the desired DNA sequence from the damaged cells, replicate it, and then inject it into a bacterial genome to create the vectors. Finally, the final step is to insert the transgenic vector into the animal. This is the fundamental process used to create and extract transgenes. Various techniques have been used to insert transgenes into many vertebrate and invertebrate gametes. These transgenes were initially introduced through microinjections, pronuclei, or mass gene transfer in mice. Other methods have also been used, such as ESCs, SMGTs, SCNTs, IVPs, TGMs, and RTDs. Validation of the effectiveness of the transgenesis is done using Western and Southern blots PCR and ELISA.

Different procedures have been used for the transfer of DNA into animal cells/embryos in addition to figure 5.6, which are as follows:

- Calcium phosphate precipitation.
- DEAE-dextran-mediated transfection.
- Direct microinjection.
- Pronuclear microinjection.
- Embryonic stem cells.
- Gene transfers using gametes.
- Sperm-mediated nuclear transfer (SGMT).
- Testis-mediated gene transfer (TGMT).
- Somatic cell nuclear transfer (SCNT).
- Induced pluripotent stem cells (IPCs).
- Lentiviral transduction.

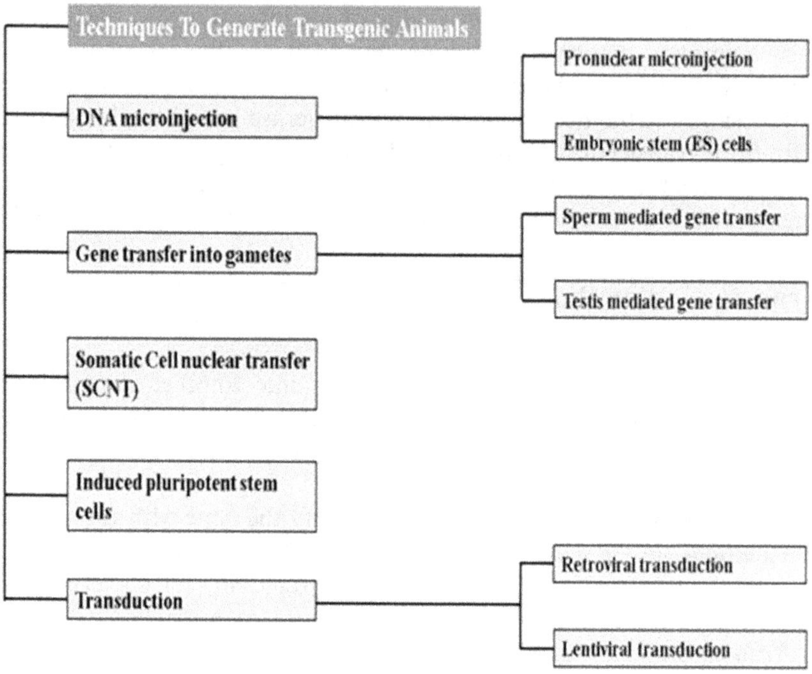

Figure 5.6. Techniques to generate transgenic animals.

- Electroporation.
- Fusion with bacterial protoplasts.
- Lipofection.
- Particle gun delivery.
- Retrovirus infection.

Moreover, transgenic mice are frequently produced by the technique of ES cell transfer (figure 5.9); this is the only alternative that allows targeted gene transfers (section 5.10).

5.7.1 Calcium phosphate-mediated transfection of eukaryotic cells

In this technique, the DNA sample to be used for transfection is initially mixed with a calcium chloride solution. This preparation is then added gradually, with mixing, to a phosphate buffer. This results in the formation of insoluble calcium phosphate, which co-precipitates with the DNA. This final preparation is left undisturbed for 30 min for proper precipitation. It is then allowed to interact with the cells to be transfected. The precipitate particles are taken in by the cells. This process is called phagocytosis (figure 5.6). Initially, 1%–2% of the cells were transfected by this approach. However, the method has now been modified to achieve transfection of up to 20% of the cells. In a small percentage of the transfected cells, the DNA becomes integrated into the cell genome producing stable or permanent transfection. The most favorable final concentration of DNA in the precipitate mixture is around

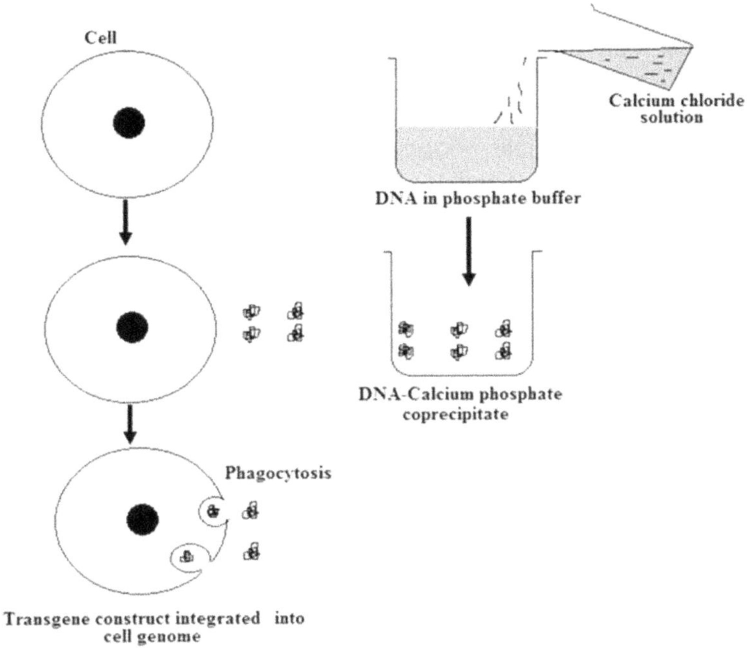

Figure 5.7. A diagrammatic representation of transfection by calcium phosphate precipitation.

20 mg ml^{-1}. This universal approach can be applied to nearly all mammalian cells; moreover, a very large number of cells can be treated with little effort. However, various cell lines do not like the calcium phosphate precipitate adhering to their surfaces or to their substrate (the surface of culture vessels). This is one of the disadvantages of this method (figure 5.7).

Recently this procedure has been utilized by Xu *et al* for SiRNA delivery. Despite the vast therapeutic potential of siRNA as a treatment approach, delivery is still a problem owing to adverse biodistribution profiles and poor intracellular bioavailability [18]. Calcium phosphate (CaP) co-precipitate has been used for almost 40 years for *in vitro* transfection because of its non-toxic nature and ease of preparation [18]. As a result of surface modification CaP will be tuned positive, which is significant for siRNA loading and crossing cell membranes without enzymatic degradation [18].

5.7.2 Transfection using DEAE-dextran

Transfection of cultured mammalian cells using DEAE-dextran/DNA can be a striking alternative to other transfection methods in many conditions. The main merits of this technique are its relative speed and simplicity, limited expense, and extraordinarily reproducible inter experimental and intra experimental transfection competence [19]. Disadvantages include inhibition of cell growth and induction of heterogeneous morphological changes in cells. In addition, the concentration of serum in the culture medium must be quickly reduced during the transfection [19]. Usually, DEAE-dextran DNA transfection is best for transient transfections with promoter/reporter plasmids in analyses of promoter and enhancer functions. In addition it is also suitable for overexpression of recombinant proteins in transient transfections or for the production of stable cell lines using vectors designed to exist in the cell as episomes [19]. Chemically, DEAE-dextran is water soluble and polycationic, i.e. has multiple positive charges. It is added to the transfection solution with DNA. In some unknown way, DEAE-dextran brings about DNA uptake by cells through endocytosis. Perhaps its interaction with negatively charged DNA molecules and with the components of cell surfaces plays a significant role. This protocol is highly suitable for the transient transfection used for different molecular biology investigations mainly using COS cell lines. However, again for some unknown reason, it is not suitable for producing stable transfection.

5.7.3 Lipofection (lipid-mediated DNA transfection method)

A DNA transfection procedure has been developed for delivery of DNA into cells using liposomes that makes use of a synthetic cationic lipid, N-[1-(2,3-dioleyloxy) propyl]-N,N,N-trimethylammonium chloride (DOTMA) [20]. Small unilamellar liposomes containing N-[1-(2,3-dioleyloxy)propyl]-N,N,N-trimethylammonium chloride interact impulsively with DNA to form lipid–DNA complexes, which results in 100% entrapment of the DNA [20]. This synthetic cationic lipid DOTMA allows fusion of the complex with the plasma membrane of tissue culture cells, resulting in both uptake and expression of the DNA. The procedure is simple, highly reproducible and effective for both transient and stable expression of transfected DNA. In this procedure of lipofection, delivery of DNA into cells is achieved using liposomes. Liposomes are small vesicles fabricated from a suitable lipid. In the beginning, non-ionic lipids were used to fabricate liposomes, which required specific DNA encapsulation protocols. Liposome preparation from cationic lipids allows spontaneous and efficient DNA complexation with them. Cationic liposomes have a single lipid bilayer membrane (unilamellar), and they bind to the cells efficiently. Perhaps they bind with the plasma membrane and thus deliver the DNA (complexed with them) into the cells, which brings about transfection [21]. Cationic liposomes complexed with DNA have been used widely as non-viral vectors for the intracellular delivery of reporter or therapeutic genes in culture and *in vivo* [21]. However, the association between the features of the lipid–DNA complexes ('lipoplexes') and their mode of interaction with cells, the efficiency of gene transfer and gene expression remain to be clarified.

Lipofection has different applications for targeting genes to specific human tissues for gene therapy. There are at least eight protocols utilized for preparing liposomes for DNA delivery:

- In one procedure animal virus particles are enclosed in lipoprotein envelopes. In this procedure the desired DNA can be inserted into a viral envelope which is separated from capsid proteins and viral genomes. This vacated space is utilized to pack the desired DNA. The prepared particles are called virosomes. Virosomes have been used to transfect cells *in vitro*, but in most cases the virosomes end up in lysosomes that result in the degradation of up to 80% of the DNA [22].

- Polycationic reagents, e.g. cationic lipids and poly-L-lysine, are extensively used for gene transfer into cells *in vitro* and show promise as vectors for *in vivo* gene therapy applications as non-viral gene transfer techniques [23]. In this procedure DNA is bound with a cationic peptide, e.g. gramicidin, which interacts with lipid membranes in a specific manner. Integration of dioleoyl phosphatidylethanolamine (DOPE) into the complex improves transfection frequency. This method is about ten times more proficient than using cationic lipid liposomes, which itself is about ten times more efficient than pH-sensitive or ionizable liposomes.
- However, other techniques allow the entrapment of large DNA sequences into liposomes, e.g. exposure of the anionic lipid phosphatidyl serine (PS) to Ca2+, and two-phase techniques.

Liposomes prepared by the above two approaches are phagocytosed by the cell. The phagocytosis vesicles thus produced ordinarily fuse with lysosomes leading to DNA degradation and low transfection frequencies.

- The fusion protein of the Sendai virus is inserted into the liposome membrane; this allows the fusion of liposomes with the plasmalemma and thus a direct delivery of DNA into the cytoplasm [24]. A receptor protein is also integrated, which facilitates a controlled delivery of the DNA into the target cells.
- Another way is to target liposomes against cell surface receptors by the insertion of ligand proteins into the liposome membrane. This is possible with the liposomes containing DNA inside the vesicle excluding cationic lipid and cationic peptide-DNA complexes. It has been recently proposed to use biotinylated bis anthracycline (which intercalates in dsDNA) for attachment of specific ligand proteins via avidin to the DNA for delivering cationic lipid/peptide-complexed DNA into specific target cells.
- The use of ionizable lipids that undergo phase change in response to the pH of cytoplasm, e.g. DOPE [25], to construct liposomes (usually, a mixture of DOPE and PC is used), which release DNA into the cytoplasm once they are phagocytosed [25].
- Utilization of cationic liposomes to which DNA binds on the outside by electrostatic attraction is also an excellent strategy. These liposomes cause perturbations in the plasma membrane due to which they attach to them later, and the DNA enters the cytoplasm. Cationic liposomes are available commercially (marketed as 'Lipofectin' by Gibco-BRL). There is a definite development in transfection frequency when a polycationic lipid (Lipofectamine) is utilized in the place of monocationic lipids.
- Generally, liposomes are fabricated by dispersion of a phospholipid-like phosphatidylcholine in water by mechanical methods, such as sonication. DNA of sizes up to 1 kb has been incorporated into small sonicated liposomes.

Viral envelope glycoproteins attach to specific cellular receptors and start fusion with the cell membrane, which permits the penetration of the viral genome into host cells. These two functions, binding and fusion, are mediated by one or multiple envelope glycoproteins [26]. The Sendai viral envelope contains fusion glycoprotein (F-protein) and a haemagglutinin-neuraminidase protein (HN protein). After removal of the HN protein the Sendai virus envelope is reconstituted, because this HN protein targets the envelope of almost all cell types. This reconstituted envelope contains only F-protein; as a result, it is called F-virosome. F-virosomes also have potential in targeted drug delivery to the liver cells. The F-protein arbitrates the fusion of the viral envelope with the cell plasma membrane. Moreover, it confers on F-virosomes a very high specificity for the liver parenchyma cells as they include receptors specific for the F-protein. F-virosomes have been used to transport the reporter genes (chloramphenicol acetyltransferase and firefly luciferase), particularly into the liver parenchyma of mice. The transgenes showed multiple copy random integration, were expressed producing mRNAs and proteins, and have been maintained for six months. F-virosomes transport the DNA directly into the cytoplasm via fusion with cell plasma membranes, and appear 10–12 times more efficient than cationic liposomes in addition to being liver-specific in delivery. Recently, it has been reported that quantitatively reconstituted F-proteins in liposomes (F-virosomes) are very efficient in delivering antineoplastic drugs into tumor cells [27].

Lipofection is the technique of preference for transfection of mammalian cells *in vitro*. It has also been used to transport DNA into live animals by direct injection or intravenous injection. Cationic liposomes have been used for intravenous or intratracheal injection in mice for the expression of marker genes in lungs. Targeted delivery has also been established by inserting specific ligand proteins into the liposome membranes. Efforts are also being made to transport the cystic fibrosis gene via nasal or bronchial tissue for stimulating a cytotoxic T-lymphocyte response in human patients. The actual mechanism of movement of the DNA from the cell cytoplasm into the nucleus is not reported. In a number of cases, DNA movement to the nucleus is greatly assisted by making DNA constructs that are capable of cytoplasmic translation, and by binding them with RNA polymerase or with a gene that fabricates RNA polymerase.

5.7.4 Bacterial protoplast fusion

In bacteria protoplasts can be obtained. Fusion can be carried out with low frequency in some gram positive organisms, while for gram negative bacteria it is possible to obtain protoplasts but regeneration is quite difficult [28]. Bacterial cell walls are removed using lysozyme treatment. Protoplasts fuse to the mammalian cells. In this procedure DNA purification is not required. Bacteria are used to produce plasmids containing the human GOI [28]. The cell walls are removed using lysozyme, resulting in the formation of protoplasts. The protoplasts are brought into contact with the mammalian cells, resulting in protoplast fusion to mammalian cells, using PEG [28]. A schematic presentation of PEG-mediated fusion of protoplasts is depicted in figure 5.8.

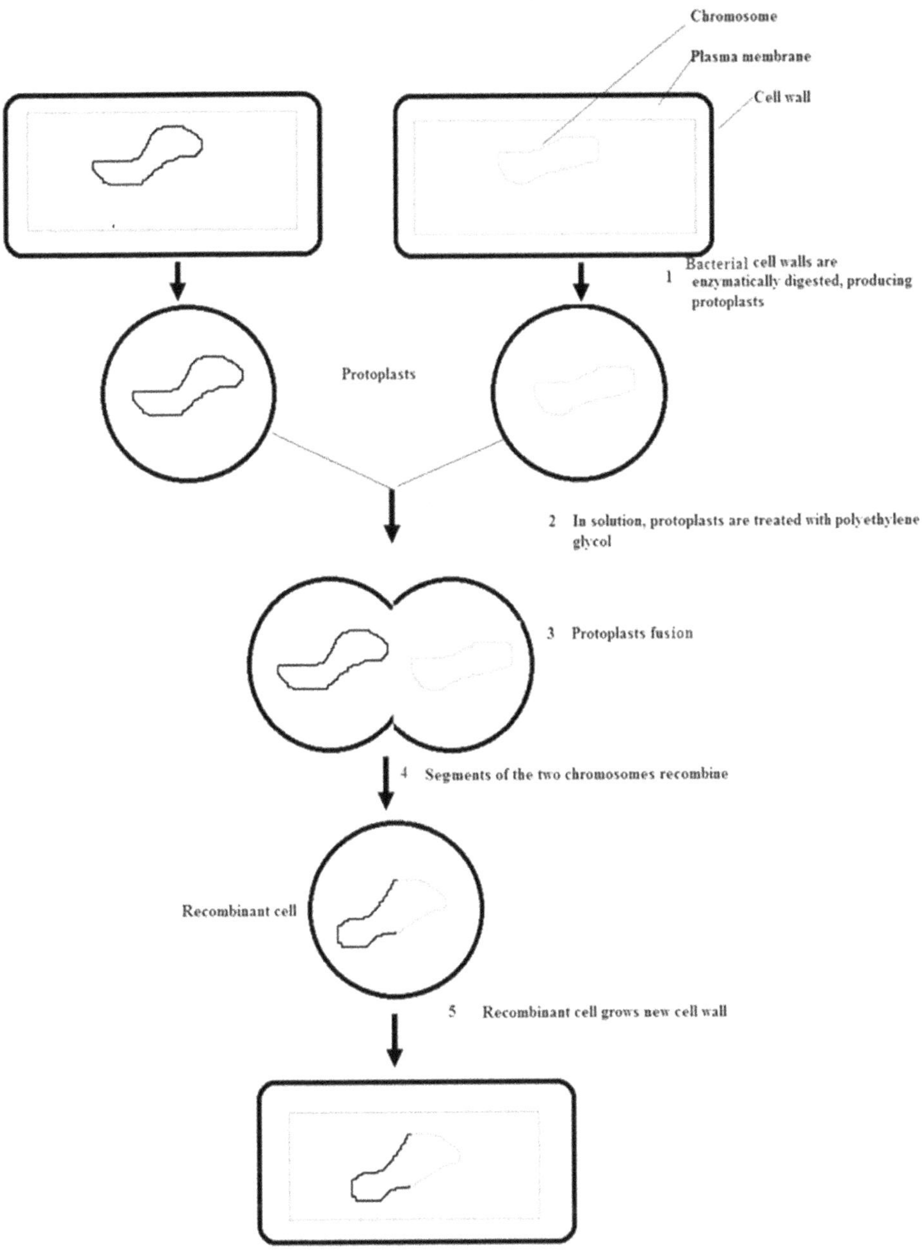

Figure 5.8. PEG-mediated fusion of protoplasts.

5.7.5 Gene transfer by electroporation

In this technique, target cells are exposed (for a very brief period, i.e. a few milliseconds) to short electric pulses of high voltage (e.g. 4000–8000 V cm^{-1}) which leads to the formation of temporary small pores in the cell membrane [29–31]. These pores facilitate the intake of DNA into the protoplast of cells. This procedure is normally performed at room temperature, but the cells are then kept on ice to let the membrane pores remain open for a longer time. This induces transient pores in the cell membranes through which DNA seems to enter the cells. It has been observed that the treatment of cells with colcemid (also known as demecolcine, which is related to colchicine but is less toxic), before they are electroporated enhances the rate of transfection [29–31]. This is most likely owing to the arrest of cells at metaphase and the related absence of a nuclear envelope or to a strange permeability of the plasma membranes. It has also been suggested that linearized DNA is far more competent in transfection than circular supercoiled DNA, perhaps due to the higher rate of integration of linear DNA into the genome. Usually, DNA integration takes place in a low copy number, whereas chemical methods typically result in multiple copy integration per genome. The electroporation method has a general applicability, and many animal cell types that could not be transfected by other techniques were effectively transfected by this approach [29–31].

A single cell electroporation microarray based on a silicon chip of 1 cm^2 has been developed. The chip has 60 circular, cell-sized (20 pm diameter) microelectrodes, each one of which is contacted by a dedicated neutral line [32]. The silicon chip is placed in a plastic chamber designed to hold culture medium. The cells are propagated on the chip surface, and can be individually electroporated by a PC-driven control system. The DNA can be delivered to a number of preselected individual cells within the same culture, at arbitrarily chosen time points, and even sequentially to the same cell. Fujimoto *et al* reported an electroporation microarray for parallel transfer of small interfering RNA into mammalian cells [32]. A schematic presentation of electroporation is demonstrated in figure 5.9.

5.7.6 DNA microinjection

Microinjection is the most common technique used to create transgenic animals. It was first used to create rabbits, pigs and sheep (1980s) before being used to create goats and cows [33]. In biological research, microinjection was first introduced

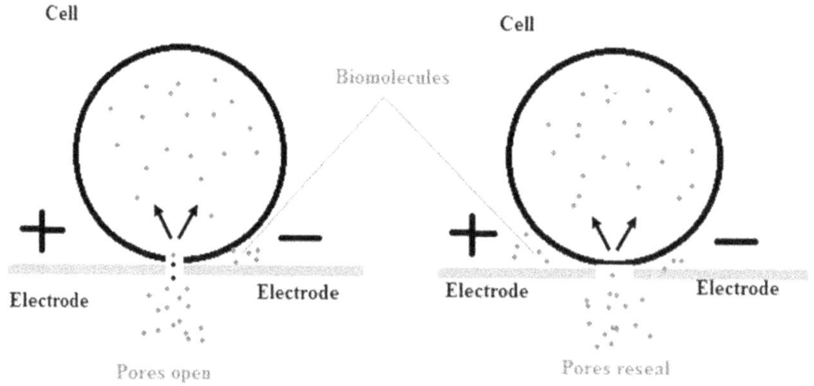

Figure 5.9. Electroporation.

with the addition of a complementary approach (DNA transfection) as it was the most viable method for introducing non-homologous large molecules into living cells. Microneedle injections were introduced into amebae in the late 1800s, Hawkins and Jeon in 1969, and mouse embryos in the late 1950s [34]. This method was later modified to include genetic molecules and was used for other biological studies of organisms. There are two types of microinjection: pronuclear (injecting the desired gene into pronuclei) or embryonic (injecting it into embryo stem cells).

Before talking about microinjection in detail we need to first understand how a transgene is created. A transgene is created in the laboratory using recombinant DNA technology discovered in the 1970s, which involves isolation and modification of genetic material of interest. The transgene is then purified and loaded in a fine glass micropipette, essentially a thin needle. This micropipette's tip is comparable to the point of a needle, making it small enough to pierce the pronucleus' membrane without severely damaging the cell. This is the process of microinjection. The success rate of the DNA microinjection technique is low and varies between organisms.

The nucleic acid delivery to protoplasts or intact cells via microinjection is a labor-intensive protocol that demands pumps, special capillary needles, inverted microscopes, micromanipulators and other equipment. Nevertheless, injection into the nucleus or cytoplasm is possible and cells can be cultured individually. For animal cells, the cells need to be immobilized first (figure 5.10(A)).

The cells are immobilized by:

- The use of a holding pipette which holds the cells using vacuum.
- Attachment of cells to poly-L-lysine coated coverslips.
- Embedding the cells in agarose, agar or sodium alginate.

A glass micropipette is used, with openings of about 0.3 μM in diameter, and is inserted into the animal cell cytoplasm and nucleus with the aid of a micromanipulator device. A syringe-like device is used for the controlled delivery of volume into the animal cell.

At present, the most extensively used technique for producing transgenic mice is the pronuclear microinjection method [35]. In this procedure, a transgenic DNA construct is physically microinjected into the pronucleus of a fertilized egg. The injected embryos are then transferred into the oviducts of pseudo-pregnant surrogate mothers. In this method, the optimum DNA solution is injected directly into the nucleus of a cell or into the male pronucleus of a fertilized one—to two-cell ovum. In general, microinjection equipment consists of a low-power stereoscopic dissecting microscope (to examine the ovum and the complete course of development) and two micromanipulators (one for a glass micropipette to grasp the ovum by partial suction and the other for a glass injection needle to insert the DNA into the male pronucleus). The male pronucleus is selected for microinjection as it is much larger than the female pronucleus of fertilized mammalian ova. However, in fish ova, the DNA is introduced into the egg cytoplasm. The usual protocol for microinjection is as follows (figure 5.11(A)) [36]. Donor females are encouraged to superovulate using

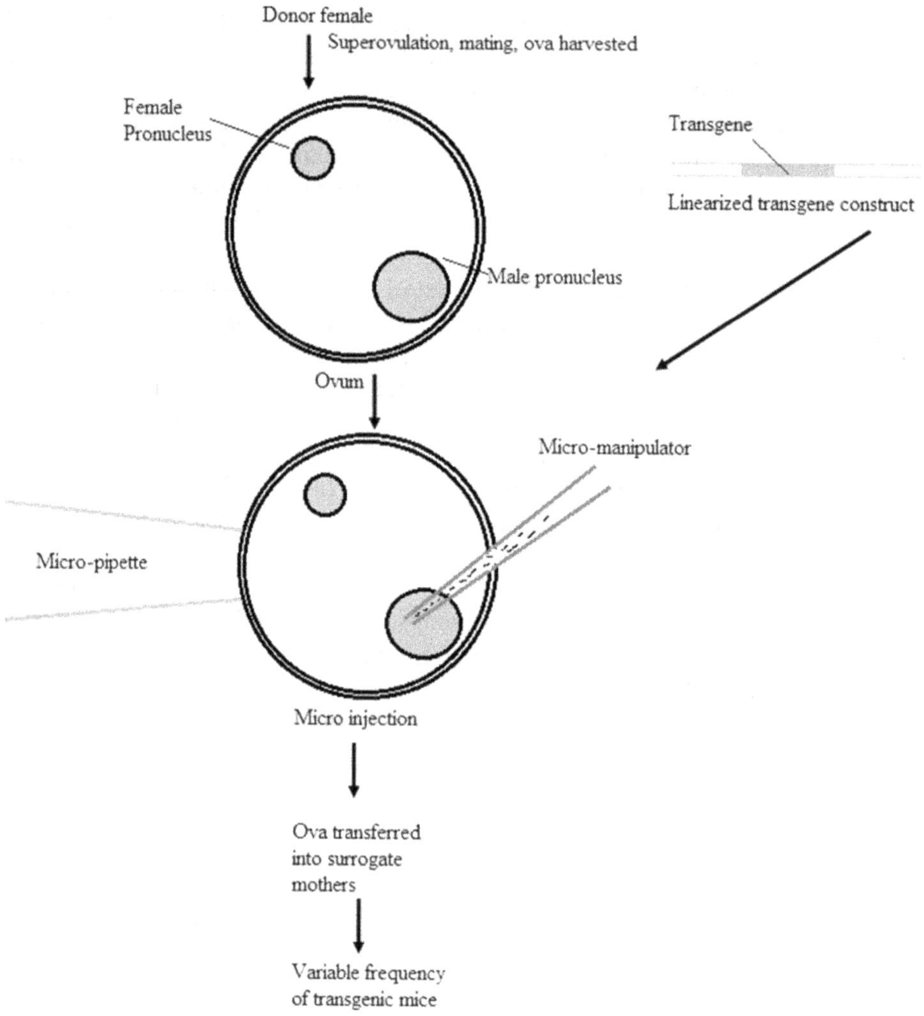

Figure 5.10. (A) Simple representation of the microinjection technique of transfection for producing transgenic animals. (B) Pronuclear microinjection in a fertilized oocyte, similar to microinjection.

suitable hormonal therapy. Female mice are subjected to a regime of pregnant mare serum gonadotropin, which encourages growth and development of follicles that contain the developing oocytes. Ovulation is stimulated by consequent treatment with hCG [36]. The superovulated females are then mated with fertile males, and large numbers of fertilized one—to two-cell ova/embryos are collected surgically. Alternatively, unfertilized ova are collected from superovulated females and the ova are then fertilized *in vitro*. The transgene construct (consisting of the promoter, intron, protein coding sequence (cDNA) from a GOI, poly (A) sequence and enhancer sequences) is prepared in a buffer solution and then introduced into the male pronuclei of fertilized eggs using a microinjection assembly. Normally, 2 pl (1 pl $= 10^{-9}$ ml) of the DNA solution is incorporated into a pronucleus. But in the

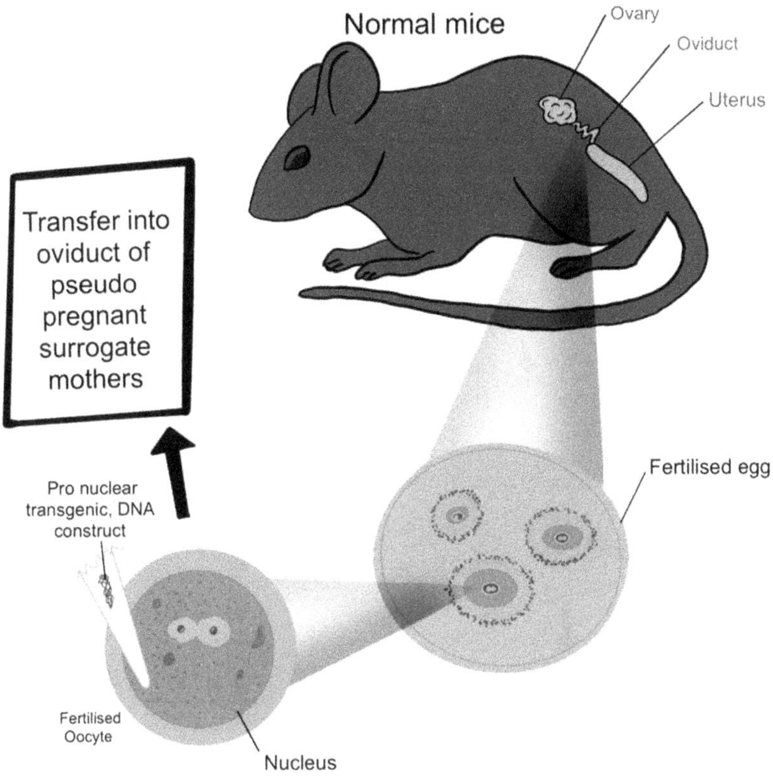

Figure 5.10. (Continued.)

case of fish, 20 nl (1 nl = 10^{-6} ml) of DNA solution, containing 10^6–10^8 linearized transgene constructs, is introduced into the cytoplasm of a single ovum. In the case of mice, the microinjected embryos are initially propagated *in vitro* up to the morula or blastocyst stage. The existing embryos are then shifted into the uterus of surrogate mothers (i.e. females which have been made receptive or synchronized by hormonal therapy); these embryos develop to full term and develop into normal mice (figure 5.8). A proportion of the progeny produced will be transgenic, in that all their cells will contain the transgene stably integrated into their genomes. In the case of fish, the microinjected embryos are incubated in water until hatching.

Microinjection of bacterial plasmids or linear copies of genes into the nuclei of mammalian cells is the most effective way of transferring new genes. Since this breakthrough in the early 1990s, the use of virus vectors has not become prevalent. Gordon *et al* [37] reported a recombinant plasmid composed of segments of HSV and SV40 viral DNA which was inserted into the bacterial plasmid pBR322 and then further microinjected into the pronuclei of fertilized mouse oocytes.

In mice, an average of about 3%–6% (range 3%–40%) of the progeny derived from microinjected embryos are transgenic; the frequency is much lower in other animals, e.g. it is <1% in sheep and pigs. In the case of fish, about 35%–80% of the

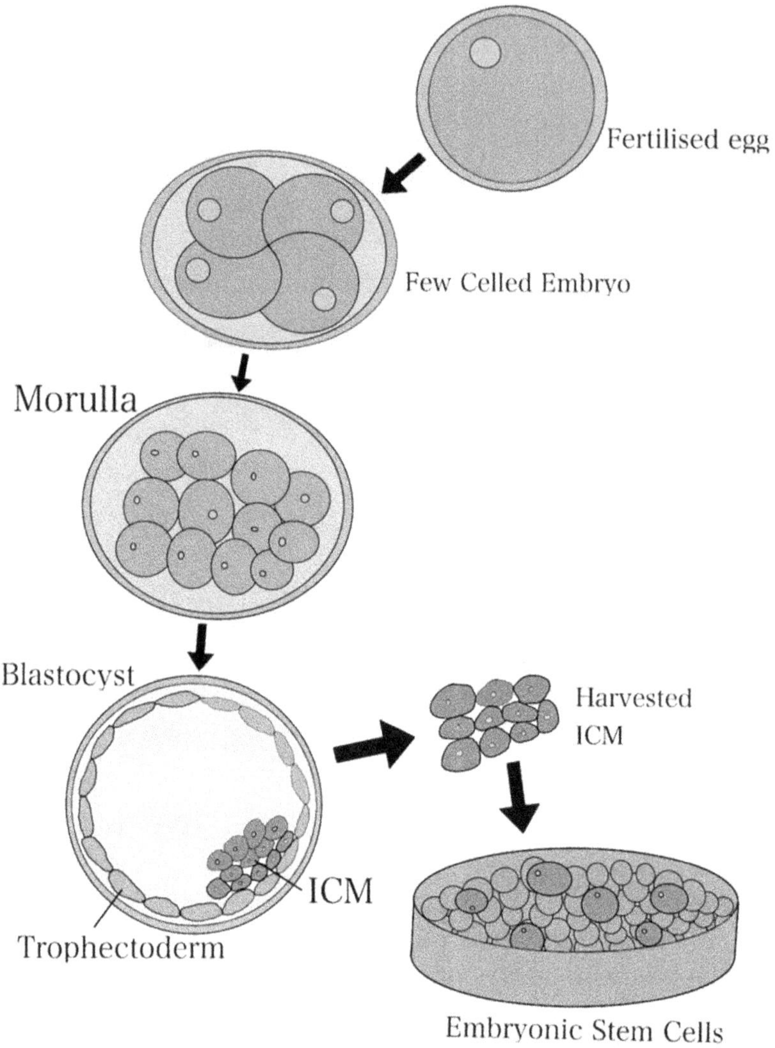

Figure 5.11. Culturing of Embryonic stem cells from inner mass cell(ICM).

embryos survive microinjection, of which 10%–70% may be transgenic. The transgenic animals contain the transgene in their germ cells and, as a consequence, pass it on to their progeny; transgenes show typical Mendelian inheritance.

The transgene incorporation takes place at random sites in the genome, but in a given cell or embryo generally only a single chromosomal site is involved. Nevertheless, there is usually a broad variation in the number of copies incorporated, ranging from the common single copy to several hundreds of copies. The several copies are incorporated at a single site in a head-to-tail arrangement. As a result, the site of addition of a transgene in different transgenic animals varies significantly and may occupy diverse sites of the same chromosome or different chromosomes. The transgene integration takes place at an early stage of embryo development following microinjection, and generally all the cells of an embryo are involved. However, often the integration may be postponed, and the transgene remains in the extrachromosomal state during this period. Afterwards, transgene integration takes place only in some cells of the embryo which results in chimeric progeny.

All the transfection techniques apply to cultured animal cells, but microinjection is normally not used owing to the tediousness of the technique and the inadequate number of cells that can be handled. For the transfection of mice embryos, the ideal techniques are microinjection, retroviral infection, and ES cell technology; however, microinjection is the most commonly used. The benefit of using the microinjection technique is that there is no limit to the size of the DNA fragment that can be injected. This allows even a small and accurate amount of foreign DNA into the genome. The limitation of using this technique is that it is highly labor intensive. Embryos of other animals are generally transfected by the microinjection techniques. In the case of fish embryos, microinjection and electroporation are routinely employed.

5.7.7 Pronuclear microinjection (PM)

PM is a powerful tool that has significantly advanced our understanding of genetics and facilitated many applications in biotechnology and scientific research. It is a highly precise technique used in introducing foreign genes, known as transgenes into the genome of an organism. This method was widely used for the production of transgenic mice. It was discovered in the early 1900s by Barber. Recent development in technology has helped us to successfully generate transgenic, knockout, conditional knockout, and knock-in mice to elucidate the precise functions of desired genes implicating diseases and developments [38]. The essence of this technique is the physical injection of a transgenic DNA construct into the pronucleus of a fertilized oocyte. The injected embryos are then transferred into the oviducts of the pseudopregnant surrogates' mothers for development into viable individuals, as shown in figure 5.10(B).

The process begins with the fertilization of an egg cell or ovum. After fertilization, two distinct pronuclei are formed in the zygote, one in sperm and another in the ovum. Each nucleus belongs to the parental gametes, containing half of the genetic information for the development of the organism [39]. Generation of transgenic mice from pronuclear microinjection technique involves five basic steps:

1. Purification (gel-purification method).
2. Harvesting.
3. Pronuclear microinjection.
4. Implantation.
5. Genotyping and analysis of transgene.

Step 1. Purification of transgenic construct

- Preparation of a clean DNA sample for better health of embryo and DNA integration efficiency.

- Make sure the DNA fragment that is going to be microinjected is without any trace of vector sequence.
- Similarly, chemical residues that remain in the final DNA solution are generally toxic to mouse zygotes, as they lead to embryonic death and reduced efficiency in producing transgenic mice.
- Dissolve the final purified DNA in the microinjection buffer and centrifuge to remove any impurities right before the microinjection of the sample.
- In case of larger DNA constructs such as Bacterial artificial chromosomes (BAC) use a specialized buffer solution.
- For DNA purification largely sucrose gradient or gel purification method is used.

Step 2. Harvesting donor zygotes

- To obtain the maximum number of donor zygotes all egg-donor female mice need to be superovulated.
- These female mice are injected with PMSG (pregnant mare serum gonadotropin) and HCG (human chorionic gonadotropin) before mating with breeding mice.
- This routine helps in harvesting 17 zygotes from 1 superovulated female mouse.
- The donor mouse strain we usually use is FVB/N.

Step 3. Microinjection of transgenic construct

For increased chance of integration into the host genome and successful transfer of foreign DNA, these steps should be evaluated carefully.

- Dilute the purified DNA to obtain optimal DNA concentration.
- Use an appropriate concentration of DNA for the microinjection, because if the concentration is too high it may cause zygotes to lyse, and if the DNA concentration is too low it may yield poor or no integration of DNA.
- The injection pressure should be low enough not to damage the DNA.
- Constant flow rate is important to deliver the DNA using an automated microinjector since it shows many benefits.
- Gently inject the DNA to minimize the trauma to the zygote.
- As soon as you can, puncture the membranes surrounding the zygote and pronucleus to prevent introducing DNA into the cytoplasm.
- The timing of microinjection should be approximately 12 h after conception to allow sufficient time for the pronuclei of the microinjected fertilized eggs to prepare for fusion to begin the first round of cell division.

Step 4. Implantation of microinjected zygotes into the pseudo-pregnant mice

- Locate the funnel, which is the opening of the fallopian tube into which the microinjected fertilized egg must be carefully transferred.
- Avoid rupturing the blood vessels and for successful embryo transfer.
- The embryo transfer can be done on the harvesting day too after culturing zygotes to the two-cell stage overnight.

Step 5. Genotyping and analysis of transgene expression in founder mice

- The pregnant mice are now ready to deliver the pups within 20 days.
- For individual analysis of transgene, all the mice are kept separately before day 17.
- After the birth of pups they should be monitored regularly for any abnormal growth.
- After 10 days postpartum, a tissue biopsy, either a small piece of tail or a piece of ear, will need to be performed for genotyping purposes to identify the transgenic mice.
- To identify the tissue of the mouse, the mouse finger is pierced with a 30-G needle that has been dyed with tattoo paste.

This is how the pronuclear microinjection is performed. The benefits of using pronuclear microinjection are:

1) It has a highly precise delivery of a small amount of DNA in the germline.
2) There is no limitation on the length of DNA injected.

5.7.7.1 Limitations

1) It is a highly challenging technique and labor intensive.
2) It can only be used for small-scale production since the whole work is done in the laboratory (*in vitro*) by specialized professionals.
3) It is not as efficient as other discovered techniques in comparison with them.

5.7.7.2 Conclusion

To complete the above steps, pronuclear injection involves harvesting the zygote while it is still in the zygote stage. Using a very fine glass microinjection needle, a picoliter of injection solution is injected into one of the pronuclei. The injected embryos are then transferred into the fallopian tubes of the surrogate mother of the transgenic animal. The time required for PM is typically between 1 h and 1 day after fertilization [34]. The successful development of pronuclear microinjection methods has been cited as a perfect example of the integration of recombinant DNA technology with the culture and manipulation of mammalian embryos. Microinjection using an injector uses a constant flow feature because as long as the injection time is the same for each zygote, it can ensure that each zygote receives the same amount of DNA solution. This is also helpful for the operator, as he does not have to press the injection button every time for each fertilized egg. This approach requires a lot of patience and practice to produce transgenic mice competently and effectively.

5.7.8 Embryonic stem cells (ES cells)

Embryonic stem cells are simply undifferentiated cells that can develop into all three embryonic tissue layers (somatic and germ cells), leading to the formation of a complete organism [40]. These stem cells dwell within the cell mass interior of an animal's blastocyst, an early stage of embryonic improvement that keeps going four to seven days after fertilization. ES cells are removed from the internal mass at the blastocyst stage and can be cultured in the laboratory under *in vitro* conditions, facilitating long-term storage (figure 5.11).

Historically, the discovery of ES cells was made by chance in 1974 when researchers Martin and Evans were studying pluripotent embryonal cancer. A few years later, in 1989, Capech's ES cells were used for gene targeting in homologous recombination. This technique has proven to be the most powerful transgenic technique as it allows mutagenesis of all genes in the genome.

The technical requirements of an ES cell technique are a dissecting microscope equipped with both a transmit and incident light source, some basic fine surgical instruments, and a germline-compatible ES cell line. And once the culture is made it is stored in appropriate conditions since it shows a remarkable ability to self-renew continuously. The culture conditions of ES cells do not require any specific medium or solution, it has a standardized solution preparation. Though the support of an ES cell culture requires customary passaging and part in particular proportions onto unused tissue culture plates.

To make the ES cell culture we need high glucose supplemented with 2 mM L − glutamine + 100μM β− mercaptoethanol + 1 mM sodium pyruvate + 0.1 mM non-essential amino acid + 15% fetal calf serum + 1000 U ml^{-1} LIF. The following procedure is for a 10-cm-diameter tissue culture plate.

Step 1 Preparation of culture media

- Aspirate the ES cell medium from the plate and then wash the plate with a phosphate-buffer solution.
- Replace PBS with trypsin solution and incubate the plate for 5 min at 37 °C. During this time the clumps should lift up from the bottom of the plate and the cells become loosely connected.
- Stop the action of trypsin by adding ES cell medium to the plate and transferring the cells to a centrifuge tube.
- Centrifuge them for 5 min.
- Aspirate the supernatant and gently introduce the residue into 5–7 ml ES cells.
- Divide the cell suspension into prepared tissue culture medium—at a ratio of 1:5 to 1:7.
- Place the plates back into a humidified C02 incubator for culture.
- Repeat steps 1–7 every other day or every 3 days, depending on the particular medium. Plates contain 10 ml of ES medium.

Step 2 Introducing DNA into and selecting for genetically altered ES cells

- The simplest approach for producing genetically modified ES cells requires electroporating exogenous DNA into the cells and then choosing an integration into the genome.
- We usually need 100,000,000–1,000,000,000 cells ES cells, depending on the project.

- Prepare vector DNA, linearize, purify by ethanol precipitation, and adjust concentration to 1 ml of water.
- Trypsinize the cells as for passaging, but resuspend the final pellet in ice-cold PBS. Count cells and adjust their concentration to 7×10^6 ml^{-1} in PBS.
- Add 10–40 pl DNA and 790–760 pl cell suspension into a 0.8-ml electroporation cuvette.
- Repeat step 5 depending on the number of planned electroporations.
- Typically, this number is 1 or 2 for regular gene transfer and 10–15 for gene targeting or gene trap experiments. Using an electroporator, such as the Bio-Rad GenePulser, discharge 500 pF at 250 V through the cuvette.
- Place the cuvette on ice for 15–20 min. Transfer the cell suspension from the cuvette to the ES cell medium and plate one cell cuvette onto two 10 cm tissue culture plates. The plate may be a gelatinized or drug-resistant feeder cell plate. Culture the cells for 1 or 2 days in a normal ES cell medium.
- Begin selection by adding selection agents to the medium. The concentration of drug should be the lowest concentration that completely kills non-resistant cells

Pro tip: when LIF is added to the culture stem cells stay undifferentiated. When LIF is not added to the culture stem cells can differentiate into any type of cell.

This technique was successfully used in producing many transgenic animals including a chimera monkey produced through embryonic stem cells with fluorescent fingertips in 2023. Major benefits of using the ES cell technique are:

(1) Modification can be done directly in the genome *in vitro* to introduce changes.
(2) Approachable technique for mutagenesis used in embryonic development and disease conditions study.
(3) Gives the advantage of transferring ES cells by surgical or non-surgical methods.

5.7.8.1 Limitations

1. Microinjection of ES cells into embryos is often characterized by low efficiency. Not all injected cells may successfully integrate into the host embryo, leading to a low percentage of animals that actually become transgenic.
2. Microinjection can result in mosaic animals where only a subset of cells carry the transgene. This variability can affect the reliability and consistency of transgene expression in the generated animals.

5.7.8.2 Conclusion

To conclude the whole technique you need to start with the preparation of the ES culture medium, then wash the ES cells off. After washing, we need to dissociate the ES cells with trypsin. Right after dissociating, we need to immediately freeze them for the long run. To manipulate embryos on the bench we need to make an M2 medium. To culture embryos, we need to extract them from the M16 medium. Finally, we need to remove zona pellucida with the help of acid tyrodes. After following these protocols our embryonic stem cells are ready for transfer to a host organism for producing transgenic animals.

5.7.9 Mass gene transfer using gametes

Gametes are presented since they are normally secured against foreign invasion. After all, certain proteins within the plasma or plasma layer avoid the passage of remote qualities into sperm. Mass gene transfer using gametes involves using sperm to carry a gene construct into an ovum during fertilization. Gametes would develop some kind of mechanisms that modify the expression of transgenes, or that block the expression of transgenes. The concept of mass gene transfer has been around for centuries, but it was not until the 20th century that scientists began to understand the mechanisms involved.

In 1928, Frederick Griffiths helped in the discovery of horizontal gene transfer by conducting a series of experiments showing that bacteria could transmit genetic information to each other through a process called transformation. Horizontal gene transfer (HGT), is the method by which hereditary material is exchanged between living beings by means other than sexual reproduction.

HGT occurs through different mechanisms such as transformation, conjugation, and transduction. Transformation occurs when naked DNA is introduced into a recipient cell. Conjugation occurs when two cells form a physical connection and pass genetic material to each other. During transduction, bacteria (viruses that infect bacteria) transfer genetic material from one bacterium to another. HGT is a common phenomenon in the natural world and has played a major role in the evolution of all forms of life. It is estimated that up to 20% of the genes in the human genome have been acquired through HGT.

5.7.9.1 Involvement of mass gene transfer

Mass gene transfer is the process of transferring large amounts of genetic material from one organism to another. This can be done through a variety of methods, including:

- **Electroporation:** This method uses electrical pulses to create pores in the cell membrane, allowing DNA to enter the cell.
- **Microinjection:** This method uses a needle to inject DNA directly into the cell.
- **Lipofection:** This method uses liposomes, which are small vesicles made of lipids, to deliver DNA into the cell.

Viral vectors: This method uses viruses to deliver DNA into the cell.

The procedure for mass gene transfer varies depending on the method used. However, the general steps are as follows:

- Prepare the DNA: The DNA that will be transferred must be prepared in a way that makes it suitable for the chosen method. This may involve purifying the DNA, fragmenting it, or attaching it to a carrier molecule.

- Prepare the recipient cells: The recipient cells must be prepared to receive the DNA. This may involve making them more permeable to DNA or making them more susceptible to infection by viruses.
- Transfer the DNA: The DNA is transferred to the recipient cells using the chosen method.
- Select for successful gene transfer: The recipient cells are then selected for those that have successfully taken up the DNA. This can be done using a variety of methods, such as antibiotic selection or genetic screening.

The success rate of mass gene transfer varies depending on the method used and the type of cells being transfected. However, in general, the success rate is relatively low. This is because DNA is a large molecule that is difficult to get into cells. Additionally, the cells must be in the right state to receive the DNA.

Despite the low success rate, mass gene transfer is a powerful tool for genetic engineering. It allows scientists to introduce new genes into cells, which can be used to study gene function, develop new therapies, and create new organisms.

MGT (metagenomics) is a powerful tool for studying the microbiome, the community of microorganisms that live in and on our bodies. It has several major benefits, like an unbiased view of the microbiome: MGT does not require prior knowledge of the organisms present in a sample, so it can provide an unbiased view of the microbiome. This is in contrast to traditional culture-based methods, which can only detect organisms that can grow in the laboratory. MGT can detect very low levels of organisms, making it a valuable tool for studying rare or unculturable microorganisms. It can be used to study any environment: MGT can be used to study the microbiome of any environment, including the human body, soil, water, and air. It can provide insights into the role of the microbiome in health and disease: MGT has been used to study the role of the microbiome in a variety of diseases, including cancer, inflammatory bowel disease, and autism.

5.7.9.2 Limitations

Despite its many benefits, there are also some limitations to MGT. These include:

1. High cost: MGT is a relatively expensive technique, which can make it difficult to use for large-scale studies.
2. Complex data analysis: MGT generates a large amount of data, which can be difficult to analyze.
3. Potential for bias: MGT can be biased by the methods used to collect and prepare samples.

5.7.9.3 Conclusion

MGT is a powerful tool for studying the microbiome, with a number of major benefits. However, it is important to be aware of its limitations. As the cost of MGT decreases and data analysis methods improve, it is likely to become an even more valuable tool for understanding the role of the microbiome in health and disease.

5.7.10 Sperm-mediated gene transfer

Sperm-mediated gene transfer (SMGT) was developed as an alternative technique for the production of transgenic animals. This method is predicated on the sperm's capacity to *in vitro* ensnare target exogenous genes as DNA molecules and transfer them to the fertilized egg cell [41]. Thus, it is possible to introduce new genetic material into the embryo's genome to alter how particular genes are expressed in the progeny and in future generations. Sperm DNA absorption is a highly specialized and tightly controlled process.

SMGT was developed in 1989 as an alternative technique for producing transgenic animals [42]. It has been successfully used in several species, including echinoids and mammals. Sperm cells can function as vectors in an external genetic sequence, according to recent advancements in SMGT. The ultimate destiny of the foreign sequences transported by sperm is not always predictable, despite a substantial body of research suggesting that SMGT may be useful in animal transgenesis.

In certain cases, integrated foreign sequences have been found through analysis of SMGT-derived offspring, but in other cases, stable genome modifications are hard to find. It is possible that inheritance is extrachromosomal due to the occurrence of SMGT-derived modified offspring and the rarity of actual genome modification. Different steps in SMGT are mediated by a number of distinct factors that have been identified. Among them, an endogenous reverse transcriptase with retrotransposon origin plays a significant role. Although mature spermatozoa are naturally shielded from foreign nucleic acid molecules, certain environmental factors, like those present during human-assisted reproduction, can eliminate this defense. It is important to give careful thought to the possibility that sperm cells in these circumstances harbor genetic sequences that compromise the identity or integrity of the host genome. These considerations further suggest the possibility that SMGT events may occasionally take place in Nature, with profound implications for evolutionary processes [43].

It involves the development of an alternative technique for the production of transgenic animals.

There are four steps in the gene transfer:

1. Isolation (by PCR).
2. Digestion (by restriction endonuclease).
3. Ligation (by DNA ligase).
4. Selection and expression.

Step 1: Isolating gene and vector

- Extraction of DNA from cells with the help of centrifugation.
- Amplify the gene of interest by PCR.
- Reverse transcriptase is used to create gene sequences from mRNA; these DNA sequences, or cDNA, are devoid of introns.
- A DNA molecule called a vector is employed to transfer an gene of interest into an alien cell.
- Because bacterial plasmids can replicate and express themselves on their own, they are frequently utilized as vectors.
- Other types of vectors include modified viruses and artificial chromosomes.

- For additional functionality, these plasmids can be altered (e.g. selection markers, reporter genes, inducible expression promoters).

Step 2: Digestion with restriction enzymes

- The sugar-phosphate backbone is broken down by restriction enzymes to produce sticky or blunt ends (complementary overhangs).
- In order to guarantee that the gene is inserted in the right orientation and to stop the vector from re-annealing without the required insert, scientists frequently cleave the vector and gene using two distinct 'sticky end' restriction endonucleases (double digestion).

Step 3: Ligation of vector and insert

- Using the same restriction endonucleases, the target gene is introduced into a plasmid vector.
- This happens as a result of complementary base pairing between the sticky ends of the gene and the vector.
- The recombinant construct is created by splicing the gene and vector together using the DNA ligase enzyme.
- DNA ligase forms a covalent phosphodiester connection between the sugar-phosphate backbones of the vector and the gene to bind them together.

Step 4: Selection and expression

- The intended gene-containing recombinant construct is then introduced into the appropriate host cell or organism.
- This process, known as transformation in prokaryotes or transfection in eukaryotes, can be accomplished in a number of ways.
- To determine whether cells have effectively assimilated the recombinant design, antibiotic selection is frequently employed.
- Antibiotic-resistant genes are present in the plasmid vector, which means that only transgenic cells will proliferate when antibiotics are present.
- After being separated and refined, transgenic cells ought to start expressing the desired characteristic that the target gene encodes.

The success rate of the mice experiment would be controversial because, from a number of experiments, 13 host mice produced only a total of 7.4% of fetuses, which was still considered to be a success.

5.7.10.1 Limitations

1. Although the effectiveness of sperm-mediated DNA transfer in mice has been questioned, it has the potential to significantly simplify the generation of transgenic animals.
2. We conducted a comprehensive, cooperative study of sperm-mediated DNA transfer to mouse eggs in well-established laboratory conditions for *in vitro* fertilization and offspring development after embryo transfer in order to identify the fundamental causes of the variability of the process in mice [44].

5.7.10.2 Conclusion

First thought was given to the idea of utilizing sperm to introduce foreign DNA into an oocyte during fertilization. Following DNA uptake, Brackett and colleagues showed how spermatozoa can transfer viral DNA into rabbit oocytes. Since sperm is used as a DNA carrier to create transgenic animals in a variety of species, the argument has become less contentious. These consist of *Xenopus*, cattle, chicken, fish, pigs, and mice. For sperm-mediated gene transfer to successfully produce transgenic animals, three essential steps must be followed. DNA binds to the sperm cell surface in the first step, then foreign DNA is internalized into the nucleus, and lastly exogenous DNA is integrated. The process has been better understood in recent years despite the fact that the mechanics behind each phase are still not entirely known [45].

5.7.11 Testis-mediated gene transfer (TMGT)

Using testis-mediated gene transfer (TMGT) [46], foreign DNA can be directly inserted into the testes, enabling mass gene transfer to progeny through mating. In this study, we combined plasmid DNA (pEGFP-N1) with liposome (Lipofectin), dimethyl sulfoxide (DMSO), or N, N-dimethylacetamide (DMA) in an effort to enhance TMGT. To produce F0 progeny, males who had successive injections of DNA complexes were mated to females who were normal. RT-PCR, PCR, and *in vivo* assessment of EGFP expression were utilized to find exogenous DNA expression and presence in the progeny. Histological techniques were also used to assess potential testicular damage. The PCR and RT-PCR data demonstrated that liposome and DMSO increased the rate of TMGT. Histological analyses revealed that spermatogenesis can be impacted by four consecutive injections of DNA complexes. Of the reagents tested, DMSO was the most harmful. In this investigation, we found that the progeny had a transgene and that blood cells expressed the gene.

In past years [46], the use of spermatozoa for gene transfer in transgenic animal technologies has been investigated, and many methods have been employed around it. The first report by Brackett *et al* that foreign DNA might be inserted into sperm around 1971. According to a number of studies conducted on various species, spermatozoa can be used as vectors to transfer foreign DNA to the ova in order to create transgenic animals. TMGT, which enables spontaneous mating and mass gene transfer, is one method of SMGT. It involves directly inserting foreign DNA into the testes. The utilization of other techniques like embryo transfer (ET) and *in vitro* fertilization (IVF) is excluded by this technique. By directly injecting a DNA solution into the testes surgically and then using '*in vivo* ' electroporation to enhance the uptake of foreign DNA by epididymal epithelial cells, Vasicek *et al* [47] demonstrated this technique. De Los Campos *et al* [48] used TMGT to show how the present generation of mice and rabbits is produced. DMSO/DNA combination is surgically injected into the testes to enhance sperm cell uptake of foreign DNA. In addition, transgenesis was demonstrated by

Dhup and Majumdar [49] via permanent integration of genes in repopulating mice spermatogonial cells *in vivo.*

5.7.11.1 Animals

Five sets of three to six-month-old male BALB/c mice were employed. Following therapy, each male paired up with two BALB/c females [46].

5.7.11.2 Transfection solutions

Twenty micrograms of circular eukaryotic expression vector pEGFP-N1 (Clontech, USA) complexed with three different transfectants: DMSO 3%, DMA 3%, and Lipofectin 3%, all diluted in phosphate-buffered saline (PBS), pH 7.2, were used.

5.7.11.3 Non-surgical testis injection

Before the testis was injected, the animals were sedated. The testes were revealed in the scrotal sack by digital pressure in the abdomen, and the points of the fangs were secured to avoid retraction during the injection. 70% ethanol was used to accomplish the scrotal sack asepsis. To put it briefly, each testis was progressively injected with 30 μl of each previously described solution using a 30-G needle into the scrotal sack at a depth of 3–5 mm. The needle was linked to a 1-ml plastic disposable syringe. To prevent injection fluid leaking, the needle was carefully removed after injection. The two tests had injections. Each male mated with two BALB/c females for one week without superovulation, starting twenty-four hours after injection. The same men underwent this process three times a week, but this time they mated with different females. detection of pEGFP vectors Blood was drawn 60 days postpartum using the PureLinkTM Genomic DNA Purification Kit (Invitrogen®, USA) to extract DNA. A 500 bp segment was amplified using EGFP-specific oligonucleotides (5′-CG ACTTTCCAAAATGT CG-3′and 5′-GAAGATGGTGCGCTCCTGGA-3′) in a polymerase chain reaction to identify the presence of vector DNA.

5.7.11.4 Detection of EGFP expression

Using the GFsP-5 mining lamp and goggles (BLS, Hungary), which are goggle systems with a filter set to detect EGFP fluorescence and a light to excite protein fluorescence (excitation maximum = 488 nm; emission maximum = 507 nm), *in vivo* EGFP fluorescence was measured after birth. Moreover, EGFP expression was assessed by RT-PCR. RNA extraction was done on blood samples that were obtained for PCR analysis. Before being analyzed, the blood was frozen and kept in liquid nitrogen. The methods for cDNA synthesis and total RNA extraction were as previously mentioned [50]. TRIzol Reagent was used to isolate RNA samples from bedding and samples were DNase-treated with the manufacturer's instructions using a DNA-free® kit. The manufacturer's instructions were followed to perform first-strand cDNA synthesis using a High Capacity cDNA Reverse Transcription Kit and 200 ng of RNA. Two primer sets were utilized in RT-PCR reactions: EGFP (5′ CACGTCATTTTCCTGCTGCAT3′ and 5′ GCATAGCGGCTCGTAGAGGTA 3′—product with 209 bp) and β-actin (5′TCGCTGCGCTGGTCGTCG3′ and 5′ GCCAGATCTTCTCCATGTCGTCCCA 3′—product with 246 bp).

5.7.11.5 Damage analyses

The males were sacrificed seven days following the last injection, and the testes were removed. They were then fixed in Bouin's fixative for twenty-four hours at four degrees Celsius, and the normal histology protocol was followed. Each testis was sectioned into 5–6 μm thick sections and stained with hematoxylin-eosin (HE). Each of the three testis regions and each of the three slides was assessed.

PCR analysis indicated the presence of a pEGFP-N1 vector in all the treatments administered to multiple mice that were born after being mated with males subjected to TMGT [46]. Greater gene transfer was achieved with liposomes and DMSO than with DNA by itself with DMA. In the PCR assay, none of the mice born in the control group had pEGFP-N1 vector presence. No mice were found to exhibit *in vivo* EGFP fluorescence; yet, RT-PCR examination of PCR-positive animals revealed EGFP expression in blood samples in several animals across all treatment groups. The lipofection group had a higher ratio of animals expressing EGFP in comparison to other groups.

The major benefits of utilizing TMGT are that it empowers the distinguishing proof of unused medicate targets and moves forward the approval of existing targets. Typically TMGT can give experiences into the atomic components of illness and distinguish medicate targets that are likely to be viable. Progressed medication disclosure and improvement: TMGT can be utilized to progress the sedate revelation preparation by distinguishing new drug candidates and optimizing existing drugs. Usually, TMGT can give data about the structure and work of medicate targets, which can be utilized to plan drugs that are more successful and have fewer side impacts.

Personalized medication: TMGT can be utilized to create personalized medication approaches by distinguishing hereditary and molecular varieties that can be utilized to anticipate a patient's reaction to treatment. Usually, since TMGT can give data approximately for the atomic premise of a malady, it can be utilized to create focused treatments.

5.7.11.6 Limitations

1. Technical challenges: TMGT is a complex technology that can be challenging to implement and use. This is because TMGT requires a deep understanding of molecular biology and bioinformatics.
2. Cost: TMGT can be a costly technology to implement and use. This is because it requires specialized equipment and software.
3. Data limitations: The effectiveness of TMGT is limited by the availability of data. This is because TMGT requires large amounts of data to be effective.

5.7.11.7 Conclusion

TMGT is a powerful tool that can be used to improve target identification and validation, drug discovery and development, and personalized medicine. However, TMGT is a complex technology that can be challenging to implement and use, and it is limited by the availability of data.

5.7.12 Somatic cell nuclear transfer (SCNT)

Somatic cell nuclear transfer (SCNT), nuclear transfer cloning, is a biological process that involves transferring the nucleus of a non-reproductive somatic cell into an enucleated egg cell, which is an oocyte with its core removed. The encoded egg is then stimulated to develop, creating an embryo that is genetically identical to the donor's somatic cells. This technique has the potential to revolutionize the fields of medicine, agriculture and conservation.

The concept of SCNT was first proposed in the 1950s, but it was not until the 1990s that the technique was successfully applied to mammals. In 1996, Dolly the sheep became the first mammal cloned by SCNT. This breakthrough sparked renewed interest in SCNT and its potential applications. The SCNT procedure involves the following steps:

1. **Nucleus removal**: The nucleus is removed from the donor somatic cell.
2. **Enucleation**: The nucleus is removed from the egg cell.
3. **Nuclear transfer**: The enucleated egg cell receives the nucleus from the donor somatic cell.
4. **Activation:** The reconstructed embryo is stimulated to develop.

The success rate of SCNT is relatively low, with only a small percentage of attempts resulting in a viable embryo. This is due to a number of factors, including the difficulty of reprogramming the somatic cell nucleus and the sensitivity of the reconstructed embryo to developmental abnormalities.

SCNT has a number of potential benefits, including:

- Therapeutic cloning: SCNT can be used to generate ES cells that are genetically identical to a patient. These could be used to grow tissues and organs that are compatible with the patient, potentially eliminating the risk of rejection.
- Reproductive cloning: SCNT could be used to clone endangered species or to create genetically identical animals for research purposes.
- Preservation of genetic diversity: SCNT could be used to preserve the genetic diversity of endangered species or to create clones of animals with desirable traits.

5.7.12.1 Limitations

SCNT also has a number of limitations, including:

- Low success rate: The success rate of SCNT is relatively low, making it impractical for some applications.
- Ethical concerns: There are ethical concerns about the use of SCNT, particularly for reproductive cloning.
- Technical challenges: There are technical challenges associated with SCNT, such as the difficulty of reprogramming the somatic cell nucleus.

5.7.12.2 Conclusion

SCNT could be an effective method with the potential to revolutionize the areas of medicine, agriculture, and preservation. Be that as it may, a few challenges need to be overcome before SCNT can be widely applied. As the technology develops, we will see more energizing applications for SCNT in the future.

5.7.13 Induced pluripotent stem cells

One kind of pluripotent stem cell that can be produced straight from a somatic cell is called an induced pluripotent stem cell (iPSC). Somatic cells are differentiated cells, like skin or blood cells, that have already assumed a particular role in the body. Conversely, undifferentiated pluripotent stem cells have the ability to differentiate into any kind of bodily cell. This makes them an important tool in the field of regenerative medicine, which is focused on replacing or repairing diseased or damaged tissues.

In 2006, researchers Shinya Yamanaka and colleagues at Kyoto University in Japan made the initial discovery of iPSCs. By inserting four particular genes into the mouse skin cells, Yamanaka and his colleagues were able to reprogram the cells into pluripotent stem cells. These genes are involved in the regulation of gene expression and are referred to as transcription factors.

5.7.13.1 iPSC technology

The technology for reprogramming somatic cells into iPSCs has advanced rapidly since 2006, and there are now a number of different methods available. The most common method involves introducing the four Yamanaka factors into the cells using a virus. However, there are also methods that do not involve viruses, such as using small molecules or microRNAs.

The procedure for generating iPSCs is typically as follows:

1. Somatic cells are collected from an unknown patient.
2. The somatic cells are reprogrammed into iPSCs using one of the available methods.
3. The iPSCs are then characterized to ensure that they are pluripotent.
4. The iPSCs can then be differentiated into any type of cell in the body.

iPSCs have several potential benefits over ES cells, which are another type of pluripotent stem cell. ES cells are derived from embryos, which can raise ethical concerns. iPSCs, on the other hand, can be derived from a patient's cells, which eliminates the ethical concerns and also reduces the risk of rejection.

In addition, iPSCs can be used to create patient-specific cell lines, which can be used to model diseases and develop personalized therapies.

5.7.13.2 Limitations of iPSCs

Despite their potential benefits, there are also some limitations to iPSCs. One limitation is that the reprogramming process can be inefficient, and not all somatic cells can be reprogrammed into iPSCs. Another limitation is that there is a risk that iPSCs may contain genetic abnormalities, which could make them unsafe for use in therapy.

5.7.14 Lentiviral transduction

Transduction plays a pivotal role in the successful integration of foreign genes into the host organism's genome. The concept of transduction in transgenesis stems from the broader field of molecular genetics and gene transfer. The term 'transduction' was first coined by Nobel laureate Joshua Lederberg in the late 1940s to describe the transfer of genetic material from one bacterium to another through a virus (bacteriophage). Over the years, researchers adapted and expanded this concept to apply to eukaryotic organisms, leading to the development of transgenic technologies.

Transduction in transgenesis involves the use of vectors or carriers to deliver foreign genes into the target organism's cells. These vectors can be viral or non-viral, each with its own set of advantages and limitations.

5.7.14.1 Viral vectors

- Retroviruses: These are RNA viruses that can reverse transcribe their RNA into DNA, which integrates into the host genome. This feature makes retroviruses effective for stable, long-term gene expression.
- Adenoviruses: These DNA viruses do not integrate into the host genome but efficiently deliver genes into a wide range of cells. Adenoviral transduction is particularly useful for short-term expression studies.

5.7.14.2 Non-viral vectors

- Plasmids: Circular DNA molecules that can replicate independently of the host genome. Plasmids are versatile and commonly used for transient gene expression.
- Liposomes: Lipid-based vesicles that can encapsulate and deliver genetic material. Liposome-mediated transduction is suitable for certain cell types and avoids the potential immune responses associated with viral vectors.

Lentiviral transduction is a powerful and versatile technique in transgenesis, allowing for the introduction of foreign genes into a host organism's genome using lentiviruses as vectors [51]. The term 'lentivirus' is derived from the Latin word 'lente,' meaning slowly, reflecting the slow progression of diseases caused by these viruses. This technique has grown in popularity in several domains, such as gene therapy, research, and the creation of transgenic species. Because of their special ability to infect both dividing and non-dividing cells, lentiviruses are useful instruments for obtaining steady and persistent gene expression.

Lentiviruses belong to the retrovirus family and were initially discovered in the late 20th century. The basis for lentiviruses' application as gene delivery vectors was established by their discovery, which includes the well-known human immunodeficiency virus (HIV).

Lentiviral transduction involves a multi-step procedure to introduce foreign genes into the target organism's cells. The are five steps in the procedure:

1. Vector Construction.
2. Packaging.
3. Transduction.

4. Integration.
5. Expression.

Step 1 Vector Construction:

- The process begins with the construction of the lentiviral vector. This involves incorporating the desired genetic material, typically a transgene, into the viral genome.
- The vector is designed to include elements necessary for viral replication, packaging, and integration into the host genome.

Step 2 Packaging:

- The engineered lentiviral vector is then transfected into packaging cells, which provide the necessary components for viral particle formation. These particles encapsulate the vector and can infect target cells.

Step 3 Transduction:

- The lentiviral particles are harvested from the packaging cells and applied to the target cells.
- The viral particles enter the target cells, and the enzyme reverse transcriptase initiates the reverse transcriptase mechanism of lentiviral RNA into DNA.

Step 4 Integration:

- The synthesized DNA integrates into the host genome. This integration is facilitated by the viral integrase enzyme, leading to stable and long-term expression of the transgene in the host cells.

Step 5 Expression:

- The integrated transgene is now under the control of the host cell's regulatory machinery, resulting in the expression of the foreign gene. This expression can persist over multiple cell divisions, providing a durable and heritable effect.

Lentiviral transduction can effectively transduce a wide variety of cell types, including dividing and non-dividing cells, and several factors influence its success rate. It depends on the specific properties of the target cells, the design of the lentiviral vector, the choice of promoter placement, the administrative components that influence the success of transduction and the transgene itself, the concentration of lentiviral particles used for transduction, the so-called titer, and total dose are important factors. It is important to optimize the vector plan for your target application. Doses that are too high may result in cytotoxicity, and doses that are too low may result in inappropriate transduction. In general, lentiviral transduction is known to have a relatively high success rate, especially when compared to other gene transfer methods. The ability to achieve stable, long-term gene expression in a variety of cell types makes it a valuable tool for both research and therapeutic applications. The advantage of this technique is that it is highly effective for initial embryo transfer.

5.7.14.3 Limitation

Despite its many advantages, lentiviral transduction has some limitations that need to be considered:

1. The lentiviral vector can only accept transgenes that are 10 kb or smaller.
2. The virus has the potential to infect humans and animals, so safety levels need to be higher.
3. The high transduction efficiency of lentiviruses often results in the insertion of several copies of the transgene into several genomic loci.

5.7.14.4 Conclusion

To conclude this technique, lentiviral transduction provides a potent and effective way to insert foreign genes into the genome of a host organism. Due to its unusual capacity to infect both dividing and non-dividing cells as well as its stable and long-lasting transgene expression, it has been used extensively in both therapeutic and research settings. The precision, safety, and versatility of lentiviral transduction are being improved by continuing research and technical breakthroughs, despite certain limitations and constraints. The future of genetic engineering and biotechnology is expected to be significantly shaped by this technique as our understanding of lentiviral biology expands.

5.8 *Xenopus* oocytes as a heterologous expression system

Oocytes of the South African toad, *Xenopus laevis*, have been reported as a versatile and dominant heterologous expression system for eukaryotic genes and characterization of different types of proteins, including ion channels and membrane receptors. The large size and toughness of these oocytes make them easy to handle and microinject with different molecules such as natural mRNAs, cRNAs, and antibodies. Several methods can then be utilized to check the expression of the proteins encoded by the microinjected mRNA/cRNA and to perform a functional characterization of the heterologous polypeptides. *Xenopus* oocytes can be obtained in large quantities by exclusion of the ovary of the adult female. Every mature oocyte is 0.8–1.2 mm in diameter; it has a large nucleus known as a germinal vesicle sited in the darkly pigmented hemisphere of the oocyte. The oocyte nucleus is arrested at the first meiotic prophase. The oocyte presents as an important expression system for a wide variety of both animal and plant proteins. It can be utilized for the expression of the following.

- Eukaryotic mRNAs isolated from various tissues.
- mRNAs derived by *in vitro* transcription of eukaryotic genes using T7 RNA polymerase. Obviously, the gene has to be driven by the T7 promoter, and the mRNA molecules must be capped at their 5′-ends and polyadenylated at their 3′-ends.
- Extracellular DNA can be microinjected into the nucleus, where it is transcribed and the transcripts are processed, e.g. cDNA linked to a suitable promoter such as a mammalian virus promoter has been transcribed and translated.

The foreign proteins are normally subjected to relevant post-translational modifications such as alkylation, phosphorylation and accurate assembly of multi-subunit proteins. Moreover, the proteins are directed to their correct cellular compartment, e.g. plasma membrane, lysosome, etc. In reality, *Xenopus* oocytes have become a standard heterologous expression system for plasma-membrane steins, including ion channels, carriers and receptors. However, some foreign channels and receptors may be non-functional in this system for various reasons. *Xenopus* oocyte expression systems can be used to accomplish a variety of objectives, which are mentioned below.

- Production of transgenic *Xenopus*. A quantity of the microinjected DNA becomes incorporated into the *Xenopus* genome to generate transgenic individuals.
- Investigation of the roles of various DNA sequences such as promoters, enhancers, etc
- Investigation of the developmental effects of overexpressing normal gene products or of altered gene products. This may be accomplished by transcribing the concerned gene *in vitro*, capping the mRNA and microinjecting this mRNA into dejellied, fertilized eggs at the one—or two-cell stage. The mRNA is distributed more-or-less evenly among the descendants of the microinjected cell where it is expressed. On the other hand, the gene may be incorporated into a suitable expression vector and rDNA microinjected into the dejellied, fertilized eggs of the one- or two-cell stage. The plasmid DNA may amplify, in some cases to up to 50- or 100-fold, by the gastrula stage. But it is later on lost, and the only rDNA that persists is the one that is integrated into the *Xenopus* genome. However, the injected DNA is expressed in a mosaic pattern; this remains a serious drawback.
- Isolation of a specific gene from a cDNA library. This is achieved when the function/presence of the protein product of interest is explicitly assayed. The cDNA clones are separately transcribed *in vitro*, the mRNAs are translated in oocytes and the function of the desired gene product is assayed. The cDNA clones are consecutively subdivided using this assay system until a single cDNA clone encoding the function is found. This approach is frequently applicable to monomeric proteins. However, modified approaches have been planned to house heteromultimeric proteins.
- To study the protein product of a gene and the function of this product.

5.9 ES cell-mediated gene transfer (continued)

ES cells of mice are pluripotent cultured cells obtained from the early preimplanted embryonic stage, e.g. the inner cell mass of a blastocyst embryo. In this method cells are cultured on a feeder layer of fibroblasts or in the presence of leukemia inhibitory factor. These conditions facilitate the stem cells' growth but remain pluripotent so that they can afterward develop into a range of cell lineages, e.g. blood vessels, myoblasts, germ cells, myocardium and nerve cells. These cells can be retained and

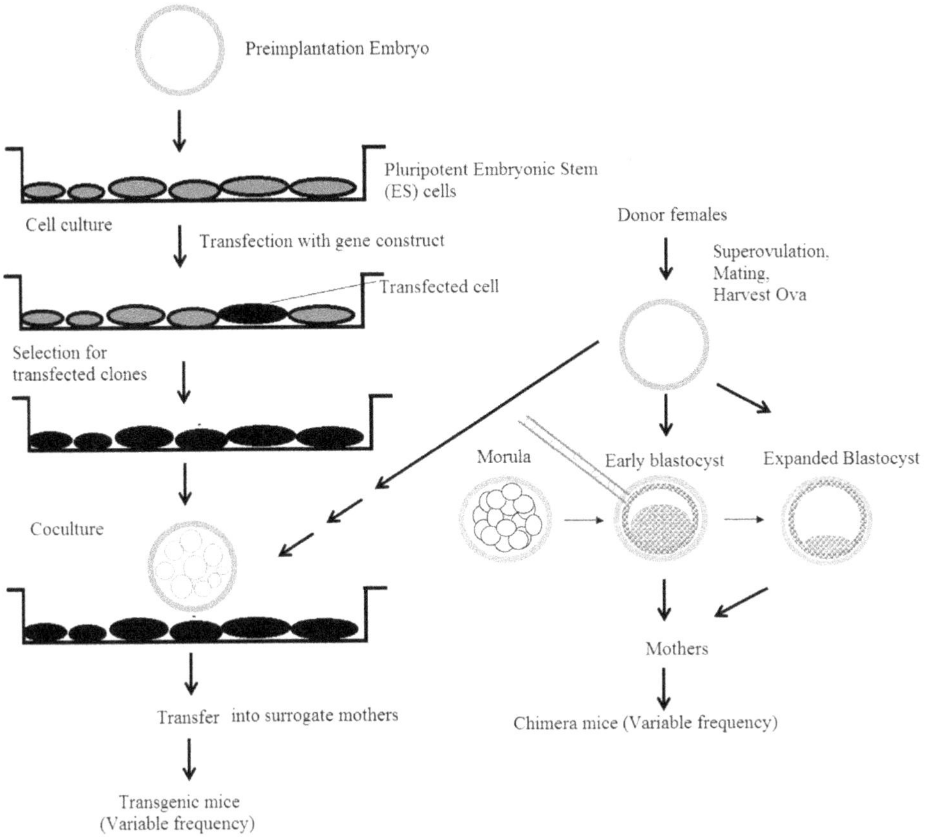

Figure 5.12. Schematic representation of ES cell transfer technology.

proliferated *in vitro* long enough to allow the different manipulations for gene transfer. A simple representation of the ES cell technique is as follows (figure 5.12). Initially, cultured pluripotent ES cells are transfected with a suitable transgene construct by the transfection technique. Transfected ES cells are identified and selected, typically by utilizing a selectable marker gene, and are cloned. The transgenic animals produced using transfected ES cell clones may be accomplished by different injection and co-culture methods:

- The cloned transgenic ES cells are injected into the blastocoel of blastocyst stage embryos; the blastocysts are derived from donor females in a similar manner as are ova for microinjection.
- The zona pellucida of eight-cell to morula stage embryos is detached, and the morulae are co-cultured with the ES cells; the ES cells are favorably introduced into the inner cell mass of the developing embryo.
- It is also feasible to transplant the ES cell nucleus into an enucleated fertilized ovum (an ovum whose nuclei have been removed), however, this method is not frequently employed as it is relatively monotonous, even though all the progeny produced by this technique are transgenic.

The transgenic ES cell line is chosen with care for vital growth as the injection of vital ES cell lines maximizes the overall yield of chimeras. In addition, the introduction of XY ES cell lines into random (XX or XY) embryos leads to a large bias towards maleness due to a high contribution by the ES lines.

The embryos co-cultured or injected with transfected ES cells are implanted into surrogate mothers where they finish their growth and development. Around 30% of the progeny obtained from such embryos contain tissues derived from the ES cells, i.e. they are chimeric. The pluripotent ES cells can give rise to germ cells as well. As a result, pure transgenic mice can be recovered from the chimeric mice using an appropriate breeding scheme. As DNA integration in the genome is random, the frequency of targeted gene transfer, i.e. integration of transgenes at a specified site (section 5.10), is discouragingly low. Therefore, transfection techniques such as microinjection are not suited for targeted gene transfer. The ES cell line technique, alternatively, allows the selection of clones(s) with targeted cells or gene.

When ES cells are incorporated into blastocoel embryos, chimeric mice are obtained. However, when eight-cell to morula stage embryos are co-cultured with ES cells, non-chimeric transgenic mice are recovered. Gene transfers are selected from among several clones showing stable transfection. The preferred clone can then be used to generate transgenic animals with targeted gene transfer. At present ES cell technology is restricted to mice as the embryos of most other mammals do not survive *in vitro*, so it is very difficult to produce and maintain their ES cell lines. Even in the case of mice, ES cell lines rarely give rise to germ cells in individuals of some strains, making it virtually impossible to produce transgenic animals of these strains using this technology. At present, ES cell lines have been developed in some mammalian species other than mice, but so far chimeric individuals have not been produced using them. It may be hoped that in the near future it may become possible to apply this technology in some more mammalian species. According to reports the first human embryonic cells were developed in 1998, and currently more than 1000 hESC lines have been developed, although only 223 are available for further research [52].

5.10 Targeted gene transfer or gene therapy in mammals

In general the aim of gene therapy is to treat or stabilize a syndrome that results from the production of a mutant protein (e.g. the chloride channel protein important in cystic fibrosis) or overproduction of a normal protein (such as the products of certain oncogenes). We can accomplish this objective by substituting the defective gene or by reducing the overexpression of the desirable gene using an antisense approach, as a result reducing the production of the disease-promoting protein [53, 54]. For either technique, it is important to transfer DNA into target cells in a concentration high enough to be effective in modifying the disease. DNA must be inserted into the desired cell population in an intact state, whereby it can be competently transcribed and finally translated. The technique of gene transfer should be highly reliable and non-toxic, and the delivery system must be comparatively simple to prepare and administer [55]. There is a great deal of optimism surrounding the advancement of gene therapy as an efficient approach for the managing of numerous different human diseases. The active means used to apply gene therapy are expected to consist of oligonucleotides, ribozymes or a DNA sequence that can be transcribed into a message capable of eliciting a therapeutic response. Unlike conventional small-molecule therapeutics, however, gene therapy entails the use of a carrier system to transport the active agent directly into the target cell population. Through targeted gene transfer, the transgene integrates at the definite location of its allele existing in the genome. This is accomplished by a technique of HR in which the transgene substitutes its allele in the genome (figure 5.13). HR can be explained as the substitution of identical sections between two DNA molecules that have identical or almost identical sequences (the variations in their sequences are limited to allelic differences). In yeast, gene integration usually occurs by HR. However, in mammals random DNA integration is far more common than HR. The frequency of integration by HR appears to be only 0.1%–1% of random integration events; this allows the recovery of transgenics making targeted gene transfer quite difficult. Current advancements in the techniques used, however, have augmented this rate to 10% (routinely) or even 50% (in a few cases) of random integrations. The strategies accessible for the identification of HRs are as follows:

- If deactivation or activation of the examined gene takes place due to HR, but not by random integration, and produces a selectable phenotype, such cells

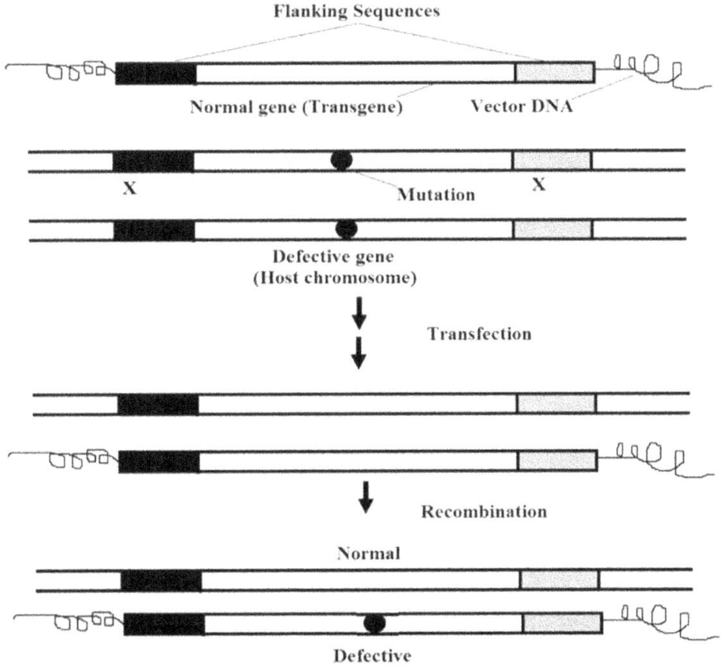

Figure 5.13. Protocol for targeted gene transfer through HR.

can be scored and selected for. However, there are not many such genes and a great majority of the GOIs do not offer a selectable phenotype.
- On the other hand, a great number of transfected cells/clones may be screened, often using PCR amplification, to recognize those with HR. As a rule, linearized gene constructs are utilized for transfection as HR between the transgene and the endogenous chromosomal gene is encouraged by the free ends of transfecting DNA.

Targeted gene transfers have the following two main applications:
- It is the perfect approach for gene therapy, i.e. the treatment of genetic diseases, by substituting the defective gene with the functional one. The transgene construct encompasses the sequences obviously present on either side of the gene it aims to replace; these sequences are known as flanking sequences. Recombination takes place in the flanking sequences, thus replacing the defective endogenous gene with the normal functional gene used for transfection (figure 5.13).
- It allows an examination of the functions of, or the effects produced by, a gene cloned and/or subjected to site-directed mutagenesis in a complete animal instead of merely in test systems such as *Xenopus* oocytes.

Gene substitution or targeted gene transfer presents two unique advantages. First, it places the functional transgene into the same context, i.e. the transgene is flanked by the same DNA sequences as the defective mutant gene it has replaced. It is well recognized that the sequences flanking a gene, even those located at substantial distances from the gene, typically influence its expression. Second, it prevents the likelihood of disruption of a significant gene, which may occur due to a random integration of the gene. However, it suffers from one weakness, that HR generally encourages the incidence of unplanned mutations in the gene.

5.10.1 Gene disruption by HR in mammals

Gene disruption or gene knockout is disruption of a target gene by the directed insertion of DNA into it using the process called recombination. In this way the gene is inactivated. This method can be used to investigate gene function. HR has been utilized to produce 'knockout' mice in which exact gene functions have been knocked out by disrupting or eliminating the relevant genes present in their genomes. A universal strategy for disrupting a chromosomal gene is illustrated in figure 5.13. The gene, e.g. gene A, to be disrupted is first isolated and cloned, and then a selectable marker gene, e.g. the bacterial gene neo, is placed within this gene. The neo gene dislocates the cloned gene A, and in addition makes the cells into which it is integrated resistant to the antibiotic G-418. This characteristic permits positive selection for the cells in which this gene construct becomes integrated. One more gene, e.g. HSV-TK, is attached to this gene construct. HSV type 1 TK forms the mice cells containing this gene, which is sensitive to the nucleoside analog GCV. Therefore HSV-TK permits a negative selection for such cells that contain this gene, i.e. the cells containing this gene are killed by GCV. This characteristic is very significant as it removes all such cells in which random integration of this gene construct has occurred (figure 5.14). This selection approach is thus known as positive-negative selection.

This gene construct is employed to transfect mouse ES cells. In a number of ES cells, HR will take place between the chromosomal (endogenous) gene A and the gene A construct transfected into them. Two concurrent recombinations, one each in the two sections of gene A located on the two sides of gene neo, will incorporate the bacterial gene neo into the chromosomal gene A, consequently disrupting it. Such ES cells will lose gene A function, will become resistant to G-418 (due to the gene neo) and will be resistant to GCV since they will not acquire the gene HSV-TK. However, in a comparatively larger number of cells, the complete gene construct will become integrated into the mouse chromosomes at random locations. These cells will be G-418 resistant, but will be sensitive to GCV owing to the HSV-TK gene; they will also have their gene A intact. As a result, when transfected ES cells are developed in a medium containing G-418 and GCV, only those cells in which HR has taken place will endure; in all such cells, gene A will be disrupted by the gene neo.

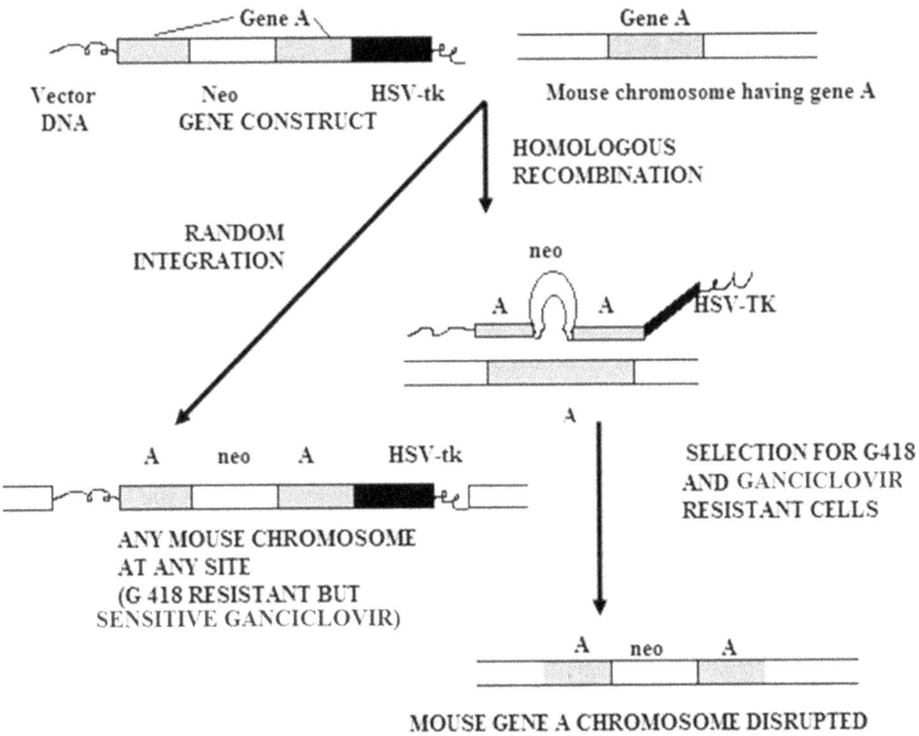

Figure 5.14. A universal method for disruption of any chromosomal gene, represented here as gene A. Gene A is first isolated, then cloned, and is disrupted by introducing a bacterial gene neo within its coding sequence.

The special ES cells are incorporated into young mouse embryos to generate chimeric mice in which gene A function has been knocked out in the ES cell-derived tissues. In 2003 Sato *et al* developed develop a gene disruption system for the hyperthermophilic euryarchaeon *Thermococcus kodakaraensis* KOD1 [56]. The gene targeting system developed in this work offers a long-needed tool in the research on hyperthermophilic archaea and will open the way to a systematic, genetic approach for the elucidation of unknown gene function in these organisms.

5.10.2 Gene targeting/replacement

Current understanding of molecular cell biology can be achieved by using certain techniques of genome mapping, protein expression and mutation. This understanding helps in the discovery of a large number of genes and their biochemical features. Analysis of these biochemical features helps in predicting their expression and encoded protein. Without their availability in mutant form it is not possible to recognize the *in vivo* roles of such genes. One approach is gene replacement, which allows replacement of particular mutated gene prepared under *in vitro* conditions with its native copy to recognize its *in vivo* function. Gene replacement is a method that entails point mutations, i.e. elimination of a gene/exons and even addition of a new gene. By means of specific gene mutation *in vitro* (develops mutant form) and then their replacement with the normal copy in the genome can be utilized to determine its *in vivo* function. There are several techniques that allow the insertion of foreign genes or their altered forms of an endogenous gene into an organism. Usually these techniques do not result in replacement of the endogenous gene, but allows the integration of additional copies of it. Such inserted genes are called transgenes and the organisms those are carrying these genes are known as transgenics. There are certain diseases that originated because of the defect in mitochondrial DNA. One of the causes behind this defect is single homoplasmic mutations [57]. Such disease can affect non-mitotic tissues present with variable phenotypes, can appear sporadically, and are untreatable. Certain examples of mtDNA abnormality based diseases are Alzheimer's, Parkinson's and type II diabetes. Researchers reported a protein transduction technology known as protofection that permits the introduction and expression of mtDNA, altered mitochondrial genome or exogenous genes into the mitochondria of living cells [58].

One major breakthrough in gene replacement was evidenced in the year of 2000, when a rapid approach for effective gene replacement in the filamentous fungus *Aspergillus nidulans* was reported. As per earlier reports gene manipulation in filamentous fungi is limited by the poor efficiency of homologous recombination in these organisms [59]. By increasing the length of homologous DNA higher recombination efficiencies can be achieved, however, this becomes a tedious process. In this study, the researchers reported a two-step technology using an *E. coli* strain expressing the phage λ functions to effectively replace the gene in the filamentous fungus *Aspergillus nidulans* [59].

After the exploration of the yeast genome sequence, attempts have been started to expose the open reading frames of yeast via targeted gene replacement using homologous recombination. One report explored a way to establish an efficient gene targeting technique in flowering plants [60]. An efficient gene targeting procedure has already been established for *Physcomitrella patens* (spreading earthmoss), which makes the moss a valuable plant-based model system. Another potential example of a valuable plant-based model system is *Arabidopsis*, due to the availability of its genomic sequence [60]. Recent research also considered CRISPR/Cas9 technology for mitochondrial gene replacement. Recent approaches are focused on the prevention of the transmission ion of mitochondrial diseases from mother to offspring. Two novel approaches may offer hope for preventing and treating mitochondrial disease: mitochondrial replacement therapy and CRISPR/Cas9 [61]. The former approach (mitochondrial replacement therapy) has the potential to prevent transmission in patients however this method is a subject of many ethical concerns. A later approach (CRISPR/Cas9 technology), also called genome editing technology, is currently considered as the simplest, most versatile and precise method of genetic manipulation. This approach can be utilized in treating individuals with disease caused by mutant mitochondrial DNA [61]. Another recent gene therapy, involving single-dose gene-replacement, has been developed for spinal muscular atrophy (progressive, monogenic motor neuron disease). Researchers have investigated the functional replacement of the mutated gene encoding survival motor neuron 1 (SMN1) in this disease.

A recent report also revealed the potential role of the human RPGR-ORF15 vector in establishing long-term dose efficacy. Gene replacement for RPGR-XLRP was hampered by the relatively slow disease development in mice [62]. Moreover, challenges in cloning the full-length RPGR-ORF15 cDNA also hampered replacement of RPGR-XLRP. Recently, several researchers have developed new stable vectors to conduct a comprehensive long-term dose-efficacy study in RPGR-knockout mice and an observed long-term efficacy study of gene replacement therapy for RPGR-associated retinal degeneration [62].

Crigler–Najjar syndrome, Dubin–Johnson syndrome, Gilbert syndrome and Rotor syndrome are inherited liver disorders of bilirubin. These disorders are due to a defect in the gene responsible for metabolism and transport of bilirubin, and can result in reduced hepatic uptake, conjugation or biliary secretion of bilirubin. This may further result in systemic accumulation of bilirubin, which can result in genetic hepatocellular jaundice. It has been reported that the defect present in the gene/protein can be corrected by gene replacement approach.

Thus, the above examples show that the gene replacement approach is considered as a potential approach to replace defective genes, which may further cure defective gene associated disease. In general, a construct made out of DNA is produced in bacteria [63]. Knockout experiments often offer a high rate of success. One of the common examples, zinc finger nuclease and homing endonuclease-mediated assembly of multigene plant transformation vectors, is described in this section. Binary vectors (a T-DNA binary system consist of a binary plasmid and a helper plasmid) are an essential component of *A. tumefaciens*-mediated plant genetic transformation systems. A limitation of this vector is that at one time it can only transfer a single GOI [63]. For the insertion of multiple genes or multiple traits another approach is required. Researchers have observed that the assembly of multitransgene binary vectors can be designed using a combination of engineered zinc finger nucleases (ZFNs) and homing endonucleases. Using this approach (multigene constructs) protoplasts of *Arabidopsis thaliana* and other plants were transiently and stably transformed. Moreover, by using this method the expression of the transformed genes was monitored across several generations.

Gene replacement experiments can also be demonstrated by the help of some knockout mouse experiments. In this procedure the gene construct is directly introduced into the mouse ES cells in culture. Selection of the cell is required to select the cells that are carrying the gene construct [64]. After selection, the selected embryo cells are inserted via embryo injection. After birth, chimeric mice are selected in which the reproductive organs are made up of modified cells, and are allowed to breed. This type of selection ensures homogeneity of the cells and retains the originally selected ES cell. Gene knockout can be potentially employed in many other organisms. So, a good understanding of the genome sequencing of several model organisms provides ease in mutating a native gene. However, for mutation in a native protein or sequenced genome the process is not easy, as shown in figure 5.15. In this case a different approach of positive-negative selection is utilized to recover ES cell lines in which homologous recombination results in the disruption of the GOI. During 1988, one researcher established positive and negative selection for gene targeting by the additional placement of the HSV thymidine kinase (HSV-tk) gene adjacent to one of the vectors arms containing targeted homology to a genetic locus [63].

On the other hand, an approach like the 'hit-and-run method' can be achieved to recover those ES cells in which a defective endogenous gene is substituted by homologous recombination. This homologous recombination (HR) by a functional gene or a normal endogenous gene is replaced with a gene modified by site-directed mutagenesis. A variation of the insertion vector approach is to generate a subtle mutation by a 'hit and run' [64]. This approach is also known as the 'in–out' method as the vector sequences are initially inserted into the genome, and then they are removed out of the genome [64].

One of the advantages of this approach is that the function of GOI is not disrupted by the neo gene, and the neo and HSV-TK genes are introduced into the vector at the side of the GOI (figure 5.15). The method of suicide gene treatment in cancerous cells is based on the concept of allowing tumor cells, by gene transfer, to convert a non-toxic pro-drug into a toxic product. This can be achieved by the insertion of the herpes simplex virus thymidine kinase (HSV-TK) gene into cancer cells followed by treatment with ganciclovir (GCV), which may ultimately allow death of HSV-TK-transduced cells by the direct cytotoxic effect of GCV-triphosphate. GCV-triphosphate is generated by HSV-TK from GCV. Since only cancerous cells possess the enzyme that converts pro-drug to active metabolites, it raises the toxicity level several fold inside the tumor while the host cells remain unaffected. Using recombinant DNA technology, it is possible to insert the desired gene in ES cells. After transfection with homologous recombination takes place between the transfected DNA and the host chromosome. This recombination allows integration of the desirable gene into the ES cell chromosome which may help in a duplication of

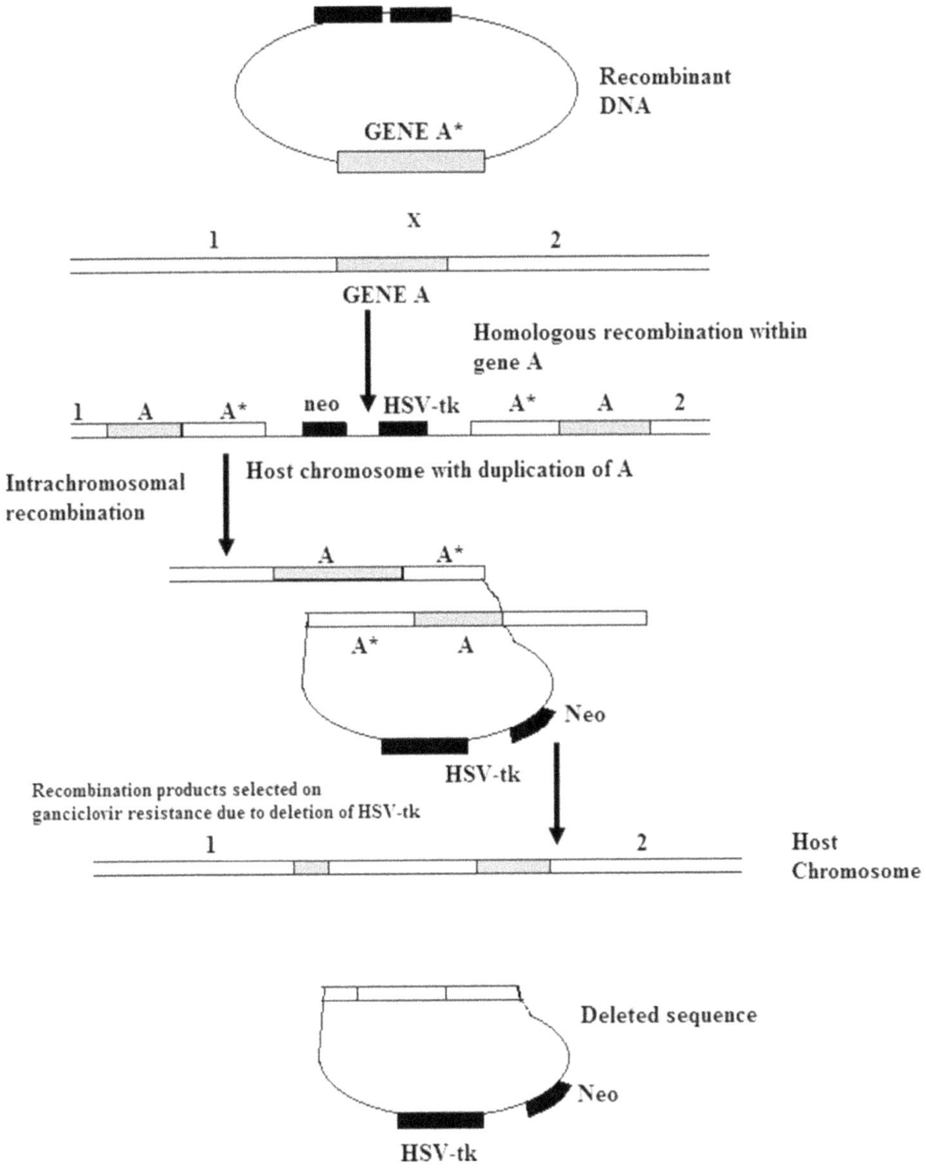

Figure 5.15. Gene replacement by HR and selection of recombination products by the hit-and-run method. 1 and 2 indicate the regions flanking the GOI, i.e. gene A. The incorporated gene A* is a tailored version and the site of change is represented by * within gene A*. X indicates the site of crossing over.

the relevant gene. By the means of selectable marker technique (antibiotic G-418) it is possible to select these cells. From such selection, transgenic cells with random integration of the transfecting DNA will be selected by G-418. The virus infected cells are first selected with G-418, mutagenized and then selected with the suicidal system anti-herpes drug acyclovir (ACV). As HSV-TK, but not the host TK, is proficient enough in converting GCV to a toxic metabolite, cells retaining the intact HSV-TK gene fail to survive, while the cells carrying a mutated HSV-TK gene or which have lost the gene can form colonies in the presence of nucleoside analog GCV, making it possible to detect the genetic defects in a positive manner. These cells will also contain the gene herpes simplex virus thymidine kinase gene (HSV-TK), also known as the negative-selection marker gene and sometimes called suicidal therapy. Afterwards, intrachromosomal recombination (between direct repeats) takes place between the two copies of the GOI in some of the transgenic cells. Such recombination will allow the elimination of one copy of the GOI plus the vector DNA and the neo and HSV-TK genes (figure 5.15). Cells expressing HSV-TK are sensitive to the nucleoside analog GCV. Therefore the cells offered by intra-chromosomal recombination will become resistant to GCV, whereas all other transgenic ES cell lines will be sensitive to this nucleoside analog. Consequently GCV is employed to select those cells that have their endogenous genes substituted by HR.

In the case of fungi, the construction of mutant fungal strains is often restricted by the poor efficiency of homologous recombination in these organisms. By increasing the length of homologous DNA flanking the transformation marker, higher recombination efficiencies can be achieved, while this is a repetitive procedure when molecular biology techniques are used for the construction of gene replacement cassettes. A quick approach for efficient gene replacement in the filamentous fungus *Aspergillus nidulans* has been reported. This approach allows the rapid establishment of mutant strains carrying gene knockouts with efficiencies >50%. It should also be suitable for the construction of fungal strains with gene fusions or promoter replacements [41].

5.11 Transgene integration, organization, and expression

A transgene is a gene or genetic material that has been transferred naturally, or by various genetic engineering techniques, from one organism to another. The incorporation of a transgene (called 'transgenesis') has the potential to alter the phenotype of an organism. In general, transgenes integrate at different sites in any of the chromosomes of the genome of host cells. Usually, in a given cell, integration takes place at a single location. As a result, various cells participate and represent transgene integration at various chromosomal sites. The number of copies incorporated per genome varies from one to several hundred. Usually, several copies are integrated when large amounts of DNA are used for transfection, whereas single copies are integrated with smaller amounts. When numerous copies are integrated, they are usually integrated at one site joined to each other head-to-tail, perhaps due to the DNA double-strand break repair system forming a concatemer, which is then integrated into the chromosome. However, in a small proportion of cases, numerous copies are located at different locations in the same genome. In some fish such as common carp and channel catfish, several copies are always integrated as single copies at multiple sites in the genome, and concatemers (elongated continuous DNA molecules that contain multiple copies of the same DNA sequences linked in series) are not found, while in others only concatemers are encountered; linearization of the gene construct appears to promote concatemer formation as well as the rate of stable transfection. When 'carrier DNA' is used, it becomes integrated into large concatemeric structures that hold segments of the carrier DNA, the selectable marker as well as the unselected DNA used for transfection. It appears that this DNA becomes fragmented and then becomes attached in random combinations to form large concatemers, which are called transgenomes. In the transformation process transgenomes appear to be formed early; later on they amalgamate into the cell genome at a random site. Usually, a single transgenome integration occurs per cell. Transgenomes are partially or more-or-less entirely removed from the genome at a comparatively high frequency. The mechanism of random integration has not been identified. The entire gene construct, including the vector DNA, becomes integrated. When two different gene constructs are mixed and used for transfection, they have a tendency to integrate together at the same site; this is known as co-transfection. Before their integration the two gene constructs become ligated together. As in the case of single gene constructs, various copies of the two constructs may be introduced at a single site. The co-transfection can potentially be used to connect two separate gene constructs.

Various gene constructs (e.g. DHFR and CDA protein gene constructs) have a tendency to become highly amplified during integration; these genes also amplify the DNA sequences linked to them. This feature can be used to attain highly amplified integration of any gene merely by linking them to such genes. Besides random integration, a very low frequency of integration occurs via HR if the gene construct has sequences that are homologous to some sequences in the host cell genome. The frequency of HR-based integration is only 0.1%–1% of that of random integrations. HR is the basis of targeted gene transfers. It is well reported that the sequences flank a gene on whichever side affects the expression of this gene. Therefore, similar transgenes integrated at different sites in the genome may demonstrate different levels of expression; this is known as the position effect. This result is supposed to arise due to:

- The general accessibility of the region for transcription.
- The regulatory elements present in the region flanking the transgene.
- The presence of cis—or trans-acting regulatory elements conferring tissue-specific expression, which will limit the expression of transgenes to particular tissues or cell types. This will create a chimera-like situation even when the transgene is present in all the cells of a transgenic animal. Transgene integration frequently results in various forms of rearrangements (e.g. duplication, deletion, etc) closer to the site of integration. If these alterations are large enough, the host gene located at the site of integration might become non-functional.

A host gene would also become non-functional if the transgene became integrated within the coding region of this gene. When incorporation of a transgene results in the loss of function of a host gene, it is called insertional mutagenesis; it frequently creates aberrant phenotypes. While insertional mutagenesis takes place by chance and cannot be regulated, it can result in accidental detection of several unsuspected genes and gene functions. Thus insertional mutagenesis is the mutagenesis of DNA by the insertion of one or more bases. It can occur naturally, by means of a virus or transposon, or can be artificially created for research reasons in the laboratory. Uren *et al* reported that retroviral insertion mutagenesis screens in mice are powerful techniques for efficient identification of oncogenic mutations in an *in vivo* setting [65]. Day *et al* recently reported that transgene integration into the same chromosome location can produce alleles that express at a predictable level, or alleles that are differentially silenced [42].

5.12 Transgene recovery in mammalian cells

Transgenic cell lines offer a potential tool for the isolation of any GOI that can be selected or recognized by its phenotypic effects in tissue culture cells. The different techniques used for the recovery of transgenes are basically variants of the 'plasmid rescue' method, which is briefly explained below using the case of the chicken TK gene (see figure 5.16):

- The total genomic DNA of chicken (containing the TK+ gene) is digested with HindIII and ligated into pBR322. The rDNA is utilized directly to transfect chicken TK+ cells, and Tle transgenic cells are selected in HAT medium.
- DNA from TK transgenic cells is isolated and used for a second round of transfection of TIC chicken cells. Transgenic TK cells are selected in HAT medium. The second round of transfection is done to remove most of the non-selected recombinant plasmid DNA, which became integrated in the first round of transfection.
- The DNA from these TK cells is isolated, cut with an appropriate restriction enzyme, e.g. EcoRI, circularized, transferred into *E. coli* and selected for plasmid-borne antibiotic resistance, e.g. ampicillin resistance in this case. The TR gene will actually be attached to the amp gene of the plasmid, which is recovered by this approach. Therefore the transgene is 'tagged' with the antibiotic resistance marker, which can be selected in *E. coli*.

The other strategies used for the recovery of the transgene follow a similar approach, with some differences in their details. Some of these approaches are as follows:

- The selected DNA for transfection is attached with an amber suppressor tRNA gene (supF) origin of integration in pBR322. Following the second round of transfection, transgenic cells are selected for the phenotype of interest, e.g. Tle in the above case. Genomic library DNA from the transgenic cells is prepared in a vector containing an amber mutation in one or more essential genes. The rDNA is plated on a non-suppressor *E. coli* host. A plaque will be formed only by the rDNA that has the supF gene and, thus, the GOI.
- The DNA used for transfection is integrated into a DNA molecule that can be used as a probe to identify the DNA insert. The DNA inserts may be

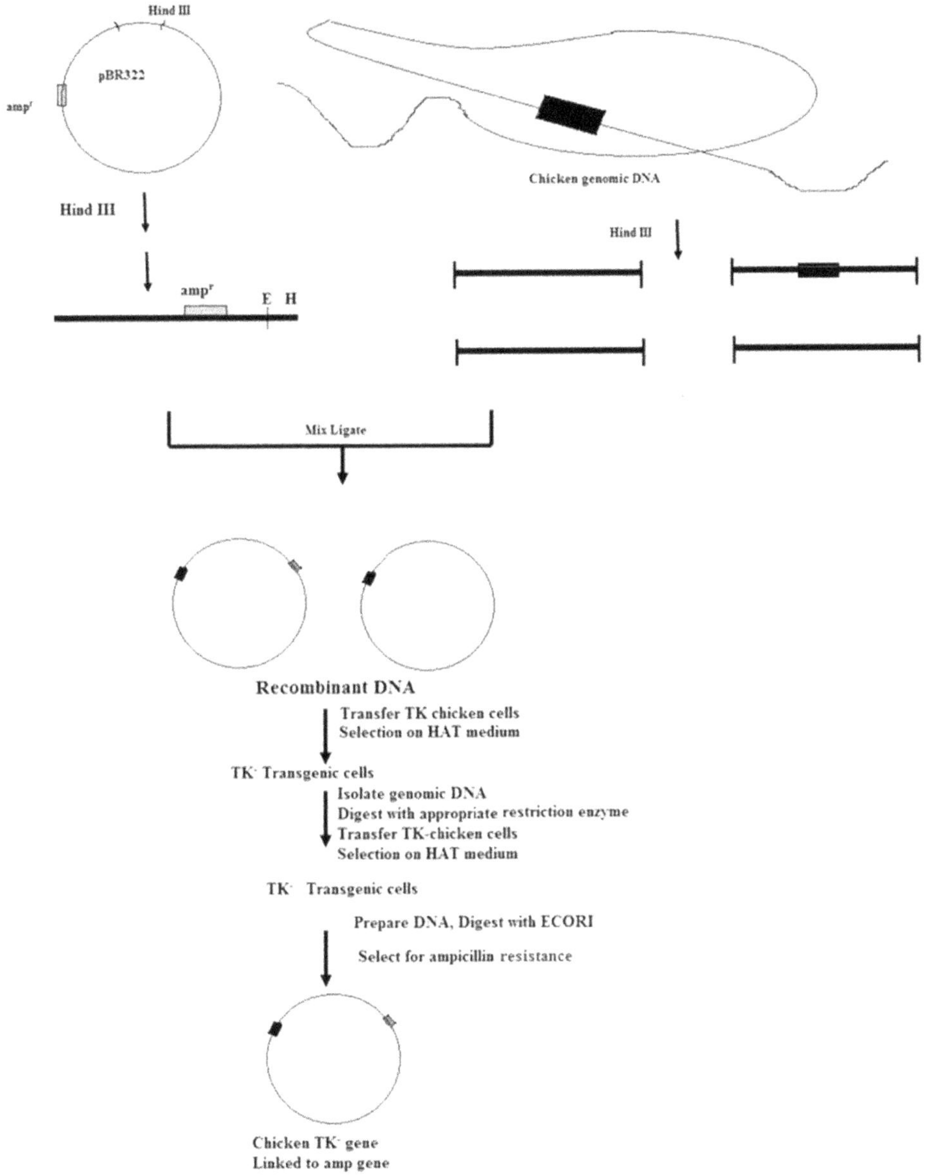

Figure 5.16. The approach of 'plasmid rescue' for gene isolation that generates the desired phenotype in the transfected cells cultured *in vitro*.

integrated into pBR322. The desired transgenic lines are recovered after the second round of transfection, and their DNA is used to prepare the genomic library in a phage λ vector. The plaques that are formed are hybridized with labeled pBR322 DNA. The positive plaques will contain the DNA insert of interest since it is physically linked to pBR322.

5.13 Cloned protein expression in mammalian cells

Animal cell technology (ACT) is defined as the expression of cloned genes in eukaryotic cells (mammalian cells) for the synthesis of recombinant proteins. It is utilized broadly for the development of biopharmaceutical products and novel therapeutics. It is a complex process which involves the entire animal cell production process, beginning with genetic investigations and cell line development to the final stages of process development and validation, involving production, purification, stability and storage [55, 56, 66–71]. Regulatory issues and development of *in vitro* models for screening and pre-clinical testing of efficacy and safety are also involved. The introduction of foreign (insert) DNA into eukaryotic cells (mammalian cells) is called transfection. It helps to investigate gene functions or gene products by manipulating specific gene expression in cells, and can also be utilized to synthesize recombinant proteins in mammalian cells. There are two types of transfection: stable and transient (figure 5.17). In stable transfection, the foreign gene is incorporated into the chromosomal DNA and is expressed stably post-host cell replication. Isolation of the stable transfected cell involves the use of selectable gene markers present on the recombinant plasmid carrying the target genes. However, transiently transfected genes are not incorporated into the genome and are expressed only for a limited period and can be lost due to several environmental factors and divisions of the cell. In transient transfection, the cell lysates derived after harvesting cells 1 day and 4 days post-transfection are standardized for expression of the target

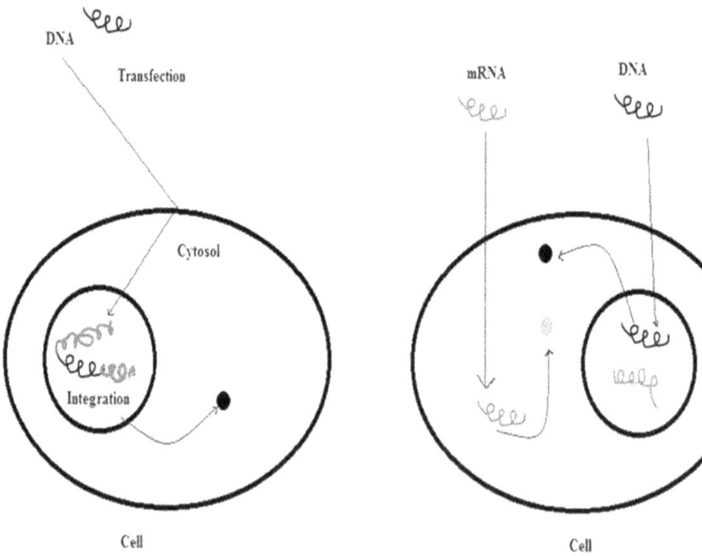

Figure 5.17. Illustration of two different transfections. (a) Stable transfection. Foreign DNA enters the nucleus, is incorporated into the host genome and is expressed sustainably. (b) Transient transfection. Foreign DNA is delivered into the nucleus but is not integrated into the genome. Foreign mRNA is also delivered into the cytosol, where it is translated. The circles are expressed proteins from transfected nucleic acids. The black arrows indicate delivery of foreign nucleic acids.

gene. Stable or permanent transfection is utilized to establish clonal cell lines in which the selected target gene is incorporated into chromosomal DNA directing synthesis of the target protein [55, 56, 66–72]. The examples of products/research areas of ACT are many, including therapeutic proteins, monoclonal antibodies, vaccines, virus-like particles (VLP), gene therapy (delivering a GOI into cells to cure a disease or improve symptoms), induced pluripotent stem cell (iPS cell) generation (involving transfection of three or four transcription factors), small interference RNA (siRNA) knockdown procedures and production of human tissue plasminogen activator in immortalized Chinese hamster ovary (CHO) cells for therapeutic purposes.

Vectors are self-replicating, extrachromosomal DNA molecules present in prokaryotes and eukaryotes that can be used for cloning of foreign DNA inserts and then, by transfection, the gene can be inserted into the host for its expression. Genetically engineered vectors contain multiple elements that include (see figure 5.18):

- An SV40 origin of replication for amplification to high copy number in COS-1 monkey cells.
- An efficient promoter for initiation of transcription.
- mRNA processing signals for post-translational modifications.
- Polylinkers containing multiple endonuclease restriction sites for insertion of foreign DNA.
- Selectable markers for identifying cells with stably integrated plasmid DNA.

A number of expression vectors for animal cells have been developed. The suitability of gene constructs for expression is generally examined by transient transformation, because it permits the examination of various alternative gene constructs in parallel. Usually, the cells are transfected, are used for standardizing

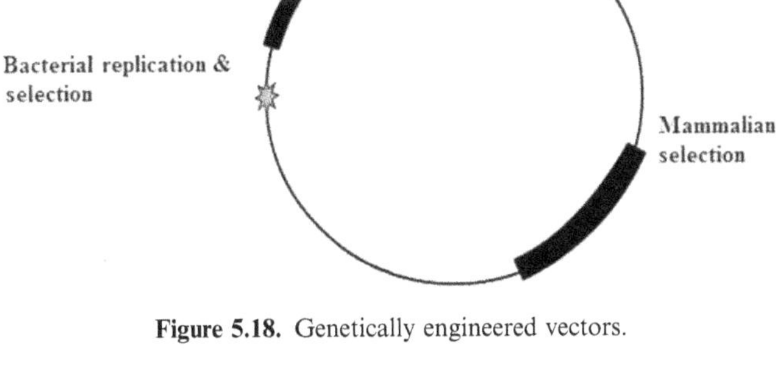

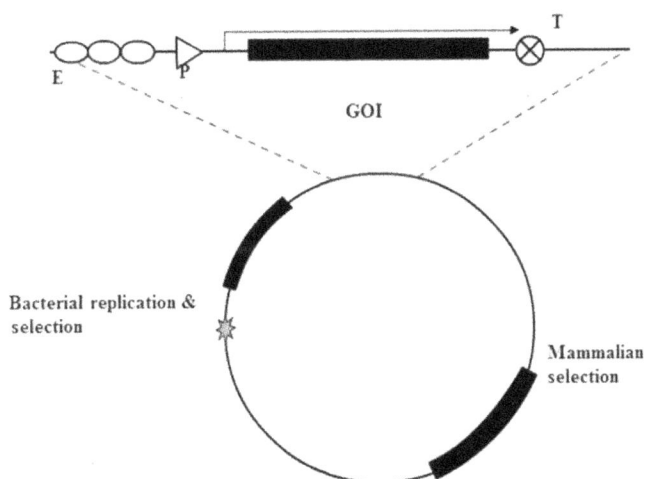

Figure 5.18. Genetically engineered vectors.

the expression of recombinant proteins after 1–2 days, and are then discarded. For this reason, the gene construct is examined using a non-replicating plasmid vector lacking an origin of replication for the concerned host. Supercoiled plasmid DNA is used for transfection since linear DNA is degraded rapidly in animal cells. Even supercoiled plasmid DNA survives only for 1–2 days; the human embryonic kidney cell line 293 can maintain such DNA for up to 80 h. Transient transformations can also be used to produce moderate amounts of the recombinant proteins. However, some transient transformation systems, e.g. plasmid vectors carrying the SV40 origin of replication, allow the harvesting of large amounts of recombinant proteins even when the percentage of transfected cells is low; this is because the transfected cells have a high copy number (up to 10^5 copies per cell) of the rDNA. A number of the expression vectors used for animal cells are described briefly below.

5.13.1 Conclusion

ACT is the process by which cloned genes are expressed in eukaryotic (mammalian) cells to produce recombinant proteins. The foreign gene is integrated into the chromosomal DNA and expresses itself steadily once the host cell replicates in a stable transfection. Isolation of the stably transfected cell involves the use of selectable gene markers present on the recombinant plasmid carrying the target genes. The cell lysates obtained from cell harvesting one day and four days post-transfection in transient transfection are standardized for target gene expression. Stable or permanent transfection is utilized to establish clonal cell lines in which the selected target gene is incorporated into chromosomal DNA directing the synthesis of the target protein [55, 56, 66–72]. After entering the nucleus, foreign DNA integrates with the host genome and expresses itself in a sustainable manner. Although it enters the nucleus, foreign DNA does not become incorporated into the genome. Vectors are self-replicating, extrachromosomal DNA molecules present in prokaryotes and eukaryotes that can be used for cloning foreign DNA inserts and then, by transfection, the gene can be inserted into the host for its expression—selectable markers for identifying cells with stably integrated plasmid DNA. Plasmid vectors carrying the SV40 origin of replication allow the harvesting of large amounts of recombinant proteins even when the percentage of transfected cells is low; this is because the transfected cells have a high copy number (up to 105 copies per cell) of the rDNA.

5.13.2 Expression vectors for mammalian cells

The expression of cloned genes in mammalian cells is an essential technique for understanding gene expression, protein structure and function, and biological regulatory mechanisms. The intensity of protein expression from heterologous genes incorporated into mammalian cells depends upon many factors such as mRNA transport, DNA copy number, mRNA processing, efficiency of transportation, mRNA stability and translational efficiency, and protein processing, transport and stability. Different genes exhibit different rate limiting steps for efficient expression. Various approaches are available to obtain high-level expression in mammalian cells. A number of expression vectors have been designed for animal cells; four such vectors are briefly discussed in the following sections.

5.13.2.1 pcDNA1.1/Amp as expression vectors

This is a highly versatile expression vector containing the following modules:

- *E. coli* phage M13 origin (generates single-stranded copies of the DNA insert).
- ColEl origin (for replication in *E. coli*).
- SV40 origin (for replication in COS cell lines).
- Polyomavirus origin (for replication in MOP-8 or WOP murine cell lines, both mouse cell lines).
- SV40 intron/polyadenylation site (PA; for enhanced transcription and poly-adenylation of mRNA).
- A polylinker or multiple cloning site (MCS; for integration of transgene/DNA insert).
- Cytomegalovirus promoter (for driving transgene transcription).
- T7 promoter (for *in vitro* transcription of the transgene).
- Ampicillin resistance gene (for selection of recombinant *E. coli* clones) (see figure 5.19).

In this procedure transgene is integrated into the MCS and is determined by the strong constitutive promoter, 'Pop', from human cytomegalovirus. The rDNA is used for transient transfection of a simian COS cell line or murine MOP-8 or WOP cell lines. The COS cell line is a derivative of African green monkey cell line CV-1.

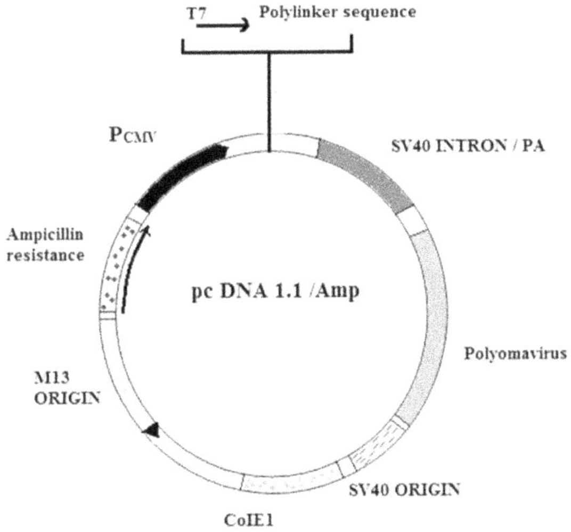

Figure 5.19. The transient expression vector pcDNA1.1/Amp. It has origins of replication from both SV40 and murine-polyomavirus. T7, *E. coli* phage T7 promoter; polylinker sequence, 5′-HindIII, BamHl, BstXl, EcPRI, BstXI, Not I, Xhol, Sphl, NsA, Xbal-3′; pCMV, human cytomegalovirus promoter; and SV40 intron/PA, SV40 intron/polyadenylation site.

This cell line contains an integrated partial copy of the SV40 genome, which comprises the entire T antigen coding sequence. Consequently, the COS cell line offers T antigens in trans and permits replication of the vector using the SV40 origin; the transfected cells contain up to 105 copies of the rDNA per genome. Similarly, the MOP-8 cell line contains an integrated polyomavirus genome so that it offers the T antigen in trans to sponsor replication using a polyomavirus origin. The WOP cell line achieves the same end by carrying a latent infection by the polyomavirus. The rDNA is used for transient transfection of a suitable cell line. The recombinant protein can then be synthesized and accumulated.

5.13.2.2 Baculovirus vectors as expression vectors

Over the past 20 years the baculovirus–insect cell expression system has become one of the most widely used systems for routine production of recombinant proteins [73–78]. In addition to producing proteins in insect cells and larvae, baculoviruses can be used for many purposes, such as by displaying foreign peptides and proteins on virus particles or by inserting cellular activity expression cassettes into baculoviruses from mammalian cells. They are used for a variety of purposes, including the efficient expression of genes in different mammals. Baculoviruses engineered to display foreign peptides or proteins on the viral surface have proven to be particularly useful as immunogens, and both surface display and capsid fusion have the potential to improve and provide additional targeting prospects for virus-mediated transduction. Baculoviruses have dsDNA genomes. They efficiently infect arthropods, chiefly insects. Baculovirus vectors are used chiefly for high-level transient protein expression in insects and insect cells. The polyhedrin gene of baculoviruses can be substituted by the transgene of interest, which is driven by the strong endogenous polyhedrin promoter, resulting in a high level of expression (up to 1 mg 10^{-6} cells). Baculoviruses AcMNPV and BmNPV have been widely used for development of vectors. AcMNPV is a reliable vector not only for *in vitro* gene delivery, but also for *ex vivo* and *in vivo* gene delivery. AcMNPV vectors are widely used for recombinant protein production in insect cell lines, mainly those derived from *Spodoptera frugiperda*, e.g. sf9, sf21, etc. BmNPV vectors have been used for recombinant protein production silkworm larvae. The high level of gene expression requires the polyhedrin promoter, the 5′-untranslated region of the polyhedrin gene sequence, and the first 30 codons of the polyhedrin gene since this region contains some regulatory sequences. Mutation of the polyhedrin initiation codon has allowed the use of the first 30 codons of the gene as part of the 5′-untranslated region of the transgene. The production of the baculovirus expression vector involves the insertion of the transgene downstream of the polyhedrin promoter plus the regulatory sequences of the 5′-untranslated region. This is typically attained by HR. A competent recombination approach is as follows. One component of this system consists of a linear derivative of the wild-type baculovirus genome containing large deletions, which can be repaired only by HR with a targeting vector (see figure 5.20). The second component is the targeting vector that spans the deletion in the first component; it also has enough flanking homologous sequences to sponsor recombination between the two components. This approach yields up to 90% recombinant plaques in insect cell lines. Another approach uses Tn7

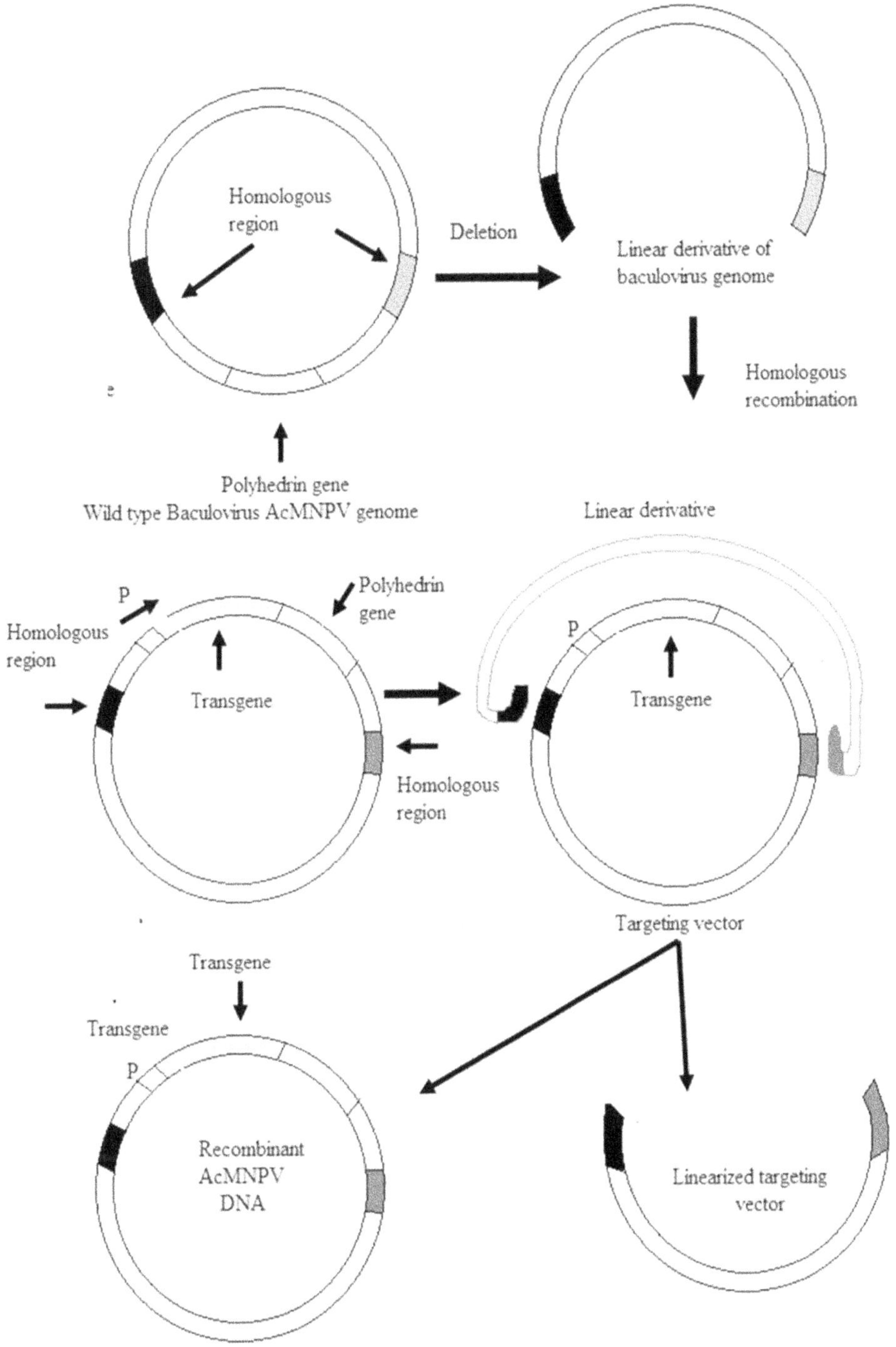

Figure 5.20. A basic depiction of the construction of baculovirus rDNA by HR. P, promoter region of polyhedrin gene.

repeat sequences, a Tn7 target site and Tn7 transposase to exploit site-specific recombination for constructing recombinant baculovirus DNA; this technology has been patented. The main limitation of the baculovirus expression system is that the glycosylation pathway of insects differs from that of mammals. This difficulty can be resolved as follows:

- A transgenic cell line may be developed that expresses a suitable enzyme for glycosylation.
- An insect cell line may be selected for its ability to carry out mammalian-type glycosylations.
- The expression vector might carry a second transgene that encodes the specific enzyme for the correct glycosylation of the recombinant protein.

All three approaches have been shown to work acceptably well.

5.13.2.3 Alphavirus vectors (communicated by insect vectors)

Alphaviruses (e.g. the Semliki forest (SF) and Sindbis viruses) are enveloped viruses with single-strand positive-sense RNA genomes which have been engineered for *in vitro* and *in vivo* expression of heterologous genes [79]. These viruses replicate in the cytoplasm and produce a large number of genomes per cell. Therefore, the transgene expression level is very high. Mutants of the SF and Sindbis viruses have been developed that show reduced cytotoxic effects. The viral genome carries only two genes: (1) a 5′-gene that encodes viral replicase and (2) a 3′-gene encoding a polyprotein. This polyprotein experiences autocatalytic cleavage to produce viral capsid proteins.

Some of the strategies used to express recombinant proteins using alphavirus vectors are as follows:

- Replication-competent vectors are synthesized by inserting another subgenomic promoter either upstream or downstream of the 3′-gene. In this procedure the transgene is inserted downstream of this promoter. Such insertion vectors are likely to be unstable and they have been almost substituted by replacement vectors.
- Replacement vectors are synthesized by replacing the 3′-gene with the transgene. The region of the first 40 codons of this gene of both the Sindbis and SF viruses contains a strong enhancer of protein synthesis. As a result, this particular region is included in the rDNA. Therefore, the recombinant protein is expressed as an N-terminal fusion protein. These vectors produce very high yields (up to 50% of total cellular protein) of the recombinant proteins.

A versatile vector based on Sindbis virus is currently marketed by Invitrogen as pSinRep5; it is a Sindbis replicon vector (figure 5.21). It contains a bacterial plasmid backbone, including a ColE1 origin, and ampicillin resistance plus the following modules:

- An SP6 promoter upstream of the replicase genes and the expression cassette for generating full-length transcripts *in vitro*.
- An expression cassette consisting of a Sindbis virus subgenomic promoter, an MCS and a polyadenylation site.

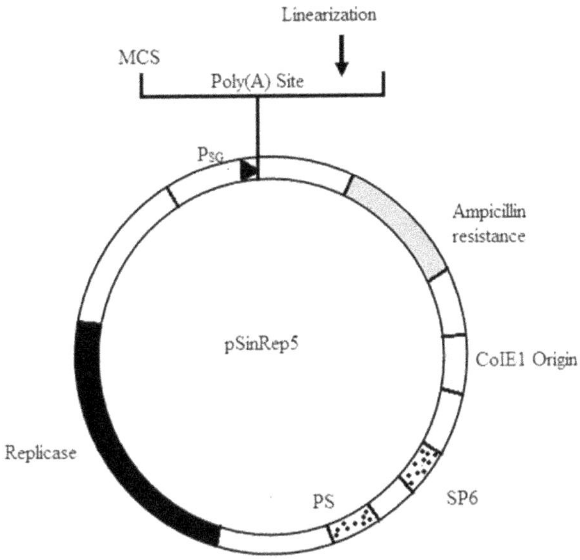

Figure 5.21. A plan representation of the pSinRep5 vector based on Sindbis virus. SP6, SP6 promoter for synthesis of *in vitro* RNA transcripts; PSG, subgenomic promoter to drive the expression of transgene; replicase; non-structural genes (nsP1–4) for *in vitro* replication of the recombinant RNA; Apal, linearization, restriction sites Pad, Noll and Xhol; MCS, Xha1, Miu1, Pm/1, Sph1, Stul and PS packaging signal allows recombinant RNA to be packaged into the virus.

- Sindbis virus packaging site (for packaging of recombinant RNA into virus particles).
- Sindbis virus replicase genes 1–4 (for *in vitro* replication of recombinant RNA).
- Three exclusive restriction sites downstream of poly(A) site.

The vector is maintained as a dsDNA copy of the RNA vector. The transgene is incorporated into the MCS of the expression cassette, and the vector is linearized and transcribed *in vitro*. The final recombinant Sindbis RNA is packaged into virus particles and used to transfect host cells from which recombinant protein is recovered.

On the other hand, the complete Sindbis or SF virus genome is placed under the control of the eukaryotic promoter and the recombinant alphavirus DNA is used for the transfection. In this procedure, the rDNA is transcribed in the nucleus and the rRNA is transported into the cytoplasm, where it directs the production of recombinant protein.

5.13.2.4 Vaccinia virus vectors (the smallpox vaccine virus)

The vaccinia virus is the smallpox vaccine virus, a virus that causes smallpox. The pox viruses have large (up to 300 kb) dsDNA genomes, which replicate in the host cell cytoplasm rather than the nucleus. Therefore, the particle contains the complete

DNA replication and transcription machinery, and the information is contained in the genome. Therefore, recombinant genomes integrated into cells by transfection are not infectious. These recombinant viruses are produced by HR by targeting plasmids that are transfected into vaccinia virus-infected cells. Recently, direct ligation vectors have been developed. These vectors are transfected into cells containing a helper vaccinia virus to sustain replication and transcription of the rDNA. Recombinant vaccinia DNA is identified using one of the following approaches:

- The transgene is introduced into the viral TK gene and negative selection (using the thymidine analog 5-bromodeoxyuridine) is carried out to reduce the wild-type vaccinia virus genomes.
- The transgene is introduced into the viral haemagglutinin locus. During this procedure the transfected cells are plated and chicken erythrocytes are supplemented to the plate. The recombinant plaques remain white while the wild-type plaques turn red.
- For direct identification of the recombinants, selectable markers, e.g. neo, or screenable markers such as lacZ or gusA, can be cointegrated with the transgene.

The expression of the transgene is typically operated by an endogenous vaccinia promoter such as P7.5 and P4b. A synthetic promoter maintains the production of up to 2 pg recombinant protein per 10^6 cells. It has also been noticed that vaccinia virus vectors cannot be utilized to express genes with introns (they are transcribed in the cytoplasm and there is no splicing facility in the cytoplasm). Moreover, the transgene sequence must not contain TTTTTNT as this virus uses this sequence as a transcription termination signal. A binary expression system has been developed. In this method, one vaccinia vector has the transgene to be expressed under the regulation of a strong T7 (*E. coli* phage) promoter. The other vaccinia vector has the gene encoding T7 RNA polymerase driven by a vaccinia virus promoter. Both the rDNAs are used together to transfect host cells. A cell transfected by both rDNAs produces T7 polymerase, which transcribes the T7 promoter-driven transgene; this approach produces the recombinant protein up to 10% of the total cellular protein. Recombinant vaccinia virus DNA has been constructed to express a variety of such significant proteins e.g. hepatitis B surface antigen, HIV and HTLV III envelope proteins (HBsAg), etc

5.13.3 Enhanced production of recombinant proteins

Recombinant protein production in microbial hosts and animal cell cultures has transformed the pharmaceutical and industrial enzyme-based industries. Animal hosts for the production of recombinant proteins are being actively pursued, taking advantage of their distinctive features. The solution to cost-efficient production in any system is the intensity of protein accumulation, which is inversely proportional to the cost [80]. High-level expression of transgenes in cultured animal cells has been observed to be exploited for the production of therapeutic recombinant proteins. Expression in mammalian cells is particularly desirable when typical mammalian glycosylation of the protein is essential for therapeutic applications. The following factors contribute to a high-level expression:

- Use of a strong enhancer/promoter, e.g. SV40 enhancer/early promoter, etc
- The sequence around the initiation codon should conform to Kozak's rules. Of these rules the most significant is the presence of a purine at the −3 position and a G at the +4 position. The A of the AUG initiation codon is counted as +1, U as +2 and so on.
- A lack of AU-rich sequences in the 3′-untranslated region of mRNA as this sequence reduces mRNA stability.
- In view of the second and third points above, the 5′-untranslated region of mRNA should be as short as possible.
- The absence of a secondary structure within the 5′-untranslated region of the mRNA.
- The absence of a correct initiation codon in the 5′-untranslated region, i.e. before the correct codon.

The different approaches for maximizing transgene expression are briefly discussed in the following sections.

5.13.3.1 Robust constitutive promoter for ectopic gene expression

Constitutive promoters are usually used to drive ectopic gene expression. A range of cellular and viral constitutive promoters have been used in expression vectors to insert exogenous genes into cells. These promoters have diverse advantages, e.g. cytomegalovirus (CMV) early enhancer/promoter directs a high level of transient gene expression in various cells [2–4, 81]. Nevertheless, a potential disadvantage of the CMV promoter is that it is prone to silencing over time after being transduced into the genome of host cells [4, 5, 82–85], although the activity of this promoter may vary depending on the host cells and experimental settings. Some additional constitutive promoters, including human β-actin (hACTB), human elongation factor-1α (hEF-1α), and cytomegalovirus early enhancer/chicken β-actin (CAG) promoters, have shown their qualities in sustaining stable gene expression for extended periods of time [2–5, 82, 86–89]. Nevertheless, most of the investigations characterizing constitutive promoters within expression vectors have been performed using plasmid, adenoviral, retroviral or lentiviral vectors as a platform for experiments. The use of strong (very active) promoters is a very promising potential approach to further improve transgene expression. In the case of viral vectors, transgenes are typically determined by very strong promoters, e.g. polyhedrin promoter (baculovirus vectors), p7.5 promoter (vaccinia virus vectors), El promoter (adenovirus vectors), etc. There are certain viruses that contain strong promoters and enhancers; some of these have been utilized to drive transgenes, e.g. SV40 early promoter and enhancer, the RSV LTR promoter and enhancer, and the human cytomegalovirus promoter are the most frequently used elements to drive transgenes in mammalian cells.

5.13.3.2 Effect of intron inclusion

Intron-mediated enhancement is the capability of an intron sequence to trigger the expression of a gene containing that intron. In particular, the intron must be present in the transcribed region of the gene for enhancement to occur, distinguishing intron-mediated augmentation from the action of typical transcriptional enhancers [84, 85]. The occurrence of an intron in an eukaryotic expression unit typically promotes transgene expression. Consequently, the majority of mammalian expression vectors in current use contain a heterologous intron, e.g. the SV40 small T antigen intron or the human GH intron. Modified hybrid introns that match the consensus splice donor and acceptor-site sequences have also been designed and used. The existence of an intron is very significant in constructs that are to be expressed in transgenic animals. However, introns may not be used in some expression vector systems, such as vaccinia virus vectors [84, 85].

5.13.3.3 Polyadenylation signals to augment expression of retroviral vectors

Polyadenylation signals are an important feature of eukaryotic protein coding genes. The polyadenylation site (poly(A) site) offers the signal for generation of a defined 3′-end to the mRNA molecules, and for addition of a poly(A) tail at the 3′-end of mRNA. A poly(A) tail comprises several hundred A residues added to the 3′-end of mRNA, after transcription, by the enzyme poly(A) polymerase [89]. A poly(A) tail is essential for the transport of mRNA from the nucleus into the cytoplasm, and it also increases mRNA's stability. When the expression system is short of a poly(A) site, the transgene expression may decrease by up to 90%. In mammalian expression vectors the poly(A) sites from the SV40 early transcription unit or the mouse 13-globin gene are often used.

5.13.3.4 Exclusion of unnecessary untranslated sequences

In molecular genetics, an untranslated region is defined as either of two sections, one on each side of a coding sequence on a strand of mRNA. In cases when it is present on the 5′ side, it is known as the 5′ UTR (or leader sequence), or if it is found on the 3′ side then it is known as the 3′ UTR (or trailer sequence). mRNA is RNA that carries information from DNA to the ribosome, the site of protein synthesis (translation) within a cell. The mRNA is primarily transcribed from the subsequent DNA sequence and then translated into protein. Nevertheless, a number of regions of the mRNA are generally not translated into protein, including the 5′ and 3′ UTRs.

Eukaryotic mRNAs possess untranslated regions (UTRs) of variable lengths at their 5′-ends as well as their 3′-ends. These UTRs can affect the level of gene expression (protein production) in different ways as follows:

- Some 5′-UTRs include AUG codons upstream of the authentic translation initiation codon; often such additional AUG codons interfere with translation initiation.
- Some other 5′-UTRs contain sequences that affect mRNA stability, e.g. AU-rich sequences reduce inRNA stability, and such sequences have been discovered in some 5′-UTRs.

In addition, the 5′- and 3′-UTRs may be rich in secondary structure, which prevents efficient translation. In view of the above, the 5′- and 3′-UTR sequences are usually eliminated from transgene constructs to increase their expression and the production of recombinant proteins.

5.13.3.5 Transgene sequence optimization (for efficient translation)

To achieve the most suitable translation competence, the sequence around the translation initiation site should be 5'-CCRCCAUG G-3' (the Kozak's consensus sequence), or as close to it as possible. In this sequence, the purine at the −3 position (denoted by R) and the G at position +4 are of the greatest importance. (The adenosine A, of the AUG codon is considered as position +1.) Moreover, different organisms prefer to use different codons for the same amino acid. As a result, if a transgene is taken from another organism, it may contain codons that are not usually used in the host organism. In that case, the competence of translation will decline; this may result in truncation of the protein or even a frame-shift in the translation. This matter can be resolved by changing the base sequence of the transgene in such a manner that the codons not favored in the host are substituted by those that are often used, but if the amino acid sequence of the encoded protein remains uninterrupted this is called codon optimization. Codon optimization is now frequently used as a standard technique for protein expression, and although a variety of techniques and strategies have been developed, they do not promise improved performance for all types of applications. In other words, codon optimization is a technique that maximizes the protein expression in living organisms by improving the translational efficiency of the GOI. This is done by transforming the DNA sequence of nucleotides of one species into the DNA sequence of nucleotides of another species, e.g. plant sequence to human sequence, human sequence to bacteria or yeast sequences, etc

5.13.3.6 Inserting a targeting signal

Eukaryotic proteins are usually modified after translation to become more functional. For instance, various proteins of high therapeutic value entail authentic glycosylation patterns for their correct function, as well as for preventing an immune response in the patient. Specific types of post-translational modifications occur in particular cellular compartments. Thus, it is essential to target the recombinant protein to that exact compartment of the cell where the specified modification will be effected. For instance the proteins that are to be glycosylated must be targeted to the secretory pathway using a signal peptide. Various mammalian expression vectors contain sequences that encode specific signal peptide sequences. For instance, the Invitrogen vector pSecTag2 (figure 5.22) includes a signal sequence from the murine immunoglobulin light-chain signal peptide; the signal peptide encoded by this sequence targets the protein to the secretary pathway with a high efficiency. Moreover, the C-terminus of the recombinant protein derived by using this vector is a fusion of two different epitope tags, which allow protein purification. Various high-level expression systems are accessible. When a large-scale production system is

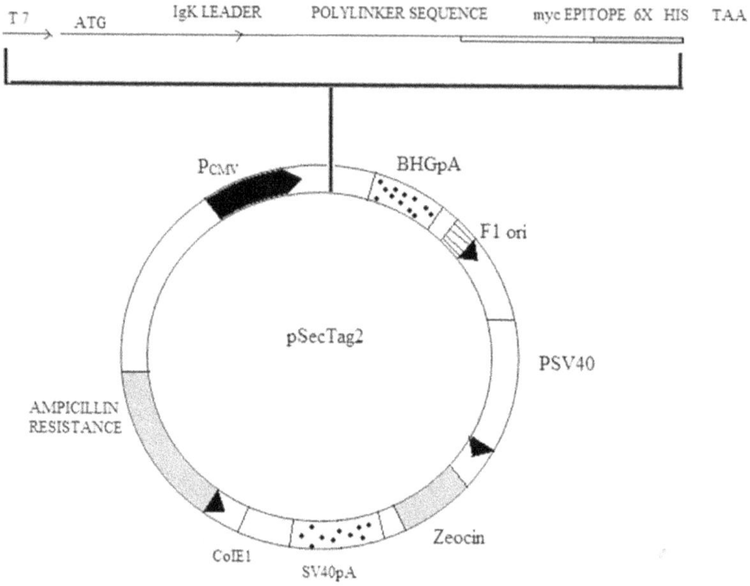

Figure 5.22. A schematic representation of the Invitrogen expression vector pSecTag2. The polylinker sequence has recognition sites for the following enzymes: Sfil, Ascl, Hrndlll, Asp718, Kpnl, BamHl, BstXI, EcoRl, Pst I, EcoRV, BstXl, Not!, Xhol, Drall and Apal. The myc epitope is recognized by the anti-myc antibody, which can be used for assaying the fusion protein using western blotting. (Other epitopes that can be used for this purpose are the polyhistidine epitope identified by the Anti-His (C-terminal) antibody, and the V5 epitope identified by the Anti-V5 antibody). pCMV, human cytomegalovirus promoter; T7, *E. coli* phage T7 promoter; bGHpA and SV40pA (polyadenylation sites); f1 ori, *E. coli* phage M13 origin of replication.

predicted, the selection of a particular system will depend on the cost of the culture system needed for stable or transient transfection, and the possible requirement for inducible expression. For therapeutic applications, a stable, permanently expressing cell line consistently yields products of reproducible quality. In the case of transient expression, the scale of the transfection step becomes important. It was observed that the maximum expression attainable may not always be required. Inducible gene expression can be achieved by using a metallothionein promoter. In this case, transcription is induced by metal ions such as cadmium and zinc. On the other hand, a promoter activated by steroid/thyroid hormone/retinoic acid may be used, e.g. mouse mammary tumor virus (MMTV) LTR has a complex promoter region that is activated by a steroid hormone.

5.13.4 Scale-up of protein purification (stages in downstream processing)

Purification of recombinant proteins is significantly facilitated by expressing them as fusion proteins with some polypeptide sequences that allow their specific isolation from the mixture of proteins produced in the cells. Such polypeptide sequences that allow protein purification are known as tags. Examples of tags include the MalE (maltose-binding) protein, glutathione-S-transferase, multiple histidine residues, myc epitope, etc. The tags allow easy purification of the recombinant proteins using affinity chromatography. The tag vectors are usually prepared in such a way that the coding sequence for an amino acid sequence cleaved by a particular protease, e.g. enterokinase, thrombin or factor Xa, is inserted between the coding sequence for the tag and the gene being expressed. Thus the tag protein can be cleaved off using the relevant protease after the fusion protein has been purified. Moreover, a sequence that can be examined easily may be placed within the tag protein; this will facilitate an easy assay of the recombinant protein when its function is not known or the assay is difficult. The use of some of the tags is briefly outlined below.

Polyhistidine affinity tags are usually placed on either the N- or the C-terminus of recombinant proteins. Optimal placement of the tag is protein-specific. A potential problem is inaccessibility of the protein tag to the immobilized metal due to occlusion of the tag in the folded protein.

5.13.4.1 Histidine-tagged protein purification

A polyhistidine tag, an amino acid motif in proteins, consists of at least six histidine (His) residues, often at the N- or C-terminus of the protein. The tag protein consists of six histidine residues; it may be located either at the N-terminal end (e.g. in vector pBAD/His (A, B, C) of Invitrogen) or the C-terminus (e.g. pSecTag2 vector of Invitrogen; figure 5.23) of the recombinant protein. The GOI is first inserted into the chosen vector, and the rDNA is introduced into the appropriate cell line. After synthesis and accumulation of the fusion protein, the cells are lysed. The viscosity of the lysate is reduced by nuclease treatment to digest both DNA and RNA. The lysate is then subjected to column chromatography; the column contains immobilized divalent nickel, which selectively binds to the polyhistidine tag [84]. The contaminating proteins are washed from the column leaving the fusion protein, which is then treated with the appropriate protease, say, enterokinase. This frees the recombinant protein from the tag, and it is then eluted from the column, leaving the tag bound to the divalent nickel column (figure 5.24). The two drawbacks of all such purification strategies are as follows: (1) the need for use of a protease for cleavage of the tag and (2) the necessity for removal of the protease from the recombinant protein.

5.13.4.2 Protein affinity purification using intein and chitin-binding protein sequences

An intein is a protein segment that is able to excise itself and join the remaining portions (the exteins) with a peptide bond in a process termed protein splicing. Introns have also been known as 'protein introns'. The CBD from *Bacillus circulans* is a small molecule of 5 kDa; it has a high affinity for chitin columns. The CBD encoding DNA sequence is placed at the downstream end of the transgene so that the CBD forms the C-terminus of the fusion protein. An intein encoding sequence is placed between the transgene and the CBD sequence. Intein is a protein splicing element, which is cleaved out from a precursor protein (a process called protein splicing); the two sequences flanking the inteins become ligated together to form the

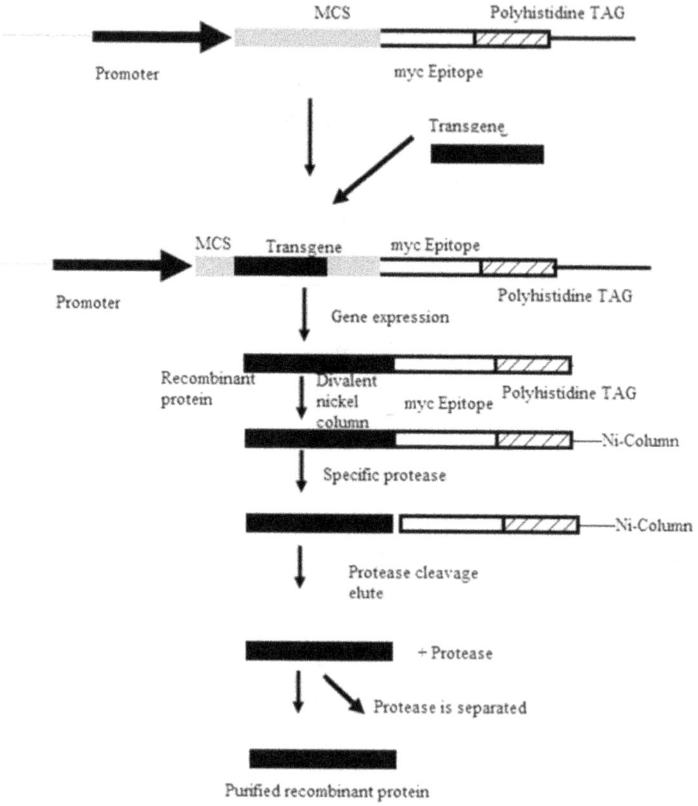

Figure 5.23. A simplified schematic representation of purification of a recombinant protein using a polyhistidine tag. This tag can be at the N-terminal end of the recombinant protein as well. A sequence identified by a specific protease is placed between the transgene and the tag (in this case, between the myc epitope and the transgene).

mature protein (the sequences flanking the intein are exteins). The intein sequence is obtained from the VMA1 gene of *Saccharomyces cerevisiae* and is modified in such a way that the intein undergoes self-cleavage at its N-terminus at low temperatures in the presence of thiols such as cysteine, dithiothreitol or P-mercaptoethanol.

5.13.4.3 Conclusion

To conclude, the protein affinity purification using intein and CBD encoding DNA sequence is placed at the downstream end of the transgene so that the CBD forms the C-terminus of the fusion protein. The transgene and the CBD sequence are separated by an intein encoding sequence. Intein is a protein splicing element, which is cleaved out from a precursor protein (a process called protein splicing). The mature protein is formed by the ligation of the two sequences (exteins) that flank the inteins together.

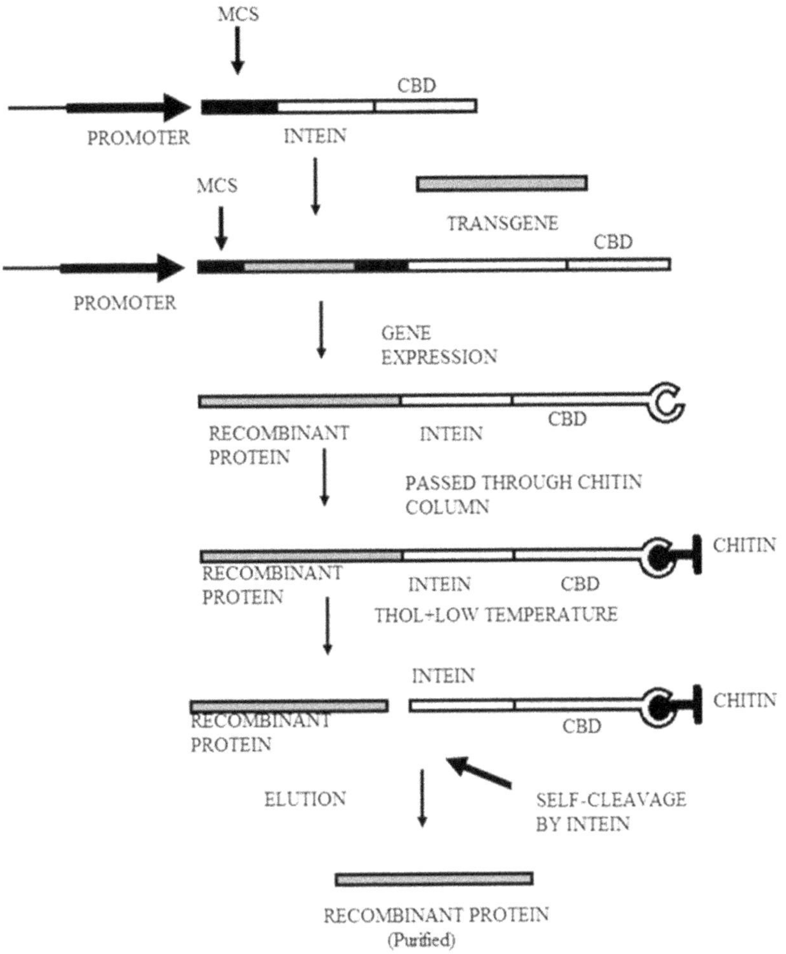

Figure 5.24. A schematic representation of purification of a recombinant protein using modified yeast intein and bacterial chitin-binding domain (CBD) sequences at the C-terminal end as a tag. In fact, the CBD functions as a tag, while the intein element serves as a specific protease that effects self-cleavage at its N-terminal end.

5.14 Applications of using these approaches

Practical applications of genetic modification in livestock production include higher disease resistance, better milk production and composition, better growth rates and feed conversion, better fertility and reproductive performance, and improved carcass composition [90]. One of the most important candidate genes for creating transgenic livestock that promotes growth and produces more milk is growth hormone.

Transgenic animals have widespread applications in numerous fields, including biotechnology, medicine, agriculture, and environment conservation.

1. Biomedical research: Transgenic animals are essential for understanding gene function, modeling human diseases, and testing potential therapies. Mice with humanized immune systems help advance the development of vaccines and treatments for diseases like HIV and cancer.
2. Agriculture: In agriculture, transgenic animals are used to improve livestock and poultry breeding. For instance, cows have been modified to produce more milk, and pigs have been engineered to have leaner meat, leading to increased food production and economic benefits.
3. Pharmaceutical production: Transgenic animals are also used in the production of biopharmaceuticals. Some animals are engineered to produce valuable proteins such as insulin and clotting factors that can be harvested for medical purposes.
4. Environmental protection: Transgenic animals can play a role in environmental protection efforts. For example, researchers have been working on genetically modifying mosquitoes to curb the spread of diseases such as malaria and dengue fever.
5. Biomarker identification: Transgenic animals can help identify biomarkers and pathways associated with various diseases, supporting the development of diagnostic tools and targeted therapies.

In conclusion, transgenic animals represent a remarkable fusion of biology and biotechnology, offering immense potential for scientific research, agriculture, and medical advancements. The ability to manipulate an organism's genetic code has opened new frontiers in our understanding of life and has far-reaching implications for improving human health and our environment. As biotechnology continues to advance, the role of transgenic animals in shaping our world is likely to become increasingly significant.

References

[1] Brinster R L and Palmiter R D 1984 Transgenic mice containing growth hormone fusion genes *Phil. Trans. R. Soc. Lond.* B*307 309–12*

[2] Qin J Y 2010 Systematic comparison of constitutive promoters and the doxycycline-inducible promoter *PLoS One* **5** e10611

[3] Chen C M, Krohn J, Bhattacharya S and Davies B 2011 A comparison of exogenous promoter activity at the ROSA26 locus using a PhiiC31 integrase mediated cassette exchange approach in mouse ES cells *PLoS One* **6** e23376

[4] Kang J, Wither J and Hozumi N 1990 Long-term expression of a T-cell receptor beta-chain gene in mice reconstituted with retrovirus-infected hematopoietic stem cells *Proc. Natl Acad. Sci. USA* **87** 9803–7

[5] Morishita H, Nakamura N, Yamakawa T, Ogino H and Kanamori T 1991 Stable expression of human tissue-type plasminogen activator regulated by beta-actin promoter in three human cell lines: HeLa, WI-38 VA13 and KMS-5 *Biochim. Biophys. Acta* **1090** 216–22

[6] Kost T A, Condreay J P and Jarvis D L 2005 Baculovirus as versatile vectors for protein expression in insect and mammalian cells *Nat. Biotechnol.* **23** 567–75

[7] Khan F A 2011 *Biotechnology Fundamentals* (Boca Raton, FL: CRC Press) p 108

[8] Robert-Guroff M 2007 Replicating and non-replicating viral vectors for vaccine development *Curr. Opin. Biotechnol.* **18** 546–56
[9] DiMaio D, Treisman R and Maniatis T 1982 Bovine papillomavirus vector that propagates as a plasmid in both mouse and bacterial cells *Proc. Natl Acad. Sci. USA* **79** 4030–4
[10] Kakeda M, Hiratsuka M, Nagata K, Kuroiwa Y, Kakitani M, Katoh M, Oshimura M and Tomizuka K 2005 Human artificial chromosome (HAC) vector provides long-term therapeutic transgene expression in normal human primary fibroblasts *Gene Ther.* **12** 852–6
[11] D'haeseleer P 2006 What are DNA sequence motifs? *Nat. Biotechnol.* **24** 423–5
[12] Aufderklamm S, Todenhöfer T, Gakis G, Kruck S, Hennenlotter J, Stenzl A and Schwentner C 2012 Thymidine kinase and cancer monitoring *Cancer Lett.* **316** 6106–10
[13] Morales C, García M J, Ribas M, Miró R, Muñoz M, Caldas C and Peinado M A 2009 Dihydrofolate reductase amplification and sensitization to methotrexate of methotrexate-resistant colon cancer cells *Mol. Cancer Ther.* **8** 424–32
[14] Martin S A, McCarthy A, Barber L J, Burgess D J, Parry S, Lord C J and Ashworth A 2009 Methotrexate induces oxidative DNA damage and is selectively lethal to tumor cells with defects in the DNA mismatch repair gene MSH2 *EMBO Mol. Med.* **1** 323–37
[15] Mucciolo E, Bertoni L, Mondello C and Giulotto E 2000 Late onset of CAD gene amplification in unamplified PALA resistant Chinese hamster mutants *Cancer Lett.* **150** 119–27
[16] Wahl G M, Vitto L and Rubnitz J 1983 Co-amplification of rRNA genes with CAD genes in N-(phosphonacetyl)-L-aspartate-resistant Syrian hamster cells *Mol. Cell. Biol.* **3** 2066–75
[17] Mulligan R C and Berg P 1981 Selection for animal cells that express the *Escherichia coli* gene coding for xanthine-guanine phosphoribosyltransferase *Proc. Natl Acad. Sci. USA* **78** 2072–6
[18] Xu X, Li Z, Zhao X, Keen L and Kong X 2016 Calcium phosphate nanoparticles-based systems for siRNA delivery *Regen. Biomater.* **3** 187–95
[19] Gulick T 2001 Transfection using DEAE-dextran *Curr. Protoc. Neurosci.* **2001** May appendix 1:Appendix 1D
[20] Felgner P L, Gadek T R, Holm M, Roman R, Chan H W, Wenz M, Northrop J P, Ringold G M and Danielsen M 1987 Lipofection: a highly efficient, lipid-mediated DNA-transfection procedure *Proc. Natl Acad. Sci. USA* **84** 7413–7
[21] de Lima M C, Simões S, Pires P, Gaspar R, Slepushkin V and Düzgüneş N 1999 Gene delivery mediated by cationic liposomes: from biophysical aspects to enhancement of transfection *Mol. Membr. Biol.* **16** 103–9
[22] Kaneda Y 2000 Virosomes: evolution of the liposome as a targeted drug delivery system *Adv. Drug Deliv. Rev.* **43** 197–205
[23] Niidome T, Ohmori N, Ichinose A, Wada A, Mihara H, Hirayama T and Aoyagi H 1997 Binding of cationic α-helical peptides to plasmid DNA and their gene transfer abilities into cells *J. Biol. Chem.* **272** 15307–12
[24] Haywood A M and Boyer B P 1985 Fusion of influenza virus membranes with liposomes at pH 7.5 *Proc. Natl Acad. Sci. USA* **82** 4611–15
[25] Hafez I M, Ansell S and Cullis P R 2000 Tunable pH-sensitive liposomes composed of mixtures of cationic and anionic lipids *Biophys. J.* **79** 1438–46
[26] Takimoto T, Taylor G L, Connaris H C, Crennell S J and Portner A 2002 Role of the hemagglutinin-neuraminidase protein in the mechanism of paramyxovirus-cell membrane *Fusion J. Virol.* **76** 13028–33

[27] Cho J E, Kim H S, Ahn W S and Park Y S 2001 Enhanced cytotoxicity of doxorubicin encapsulated in liposomes with reconstituted Sendai F-proteins *J. Microencapsul.* **18** 421–31

[28] Schaeffer P, Cami B and Hotchkiss R D 1976 Fusion of bacterial protoplasts *Proc. Natl Acad. Sci. USA* **73** 2151–5

[29] Genga T and Lu C 2013 Microfluidic electroporation for cellular analysis and delivery *Lab Chip* **13** 3803–21

[30] Gehl J 2003 Electroporation: theory and methods, perspectives for drug delivery, gene therapy and research *Acta Physiol. Scand.* **177** 437–47

[31] Tsong T Y 1991 Electroporation of cell membranes *Biophys. J.* **60** 297–306

[32] Fujimoto H, Kato K and Iwata H 2008 Electroporation microarray for parallel transfer of small interfering RNA into mammalian cells *Anal Bioanal. Chem.* **392** 1309–16

[33] Feramisco J, Perona R and Lacal J C 1999 Needle microinjection: a brief history In: J C Lacal, J Feramisco and R Perona *Microinjection. Methods and Tools in Biosciences and Medicine* (Basel: Birkhäuser)

[34] Lin T P 1966 Microinjection of mouse eggs *Science.* **151** 333–7

[35] Liu C, Xie W, Gui C and Du Y 2013 Pronuclear microinjection and oviduct transfer procedures for transgenic mouse production *Methods Mol. Biol.* **1027** 10

[36] Shen Y M, Hirschhorn R R, Mercer W E, Surmacz E, Tsutsui Y, Soprano K J and Baserga R 1982 Gene transfer: DNA microinjection compared with DNA transfection with a very high efficiency *Mol. Cell. Biol.* **2** 1145–54

[37] Gordon J W, Scangos G A, Plotkin D J, Barbosa J A and Ruddle F H 1980 Genetic transformation of mouse embryos by microinjection of purified DNA *Proc. Natl Acad. Sci. USA* **77** 7380–4

[38] Liu C, Xie W, Gui C and Du Y 2013 Pronuclear microinjection and oviduct transfer procedures for transgenic mouse production *Methods Mol. Biol.* **1027** 217–32

[39] Cho A, Haruyama N and Kulkarni A B 2009 Generation of transgenic mice *Curr. Protoc. Cell Biol.* **42** 19.11.1–22

[40] National Research Council (US) and Institute of Medicine (US) Committee on the Biological and Biomedical Applications of Stem Cell Research 2002 Embryonic stem cells *Stem Cells and the Future of Regenerative Medicine* (Washington, DC: National Academies Press (US)) ch 3

[41] Hölker M, Ghanem N, Tesfaye D and Schellander K 2012 Sperm-Mediated Gene Transfer: Implications for Biotechnology and Medicine *Sperm-Mediated Gene Transfer: Concepts and Controversies* (Bentham Books) 33–42

[42] Lavitrano M, Busnelli M, Cerrito M G, Giovannoni R, Manzini S and Vargiolu A 2006 Sperm-mediated gene transfer *Reprod. Fertil. Dev.* **18** 19–23

[43] Barbero G, de Sousa Serro M G, Lujan C P, Vitullo A D, González C R and González B 2023 Transcriptome profiling of histone writers/erasers enzymes across spermatogenesis, mature sperm and pre-cleavage embryo: Implications in paternal epigenome transitions and inheritance mechanisms *Front. Cell Develop. Biol.* **11** 1086573

[44] Maione B, Lavitrano M, Spadafora C and Kiessling A A 1998 Sperm-mediated gene transfer in mice *Mol. Reprod. Dev* **50** 406–9

[45] Atkinson P W, Hines E R, Beaton S, Matthaei K I, Reed K C and Bradley M P 1991 Association of exogenous DNA with cattle and insect spermatozoa *in vitro Mol. Reprod. Dev.* **29** 1–5

[46] Amaral M G, Campos V F, Seixas F K, Cavalcanti P V, Selau L P, Deschamps J C and Collares T 2011 Testis-mediated gene transfer in mice: comparison of transfection reagents regarding transgene transmission and testicular damage *Biol. Res.* **44** 229–34
[47] Vasicek D *et al* 2010 Effective generation of genetically modified rabbits by sperm mediated gene transfer *World Rabbit Sci.* **151** 161–6
[48] De Los Campos G *et al* 2010 Semi-parametric genomic-enabled prediction of genetic values using reproducing kernel Hilbert spaces methods *Genet. Res.* **92** 295–308
[49] Dhup S and Majumdar S S 2008 Transgenesis via permanent integration of genes in repopulating spermatogonial cells in Vivo *Nat. Methods* **5** 601–3
[50] Bourgard C *et al* 2021 A suitable RNA preparation methodology for whole transcriptome shotgun sequencing harvested from plasmodium vivax-infected patients *Sci. Rep.* **11** 5089
[51] Nakagawa T and Hoogenraad C C 2011 Lentiviral transgenesis *Methods Mol. Biol.* **693** 117–42
[52] Zeng X, Chen J, Sanchez J F, Coggiano M and Dillon-Carter O 2003 Stable expression of hrGFP by mouse embryonic stem cells: promoter activity in the undifferentiated state and during dopaminergic neural differentiation *Stem Cells* **21** 647–53
[53] Bossi E, Fabbrini M S and Ceriotti A 2007 Exogenous protein expression in *Xenopus* oocytes: basic procedures *Methods Mol. Biol.* **375** 107–31
[54] Sokol D L and Gewirtz A M 1996 Gene therapy: basic concepts and recent advances *Crit. Rev. Euk. Gene Express.* **6** 29–57
[55] Roth J A and Cristiano R J 1991 Gene therapy for cancer: what have we done and where are we going? *J. Natl Cancer Inst.* **89** 21–39
[56] Bertling W A, Gareis M, Paspaleeva V, Zimmer A, Kreuter J, Numberg E and Harrer P 1991 Use of liposomes, viral capsids and nanoparticles as DNA carriers *Biotech. Appl. Biochem.* **13** 390–405
[57] Spradling A C and Rubin G M 1982 Transposition of cloned P elements into *Drosophila* germ line chromosomes *Science* **218** 341–7
[58] Engels W R 1984 A trans-acting product needed for P factor transposition in *Drosophila Science* **226** 1194–6
[59] Chaveroche M K, Ghigo J M and d'Enferta C 2000 A rapid method for efficient gene replacement in the filamentous fungus *Aspergillus nidulans Nucleic Acids Res.* **28** e97
[60] Puchta H 2002 Gene replacement by homologous recombination in plants *Plant Mol. Biol.* **1–2** 173–82
[61] Fogleman S, Santana C, Bishop C, Miller A and Capco D G 2016 CRISPR/Cas9 and mitochondrial gene replacement therapy: promising techniques and ethical considerations *Am. J. Stem Cells* **5** 39–52
[62] Wu Z 2015 A long-term efficacy study of gene replacement therapy for RPGR-associated retinal degeneration *Hum. Mol. Genet.* **24** 3956–70
[63] Mansour S L, Thomas K R and Capecchi M R 1988 Disruption of the proto-oncogene int-2 in mouse embryo-derived stem cells: a general strategy for targeting mutations to non-selectable genes *Nature* **336** 348–52
[64] Valancius V and Smithies O 1991 Testing an 'in–out' targeting procedure for making subtle genomic modifications in mouse embryonic stem cells *Mol. Cell. Biol.* **11** 402–8
[65] Liew C G, Draper J S, Walsh J, Moore H and Andrews P W 2007 Transient and stable transgene expression in human embryonic stem cells *Stem Cells* **25** 1521–8

[66] Sato T, Fukui T, Atomi H and Imanaka T 2003 Targeted gene disruption by homologous recombination in the hyperthermophilic archaeon *Thermococcus kodakaraensis* KOD *J. Bacteriol.* **185** 210–20
[67] Chaveroche M K, Ghigo J M and d'Enferta C 2000 A rapid method for efficient gene replacement in the filamentous fungus *Aspergillus nidulans Nucleic Acids Res.* **28** e97
[68] Day C D, Lee E, Kobayashi J, Holappa L D, Albert H and Ow D W 2000 Transgene integration into the same chromosome location can produce alleles that express at a predictable level, or alleles that are differentially silenced *Genes Dev.* **14** 2869–80
[69] Glick B R and Pasternak J J 2003 *Molecular Biotechnology—Principles and Applications of Recombinant DNA* (Washington, DC: ASM)
[70] Castilho L R, Moraes A M, Augusto E F P and Butler M (ed) 2007 *Animal Cell Technology: From Biopharmaceuticals to Gene Therapy* (New York: Taylor and Francis)
[71] Primrose S B and Twyman R 2006 *Principles of Gene Manipulation* 6th edn (Malden, MA: Blackwell Science)
[72] Mueller P P, Wirth D, Unsinger J and Hauser H 2013 *Genetic Approaches to Recombinant Protein Production in Mammalian Cells* (New York: Humana) pp 21–49
[73] Palomares L A, Estrada-Mondaca S and Ramírez O T 2004 Production of recombinant proteins *Methods Mol. Biol.* **267** 15–52
[74] Kim T K and Eberwine J H 2010 Mammalian cell transfection: the present and the future *Trends Anal. Bioanal. Chem.* **397** 3173–8
[75] Khan K H 2013 Gene expression in mammalian cells and its applications *Adv. Pharm. Bull.* **3** 257–63
[76] Kaufman R J 2000 Overview of vector design for mammalian gene expression *Mol. Biotechnol.* **16** 151–60
[77] Luckow V L and Summers M D 1988 Trends in the development of baculovirus expression vectors *Nat. Biotechnol.* **6** 47–55
[78] O'Reilly D R, Miller L K and Luckow V A 1992 *Baculovirus Expression Vectors: A Laboratory Manual* (New York: Freeman)
[79] Lundstrom K 2016 Alphavirus vectors as tools in neuroscience and gene therapy *Virus Res.* **216** 16–25
[80] Egelkrout E, Rajan V and Howard J A 2012 Overproduction of recombinant proteins in plants *Plant Sci.* **184** 83–101
[81] Norrman K, Fischer Y, Bonnamy B, Wolfhagen Sand F and Ravassard P 2010 Quantitative comparison of constitutive promoters in human ES cells *PLoS One* **5** e12413
[82] Nakagawa K, Yajima K, Yamashita K, Ikenaka Y and Yokota S 1991 Constitutive high-level production of human lymphotoxin by CHO-K1 cells transformed with the human lymphotoxin gene controlled by a human beta-actin promoter *Agric. Biol. Chem.* **55** 501–8
[83] Kim D W H T S I M T 1993 An efficient expression vector for stable expression in human liver cells *Gene* **134** 307–8
[84] Najjar S M and Lewis R E 1999 Persistent expression of foreign genes in cultured hepatocytes: expression vectors *Gene* **230** 41–5
[85] Kosuga M, Enosawa S, Li X K, Suzuki S and Matsuo N 2000 Strong, long-term transgene expression in rat liver using chicken beta-actin promoter associated with cytomegalovirus immediate-early enhancer (CAG promoter) *Cell Transplant* **9** 675–80

[86] Sakurai F, Kawabata K, Yamaguchi T, Hayakawa T and Mizuguchi H 2005 Optimization of adenovirus serotype 35 vectors for efficient transduction in human hematopoietic progenitors: comparison of promoter activities *Gene Ther.* **12** 1424–33

[87] Liu J W, Pernod G, Dunoyer-Geindre S, Fish R J and Yang H 2006 Promoter dependence of transgene expression by lentivirus-transduced human blood-derived endothelial progenitor cells *Stem Cells* **24** 199–208

[88] Damdindorj L, Karnan S, Ota A, Takahashi M and Konishi Y 2012 Assessment of the long-term transcriptional activity of a 550-bp-long human beta-actin promoter region *Plasmid* **68** 195–200

[89] Gopalkrishnan R V, Christiansen K A, Goldstein N I, DePinho R A and Fisher P B 1999 Use of the human EF-1α promoter for expression can significantly increase success in establishing stable cell lines with consistent expression: a study using the tetracycline-inducible system in human cancer cells *Nucleic Acids Res.* **27** 4775–82

[90] Shakweer W M E, Krivoruchko A Y, Dessouki S M and Khattab A A 2023 A review of transgenic animal techniques and their applications *J. Genet. Eng. Biotechnol.* **21** 55

www.ingramcontent.com/pod-product-compliance
Lightning Source LLC
Chambersburg PA
CBHW082122210326
41599CB00031B/5842